# Neural Development and Regeneration

Cellular and Molecular Aspects

# NATO ASI Series

## Advanced Science Institutes Series

*A series presenting the results of activities sponsored by the NATO Science Committee, which aims at the dissemination of advanced scientific and technological knowledge, with a view to strengthening links between scientific communities.*

The Series is published by an international board of publishers in conjunction with the NATO Scientific Affairs Division

| | |
|---|---|
| A Life Sciences<br>B Physics | Plenum Publishing Corporation<br>London and New York |
| C Mathematical and Physical Sciences<br>D Behavioural and Social Sciences<br>E Applied Sciences | Kluwer Academic Publishers<br>Dordrecht, Boston and London |
| F Computer and Systems Sciences<br>G Ecological Sciences<br>H Cell Biology | Springer-Verlag<br>Berlin Heidelberg New York<br>London Paris Tokyo |

Series H: Cell Biology Vol. 22

# Neural Development and Regeneration

## Cellular and Molecular Aspects

Edited by

A. Gorio

Istituto di Scienze Farmacologiche
Facoltà di Farmacia
Università di Milano
Via Balzaretti 9, 20129 Milano, Italy

J. R. Perez-Polo

Department of Human Biological Chemistry and Genetics
Marine Biomedical Institute
University of Texas Medical Branch
Galveston, TX 77550, USA

J. de Vellis

Mental Retardation Research Center #68-177
Department of Anatomy and Department of Psychiatry
and Biobehavioral Science
University of California, LA
760 Westwood Plaza, Los Angeles, CA 90024, USA

B. Haber

Department of Human Biological
Chemistry and Genetics and Department of Neurology
Marine Biomedical Institute
University of Texas Medical Branch
200 University Blvd., #519, Galveston, TX 77550, USA

Springer-Verlag
Berlin Heidelberg New York London Paris Tokyo
Published in cooperation with NATO Scientific Affairs Division

Proceedings of the NATO Advanced Research Workshop on Cellular and Molecular Aspects of Neural Development and Regeneration held at Sheraton Bal Harbour, Bal Harbour, Florida, USA, May 21–25, 1987

Satellite, First Joint Meeting of the American Society for Neurochemistry and the International Society for Neurochemistry

Co-Sponsored by:
National Science Foundation
University of Miami, School of Medicine
Marine Biomedical Institute, University of Texas Medical Branch
Institute of Pharmacological Sciences, School of Pharmacy, University of Milano

This workshop was made possible by the generous contributions of the following sponsors:
ELLEM S.p.A., CRINOS S.p.A., FIDIA S.p.A., CYANAMID S.p.A., SIGMA TAU S.p.A., BOERINGHER INGELHEIM DE ANGELIS S.p.A.
and
AMERICAN PARALYSIS ASSOCIATION (APA)
KENT WALDREP NATIONAL PARALYSIS ASSOCIATION
THE NATIONAL SPINAL CORD INJURY ASSOCIATION
THE MIAMI PROJECT
THE DANIEL HEUMANN FUND FOR SPINAL CORD RESEARCH



ISBN 3-540-18553-4 Springer-Verlag Berlin Heidelberg New York
ISBN 0-387-18553-4 Springer-Verlag New York Berlin Heidelberg

Library of Congress Cataloging-in-Publication Data. NATO Advanced Research Workshop on Cellular and Molecular Aspects of Neural Development and Regeneration (1987 : Bal Harbour, Fla.) Neural development and regeneration : cellular and molecular aspects / edited by A. Gorio ... [et al.]. p. cm.—(NATO ASI series. Series H, Cell biology ; vol. 22) "Proceedings of the NATO Advanced Research Workshop on Cellular and Molecular Aspects of Neural Development and Regeneration, held at Sheraton Bal Harbour, Bal Harbour, Florida, USA, May 21–25, 1987"—T.p. verso. "Satellite, first joint meeting of the American Society for Neurochemistry and the International Society for Neurochemistry"–T.p. verso. Co-sponsored by the National Science Foundation and others. "Published in cooperation with NATO Scientific Affairs Division." Includes index.
ISBN 0-387-18553-4 (U.S.)
1. Nerves—Growth—Congresses. 2. Nerves—Regeneration—Congresses. 3. Nerve growth factor—Physiological effect—Congresses. I. Gorio, Alfredo. II. American Society for Neurochemistry. III. International Society for Neurochemistry. IV. National Science Foundation (U.S.) V. North Atlantic Treaty Organization. Scientific Affairs Division. VI. Title. VII. Series. [DNLM: 1. Nerve Growth Factors—congresses. 2. Nerve Regeneration—congresses. 3. Nervous System—growth & development—congresses. 4. Neurons—congresses. WL 102 N2785n 1987] QP363.5.N35 1987 599'.0188—dc 19 DNLM/DLC for Library of Congress 88-15951


Printed in Germany

Printing: Druckhaus Beltz, Hemsbach; Binding: J. Schäffer GmbH & Co. KG, Grünstadt
2131/3140-543210

TABLE OF CONTENTS

Theme I: (Cont.)

Theme II: (Cont.)

## POSTER ABSTRACTS

PARTICIPANTS

H. C. Agrawal, Ph.D.
Department of Pediatrics
Washington University School of Medicine
400 S. Kingshighway
St. Louis, MO 63110

Ms. L. Allison
Kent Waldrep National Paralysis Foundation
5050 Quorum Drive, Suite 450
Dallas, TX 75240

D. J. Anderson, Ph.D.
Department of Biology
California Institute of Technology
Division of Biology 216-76
Pasadena, CA 91125

L. Angelucci, M.D.
Department of Pharmacology
University of Rome "La Sapienza"
Facolta di Medicina
P. le A. Moro 2
Roma 00185
Italy

D. R. Archer, Ph.D.
Department of Pharmacology
P. O. Box 147
Liverpool, L69 3BX
United Kingdom

R. Avalo, Ph.D.
Institute of Biological Chemistry
University of Catania
Viale Andrea Doria 6
95125 Catania
Italy

R. R. Baichwal
Department of Biochemistry & Molecular Biophysics
Box 614 MCV Station
Richmond, VA 23298

J. Barret, Ph.D.
Department of Physiology and Biophysics
University of Miami Medical School
P. O. Box 016430
Miami, FL 33101

C. F. Baxter, Ph.D.
Neurochemistry Laboratory
VA Medical Center (151B-2)
16111 Plummer Street
Sepulveda, CA 91343

C. Beck
Department of Human Biological Chemistry
and Genetics
432 Gail Borden Bldg.
University of Texas Medical Branch
Galveston, TX 77550

J. Bernstein, Ph.D.
Laboratory of Central Nervous System Injury
and Regeneration
Veterans Administration Medical Center
Washington, DC 20422

A. Blight, Ph.D.
Dept. of Neurosurgery, Physiology, and Biophysics
New York University Medical Center
550 1st Avenue
New York, NY 10016

E. Bock, M.D.
The Protein Laboratory
University of Copenhagen
34, Sigurdsgade
DK-2200 Copenhagen N
Denmark

J. Bottenstein, Ph.D.
Marine Biomedical Institute
Department of Human Biological Chemistry
and Genetics
University of Texas Medical Branch
200 University Blvd.
Galveston, TX 77550

S. Brady, Ph.D.
Department of Cell Biology
University of Texas Health Science Center
5323 Harry Hines Blvd.
Dallas, TX 75235

J. S. Brugge, Ph.D.
Department of Microbiology
State University of New York
Stony Brook, NY 11794-8621

K. Bulloch, Ph.D.
Neuroimmune Physiology Laboratory
The Helicon Foundation
4622 Santa Fe St.
San Diego, CA 92109

P.Calissano, M.D., Ph.D.
Laboratorio de Biologia Cellulare
Consiglio Nazionale delle Richerche
00196 Rome
Italy

F. Cattabeni, Ph.D.
Department of Applied Pharmacology
School of Pharmacology
Universita di Milano
Via Balzaretti 9
20133 Milano
Italy

K. Y. Chan, Ph.D.
Department of Ophthalmology, RJ10
University of Washington
School of Medicine
Seattle, WA 98195

G. Ciment, Ph.D.
Department of Cell Biology and Anatomy
Oregon Health Sciences University
Portland, OR 97201

J. A. Clemens, Ph.D.
Lilly Research Laboratories, MC904
Lilly Corporate Center
Indianapolis, IN 46285

F. Clementi, M.D.
Department of Pharmacology
University of Milano
Via Vanvitelli 41
Milano 20129
Italy

R. Coggeshall, M.D.
Department of Anatomy & Neurosciences and of Physiology & Biophysics
University of Texas Medical Branch
Member, Marine Biomedical Institute
200 University Blvd, #532
Galveston, TX 77550

D. R. Colman, Ph.D.
Department of Cell Biology
New York University Medical School
550 First Avenue
New York, NY 10016

C. Cotman, Ph.D.
Department of Psychobiology
University of California, Irvine
Irvine, CA 92717

P. Davies, Ph.D.
Department of Neuroscience & Pathology
Albert Einstein College of Medicine
1300 Morris Park Avenue
Bronx, NY 10461

E. De Robertis, M.D., Ph.D.
Department of Biological Chemistry
University of California
School of Medicine
Los Angeles, CA 90024

J. de Vellis, Ph.D.
Mental Retardation Research Center
#68-177
Dept. of Anatomy and Dept. of Psychiatry
and Biobehavioral Science
University of California, LA
760 Westwood Plaza
Los Angeles, CA 90024

S. K. de Waegh, Ph.D.
Department of Cell Biology
University of Texas Health Science
Center at Dallas
5323 Harry Hines Blvd.
Dallas, TX 75234

A. M. di Giulio, Ph.D.
Department of Medical Pharmacology
Universita di Milano
Via Vanvitelli 32
20129 Milano
Italy

T. Ebendal, Ph.D.
Department of Zoology
Uppsala University
Box 561
S-751 22 Uppsala
Sweden

Mr. M. Ergas
American Paralysis Association (APA)
55 Morris Avenue
Suite 309
Springfield, NY 07081

P. Foresta, Ph.D.
Sigma Tau S.P.A.
Via Pontina KM. 30.400
00040 Pomezia
Italy

K. Frei, Ph.D.
Section of Clinical Immunology
Department of Internal Medicine
University Hospital
Haldeliweg 4
CH-8044 Zurich
Switzerland

O. Ghirardi, Ph.D.
Sigma Tau S.P.A.
Via Pontina KM. 30.400
00040 Pomezia
Italy

A. M. Giuffrida Stella, Ph.D.
Instituto di Chimica Biologica
Universita di Catania
Via Andrea Doria, 6
95125 Catania
Italy

D. Giulian, Ph.D.
Dept. of Neurology
Baylor College of Medicine
Houston, TX 77030

M. E. Goldberger, Ph.D.
Department of Anatomy
The Medical College of Pennsylvania/
EPPI Division
3200 Henry Avenue
Philadelphia, PA 19129

M. Goldstein, D.O., MPh
National Institutes of Health
Bldg. 31, Room 8A52
Bethesda, MD 20205

A. Gorio, Ph.D.
Department of Cellular Pharmacology
School of Pharmacology
Universita di Milano
Istituto di Farmacologia
E di Farmacognosia
Via Balzaretti 9
20129 Milano
Italy

B. Grafstein, Ph.D.
Department of Physiology
Cornell University Medical College
1300 York Avenue
New York, NY 10021

B. Green, M.D.
Department of Neurological Surgery
School of Medicine (D-4-6)
University of Miami
P. O. Box 016960
Miami, FL 33101

B. Haber, Ph.D.
Department of Human Biological
Chemistry and Genetics and
Department of Neurology
Member, Marine Biomedical Institute
University of Texas Medical Branch
200 University Blvd., #519
Galveston, TX 77550

N. Hall, Ph.D.
Department of Biochemistry
George Washington University Sch. of Med.
2300 Eye Street Bldg. D03
Washington, D.C. 20037

E. Hansson, Ph.D.
Institute of Neurobiology
University of Goteborg
P. O. Box 33031
S-400 33 Goteborg
Sweden

H. Hatanaka, Ph.D.
Department of Neuroscience
Mitsubishi-Kasei Institute of Life Sciences
11 Minamiooya, Machida-shi
Tokyo 194
JAPAN

F. Hefti, Ph.D.
Department of Neurology and
Pharmacology
University of Miami School of Medicine
P. O. Box 016960
Miami, FL 33101

H. Herschman, Ph.D.
Department of Biological Chemistry
UCLA School of Medicine
University of California, Los Angeles
Los Angeles, CA 90024

L. Hertz, M.D., D.Sc.
Department of Pharmacology
University of Saskatchewan
Saskatoon, Saskatchewan
S7N OWO
CANADA

Mrs. M. Heumann
The Daniel Heumann Fund for Spinal
Cord Research, Inc.
150 Broadway
New York, NY 10038

R. Heumann, Ph.D.
Max-Planck-Institut fur Psychiatrie
Abteilung Neurochemie
Am Klopferspitz 18A
8033 Planegg-Martinsried
Munchen
Federal Republic of Germany

Mr. W. Heumann
The Daniel Heumann Fund for Spinal
Cord Research, Inc.
150 Broadway
New York, NY 10038

R. Hogue Angeletti, Ph.D.
Laboratory of Neuropathology
University of Pennsylvania School of Medicine
Philadelphia, PA 19104-6079

E. Holmes
Laboratory of Biomedical and Environmental Sciences
900 Veteran Avenue
Los Angeles, CA 90024

A-P. Holtorf
Institut fur Anatomie and Zallbiologie
Philipps Universitat Marburg
Robert Koch Str. 6
D-3550 Marburg
Federal Republic of Germany

K. R. Huff
University of Southern California
School of Medicine
4650 Sunset Blvd.
Los Angeles, CA 90027

C. Hulsebosch, Ph.D.
Department of Anatomy & Neurosciences
Marine Biomedical Institute
University of Texas Medical Branch
200 University Blvd.
Galveston, TX 77550

N. A. Ingoglia
Department of Physiology
New Jersey Medical School
185 South Orange Avenue
Newark, NJ 07103-2757

K. Kelley, Ph.D.
Department of Animal Sciences
University of Illinois at Urbana-Champaign
162ASL, 1207 West Gregory Drive
Urbana, IL 61801

M. Kletzkin, Ph.D.
Sigma Tau
723 North Bears St.
Holmdale, NJ 07733

J. Lauder, Ph.D.
Department of Anatomy
108 Swing Bldg, 217H
University of North Carolina School of Medicine
Chapel Hill, NC 27514

G. Levi, M.D.
Department of Organ and System Pathophysiology
Istituto Superiore di Sanita
Viale Regina Elena 299
I-00161 Roma
Italy

Y. P. Loh, Ph.D.
National Institutes of Health
Bldg. 36, Room 2A-21
Bethesda, MD 20892

R. Loy, Ph.D.
Department of Neurobiology and Anatomy
University of Rochester
School of Medicine and Dentistry, Box 603
601 Elmwood Avenue
Rochester, NY 14642

V. H. Mah
Department of Pathology
UCLA Center for the Health Sciences
10833 Le Conte Avenue
Los Angeles, CA 90024

T. Martin, Ph.D.
Bristrol-Myers Company
5 Research Parkway
Wallingford, CT 06492

P. W. Mason
Dept. of Biochemistry and Molecular
Biophysics
Box 614 MCV Station
Richmond, VA 23298

D. Maysinger
Department of Pharmacology and Therapeutics
McGill University
3655 Drummond St.
Montreal H3G 1Y6
CANADA

L. Mendelsohn, Ph.D.
CNS Research (M907)
Lilly Corporate Center
Indianapolis, IN 46285

A. Michler, Ph.D.
Department of Clinical Anatomy &
Developmental Neurobiology
Center of Anatomy
University of Goettingen
Kreuzbergring 3G
3400 Goettingen
Federal Republic of Germany

T. P. Misko, Ph.D.
Department of Neurobiology
Stanford University School of Medicine
Stanford, CA 94305

D. Monard, Ph.D.
Friedrich Miescher Institut
P. O. Box 2543
Ch-4002 Basel
Switzerland

N. E. Naftchi, Ph.D.
New York University Medical Center
400 E. 34th Street
New York, NY 10016

Mr. J. Nichols
Kent Waldrep National Paralysis Foundation
5050 Quorum Drive
Suite 450
Dallas, TX 75240

R. N. Nishimura, M.D.
Department of Neurology, RNRC 4231
UCLA
Los Angeles, CA 90024-1769

M. Noble, Ph.D.
Cellular Neurobiology
Ludwig Institute for Cancer Research in the
Courtold Institute for Biochemistry
at the University and Molecular Hospital School
of Medicine of the University of London
Mortimer St.
London WI
England

M. Norenberg, M.D.
Department of Pathology (D33)
University of Miami School of Medicine
P. O. Box 016960
Miami, FL 33101

R. Paoletti, M.D.
Istituto di Farmacologia
Universita di Milano
Via Andrea del Sarto 21
I-20129 Milano
Italy

H. M. Pappius, Ph.D.
Montreal Neurological Institute
3801 University Street
Montreal, Quebec
Canada H3A 2B4

J. R. Perez-Polo, Ph.D.
Department of Human Biological
Chemistry and Genetics
Adjunct Member, Marine Biomedical Institute
University of Texas Medical Branch
Galveston, TX 77550

G. W. Perry
Department of Physiology and Biophysics
University of Miami School of Medicine
P. O. Box 016430
Miami, FL 33010

Ms. L. Phillips
National Spinal Cord Injury Association
National Office
149 California St.
Newton, MA 02158-1063

N. Pitts, Ph.D.
National Science Foundation
1800 G Street, NW
Washington, D.C. 20550

A. Privat, M.D., D.B.H.
Institut de biologie
Laboratory of Medicine Experimentale
Faculty of Medicine
University of Montpellier
Boulevard Henry IV
34060 Montpellier
France

P. J. Reier, Ph.D.
Departments of Neurological Surgery
and Neuroscience
University of Florida
Box J-265
JHM Health Center
Gainesville, Florida 32610

L. Ronback, Ph.D.
Institute of Neurobiology
University of Goteborg
P. O. Box 33031
S-400 33 Goteborg
Sweden

R. Saneto, Ph.D.
Oregon Regional Primate Research Center
Division Neuroscience
505 NW 185th Avenue
Beaverton, Oregon 97006

A. Schousboe, Ph.D., D.Sc.
Department of Biochemistry A
Panum Institute
University of Copenhagen
DK-2200 Copenhagen N
Denmark

M. Schwartz, Ph.D.
Department of Neurobiology
Weizmann Institute of Science
Rehovot 76100
Israel

W. Seifert, Ph.D.
Laboratory for Molecular
Neurobiology
Max-Planck-Inst. Biophys. Chemie
P. O. Box 2841
3400 Gottingen
West Germany

F. J. Seil, M.D.
Office of Regeneration Research
Programs (151N)
VA Medical Center
Portland, OR 97201

A. Shahar, Ph.D.
Electromicroscopy Section
The Israel Institute for Biological Research
P.O.B. 19
Ness-Ziona 70450
Israel

D. Shine, Ph.D.
Department of Neuroscience
Children's Hospital and
Harvard School of Medicine
300 Longwood Avenue
Boston, MA 02115

R. Small, Ph.D.
Department of Zoology and Cell Biology
University College of London
London WC1E 6BT
England

D. Soifer, Ph.D.
Laboratory of Cell Biology
New York State Institute for Basic Research
in Mental Retardation
Staten Island, NY 10314

H. E. Spiegel, Ph.D.
American Paralysis Association (APA)
55 Morris Avenue
Suite 309
Springfield, NJ 07081

J. Springer, Ph.D.
Department of Neurobiology and Anatomy
University of Rochester Medical Center
Rochester, NY 14642

L. Sternberger, M.D.
Department of Neurology, Pathology, and Anatomy
University of Maryland School of Medicine
22 South Greene Street
Baltimore, MD 21201

N. Sternberger, Ph.D.
Department of Anatomy
University of Maryland School of Medicine
655 W. Baltimore St.
Baltimore, MD 21201

O. Steward, M.D., Ph.D.
Departments of Neuroscience
and Neurological Surgery
University of Virginia School of Medicine
Charlottesville, VA 22908

L. W. Thorpe, Ph.D.
Department of Human Biological Chemistry & Genetics
432 Gail Borden Bldg., D03
University of Texas Medical Branch
Galveston, TX 77550

D. B. Tower, M.D., Ph.D., D.Sc.(hon)
7105 Brennon Lane
Chevy Chase, Maryland 20815

M. Trachtenberg, Ph.d.
Matrix Corp.
18543 Prince William
Nassau Bay, TX 77058

K. Unsicker, M.D.
Department of Anatomy and Cell Biology
University of Marburg
West Germany

S. Varon, M.D., Engin.D.
Department of Biology
School of Medicine
M-001
University of California, San Diego
La Jolla, CA 92093

A. Vernadakis, Ph.D.
Departments of Psychiatry and Pharmacology
University of Colorado
School of Medicine
Denver, CO 80262

Z. Vogel, Ph.D.
Neurobiology Department
Weizmann Institute
Rehovot 76100
Israel

Mrs. L. Waldrep
Kent Waldrep National Paralysis Foundation
5050 Quorum Drive, Suite 450
Dallas, TX 75240

Mr. K. Waldrep
Kent Waldrep National Paralysis Foundation
5050 Quorum Drive, Suite 450
Dallas, TX 75240

M. J. Weber, Ph.D.
Centre National de la Recherche Scientifique
Laboratoire de Pharmacologie et Toxicologie Fondamentales
205 route de Narbonne
31077 Toulouse Cedex
FRANCE

S. R. Whittemore, Ph.D.
Department of Neurological Surgery
University of Miami School of Medicine
1600 NW 10th Avenue - R48
Miami, FL 33136

L. R. Williams, Ph.D.
The Upjohn Company
Unit 7251 - 209 - 5
Kalamazoo, MI 49001

H. Wisniewski, M.D., Ph.D.
New York State Institute for Basic Research
In Mental Retardation
1050 Forest Hill Road
Staten Island, NY 10314

T. Wood
Department of Neurobiology and Behavior
SUNY/Stony Brook
Stony Brook, NY 11794

W.Young, M.D., Ph.D.
Department of Neurosurgery and Physiology & Biophysics
New York University Medical Center
New York, NY 10016

J. E. Yoshino, Ph.D.
Department of Biochemistry
Box 614 MCV Station
Richmond, VA 23298

# T H E M E I

## GROWTH FACTORS AND HORMONES IN DEVELOPMENT AND AGING OF NEURONS AND GLIA

## Theme I - INTRODUCTION

The hypothesis that growth factors and hormones determine or permit the expression of the phenotypic properties that characterize different neuroendocrine cell types has gained universal acceptance. Much of the earlier work in the development of neuronal culture systems relying on different defined media and the purification of neuronotrophic factors has led to more recent advances in the separation and in vitro study of different glial populations. Our understanding of neural cell lineage and the factors that govern passage of cells to different end points of development is now more molecular as the external signals that control cellular development are isolated and analyzed in vivo and in vitro. Lastly, neurotransmitters have been shown to have trophic and tropic effects on neuronal structures that go beyond their previously recognized signalling role.

# DEVELOPMENTAL BIOLOGY OF THE OPTIC NERVE

Mark Noble
Ludwig Institute for Cancer Research
91 Riding House Street, London, W1P 8BT
England

Any attempt to determine the rules involved in building the nervous system might best begin with a simple region of this complex tissue. Some laboratories have developed approaches which utilize simple organisms in their investigations. Others, such as ourselves, have decided to work within the simplest regions of the mammalian nervous system.

For many reasons, the simplest portion of the mammalian nervous system is the optic nerve. First, no neurons develop in this tissue, and all of the nerve cell processes which pass through the optic nerve emanate from cell bodies located elsewhere in the CNS. Thus, by concentrating on the optic nerve one is able to focus on the majority cellular population in the CNS, the glia. The optic nerve is also simple in being entirely a white matter (myelinated) tract, and has the advantage of being seemingly homogeneous in construction along most of its length. The developmental anatomy of the optic nerve has been well described, thus offering important observations about development in vivo. Finally, this tissue is readily accessible, both for dissection and for experimental manipulation. For these reasons, we have spent the last several years trying to understand the cellular biological principles which underly the creation of the optic nerve.

To study the cell biology of the optic nerve, it was first necessary to identify the cells which make up this tissue. Anatomical studies indicated long ago that the optic nerve contained astrocytes, the most numerous individual glial cell-type, and oligodendrocytes, the myelin-forming cells of the CNS. These

NATO ASI Series, Vol. H22
Neural Development and Regeneration
Edited by A. Gorio et al.

cells can be specifically identified in tissue culture using cell-type specific antibodies (Raff et al, 1979): antibodies against glial fibrillary acidic protein (GFAP) label astrocytes (Bignami et al, 1972) and antibodies against galactoceroside, a myelin-specific glycolipid, specifically label oligodendrocytes (Raff et al, 1978). With the ability to specifically identify cells of interest, it is then possible to use tissue culture techniques to examine, and manipulate, the development of individual cells.

Two types of astrocytes. Contrary to earlier beliefs, the optic nerve contains at least three distinct glial populations instead of two. Several years ago, studies on the astrocytes of the optic nerve began to indicate that this tissue, and other white matter tracts, contains two distinct populations of astrocytes which differ in antigenic phenotype, morphology, developmental histories, function and lineage. Initially, these two populations were distinguished by morphology and by labelling with the A2B5 monoclonal antibody (Eisenbarth, et al, 1979) or with tetanus toxin (TTX). Type 1 astrocytes have large fibroblast-like cell bodies, and are A2B5$^-$ and TTX$^-$. Type 2 astrocytes, in contrast, are process-bearing cells with small cell bodies and are both A2B5$^+$ and TTX$^+$ (Raff et al, 1983a). Type 1 astrocytes appear in the optic nerve at about the 15th day of embryonic development, while type 2 astrocytes are not found in the nerve until the second week after birth (Miller and Raff, 1984). Oligodendrocytes, the third glial population of the optic nerve, appear in the rat optic nerve around the time of birth (Miller et al, 1985).

The oligodendrocyte-type 2 (0-2A) progenitor cell. Shortly after the discovery of type 2 astrocyes, we found that optic nerves of neonatal rats contain a bipotential progenitor cell which can be induced in tissue culture to give rise either to type 2 astrocytes or to oligodendrocytes, but not to type 1 astrocytes (Raff et al, 1983b). When grown in the presence of fetal calf serum, or fetal sera from other species, 0-2A progenitor cells differentatiate into type 2 astrocytes within 48-72h; grown in the absence of serum, in chemically-defined medium, this same progenitor cell differentiates into an oligodendrocyte, again within 48-72h. The

0-2A progenitor cell, along with being the first progenitor cell to be identified in the CNS, is one of a small number of bipotential progenitors which can be readily identified and isolated for detailed study.

The discovery of the 0-2A progenitor cell initiated a major shift in our thinking about glial lineages. Previous discussion had focused on the question of whether a common progenitor cell gave rise to both oligodendrocytes and astrocytes, or whether these two cell-types were separately derived from astroblasts and oligodendroblasts. In fact, it appears that both of these views are right and both are wrong: a common progenitor exists for oligodendrocytes and type 2 astrocytes, and this cell is distinct from the precursor which gives rise to type 1 astrocytes.

Astrocytes and neuronal growth: the adhesion gradient hypothesis. Having identified the major cell-types of the optic nerve, we began to explore the cell-cell interactions which might play a role in the formation of this tissue. The earliest cell-cell interaction we examined was that between astrocytes and growing neurons. As the glial precursors found in the embryonic optic nerve at the earliest stages of axonal growth appear to be precursors of only type 1 astrocytes (Small et al, 1987; see also below), it is the properties of type 1 astrocytes that I will discuss in this regard.

To examine interactions between neurons and type 1 astrocytes, we compared the growth of dissociated CNS neurons on monolayers of astrocytes, schwann cells, skin fibroblasts, meningeal cells and cardiac myocytes. Purified cortical astrocytes, with the characteristics of type 1 astrocytes, and other cell-types were prepared as described previously (Noble et al, 1984).

Dissociated neurons plated onto astrocytes grew as if they preferred the astrocytic surface to any other surface available. The neurons, plated as a suspension of single cells, remained as single cells and their neurites grow as isolated processes. We saw extensive crossing over of neuronal processes, and occasional instances of processes running in parallel for short distances. We did not see neurites growing in fascicles, or neuronal cell bodies packed together in multineuronal aggregates.

In contrast to the pattern of growth expressed by neurons on astrocytes, when these same single-cell suspensions were plated onto fibroblasts, meningeal cells, or cardiac myocytes the neurons rapidly coalesced into multineuronal aggregates, and almost all neurite outgrowth occurred in multineuritic fascicles. Thus, when grown on non-glia, neurons appeared to prefer to adhere to each other in preference to the cellular substrate offered to them. In addition, where we found neurons growing in isolation, neuritic extension was greatly reduced on the non-glial monolayers as compared with growth on astrocytes.

We also found that CNS neurons plated onto schwann cells behaved similarly to neurons growing on astrocyte monolayers. In these cultures also, neurons grew as single cells and neurites grew as single processes. Even neurons from the cerebellum, which never ordinarily encounter schwann cells, grew in a manner which suggested that there are striking common properties shared by the surfaces of schwann cells and astrocytes. In further experiments we found that the glial properties seemed to reflect an intrinsic characteristic of the cell surface, and that even heat-killed astrocytes supported the growth of CNS neurons in a manner indistinguishable from living astrocytes.

The nature of neuritic outgrowth on glia and non-glia suggested a simple hypothesis: Neurons adhere more strongly to glia than to other neurons, but are more adherent to other neurons than to non-glia. The idea that glia offer a preferred substrate for neurite outgrowth was subsequently extended to consider neurons of the peripheral nervous system by Fallon (1985), whose interpretations were identical to our own previous conclusions.

<u>Neuron-glia adhesion, the maintenance of order in fiber tracts, and the control of fasiculation.</u> One of the striking aspects of the development of the axon tracts of the optic nerve is that fibres largely remain in order (Silver, 1984), even though there seems to be little positional information within the optic nerve itself. Despite the position-dependent properties of retinal axons and their growth cones observed in vitro by Bonheoffer and Huf (1985), neurons which are growing in the wrong position within

the optic nerve, for example due to the injection of anti-NCAM antibodies into the optic cup (Silver and Rutishauser, 1984), do not reorient to their correct location until they reach the optic tectum. How then are these fibres maintained in the correct order in the developing optic nerve?

If the glia of the embryonic optic nerve offer a preferred substrate for neuritic outgrowth, then the maintenance of order in the optic nerve may be simple to understand. Numerous investigators have observed that, at least in the optic nerve, neuronal growth cones are almost always found at the interface between fascicles and glial endfeet (for review, see also Noble, 1986), suggesting that it is along the glial endfeet that new axons are added to individual axons. Older axons would thus be pushed furthest away from the glial endfeet. As axons entering the optic nerve appear to be generated in a strict sequential order within the retina (see Silver and Sapiro, 1981), such an adhesion interaction would maintain order in individual fascicles. Whether neurons in individual fascicles can recognize each other's surfaces is not known, but the observation that incorrectly located axons grow in their new location until reaching the tectum suggests that the cellular properties of the optic nerve help to keep axons in the same location in which they are found when they first enter the nerve.

On a larger scale, the location of fascicles within the optic nerve, and the control of fasiculation itself, may also be largely the result of preferred adhesion of neurites to glia. For example, in the optic nerves of pigmented rodents, there is a region of pigmented cells which extends centrally from the eye along the dorsal surface of the nerve during embryonic development (Silver and Sapiro, 1981). No fascicles occur along this surface; instead, they all grow along the glial endfeet on the ventral surface. In the chick optic nerve, which has no pigmented cells, fibres are found all along the circumference of the nerve. Finally, in the frog optic nerve, which seems to be initially composed entirely of pigmented epithelial cells, all neurites are found in a single large fascicle in the core of the optic nerve trunk (Silver and Sapiro, 1981). Thus, the formation of fascicles is tightly correlated with the presence or absence of surrounding glial cells.

Glial NCAM and neuron-glial adhesion. We do not yet know the molecules responsible for the adhesive characteristics of the glial surface. However, two pieces of evidence suggest that the neural cell adhesion molecule (NCAM) may be of importance. First, glial cells express NCAM (Noble, et al, 1985); neurons also express NCAM and, as NCAM is thought to bind to other NCAM polypeptides (for review, see Rutishauser, 1984), any two NCAM-expressing cells should bind to each other in an interaction mediated by these molecules. Glial endfeet in the optic nerve also express NCAM, and injection of anti-NCAM antibodies into the eyecup of developing chicks results in a separation of axonal fasicles from the glial endfeet (Silver and Rutishauser, 1984).

Type 1 astrocytes and control of 0-2A progenitor division. Positing a role for type 1 astrocytes, or their precursors, in providing a suitable substrate for growth of retinal ganglion cell axons would not have surprised Cajal. However, our next identified function of type 1 astrocytes represented an entirely new insight into the role of type 1 astrocytes and the control of glial proliferation in the CNS.

In our attempts to identify the cell-cell interaction responsible for promoting division of 0-2A progenitor cells, we found that when optic nerve cells were grown on monolayers of type 1 astrocytes the 0-2A progenitors in these cultures divided extensively (Noble and Murray, 1984). Increasing numbers of progenitors and oligodendrocytes were both generated, although division only occurred in the progenitor population. Thus, in the complete absence of neurons, type 1 astrocytes were able to support both progenitor division and differentiation of dividing progenitors into oligodendrocytes. Moreover, when axons were elimated from the optic nerves of newborn rats by transection, 0-2A progenitor cells continued to synthesize DNA (David et al, 1984), suggesting that type 1 astrocytes - the first differentiated glial cell-type to appear during optic nerve development (Miller and Raff, 1984) - may be the primary source of progenitor mitogen during normal development. This mitogen is secreted into tissue culture medium (Noble and Murray, 1984) and is currently being characterized.

Type 1 astrocytes and the blood-brain barrier. Yet another function for the versatile type 1 astrocyte appears to be the induction of specialization of endothelial cells to form a blood-brain barrier (Janzer and Raff, 1987). For example, purified type 1 astrocytes, grown on the chorioallantoic membrane of embryonic chicks, attract blood vessels and then induce the endothelial cells of these blood vessels to express the characteristic properties of the endothelial cells of the CNS.

Astrocytic specializations at the nodes of Ranvier: a role for type 2 astrocytes. What is the function of type 2 astrocytes? Recent evidence suggests that these cells extend fine processes which enwrap the bare axonal membrane which lies between adjacent myelin sheaths (ffrench-Constant and Raff, 1986). This observation suggests that the entire 0-2A lineage can be viewed as specialized for the creation of the anatomical features which characterize the white matter tracts of the CNS: myelin sheaths and astrocytic specializations at nodes of Ranvier.

Migrating 0-2A progenitor cells and specialization of the neuroepithelium of the optic stalk. Given the observation that the optic nerve contains two different glial lineages, which are distinct at least as early as embryonic day 17 in the rat (Raff et al, 1984), it is of interest to determine how this occurs. Originally, the neuroepithelium of the optic stalk was thought to give rise to all of the glial cells found in the optic nerve, but not to neurons. However, recent studies suggest that this neuropithelium is even more restricted than previously thought, and gives rise only to type 1 astrocytes. These studies suggest that 0-2A progenitor cells enter the optic nerve as a wave of migratory cells during embryonic development, and have their origins in a germinal zone extrinsic to the nerve itself (Small et al, 1987).

The first 0-2A progenitors seen in the rat optic nerve appear close to the optic chiasm at day 16 of embryonic development (E16), and are not found in the mid-segment or retinal portions of the nerve until 1 or 2 days later (Small et al, 1987). A steep gradient in the number of these cells, and later of oligodendrocytes, found along the optic nerve continues until 9 days after birth. Although this observation could reflect a general wave of glial differentiation which progresses from the brain towards the eye, the differentiation of type 1 astrocytes proceeds in the opposite direction (from eye to brain).

Direct demonstration of the migratory behavior of 0-2A progenitor cells came from filming the behavior of these cells when grown in medium conditioned by type 1 astrocytes. In these experiments we found that 0-2A progenitors were highly motile cells which migrated with a top speed of over 100 um/h and with an average rate of 21 um/h. Differentiation of dividing progenitors into oligodendrocytes was associated with cessation of migration, suggesting that the migration of oligodendrocyte-related cells which has been previously observed in vivo (LaChapelle, et al, 1984) may be due to migration of 0-2A progenitors rather than of oligodendrocytes themselves.

The source of 0-2A progenitor cells for the optic nerve may be a germnal zone located in the preoptic recess of the optic chiasm (J. Altman, unpublished observations). It is interesting that migration of these cells into the optic nerve begins with the first arrival of retinal ganglion axons at the optic chiasm, suggesting that axons may provide the substrate needed to guide these cells into the optic nerve (Small, et al, 1987).

If 0-2A progenitor cells are migratory, why then do they not migrate into the eye and myelinate the retina? Over a half a century ago, Berliner (1931) proposed that the lamina cribosa, located just behind the eye, kept oligodendrocytes from entering the retina. In more recent studies, Raff and colleagues have suggested that the lamina cribrosa is formed by specialized type 1 astrocytes (ffrench-Constant et al, submitted). As previously described by Berliner, ffrench-Constant et al also found that the optic nerve of the rabbit contains no lamina cribrosa. This species, which is distinct in having a myelinated retina, also have 0-2A progenitor cells present in the retina, which presumably enter because of the lack of a lamina cribrosa. Myelination of the retinal ganglion axons in the eyes of these animals would opacify the retina; this is undoubtedly the reason why it is so difficult to teach rabbits to read.

0-2A progenitor cells in adult rats: a new cell type. In contrast to the general absence of repair of axons after neuronal damage in the CNS, repair and replacement of myelin sheaths after a demyelinating injury is effective under a variety of circumstances (for review, see McDonald, 1974). The cellular mechanisms which underly this repair are unknown, although it has been suggested that limited division of oligodendrocytes may occur follow demyelinating damage. However, the adult optic nerve also contains 0-2A progenitor cells (ffrench-Constant and Raff, 1986; Wolswijk and Noble, submitted), and it seems likely that these cells play a role in the replacement of oligodendrocytes in the adult CNS.

In the course of our studies on 0-2A progenitors of the optic nerves of adult rats, we found that these cells differ from their perinatal counterparts in antigenic phenotype, morphology, rate of division and migration and time course of differentiation into oligodendrocytes. For example, the earliest perinatal progenitors are A2B5$^{+}$ bipolar cells which express vimentin filaments, are not labelled with the 04 monoclonal antibody described by Sommer and Schachner (1981; see also below), can differentiate into oligodendrocytes or type 2 astrocytes in a timespan of less than 3 days, and divide with a cell-cycle time of about 22h (Raff et al., 1983b; Noble and Murray, 1984; Raff et al., 1985; Sommer and Noble submitted). In contrast, the progenitors isolated from the optic nerves of adult rats are both A2B5$^{+}$ and 04$^{+}$, lack vimentin filaments, have a unipolar morphology, divide with a cell-cycle time of about 60h, and require about two-and-a-half times longer to differentiate into either oligodendrocytes or type 2 astrocytes (Wolswijk and Noble, submitted).

The 0-2A$^{adult}$ progenitor: a third developmental pathway of the 0-2A$^{perinatal}$ progenitor cell. 0-2A$^{adult}$ progenitor cells seem to appear in the rat optic nerve as early as 7d after birth, and represent a substantial proportion of the progenitor population of the nerve by 21d after birth. The identification of the 0-2A$^{\underline{adult}}$ progenitor, and the finding that optic nerves of young rats contain two distinct types of 0-2A progenitor cells, raise the question of whether the 0-2A$^{\underline{adult}}$ progenitors represent a new population of progenitor cells which enter the optic nerve as a second migratory wave, or whether these cells are derived from their perinatal counterparts.

We have recently found that 0-2A$^{\underline{adult}}$ progenitors can be directly derived from 0-2A$^{\underline{perinatal}}$ progenitors (Wolswijk, et al., submitted), indicating that the cells we originally described as bipotential progenitors (Raff et al., 1983b) are actually tripotential cells which can give rise to a new type of progenitor which appears to be specialized to suit the needs of the adult animal (see below). The different properties of these cells suggest that the perinatal lineage gives rise to another progenitor cell more appropriate to the needs of the adult animal.

<u>Symmetric and asymmetric division and differentiation of 0-2A progenitors: two developmental pathways to the oligodendrocyte, and one pathway to the 0-2A$^{adult}$ progenitor cell.</u> Before discussing the derivation of 0-2A$^{\underline{adult}}$ progenitor cells from 0-2A$^{\underline{perinatal}}$ progenitors, it is first necessary to discuss oligodendrocyte differentiation.

At present we know of two distinctly different developmental strategies which can lead to the generation of oligodendrocytes. In the first, described by Temple and Raff (1986), 0-2A progenitors undergo a limited number of divisions, after which clonally related cells synchronously differentiate into oligodendrocytes. In the second pathway, which we have recently identified, progenitors divide asymmetrically, with one member of a pair of progeny differentiating into an oligodendrocyte while the other member of the pair continues on as a dividing progenitor cell (Wren, et al., submitted).

Are both patterns of oligodendrocyte development seen in vitro relevant in vivo? Regulation of differentiation by counting of cell divisions offers a simple means of generating large numbers of oligodendrocytes at well defined developmental periods (Temple and Raff, 1986). The requirement for extended progenitor division prior to differentiation may be particularly important in the 0-2A lineage during embryogenesis and early postnatal development, as asymmetric differentiation of progenitors into oligodendrocytes would reduce the capacity to generate large numbers of the migratory population which we think are necessary for the colonization of the optic nerve.

Although the needs of embryonic development may be met by families of cells which divide extensively before symmetrically generating large numbers of oligodendrocytes, such a developmental strategy is clearly not appropriate to the needs of the CNS of the healthy adult animal. Asymmetric generation of oligodendrocytes from slowly dividing progenitor cells capable of self-renewal for extended periods seems a more appropriate regulatory strategy to address such needs as the occassional replacement of dying cells within the CNS, or the ensheathment of bare axons developing due to continued lengthening of nerve tracts for some time after the initial burst of oligodendrocyte formation has ended.

In respect of the adult animal, it is of interest that the asymmetric division and differentiation of 0-2A$^{\underline{perinatal}}$ progenitor cells is associated the generation of cells with a phenotype almost identical to that of the 0-2A$^{\underline{adult}}$ progenitor.

Multiple stages in the differentiation of oligodendrocytes. Along with trying to understand the developmental biology of the optic nerve, we have also been utilizing the 0-2A progenitor as a tool for studying the regulation (and association between) division and differentiation. As I'm running out of alloted space, our work with growth factors will have to be sought out in the literature (Noble et, various papers in preparation). However, I do want to comment on the complexity of the differentiation of 0-2A progenitors into oligodendrocytes.

In our recent studies on 0-2A progenitors isolated from the optic nerves of 7d rats, we have found that we can distinguish at least 5 different bipotential phonotypes which seem to represent a developmental progression starting with the 0-2A$^{\underline{perinatal}}$ progenitor cell and ending up with a terminally committed oligodendrocyte. We have found that progenitor cells appear to go through a sequential loss of ability to dedifferentiate, ability to respond to astrocyte-derived mitogen and finally ability to respond to the GFAP-inducing factor(s) present in fetal serum before becoming a committed preoligodendrocyte (Sommer and Noble, in preparation).

Do neurons do anything? It is striking that in all of our studies on the control of division and differentiation of 0-2A progenitor cells, we have yet to identify a critical role for neurons. Purified type 1 astrocytes can promote progenitor cell division (Noble and Murray, 1984) and can support the generation of 0-2A$^{adult}$ progenitor cells from 0-2A$^{perinatal}$ progenitors (Wolswijk, et al., submitted), the correctly-timed and symmetrical differentiation of perinatal progenitors into oligodendrocytes (Raff et al., 1986; Temple and Raff, 1986), and the generation of oligodendrocytes by asymmetrical division and differentiation of both perinatal and adult progenitor cells (Wolswijk et al., submitted; Wren, et al., submitted). In addition, 0-2A progenitor cells that differentiate into oligodendrocytes in vitro go on to synthesize a full range of myelin specific lipids and proteins in the absence of neurons (Mirsky et al., 1978). The question therefore arises as to whether neurons are simply a passive partner in the interactions with the 0-2A lineage. For example, neurons may provide an appropriate substrate for migration of 0-2A progenitor cells into developing optic nerve and for the wrapping of myelin sheaths by oligodendrocytes. However, it seems more likely that the role of neurons is more dynamic than this, and it would not be surprising if neurons were soon found to induce particular differentiative events in cells of the 0-2A lineage.

Molecular studies. To probe the molecular biology of differentiation and growth control we need homogeneous population of cells. To better study migration in vivo we need marked cells which can be injected into an animal and easily recognized. To study the function of genes which may play role in the control of differentiation and proliferation, one needs a well-characterized cell-type to study. For these reasons, we have been using retrovirally-mediated gene insertion to create lines of 0-2A progenitors which are maturation arrested prior to terminal committment (MN and H. Land, in preparation). These cells, along with cell lines we are creating from other regions of the nervous system, will be of central importance in our future research.

## REFERENCES


Berliner, ML (1931) Cytologic studies on the retina. I. Normal coexistence of oligodendroglia and myelinated nerve fibers. Arch. Opthamol. 6: 740-751.

Bignami, A. Eng, LF, Dahl, D. & Uyeda, CT (1972) Localization of the glial fibrillary acidic protein in astrocytes by immunofluorescence. Brian Res. 43: 429-435.

Bonhoeffer, F & Huf, J (1985) Position-dependent properties of retinal axons and their growth cones. Nature 315: 409-410.

David, S, Miller, RH, Patel, R & Raff, MC (1984) Effects of neonatal transection on glial cell development in the optic nerve: evidence that the oligodendrocyte-fibrous astrocyte lineage depends on axons for its survival during development. J. Neurocytol. 13: 961-974.

Eisenbarth, GS, Walsh, FS and Nirenberg, M (1979) Monoclonal antibody to a plasma membrane antigen of neurons. Proc. Nat. Acad. Sci. (USA) 76: 4913-4917.

Fallon, JR (1985) Neurite guidance by non-neuronal cells in culture: Preferential outgrowth of peripheral neurites on glial as compared with noglial cell surfaces. J. Neurosci. 5: 3169-3177.

ffrench-Constant, C, Miller, RH, Burne, JF & Raff, MC. Evidence that specialized type-1 astrocytes in the lamina cribrosa region of the rat optic nerve prevent the migration of oligodendrocyte-type 2 (0-2A) progenitor cells into the retina. (submitted)

ffrench-Constant, C. & Raff, MC (1986a) Proliferating bipotential glial progenitor cells in adult rat optic nerve. Nature 319: 499-502.

ffrench-Constant, C and Raff, MC (1986b) The oligodendrocyte-type 2 astrocyte cell lineage is specialized for myelination. Nature 323: 335-338.

Janzer, RC & Raff, MC (1987) Astrocytes induce blood-brain barrier properties in endothelial cells. Nature 325: 253-257.

LaChapelle, F, Gumpel, M, Baulac, M, Jacque, C, Due, P & Baumann, N (1984) Transplantation of CNS fragments into the brain of shiverer mutant mice: extensive myelination by implanted oligodendrocytes. I. Immunological studies. Devel. Neurosci. 6: 325-334.

McDonald, WI (1974) Remyelination in relation to clinical lesions of the central nervous system. Br. Med. Bull. 30: 186-189.

Miller, RH, David, S, Patel, R, Abney, ER & Raff, MC (1985) A quantitative immnohistochemical study of macroglial cell development in the rat optic nerve: in vivo evidence for two distinct astrocyte lineages. Dev. Biol. 11:35-41.

Miller, RH & Raff, MC (1984) Fibrous and protoplasmic astrocytes are biochemically and developmentally distinct. J. Neurosci. 4: 485-492.

Mirsky, R, Winter, J, Abney, ER, Pruss, RM, Gavrilovic, J & Raff, MC (1980) Myelin-specific proteins and glycolipids in rat Schwann cells and oligodendrocytes in culture. J. Cell Biol. 84: 483-494.

Moore, MAS, Williams, N & Metcalf (1972) J. cell Physiol. 79: 283-292.

Noble, M (1986) Glial development and glial-neuronal interaction. In: Asbury, A, McKhann, G & McDonald, WI (eds) Diseases of the Nervous System. Heinemann, London, p 109-124.

Noble, M, Albrechtsen, M, Moller, C, Lyles, J, Bock, E, Goridis, C, Watanabe, M & Rutishauser, U 91985) Glial cells express N-CAM/D2-CAM-like polypeptides in vitro. Nature 316: 725-728.

Noble, M, Fok-Seang, J & Cohen, J (1984) Glia are a unique substrate for the in vitro growth of central nervous system neurons. J. Neurosci. 4: 1892-1903.

Noble, M & Murray, K (1984) Purified astrocytes promote the in vitro division of a bipotential glial progenitor cell. EMBO J. 3: 2243-2247.

Raff, MC, Abney, ER, Cohen, J, Lindsay, L & Noble, M (1983a) Two types of astrocytes in cultures of developing rat white matter: differences in morphology, surface gangliosides and growth characteristics J. Neurosci. 3: 1289-1300.

Raff, MC, Abney, ER & Miller, RH (1984a) Two glial cell lineages diverge prenatally in rat optic nerve. Develop. Biol. 106: 53-60.

Raff, MC, Fields, KL, Hakomori, S-I, Mirsky, R, Pruss, RM & winter, J (1979) Cell-type specific markers for distinguishing and identifying neurons and the major classess of glial cells in culture. Brain Res. 174: 283-308.

Raff, MC, Miller, RH & Noble, M (1983b) A glial progenitor cell that develops in vitro into an astrocyte or an oligodendrocyte depending on the culture medium. Nature 303: 390-396.

Raff, MC, Mirsky, R, Fields, KL, Lisak, RP, Dorfman, SH, Silberberg, DH, Gregson, NA, Leibowitiz, S, Kennedy, M (1978) Galactocerebroside: a specific cell surface antigenic marker for oligodendrocytes in culture. Nature 274: 813-816.

Raff, MC, Williams, BP & Miller, RH (1984b) The in vitro differentiation of a bipotential glial progenitor cell. EMBO J 3: 1857-1864.

Ranscht, B, Clapshaw, PA, Price, J, Noble, M & Seifert, W (1982) Development of oligodendrocytes and Schwann cells studies with a monoclonal antibody against galactocerebroside. Proc. Nat. Acad. Sci. (USA) 79: 2709-2713.

Rutishauser, U (1984) Development biology of a cell adhesion molecule. Nature 310: 549-554.

Silver, J (1984) Studies on the factors that govern directionality in the embryonic optic nerve and at the optic chiasm of mice. J. Comp. Neurol. 223: 238-251.

Silver, J & Rutishauser, U (1984) Guidance of optic axons in vivo by a preformed adhesive pathway on neuroepithelial endfeet. Dev. Biol. 106: 485-494.

Silver, J & Sapiro, J (1981) Axonal guidance during development of the optic nerve: the role of pigmented epithelia and other extrinsic factors. J. Comp. Neurol. 202: 521-538.

Silver, J & Sidman, RL (1979) A mechanism for the topographic patterning of retinal ganglion cell axons. J. Comp. Neurol. 189: 101-111.

Small, RK, Riddle, P & Noble, M (1987) Evidence for migration of oligodendrocyte-type 2 astrocyte progenitor cells into the developing rat optic nerve. Nature 328: 155-158.

Sommer, I & Schachner, M (1981) Monoclonal antibodies (01 to 04) for oligodendrocyte cell surfaces: an immunological study in the central nervous system. Devel. Biol. 83: 311-327.

Temple, S & Raff, MC (1986) Clonal analysis of oligodendrocyte development: Evidence for a developmental clock that counts cell dvisions. Cell 44: 773-779.

Wolswijk, G & Noble, M. Oligodendrocyte-type 2 astrocyte (0-2A) progenitor cells isolated from otpic nerves of adult rats differ from their neonatal counterparts in antigenic phenotype, morphology, rate of migration, cell cycle time and time course of differentiation in vitro. (submitted).

Wolswijk, G, Wren, D & Noble, M. Developmental studies in vivo and in vitro on the oligodendrocyte-type 2 astrocyte (0-2A)adult progenitor cells of the rat optic nerve : A third developmental pathway for the 0-2Aperinatal progenitor cell.

Wren, D, Wolswijk, G & Noble, M. Symmetric and asymmetric division and differentiation of oligodendrocyte-type 2 astrocyte progenitor cells.

# NEURAL CREST CELLS CHANGE THEIR HOMING BEHAVIOR FOLLOWING TREATMENT WITH A PHORBOL ESTER DRUG

G. Ciment and R. Sears
Department of Cell Biology and Anatomy
Oregon Health Sciences University
Portland, Oregon 97201
U.S.A.

## BACKGROUND

The neural crest is a transient embryonic structure seen at the end of neurulation during vertebrate embryogenesis. Neural crest cells originate within the neural tube, but leave the tube to migrate along characteristic pathways in the embryo, eventually giving rise to a wide variety of different cell types in the adult, including neuronal and glial cells of the peripheral nervous system, endocrine cells, pigment cells of the integument, and various connective tissue cell types in the head and neck (Le Douarin, 1982).

The pathways utilized by migrating neural crest cells have been well studied, principally in avian embryos (Weston, 1963; Noden, 1978; Le Douarin, 1982; Bronner-Fraser, 1986a). In the trunk, the majority of crest cells migrate ventrally through the anterior portion of each somite just after the somite has begun to de-epithelialize into the dermomyotome and sclerotome. These crest cells later give rise to the neurons and glial cells of the dorsal root ganglia (DRG) and sympathetic ganglia, as well as pheochromocytes of the adrenal medulla, etc. Other truncal crest cells migrate dorsad to the dermomyotome, thereby colonizing the integument and giving rise to melanocytes.

In previous work, we studied the effects of the phorbol ester drug 12-0-tetradecanoylphorbol-13-acetate (TPA) on avian neural crest development. We found

NATO ASI Series, Vol. H22
Neural Development and Regeneration.
Edited by A. Gorio et al.

that the neural crest-derived cells of quail DRG changed their differentiative behavior when cultured in the presence of TPA (Ciment et al., 1986). Whereas DRG dissected from embryos older than 4 days did not give rise to pigmented cells when cultured in the absence of TPA, DRG from embryos of 5-9 days readily gave rise to pigment cells when cultured in the presence of TPA. These cells were judged to be true melanocytes based on their ability to colonize the integument and produce normal-appearing pigmented feather primordia in *in vivo* experiments. We interpret these data to mean that neural crest cells which migrate to the DRG (and other sites where melanogenesis does not normally occur) undergo the developmental restriction of melanogenesis sometime between embryonic days 4 and 5, and that TPA somehow reverses this developmental restriction.

In work presented here, we examined the effects of TPA on the homing behavior of crest-derived cells. We report that TPA also has dramatic effects on the site of localization of DRG cells in early embryos. Whereas crest-derived cells of the DRG normally home to the host's DRG, peripheral nerves and sympathetic ganglia when back-grafted into younger embryos, we report that TPA-treated DRG cells localize in the integument and, more surprisingly, the central nervous system.

## MATERIALS AND METHODS

Dorsal root ganglia were dissected from 4.5 day embryonic quail (*Coturnix coturnix japonica)* and cultured as explants for 5-6 days at 38°C in a 10% $CO_2$, 100% humidified incubator. Culture medium consisted of 10% fetal calf serum (Gibco), 5% chicken embryo extract, 5 ng/ml nerve growth factor (Collaborative Research), 100 units/ml penicillin G, and 100 ug/ml streptomycin in Ham's F-12 nutrient medium (Gibco). Culture medium was supplemented either with 1.0 uM TPA (Sigma) and 0.1% ethanol, or with 0.1% ethanol alone as a negative control.

Heterospecific grafting was performed as described (Ciment and Weston, 1985; Ciment et al., 1986). Briefly, this involved grafting fragments of DRG explants into the neural crest migratory space at an axial level approximately 2-5 somites anterior to the unsegmented mesoderm of 2.0-2.5 day embryonic chick (White Leghorn) embryos *in ovo*. Care was taken to avoid using fragments containing pigmented cells. The host chick embryos were allowed to develop for an additional 5 days, and then were fixed, embedded in parafin, sectioned, and stained according to the Feulgen-Rosenbeck procedure, which allows one to distinguish between quail-derived (i.e., graft) and chick-derived (i.e., host) cells based on differences in nuclear staining (Le Douarin, 1973).

For this report, a total of five chimeric embryos were generated--three containing TPA-treated DRG cells, and two negative controls containing DRG cells treated with vehicle only.

## RESULTS

To determine whether TPA affects the homing behavior of early crest-derived cells, heterospecific grafting studies were performed using implants of 4.5 day embryonic quail DRG cultured in the presence or absence of TPA.

**Grafts of DRG treated with TPA in culture**

When TPA-treated DRG were grafted into the neural crest migratory space, the vast majority (>95%) of quail-derived cells were found to be pigmented, regardless of their location. The closed circles in Fig.1 represent the approximate sites of these pigmented cells, as seen in one chimeric embryo. Not surprisingly, many of the pigmented cells were found in the loose connective tissue of the dermis (e.g., Fig.2A and 2B) and had the morphological appearance of melanocytes. Other pigmented cells were observed within deeper connective tissue or adjacent to the cartilage of the nascent vertebrae (Fig.2C and 2D) -- also normal locations of melanocytes in quail. Although most pigmented cells were found ipsilateral to the graft site, other cells were seen to have crossed the dorsal midline to a small extent. These data, then, support our earlier notion that TPA-treatment in culture causes some DRG cells to undergo a metaplastic transformation into melanocytes (Ciment et al., 1986).

Surprisingly, a significant proportion of pigmented cells were also observed within the C.N.S. of these same embryos (Fig.1). Although there were some variation between embryos, in general, three C.N.S. areas were found to contain pigmented quail cells. The most common site was in the marginal zone of the nascent spinal cord adjacent to the germinal matrix zone (Fig.3C and 3D). Here, pigmented cells were seen to send processes intertwining with nearby post-mitotic neurons (arrow in Fig.3D). The second most common site was in the white matter of the dorsal half of the cord, where again, pigment-bearing processes were common (Fig.3A and 3B). The third site of localization of pigmented cells was within the germinal matrix zone in the roof of the cord (Fig.1.). At all three sites, pigmented cells were spread out along the spinal cord, and not found in clusters. As before, most pigmented cells were ipsilateral to the side in which grafting occurred.

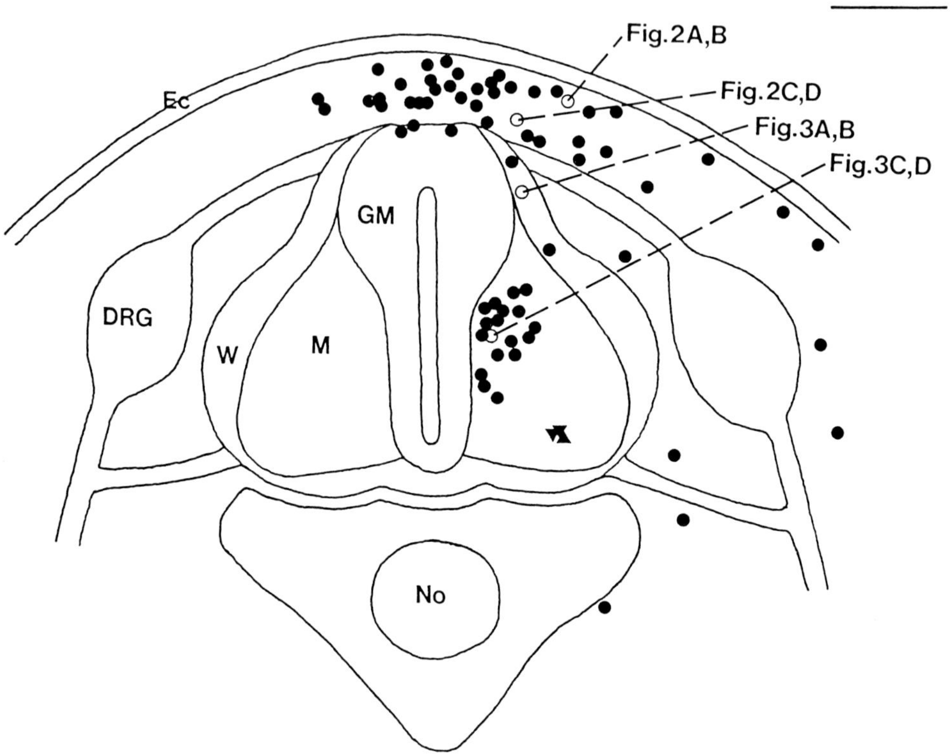


**Fig.1** - Diagramatic representation compiling the locations of TPA-treated DRG cells in one chimeric embryo. In this experiment, DRG from 4.5 day quail embryos were cultured in the presence of TPA for 5 days and then back-grafted into the neural crest migratory space of a 2.0 day chicken host, as described in the Materials and Methods. The closed circles indicate the approximate locations of pigmented quail-derived cells seen at various axial levels; open circles indicate the locations of the pigmented quail-derived cells seen in Figs. 2 and 3 (from a second embryo); closed triangles indicate the locations of the non-pigmented quail-derived cells seen in Fig.4 (also from this second embryo). The scale bar in the upper right corner corresponds approximately to 100 um. DRG, dorsal root ganglion; Ec, ectoderm; GM, germinal matrix zone; M, marginal zone; No, notocord; W, white matter.

Although encountered less frequently, non-pigmented quail-derived cells couldalso be found within the C.N.S. (Fig.4). In the two cases observed, non-pigmented cells were found in small clusters in the ventral portion of the marginal zone near the point of exit of the ventral roots. The nuclei of these cells were small (around 4 um) and did not have the morphological appearance of neurons.

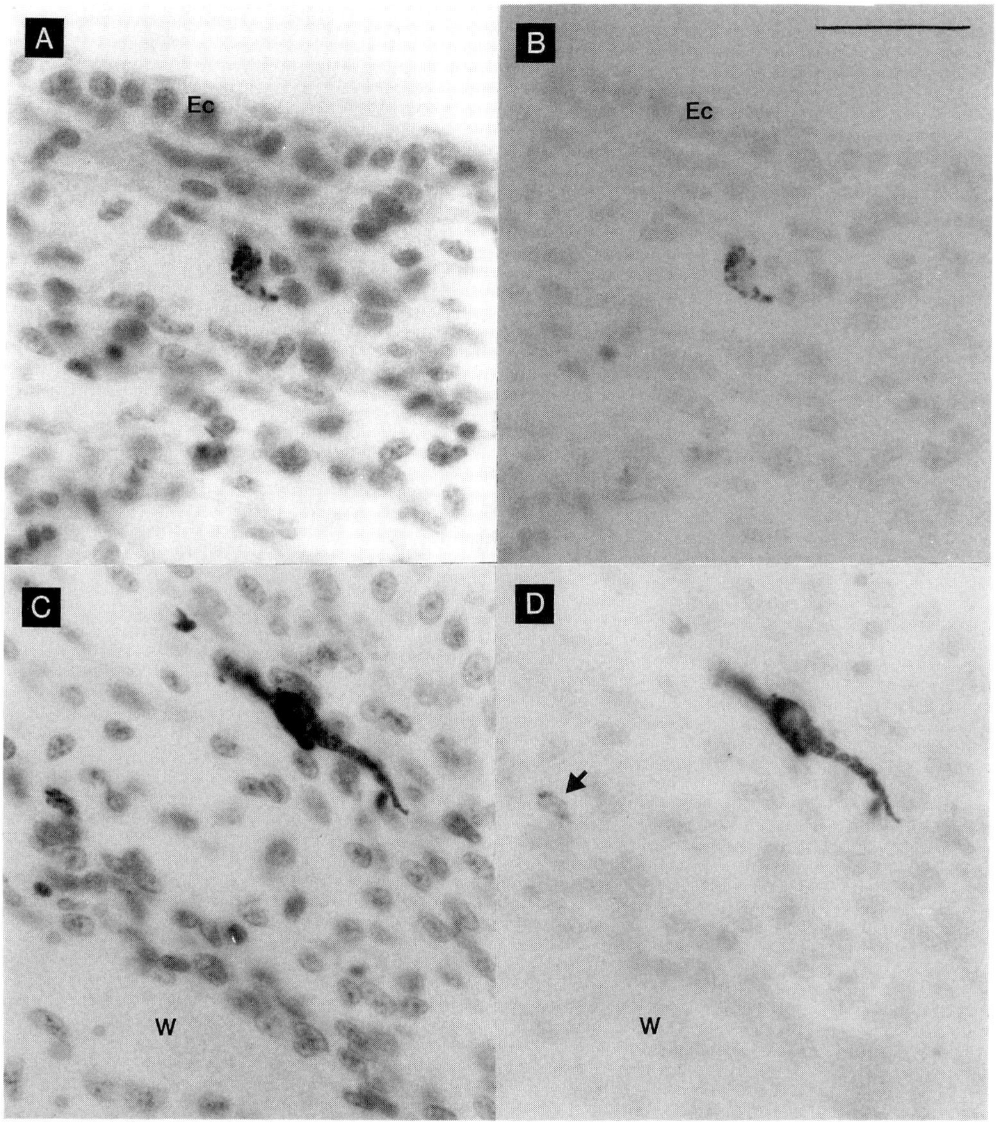


**Fig.2** - Photomicrographs showing pigmented quail-derived cells in the connective tissue of the dermis (A and B) or surrounding the spinal cord (C and D) of a chimeric embryo similar to the one represented in Fig.1. Panels A and C were photographed through a green filter to accentuate the magenta-staining nuclei of all cells; panels B and D were photographed through a red filter, allowing the opaque melanosomes to be seen more clearly. Note the melanocyte-like morphologies of these pigmented cells, and that a second, lightly pigmented cell can also be seen in panel D (at the arrow). The scale bar in the upper right corner corresponds to 25 um. Ec, ectoderm; W, white matter.

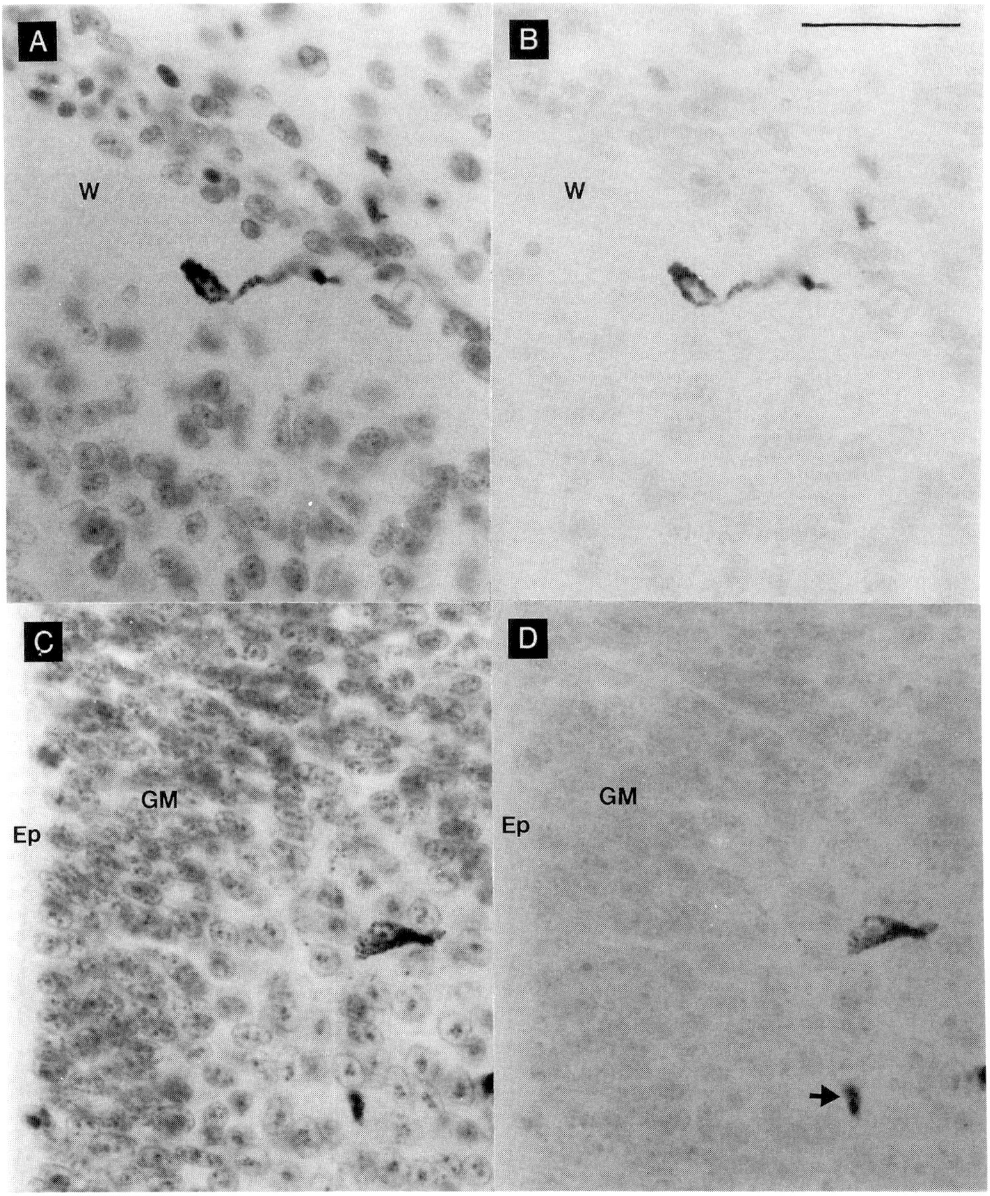


**Fig.3** - Photomicrographs showing pigmented quail-derived cells in the white matter (A and B) or marginal zone (C and D) of the spinal cord of the chimeric embryo seen in Fig.2. Again, panels A and C were photographed through a green filter, and panels B and D were photographed through a red filter. Note the pigmented processes of cells whose nuclei are in adjacent sections in panel D (at the arrows). The scale bar in the upper right corner corresponds to 25 um. Ep, ependymal surface, GM, germinal matrix zone, W, white matter.

**Grafts of DRG NOT treated with TPA in culture**

When DRG were cultured in the absence of TPA and then back-grafted into the neural crest migratory space of host chicken embryos, quail-derived cells were found in peripheral nerves, sympathetic ganglia, and in the aortic plexus (data not shown). In no case were quail cells seen in the C.N.S., nor did any of the quail-derived cells contain pigment granules. These control chimeric embryos, then, essentially re-confirm the results of earlier heterospecific grafting studies using DRG cells (Le Lievre et al., 1980; Schweizer et al., 1983).

## DISCUSSION

These and other data indicate that TPA has dramatic effects on both the differentiative and morphogenetic properties of early neural crest-derived cells. Earlier experiments showed that TPA reverses the developmental restriction of melanogenesis in DRG cells (Ciment et al., 1986), and we now show that TPA causes some DRG cells to migrate into the C.N.S. -- a site in which crest-derived cells are never seen in heterospecific grafting experiments (e.g., Erickson et al., 1980; Le Lievre et al., 1980; Le Douarin, 1982; Schweizer et al., 1983; Teillet et al., 1987).

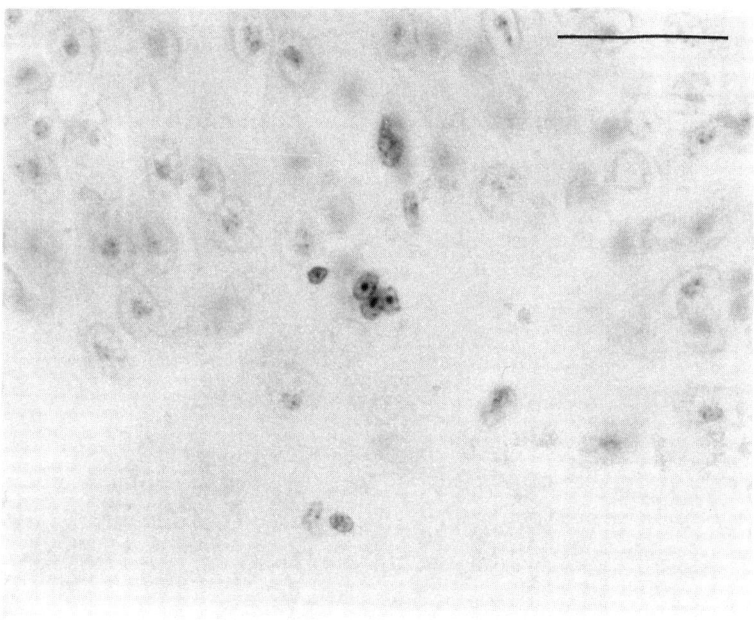

**Fig.4** - Photomicrograph showing unpigmented quail-derived cells in the marginal zone of the nascent spinal cord. The chimeric embryo is the same as that seen in Fig.2. The scale bar in the upper right corner corresponds to 25 um.

**Homing of neural crest cells is a carefully regulated morphogenetic event**

Various studies indicate that the homing behavior of neural crest cells is a carefully regulated event. First, studies examining the normal route of crest cell migration showed that crest cells migrated only along specific pathways in the embryo, even when other potential routes of migration become available to them (Weston et al., 1978; Bronner-Fraser, 1986a; Teillet et al., 1987). Second, when crest cells from one axial level were experimentally grafted to other axial levels, they migrated along crest migratory routes appropriate to their new location rather than their source (Le Douarin, 1982). And third, when various non-crested-derived cell types are grafted into the crest migratory space, they did not follow the neural crest migratory pathway, indicating that not all types of migrating cells recognize the same environmental cues (Erickson et al., 1980). Together then, these studies suggest that crest cells have an intrinsic cellular "program" which governs the route of migration, presumably by controlling the recognition of specific sets of cues in the microenvironment. It seems likely, moreover, that this program is relatively stable during early development, since both crest cells and early crest-derived cells show qualitatively similar patterns of migration and localization (Schweizer et al., 1983).

**TPA changes the homing behavior of neural crest-derived cells**

The studies reported here indicate that treatment with TPA alters the cellular programs governing both the subsequent differentiation and migration of early crest-derived cells. Not only does TPA cause DRG cells to undergo pigmentation in these chimeric embryos, but it also dramatically alters the sites to which these cells home.

A number of additional conclusions can be drawn from these experiments. First, it is clear that TPA affects the crest cells themselves, rather than the cells constituting their environment, since only grafted (i.e., crest-derived) cells were exposed to TPA in these studies. Second, it seems likely that these effects of TPA are relatively long-lasting, since this drug was not present at the time that overt differentiation and migration occurred. And third, these two TPA-induced events -- namely, pigmented formation and C.N.S. homing -- are not necessarily linked, since we also found non-pigmented quail-derived cells in the C.N.S. Indeed, Erickson et al. (1980) have essentially done the reciprocal experiment by grafting cultures of pigmented neural crest cells into the crest-migratory space of chicken hosts, and found that pigmented (but not TPA-treated) cells also did not home to the C.N.S.

Although it is not known which environmental elements are recognized as pathway cues by migrating crest cells, several studies have implicated fibronectin and/or laminin. Injection of antibodies against the cell surface receptors for either of these extracellular matrix molecules, for example, have been shown to disrupt the migration of cranial crest cells (Bronner-Fraser, 1986b). Moreover, injection of the tetrapeptide fragment believed to be the portion of the fibronectin molecule recognized by the fibronectin receptor, has similar effects (Poole and Thiery, 1986). These studies suggest that crest cells recognize these extracellular matrix molecules as pathway cues, and that substances which interfere with this recognition interfere with migration. In the context of our studies, then, it is interesting to note that neither of these matrix molecules are present at appreciable levels in the C.N.S.

The areas within the C.N.S. where TPA-treated DRG cells were found are also of interest. These sites included the marginal zone (containing differentiating post-mitotic neurons), the white matter (containing axons and growth cones), and to a lesser degree, the germinal matrix zone (containing proliferating neuroepithelial cells). It should not be surprising that there were only a few cells in the germinal matrix zone, however, since this area is one of continuous cellular movements as the nuclei of proliferating cells move back and forth between the ependymal and pial surfaces. It remains to be seen whether these various sites are "specific" (yet, of course, ectopic) targets of TPA-treated crest cells, or whether they are simply areas of the early C.N.S. where relatively less motile cells tend to accumulate.

Although it is not yet known exactly how TPA affects crest-derived cells in our experimental system, it is interesting to note that protein kinase C is considered to be the site of TPA action in other cell types (Niedel et al., 1983). In these other cells, short-term treatment with TPA increases protein kinase C activity, whereas long-term treatment (i.e., for days) causes the down-regulation of activity (Inagaki at al., 1984). Since it is also believed that protein kinase C serves as part of the mechanism by which various "growth factors" act (Nishizuka, 1984), it is interesting to speculate that these growth factors might play a role during early development governing the differentiative and homing properties of migrating neural crest cells -- a role presumably independent of their effects on proliferation.

## ACKNOWLEDGEMENTS

This work was supported by NIH grant NS23883 to GC.

## LITERATURE REFERENCES

Bronner-Fraser M (1986a) Analysis of the early stages of trunk neural crest migration in avian embryos using monoclonal antibody HNK-1. Develop Biol 115:44-55

Bronner-Fraser M (1986b) An antibody to a receptor for fibronectin and laminin perturbs cranial neural crest development *in vivo*. Develop Biol 117:528-536

Ciment G, Weston JA (1985) Segregation of developmental abilities in neural crest-derived cells: Identification of partially restricted intermediate cell types in the branchial arches of avian embryos. Develop Biol 111:73-83

Ciment G, Glimelius B, Nelson DM, Weston JA (1986) Reversal of a developmental restriction in neural crest-derived cells of avian embryos by a phorbol ester drug. Develop Biol 118:392-398

Erickson, CA, Tosney KW, Weston JA (1980) Analysis of migratory behavior of neural crest and fibroblastic cells in embryonic tissues. Develop Biol 77:142-156

Inagaki M, Hagiwara M, Saitoch M, Hidaka H (1984) Protein kinase C negatively modulated by phorbol ester. FEBS Letts 202:277-281

Le Douarin NM (1973) A biological cell labeling technique and its use in experimental embryology. Develop Biol 30:217-222

Le Douarin NM (1982) The Neural Crest. Cambridge University Press, Cambridge

Le Lievre CS, Schweizer GG, Ziller CM, Le Douarin NM (1980) Restrictions of developmental capabilities in neural crest cell derivatives as tested by *in vivo* transplantation experiments. Develop Biol 77:362-378

Niedel JE, Kuhn LJ, Vandermark GR (1983) Phorbol diester receptor copurifies with protein kinase C. Proc Natl Acad Sci (USA) 80:36-40

Nishizuka Y (1984) The role of protein kinase C in cell surface signal transduction and tumour promotion. Nature 308:693-698

Noden D (1978) An analysis of the migratory behavior of avian cephalic neural crest cells. Develop Biol 42:106-130

Poole TJ, Thiery JP (1986) Antibodies and a synthetic peptide that blocks cell-fibronectin adhesion arrest neural crest cell migration *in vivo*. In: Slavkin H (ed) Progress in Developmental Biology, Part B. Alan Liss, New York, pp 235-238

Schweizer G, Ayer-Le Lievre C, Le Douarin NM (1983) Restrictions of developmental capacities in the dorsal root ganglia during the course of development. Cell Diffn 13:191-200

Teillet M-A, Kalcheim C, Le Douarin NM (1987) Formation of the dorsal root ganglia in the avian embryo: Segmental origin and migratory behavior of neural crest progenitor cells. Develop Biol 120:329-347

Weston JA (1963) A radiographic analysis of the migration and localization of trunk neural crest cells in the chick. Develop Biol 6:279-310

Weston JA, Derby MA, Pintar JE (1978) Changes in the extra-cellular environment of neural crest cells during their early migration. Zoon 6:103-113

# DIFFERENTIATION OF GLIAL PRECURSORS IN CEREBELLAR PRIMARY CULTURES

G. Levi, F. Aloisi, V. Gallo and C. Agresti
Istituto Superiore di Sanità
Laboratorio di Fisiopatologia di Organo e di Sistema
Viale Regina Elena 299
00161 Roma
Italy

## INTRODUCTION

In the last few years we have utilized cerebellar primary cultures in order to study problems related to the differentiation, lineage and function of cerebellar glial cells.

Initially, we characterized 2 populations of astroglial cells in serum-containing cultures, obtained from the 8-day postnatal rat cerebellum (Wilkin et al. 1983; Johnstone et al. 1986). These two populations differ from each other morphologically, antigenically and functionally and appear to be the cerebellar equivalent of the type-1 and type-2 astrocytes described by Raff and collaborators in the rat optic nerve (Raff et al. 1983b).

In another set of studies (Levi et al. 1986), we have shown that when postnatal cerebellar cells are plated and cultured in a serum-free medium, only one, scarcely proliferating, astroglial cell population is present. Adopting antigenic and functional criteria, this population is composed of only type-1 astrocytes. The cultures, however, contain colonies of proliferating glial precursors which express on their surface the gangliosides recognized by the monoclonal antibodies A2B5 and LB1, (Kasai and Yu 1983; Fredman et al. 1984; Curtis et al. in press). After about a week in serum-free conditions these precursors start to differentiate into galactocerebroside$^+$ (GalC$^+$) oligodendrocytes, passing through four distinct stages (Levi et al. 1987). The first stage is characterized by A2B5-LB1 positivity. After 3-4 days in vitro, the cells enter the second stage, during which they express another surface antigen, recognized by the monoclonal antibody O4, which has been shown to label both immature and mature oligodendrocytes (Sommer and Schachner 1981). After another few days, the cells start to ex-

NATO ASI Series, Vol. H22
Neural Development and Regeneration
Edited by A. Gorio et al.

press on their surface also the mature oligodendrocyte marker GalC (Raff et al. 1978), so that, although for a short period, they become positive for all four markers, A2B5, LB1, O4 and GalC. In the fourth stage the cells stop proliferating and lose the surface gangliosides recognized by A2B5 and LB1, remaining $O4^+$ and $GalC^+$.

In agreement with the observations of Raff et al. (1983a) who used rat optic nerve cultures, we could demonstrate that the cerebellar glial precursors have a bipotential nature, namely, they differentiate into glial fibrillary acidic protein (GFAP)-positive type-2 astrocytes if serum is added to the incubation medium (Levi et al. 1986). In particular, they maintain their bipotentiality during the first two differentiation stages (A2B5-LB1 and A2B5-LB1-O4 positivity) and probably also during the short-lasting third stage (A2B5-LB1-O4-GalC positivity) (Levi et al. 1987).

In apparent contrast with the above observations, it is known that oligodendrocytes can be cultured in the presence of serum, and in some cases it has been shown that oligodendrocytes can even differentiate from precursor cells in serum-containing media (McCarthy and De Vellis 1980; Bologa-Sandru et al. 1981; Barbarese and Pfeiffer 1981; Goldman et al. 1986). On the basis of experiments on cortical glial cultures, Goldman et al. (1986) suggested that, besides serum, cellular interactions may influence the differentiation route taken by bipotential glial precursors. In order to try to clarify this problem, we monitored the antigenic development of $LB1^+$ progenitor cells in serum-containing cerebellar cultures.

## EFFECT OF CELL DENSITY ON THE DIFFERENTIATION PROFILE OF BIPOTENTIAL GLIAL PRECURSORS

In low density, serum-containing cultures ($1 \times 10^5$ cells/$cm^2$), within 5 days in vitro about 70% of the $A2B5^+$, $LB1^+$ precursors became, as previously noted (Levi et al. 1986), $GFAP^+$ (Fig. 1 A-B). However, even if not all, an elevated proportion of the $LB1^+$ precursors appeared to express GFAP after having expressed the O4 antigen (Fig. 1 C-D), generally considered to be characteristic of the oligodendroglial differentiation route, while only few $O4^+$ cells became $GalC^+$ (Fig. 1 E-F). It is therefore possible that, in the culture conditions adopted, cells that had already received in vivo the signals capable of orienting them towards an oligodendroglial differentiation are forced towards an astroglial differentiation. However, when the initial plating density was increased to $2.5 \times 10^5$ cells/$cm^2$, a lower

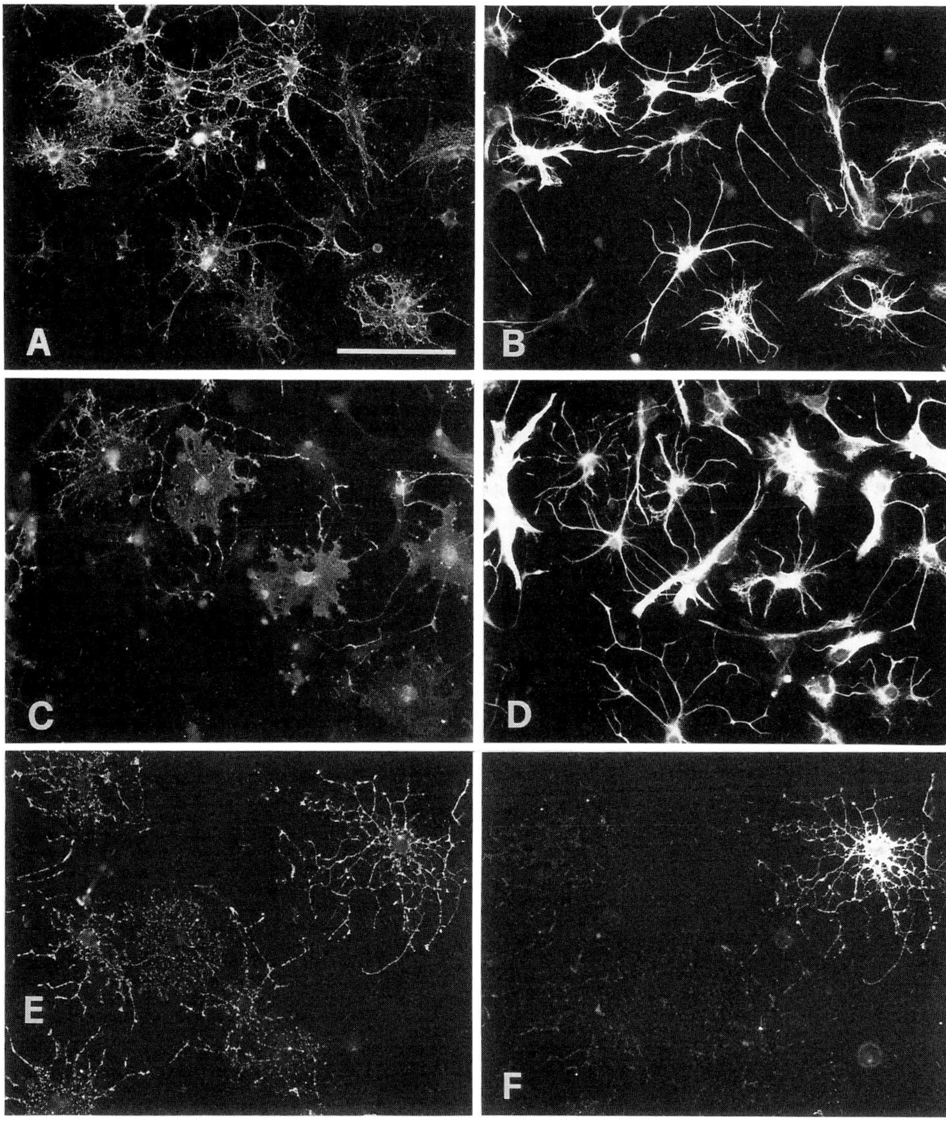


Fig. 1. Differentiation of cerebellar glial cells in serum-containing low density cultures at 5 days in vitro. Cells dissociated from 8-day postnatal rat cerebella (Levi et al. 1984) were plated at low density ($1 \times 10^5$ cells/$cm^2$) on poly-L-lysine-coated coverslips and cultured in Basal Eagle's Medium supplemented with 10% fetal calf serum. Double immunofluorescence staining was performed according to Levi et al. (1987), using the following antibodies: LB1 (A, fluorescein optics) and anti-GFAP (B, rhodamine optics); O4 (C, fluorescein optics) and anti-GFAP (D, rhodamine optics); O4 (D, fluorescein optics) and anti-GalC (E, rhodamine optics). Each couple of panels (A-B, C-D, E-F) represents the same microscopic field. Scale bar = 100 μm.

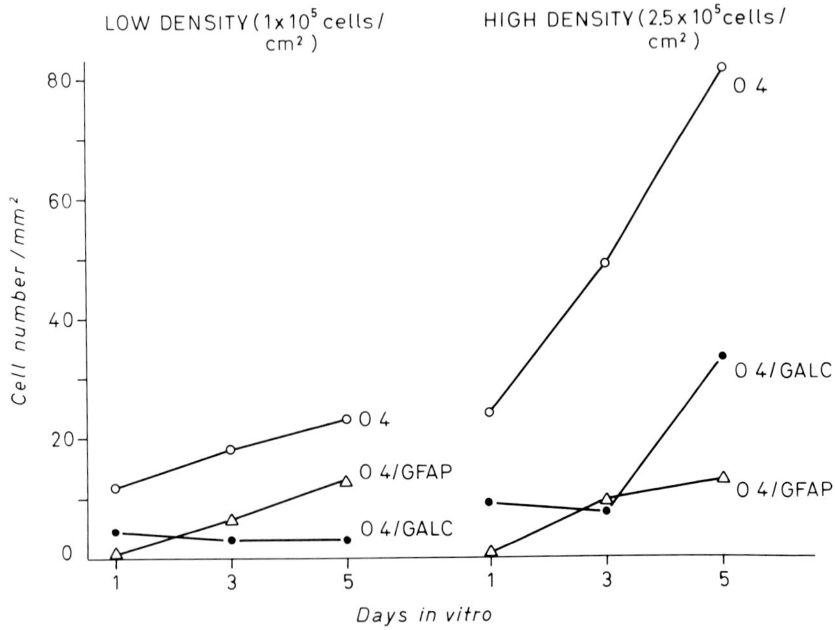


Fig. 2. Time course of expression of GFAP and GalC by $04^+$ cells in cerebellar cultures at different cell densities. Experimental details as in Fig. 1. Cells were plated at low density (left panel, 1 x $10^5$ cells/ $cm^2$) or at high density (right panel, 2.5 x $10^5$ cells/$cm^2$), cultured for up to 5 days, and double-stained with 04 and either anti-GFAP or anti-GalC antibodies. The number/$mm^2$ of total $04^+$ cells and the number of $04^+$, $GFAP^+$ and of $04^+$, $GalC^+$ cells is reported on the ordinate. Each point represents the average of cell counts obtained in 2-4 experiments (two coverslips per experiments, twenty 0.44 $mm^2$ microscopic fields per coverslip).

percentage of the $LB1^+$ or $04^+$ precursors expressed GFAP, while a substantial proportion of them became $GalC^+$. The data reported above, expressed in a quantitative form in Fig. 2, suggest that, in high density cultures, specific cell interactions are established which allow the progenitor cells to carry on their differentiation into oligodendrocytes, and render less likely the expression of an astroglial phenotype.

## EFFECT OF TYPE-1 ASTROCYTES ON THE DIFFERENTIATION OF BIPOTENTIAL GLIAL PRECURSORS

In the glial cultures used in our study, $GFAP^+$, $LB1^-$, type-1 astrocytes represent the most abundant cell population. We performed two types of

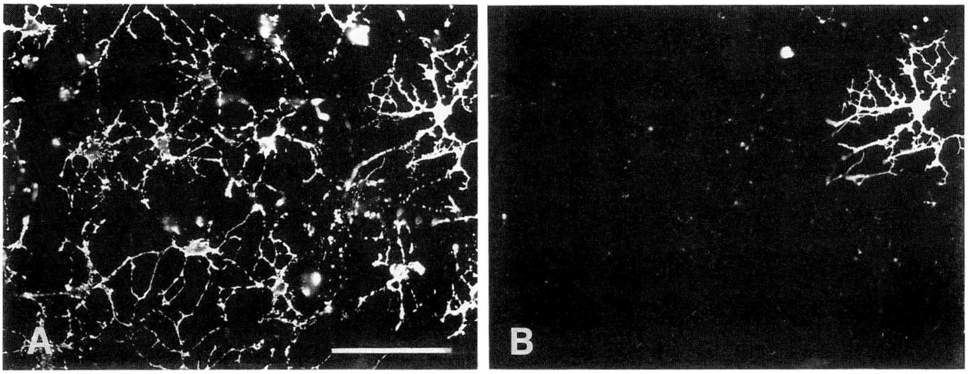


Fig. 3. Expression of GalC by $04^+$ cells in low density cerebellar cultures maintained for 5 days in type-1 astrocyte conditioned, serum-containing medium. For experimental details and quantitative evaluation, see Table 1. Double immunofluorescence staining with 04 (panel A, fluorescein optics) and anti-GalC (panel B, rhodamine optics) monoclonal antibodies. Scale bar = 100 µm.

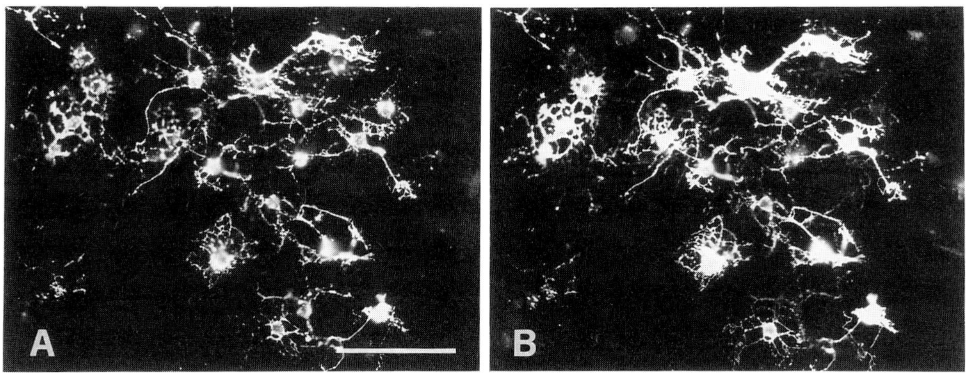


Fig. 4. Expression of GalC by $04^+$ cells in low density cerebellar cultures plated together with purified type-1 astrocytes and incubated for 5 days. For experimental details and quantitative evaluation, see Table 1. Double immunofluorescence staining with 04 (panel A, fluorescein optics) and anti-GalC (panel B, rhodamine optics) monoclonal antibodies. Scale bar = 100 µm.

experiments in order to determine whether the differentiation of bipotential glial precursors into oligodendrocytes in high density serum-containing cultures could be related to humoral factors secreted by type-1 astro-

TABLE 1. Influence of type-1 astrocytes on bipotential glial progenitor cell differentiation and proliferation in serum-containing cerebellar primary cultures.

| Plating conditions | $LB1^+$ cells per $mm^2$ | $LB1^+$ cells expressing GFAP | $04^+$ cells per $mm^2$ | $04^+$ cells expressing GalC |
|---|---|---|---|---|
| A. Low density, controls | 41 | 63% | 38 | 11% |
| B. Low density, grown in type-1 astrocyte conditioned medium. | 105 | 20% | 89 | 10% |
| C. Low density, plated with purified type-1 astrocytes | 67 | 33% | 64 | 36% |

Freshly dissociated 8-day postnatal rat cerebellar cells were cultured for 5 days in three different conditions: A: controls. The cells were plated at low density ($1 \times 10^5$ cells/$cm^2$) on poly-L-lysine coated coverslips and cultured as such. B: the cells were plated as in A, and 2h later the coverslips were transferred into plastic dishes containing a monolayer of confluent, purified type-1 astrocytes, in order to expose the freshly dissociated cells to a medium conditioned by type-1 astrocytes, and to avoid direct contact with them. C: the cerebellar cells were plated after mixing them with purified type-1 astrocytes dissociated from confluent astrocyte cultures. The density of the cells in the suspension was adjusted to plate $4 \times 10^4$ type-1 astrocytes/$cm^2$, together with $1 \times 10^5$ freshly dissociated cerebellar cells/$cm^2$. Purified type-1 astrocyte cultures were obtained by exposing cerebellar cell suspensions to A2B5 monoclonal antibodies and complement, to kill neurons and bipotential glial precursors. Line A, B and C: the cultures were processed for double immunofluorescence staining with LB1 and anti-GFAP or with 04 and anti-GalC antibodies (Levi et al. 1987), and the labelled cells were counted in 3-4 experiments (two coverslips/experiment, twenty 0.44 $mm^2$ microscopic fields/experiment). In the coculture experiments (C) counting the $LB1^+$, $GFAP^+$ cells lying on top of the $GFAP^+$ type-1 astrocytes was difficult. In this case the cells were dissociated with trypsin-EDTA, and replated at a lower density on new coverslips before immunostaining and counting.

cytes or to a direct cellular interaction with them.

In order to test for the effect of soluble factors present in astrocyte conditioned medium, the differentiation of the precursors in control low density cultures was compared to that occurring when the coverslips containing freshly plated cerebellar cells were transferred into culture dishes containing a monolayer of purified type-1 astrocytes. Table 1 shows that, after 5 days in vitro in the presence of conditioned medium, the number of $LB1^+$ or $O4^+$ precursors was much greater than in control cultures, but the proportion of $LB1^+$ cells expressing GFAP and of $O4^+$ cells (Fig. 3) expressing GalC was very low. These data suggest that the conditioned medium increases the proliferation of the bipotential precursors (an observation in accord with those of Noble and Murray (1984) and Raff et al. (1985) in optic nerve serum-free cultures) but slows down their differentiation into either direction. Incidentally, it has to be noted that the type-1 astrocytes present on the coverslips placed in conditioned medium proliferated substantially less than in control cultures (data not shown), a finding that is in keeping with our previous observations on the antiproliferative activity of serum-containing media conditioned by astroglial cells (Aloisi et al. 1987).

In the second type of experiment, cells dissociated from the cerebellum were plated at low density together with type-1 astrocytes ($4 \times 10^4$ cells/$cm^2$) dissociated from purified confluent cultures. Also in this case the population of $LB1^+$ or $O4^+$ precursors proliferated more than in low density controls, but the proportion of $O4^+$ cells differentiating into $GalC^+$ oligodendrocytes was much greater (Fig. 4), while the proportion of precursors taking the astroglial differentiation route was low (Table 1). It seems therefore reasonable to suggest that in the cocultures the direct interaction between type-1 astrocytes and glial precursors pushes the precursors towards an oligodendroglial differentiation and tends to antagonize both the serum factors facilitating their differentiation into astrocytes and the humoral, type-1 astrocyte-derived factors enhancing the proliferation, but slowing down the differentiation of the precursors.

## EXPRESSION OF THE PROTEOGLYCAN CHONDROITIN SULFATE BY CEREBELLAR GLIAL CELLS

It seems now important to understand what mediates the presumed direct interaction between type-1 astrocytes and glial precursors. Among the possible candidates, two classes of compounds might play an important role: components of the extracellular matrix and adhesion molecules. Studies in this direction are in progress in our laboratory, and so far we have analyzed in some detail the distribution of a major component of the CNS ex-

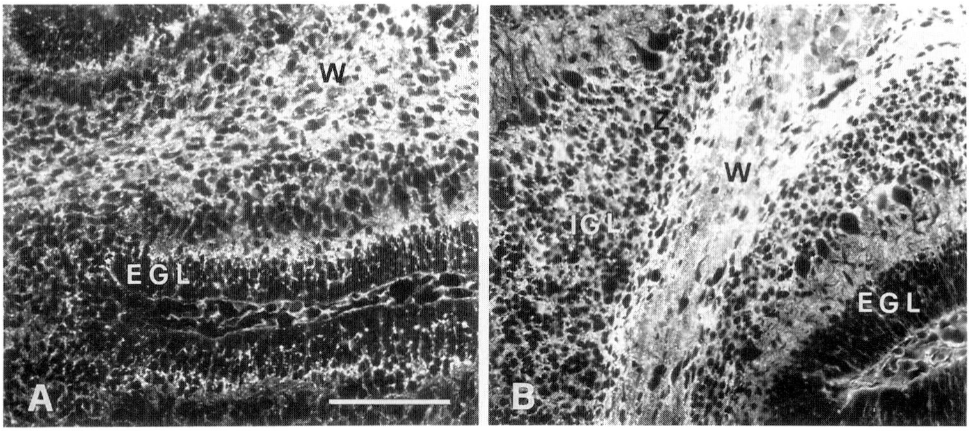


Fig. 5. Expression of chondroitin sulfate (CS) by developing rat cerebellum. Cryostat sections (5 µm thick) of perfusion-fixed cerebella were digested with chondroitinase ABC and immunostained with anti-CS antibodies (Gallo et al. 1987). Panel A: 1-day postnatal cerebellum, fluorescein-conjugated 2nd antibody. Panel B: 9-day postnatal cerebellum, rhodamine-conjugated 2nd antibody. EGL = external granule cell layer; IGL = internal granule cell layer; W = putative white matter. The sections were prepared by Drs. R. Suergiu and R. Reynolds, during a stage of RS in the laboratory of Dr. G.P. Wilkin at the Imperial College, London. Scale bar = 100 µm.

tracellular matrix, the proteoglycan chondroitin sulfate (CS). In this study, an antibody specific for the glycosaminoglycan digested with chondroitinase ABC was utilized (Bertolotto et al. 1986). In immunostained cryostat sections, CS exhibited a widespread distribution in the developing cerebellum. At the light microscopic level it was virtually impossible to determine which cell types are responsible for its synthesis, even in double immunofluorescence experiments. It was, however, interesting to note that the distribution of CS varied during development. In 1-day old cerebella (Fig. 5A), the heaviest labeling was present in the central part of the cerebellar folia, where the white matter will develop, and good labeling was observed also at the base of the external granule cell layer. In 9-day cerebella (Fig. 5B), the putative white matter was still well stained. Staining was present also in the external granule layer, where one could note radially oriented immunofluorescence between the granule cell bodies. At this age, also the internal granule cell layer exhibited a substantial staining, which further increased in adult animals (not shown). The labeling pattern obtained was not substantially different from that reported by Aquino et al. (1984), who used a different anti-CS antibody.

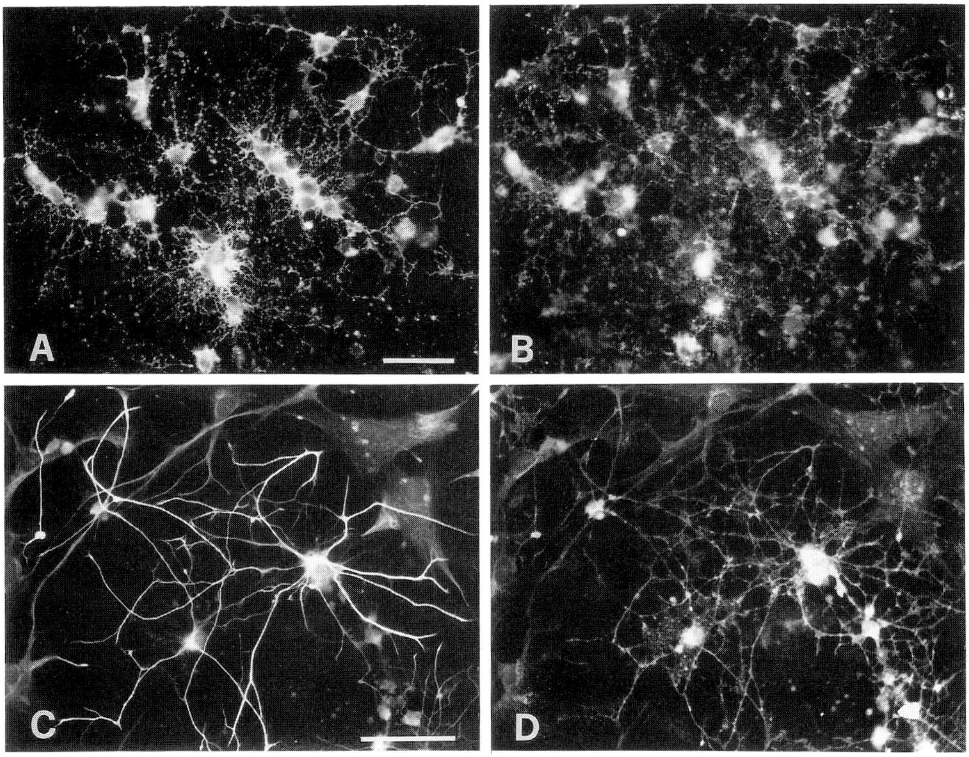


Fig. 6. Expression of chondroitin sulfate by glial precursors and type-2 astrocytes in cerebellar cell cultures. Panels A and B: cerebellar cells were cultured for 6 days in a serum-free medium, in conditions in which the $LB1^+$ bipotential glial precursors proliferate and, after 5-6 days, start to differentiate into oligodendrocytes (Levi et al. 1986). The cultures were surface-stained with both LB1 monoclonal antibodies (panel A, fluorescein optics) and anti-CS antibodies (panel B, rhodamine optics). Panels C and D: cerebellar cells were plated at low density ($1 \times 10^5$ cells/$cm^2$) and cultured in serum-containing medium for 5 days, in conditions in which the $LB1^+$ glial precursors largely differentiate into $GFAP^+$, type-2 astrocytes. Double intracellular staining with anti-GFAP monoclonal antibodies (panel C, fluorescein optics) and anti-CS antibodies (panel D, rhodamine optics). For staining procedures, see Gallo et al. (1987). Scale bars = 50 µm.

The data on the cellular distribution of CS obtained with cerebellar cultures provided a much clearer picture (Gallo et al. 1987). In all the conditions tested (different stages in vitro, culturing in the presence or in the absence of serum), the anti-CS antibodies labeled, both intracellularly and on their surface, only $LB1^+$ non neuronal cells. In serum-free cultures, about 70% of the $LB1^+$ cells was $CS^+$ (Fig. 6A-B). However, as the cells expressed the oligodendrocyte marker GalC, they rapidly became $CS^-$ (Gallo et al. 1987). In low density serum-containing cultures, in which most of the LB1$^+$ precursors differentiate into type-2 astrocytes, all the LB1$^+$ cells and about 90% of the GFAP$^+$ stellate cells were CS$^+$ (Fig. 6 C-D). This pattern of labelling is not incompatible with that observed in sections of immature cerebella where heavy staining was present in the putative white matter entering the folia. In fact, this is the location where the LB1$^+$ precursors and the in vivo equivalent of type-2 astrocytes (the fibrous astrocytes) are found in cryostat sections (Curtis et al. in press).

In summary, the presence of CS appears to be restricted, at least in culture, to bipotential glial precursors and type-2 astrocytes . We are presently trying to determine whether these or other components of the extracellular matrix, which in vitro are selectively expressed by defined glial cell populations, play a role in the establishment of those cellular interactions that seem to be important for the orientation of the developmental profile of bipotential glial precursors.

## ACKNOWLEDGEMENTS

We thank Drs. G.P. Wilkin, R. Reynolds and R. Suergiu for the immunostained cerebellar cryostat sections. We are grateful to the following collegues for gifts of antibodies or hybridoma cells: Drs. G.P. Wilkin and J. Cohen (LB1); Dr. B. Ranscht (anti-GalC); Drs. A. Bertolotto and G. Tarone (anti-CS); Dr. A. Bignami (anti-GFAP); Dr. M. Schachner (O4); Dr. S. Alemà (A2B5). This study was partly supported by Research Grant n° 86.02034.56 of the Italian National Research Council (Target Project "Preventive Medicine and Rehabilitation", subproject "Diseases of the Nervous System").

## REFERENCES

Aloisi F, Agresti C, Levi G (1987) Glial conditioned media inhibit the proliferation of cultured rat cerebellar astrocytes, Neurochem Res 12: 189-195

Aquino DA, Margolis RU, Margolis RK (1984) Immunocytochemical localization of chondroitin sulfate proteoglycan in nervous tissue. II Studies in developing brain, J Cell Biol 99: 1130-1139

Barbarese E, Pfeiffer SE (1981) Developmental regulation of myelin basic protein in dispersed cultures, Proc Natl Acad Sci USA 78: 1953-1957

Bertolotto A, Palmucci L, Gagliano A, Mongini T, Tarone G (1986) Immunohistochemical localization of chondroitin sulfate in normal and pathological human muscle, J Neurol Sci 73: 233-244

Bologa-Sandru L, Siegrist HP, Z'graggen A, Hofmann K, Wiesmann U, Dahl D, Herschkowitz N (1981) Expression of antigenic markers during the deve-

lopment of oligodendrocytes in mouse brain cell cultures, Brain Res 210: 217-229
Curtis R, Cohen J, Fok-Seang J, Hanley MR, Gregson NA, Reynolds R, Wilkin GP (1987) Use of antibodies to GD3 ganglioside, galactocerebroside and glial fibrillary acidic protein to follow the development of macroglial cells in rat cerebellum, J Neurocytol in press
Fredman P, Magnani JL, Nirenberg M, Ginsburg (1984) Monoclonal antibody A2B5 reacts with many gangliosides in neuronal tissue, Arch Biochem Biophys 233: 661-666
Gallo V, Bertolotto A, Levi G (1987) The proteoglycan chondroitin sulfate is present in a subpopulation of cultured astrocytes and in their precursors, Dev Biol in press
Goldman JE, Scott Geier S, Hirano M (1986) Differentiation of astrocytes and oligodendrocytes from germinal matrix cells in primary culture, J Neurosci 6: 52-60
Johnstone SR, Levi G, Wilkin GP, Schneider A, Ciotti MT (1986) Subpopulations of rat cerebellar astrocytes in primary culture: Morphology, cell surface antigens and $^{3}H$ GABA transport, Dev Brain Res 24: 63-75
Kasai N, Yu R (1983) Monoclonal antibody A2B5 is specific to ganglioside GQlc, Brain Res 277: 155-158
Levi G, Aloisi F, Ciotti MT, Gallo V (1984) Autoradiographic localization and depolarization-induced release of acids amino acids in differentiating cerebellar granule cell cultures, Brain Res 290: 77-86
Levi G, Gallo V, Ciotti MT (1986) Bipotential precursors of putative fibrous astrocytes and oligodendrocytes in rat cerebellar cultures express distinct surface features and "neuron-like" $\gamma$-aminobutyric acid transport, Proc Natl Acad Sci USA 83: 1504-1508
Levi G, Aloisi F, Wilkin GP (1987) Differentiation of cerebellar bipotential glial precursors into oligodendrocytes in primary culture: Developmental profile of surface antigens and mitotic activity, J Neurosci Res in press
McCarthy KD, De Vellis J (1980) Preparation of separate astroglial and oligodendroglial cell cultures from rat cerebral tissue, J Cell Biol 85; 890-902
Noble M, Murray K (1984) Purified astrocytes promote the in vitro division of a bipotential glial progenitor cell, EMBO J 3: 2243-2247
Raff MC, Mirsky R, Fields KL, Lisak RP, Dorfman SH, Silberberg DH, Gregson NA, Liebowitz S, Kennedy M (1978) Galactocerebroside: a specific cell surface antigen marker for oligodendrocytes in culture, Nature 274: 813-816
Raff MC, Miller RH, Noble M (1983a) A glial progenitor cell that develops in vitro into an astrocyte or an oligodendrocyte depending on culture medium, Nature 303: 390-396
Raff MC, Abney ER, Cohen J, Lindsay R, Noble M (1983b) Two types of astrocytes in cultures of developing rat white matter: differences in morphology, surface gangliosides and growth characteristics, J Neurosci 3: 1289-1300
Raff MC, Abney ER, Fok-Seang J (1985) Reconstitution of a developmental clock in vitro: A critical role for astrocytes in the timing of oligodendrocyte differentiation, Cell 42: 61-69
Sommer I, Schachner M (1981) Monoclonal antibodies (01 to 04) to oligodendrocyte cell surface: An immunocytological study in the central nervous system, Dev Biol 83: 311-327
Wilkin GP, Levi G, Johnstone S, Riddle PN (1983) Cerebellar astroglial cells in primary culture: Expression of different morphological appearances and differential ability to take up $[^{3}H]$D-aspartate and $[^{3}H]$ GABA, Dev Brain Res 10: 265-277

# NEUROECTODERMAL CELLS: STORAGE AND RELEASE OF GROWTH FACTORS

K. Unsicker, D. Blottner, D. Gehrke, C. Grothe, D. Heymann, F. Stögbauer, R. Westermann

Department of Anatomy and Cell Biology
University of Marburg
Robert-Koch-Str. 6
D-3550 Marburg
Federal Republic of Germany

## INTRODUCTION

Neurons and glial cells, both derived from the embryonic neuroectoderm, are the principal cellular constituents of the nervous system. Homo- and heterologous cell - cell adhesion, metabolic and trophic couplings between these partners play key roles for development, maintenance and regenerative processes of neural systems.

Neurons recruit their trophic support required to overcome developmental and lesion-induced cell death from a variety of sources the best established being their target areas and glial cells. Several laboratories have shown that astroglial and Schwann cells as well as their tumor counterparts release into the cell culture medium neuronotrophic (i.e. neuronal survival promoting) and neurite growth enhancing factors (NTFs and NPFs, respectively; Barde et al. 1978; Lindsay et al. 1982; Manthorpe et al. 1983; Rudge et al. 1985; Varon et al. 1987). Despite obvious difficulties inherent to the isolation of growth factors from sources where they occur in very small amounts the successfull recent purification of a C6 glioma cell-derived NPF (Guenther et al. 1985) underscores the potential usefulness of glial tumor cell lines for defining and characterizing trophic molecules. We have analyzed NTF activities released by C6

NATO ASI Series, Vol. H22
Neural Development and Regeneration
Edited by A. Gorio et al.

cells and describe our initial characterization of six activities that differ in terms of target neurons being supported, temporal secretory patte s and gel filtration behavior. Neurons have only recently emerged as putative sources of NTFs (Barbin et al. 1984), although stringent conceptualization of target organ regulated neuronal death would imply that neurons are storage sites of trophic molecules serving the maintenance of presynaptic partners. Again, availability of large, homogeneous cell populations is a prerequisite for an identification of neuron-derived NTFs. The second part of this report focuses on biological and molecular characteristics of NTFs that we have found in adrenal medullary chromaffin and neuroblastoma cells.

## ASSAYS FOR MONITORING NTF ACTIVITIES

Microassay systems have been developed that allow one to recognize, quantify and monitor NTF activities in monolayer cultures of embryonic and neonatal neurons (Varon et al. 1983). The rationale of the assays is based on (i) the operational definition of NTFs as substances promoting in vitro survival of selected neuron populations and (ii) similar survival behaviors and trophic factor requirements of neurons in vitro and in vivo, which are best exemplified by the NGF-dependent in vivo and in vitro survival of neonatal mouse and rat sympathetic neurons. NTF activities in samples of cell and tissue extracts and conditioned media with preferably defined protein contents can be quantified by presenting them in serial dilutions to the neurons grown in serum-free media and on substrata such as polyornithine or laminin. The titer of NTF activities in a sample is expressed in Trophic Units (TU) per mg protein or per ml, one TU being the amount of material per one ml that assures half-maximal survival ($ED_{50}$). Plateau survival is established by applying saturating amounts of purified NTFs (NGF or CNTF for peripheral neurons, pyruvate for CNS neurons, cf. Varon et al. 1987). Neurons used in our assays are listed in table 2.

## NTFs RELEASED FROM C6 GLIOMA CELLS

### Preparation of conditioned media

C6 cells (American Type Culture Collection, passages 6-30) were grown to confluence (20 x $10^6$ cells/75 $cm^2$ flask) in Dulbecco's modified Eagle's medium (DMEM) with 10% fetal calf serum (FCS), glutamine, $NaHCO_3$ and antibiotics. For obtaining conditioned medium (C6CM) confluent cultures were treated according to one of the following procedures: (i) "normal" C6CM was prepared by washing cells 3 times in serum-free medium and incubation with serum-free medium for 1, 2, 3 or 4 days. In this C6CM most of the protein corresponds to residual FCS-proteins; (ii) if cells were extensively washed and incubated with FCS-free culture medium, serum-proteins were no longer detectable ($^{-}$FCS-C6CM); (iii) as a control we conditioned C6 cells with normal culture medium (DMEM plus 10% FCS, $^{+}$FCS-C6CM). After harvesting CMs were centrifuged twice (100 x g, 5 min; 3,000 x g, 30 min) and stored at -80°C.

### Characterization of C6 cultures

Analyses using immunocytochemistry, ELISA and immunoblots indicated that C6 cells contained the glial cell-specific proteins GFAP and S-100 as well as nuclear proteins histone H1 and HMG 14. In C6CMs the cytoskeletal and nuclear proteins were not detectable which suggests that proteins in C6CM resulted from cellular release rather than cell death.

### Neuronotrophic activities in C6CM and C6 cell extracts

NTF, survival promoting activities accumulating in C6CM after 1 to 4 days of conditioning were assayed on embryonic chick peripheral neurons. In "normal" C6CM activity addressing cCG8 neurons increased from day 1 through day 4, while a reverse temporal pattern was seen for an activity supporting cDRG 8 neurons. Activity for cDRG 10 and cSG 11 neurons accumulated over the first 2 days and declined thereafter. In table 1 activities are expressed as TU/mg protein. Results for $^{+}$FCS-C6CM were identical. In contrast, virtually no NTF activities were detectable in $^{-}$FCS-C6CM, even when C6 cells were grown and conditioned with a synthetic medium (N1 supplement; Bottenstein et al. 1980). Extracts of C6 cells grown in the presence or absence of FCS lacked NTF activities as well. These data indicate that (i) FCS component(s) induce synthesis and release of NTF activities in C6 cells, and (ii) C6CM contains at least 3 NTFs differing in terms of neurons being supported and temporal secretory patterns.

NGF was detected in C6CM in very small amounts using a sensitive two-site-ELISA (about 0.5 pg/ml; Otten, personal communication, cf. Westermann et al., 1987). This amount is too small to account for an NGF-mediated effect of C6CM. Accordingly, anti-NGF antibodies failed to block the biological activity of C6CM. To further characterize NTF activities of C6CM, proteins of "normal" C6CM were precipitated with acetone, dialyzed,lyophilized and separated by gelfiltration on FPLC superose columns. NTF activities resided in three fractions: one fraction (approximately 40 kD) addressed all NGF-responsive neurons, anotherone was specific for DRG10 neurons (approximately 60 kD). A third fraction of about $M_r$ = 100 000 supported cCG8 and cDRG10 neurons. Taken together, analyses of the temporal secretory patterns of NTFs, chromatographic behaviors of C6CM proteins with NTF properties and their respective combinations of target neurons being supported suggest that C6CM contains at least 6 different NTF species.

## NTFs IN ADRENAL MEDULLARY CHROMAFFIN CELLS

Regulation of developmental death of neurons by the size of their innervation territory is an established principle in neurogenesis. Whether competition of neurons for target-derived trophic factors is restricted to target tissues such as muscle and glands, or may include neurons in their role

Table 1: Trophic activities of "normal" C6CM

Days of conditioning

| | 1 | 2 | 3 | 4 |
|---|---|---|---|---|
| $DRG_8$ | 15 | <10 | <10 | <10 |
| $DRG_{10}$ | 40 | 112 | 28 | 15 |
| $SG_{11}$ | 77 | 250 | 111 | 42 |
| $CG_8$ | 5 | 18 | 27 | 21 |

The ability of "normal" C6CM collected after 1-4 days of conditioning to support 24 - 48 h neuronal survival was assayed on 4 peripheral neuron populations (for abbreviations see table 2). Results are expressed as TU/mg protein.

as target cells for other neurons is unknown. Addressing this issue requires as well-defined neuron-neuron relationship and a large homogeneous population of neurons as a putative source of NTFs for biochemical studies. Both requirements are met by adrenal chromaffin cells, modified sympathetic neurons that receive their main nerve supply from preganglionic spinal cord neurons, and minor neuronal inputs from sympathetic and sensory neurons.

Chromaffin cells were isolated and purified in bulk from bovine adrenal medullae (Unsicker and Müller 1981; Livett 1984). The cells maintained in the absence of serum for 48h conditioned their culture medium with trophic activities that supported the in vitro-survival of several embryonic neuron populations including embryonic chick ciliary, sensory and sympathetic neurons. The sensitivities of these NTFs to trypsin and heat and the failure to block their effects by anti-NGF antibodies (cross-reacting with bovine NGF) suggested that the molecules of interest were proteins and immunologically different from NGF.

Stimulation of cultured chromaffin cells with the cholinergic agonist carbachol ($10^{-4}$M, 2h) increased the titer of NTF activities in the medium by 5- to 15-fold. Total catecholamines and chromogranin A, the major acidic protein in the transmitter storage organelle of chromaffin cells, were augmented within the same order of magnitude suggesting that there was a high probability of NTFs being stored in chromaffin vesicles. In accordance with this assumption the proteinaceous constituents of highly purified bovine chromaffin vesicles were found to carry survival promoting activity for a large number of cultured embryonic and postnatal CNS and PNS neurons (table 2; cf. Unsicker and Lietzke 1987).

Table 2: NTF activities of bovine chromaffin vesicle proteins

| | chick - rat | Age | Target neuron | Abbreviation | TU/mg protein |
|---|---|---|---|---|---|
| Peripheral Nervous System | c | E8 | ciliary ganglia | cCG8 | ~100 |
| | c | E8 | dorsal root ganglia | cDRG8 | ~100 |
| | c | E10 | dorsal root ganglia | cDRG10 | ~ 50 |
| | c | E11 | lumbar sympathetic ganglia | cSG11 | ~200 |
| | r | new-born | superior cervical ganglia | rSCGn | ~ 70 |
| | r | new-born | nodose ganglia | rNODn | no activity |
| | r | P8 | adrenal chromaffin cells | rAD8 | ~ 80 |
| CNS | c | E6 | spinal cord | cSC6 | ~ 50 |
| | r | E18 | hippocampal | rHIPP18 | ~ 50 |

Two different strategies were subsequently employed to characterize NTFs in chromaffin vesicles. The first was to test two categories of established constituents of chromaffin vesicles, chromogranins and neuropeptides for NTF activity. Polyclonal antibodies to chromogranin A, B and C (generously provided by R. Fischer-Colbrie and H. Winkler, Innsbruck) did not interfere with the survival promoting activity of chromaffin vesicle proteins for cCG8 and cDRG8 neurons. Surprisingly, however, purified chromogranin A obtained from an affinity column with a monoclonal antibody against this protein (raised by R.

Lietzke) carried NTF activity for cDRG8, but not cCG8 neurons. Studies are in progress to investigate whether the effect of chromogranin A is due to a contaminant or a fragment of chromogranin A. Porcine pancreastatin (provided by K. Tatemoto, Stanford, cf. Tatemoto et al. 1986), a protein with 70% sequence homology to bovine chromogranin A between residues 251 and 294 (Eiden 1987; Huttner and Benedum 1987), failed to promote survival of $cDRG_8$ neurons. Table 3 presents a list of neuropeptides that were tested for putative NTF activities on cCG8, cDRG8 and 10 and cSG11 neurons. Met- and leu-enkephalin as well as somatostatin supported the survival of sympathetic neurons ($ED_{50}$ = 5 x $10^{-6}$M). Leu-enkephalin and somatostatin had also weak effects on cDRG neurons reaching about 50% of the plateau obtained with saturating concentrations of NGF or CNTF. VIP and neurotensin (to an even minor extent) promoted the survival of cCG8 neurons. Although the specificity of the effects in terms of being mimicked by respective agonists and blocked by antagonists remains to be established, it is an intriguing speculation that neuropeptides might act as NTFs (cf. Brenneman et al. 1985).

Table 3: Survival promoting effects of neuropeptides

| Peptide / Neuron | MET-ENK | LEU-ENK | SOMAT. | SUBST.P | NPY | NEUROT. | VIP | BOMBESIN | SEKRETIN | PANCREA-STATIN | DYN1-13/B | MSHs |
|---|---|---|---|---|---|---|---|---|---|---|---|---|
| cCG8 | 0 | 0 | 0 | 0 | 0 | (+) | (++) | 0 | 0 | 0 | 0 | 0 |
| cDRG8 | 0 | (++) | (++) | 0 | 0 | 0 | 0 | 0 | 0 | 0 | 0 | 0 |
| cDRG10 | 0 | (++) | (++) | 0 | 0 | 0 | (++) | 0 | 0 | 0 | 0 | 0 |
| cSG11 | + | + | + | 0 | n.d. | n.d. | n.d. | n.d. | n.d. | n.d. | 0 | 0 |

Neuropeptides were assayed for survival promoting effects (24-48h) on the indicated neurons (for abbreviations see table 2).

0 = no effects; (+) = 25%, (++) = 50%, + = 100% of plateau values obtained with saturating concentrations of NGF or CNTF. Neuropeptides were supplied at a starting concentration of 2 x $10^{-5}$M. Titration curves revealed an $ED_{50}$ of 1 to 5 x $10^{-6}$M for MET-ENK, LEU-ENK, SOM and VIP.
It was not determined in these experiments, however, what fraction of the initially applied neuropeptide was actually present in the culture after 24-48 h. n.d. = not done.

As an alternative means of further characterizing the chromaffin NTFs chromatographic and electrophoretic procedures were used for an enrichment and determination of approximate molecular size of the respective molecules. Separation of chromaffin vesicle proteins on TSK W 3000 HPLC molecular sieve columns provided an activity of about $M_r$=22kD addressing cCG8 neurons. An activity supporting survival of cCG8 and cDRG8 neurons was ten-fold enriched by passing chromaffin vesicle proteins over a heparin-sepharose affinity column. Since cCG8 neurons have previously been shown to respond to the heparin-binding mitogens basic and acidic fibroblast growth factor (bFGF, aFGF) by enhanced survival and induction of choline acetyltransferase activity (Unsicker et al. 1987), we explored the possibility that FGFs might be stored in chromaffin vesicles. Vesicle proteins, like FGFs, were found to stimulate proliferation of cultured endothelial cells and contained 1-2 ng/mg protein of bFGF (detected by radioimmunoassay; P. Böhlen, Zürich). Studies are under way to evalute whether bFGF is stored in <u>and</u> released from chromaffin cells or whether its presence in chromaffin vesicles might reflect an isolation artifact and contamination of vesicles by bFGF of adrenocortical origin (cf. Gospodarowicz et al. 1986a).

A novel powerful means for the identification of NTF activities in tissue extracts (chromaffin vesicle proteins in our case) that exploits separation of proteins by SDS-PAGE, their subsequent transfer to nitrocellulose and exclusive survival of seeded cCG8 neurons on NTF-containing bands (Carnow et al. 1985) revealed 4 distinct bands with $M_r$ = 24, 34, 55 and 95 kD supporting neuronal survival. 24 kD is the molecular weight of CNTF isolated from rat sciatic nerve (Manthorpe et al. 1986).

Summing up, the above experiments suggest the presence of multiple NTFs in chromaffin vesicles. Candidates may include (i) bFGF, (ii) another heparin-binding growth factor different from bFGF and CNTF that addresses cDRG8 neurons, a population which is not supported by bFGF and CNTF (iii) CNTF, (iv) a fragment of or molecule(s) associated with chromogranin A, which is distinct from the bovine chromogranin A 251-294 sequence (pancreastatin), and (v) several neuropeptides.

## PUTATIVE IN VIVO-RELEVANCE OF ADRENAL MEDULLARY NTFs

In the previous section we have summarized several lines of evidence that suggest storage and release of multiple NTFs from the transmitter storing organelle of chromaffin cells. The putative physiological significance of these factors was assessed in a series of experiments in which we tested (i) the NTF contents of rat adrenal medulla and cortex at various developmental ages, and (ii) the effects of adrenalectomy on cholinergic preganglionic spinal cord neurons innervating the adrenal medulla. Adrenal glands were dissected from embryonic day (E) 19 through postnatal day (P) 90 rats and cortical and medullary portions carefully separated. High speed supernatants of tissue extracts were assayed for NTF activities capable to support the in vitro survival of cCG8 (as a model for cholinergic neurons), DRG8, 10 and cSG11 neurons. NTF activity for ciliary and sensory neurons was detectable in medullary, but not in cortical samples starting at P8, i.e. shortly after the onset of a functional innervation of the adrenal medulla at P5. A weak activity for sympathetic neurons was found in both medullary and cortical cell homogenates. Half-maximal effects required presentation of about 20 µg protein/ml with samples from all ages.

These results demonstrate that rat adrenal medullary cells, like those from bovine glands, contain NTFs. Furthermore, their initial expression seems to be triggered by a neuronal signal from preganglionic nerves. The latter finding would imply that growth of preganglionic nerve fibers into the adrenal medulla which is noticed from E15 onwards (Millar and Unsicker 1981) does not require detectable levels of these NTFs within the target organ of these nerves. From these results one may predict that removal of the adrenal medulla or splanchnic nerve lesions should interfere with the morphological and functional

integrity of the preganglionic neurons of the intermediolateral column (ILC) of the spinal cord innervating the adrenal medulla. In fact, adrenalectomy performed in rats at P2 caused neuronal cell losses of about 20% after 4 weeks in the ipsilateral ILC and a reduction of choline acetyltransferase activity at segmental levels Th 7 - Th 10 as compared to the unlesioned side. Studies are in progress to determine (i) the effects of splanchnicotomy on preganglionic cell bodies and NTF levels in the denervated adrenal medulla, (ii) the extent of physiological neuronal cell death in the ILC (iii) the effect of bFGF and CNTF on ILC neurons during the period of ontogenetic cell death and after adrenomedullectomy in substitution experiments.
The demonstration of NTFs in chromaffin cells and their characterization and isolation also bears on our understanding of the beneficial effects of chromaffin cells grafted into the brain. It has been argued that striatal transplants of adrenal chromaffin cells in humans and animals with a parkinsonian syndrome improve the signs of this disease by providing a growth-promoting substance(s) for unimpaired dopaminergic neurons (Moore 1987). It is conceivable that the purified molecules installed into the brain would function more effectively than medullary grafts and improve clinical handling of the disease.

## NTFs IN NEUROBLASTOMA CELLS

We have previously reported that high speed supernatants of extracts from two neuroblastoma (NB) cell lines, the mouse C1300 N2a and the human IMR 32, support in vitro survival of a spectrum of embryonic chick neurons, which is also addressed by CNTF (cCG8, cDRG10, but <u>not</u> cDRG8, cSG11 neurons; Heymann et al. 1986, 1987; Heymanns and Unsicker 1987). Promotion of survival of these neurons was dose-dependent with an $ED_{50}$ of 80 µg (IMR 32) and 140 µg (C1300) protein/ml and saturable at plateau values identical to those achieved with purified CNTF. The activity was heat- and protease-sensitive and not

blocked by anti-NGF (mouse) antibodies. Cell blots revealed exclusive survival of cCG8 neurons on two distinct bands with apparent molecular weights of 24 and 48 kD. The 24 kD band, together with the CNTF-typical spectrum of target neurons being addressed by the NB extracts, suggests the occurrence of CNTF in these NB cell lines.
Gel chromatography studies on IMR-extracts revealed an apparent $M_r$ of 21 and 45 kD for activities addressing cCG8 neurons. C1300-extracts enriched for cCG8 activity on heparin sepharose and blotted onto nitrocellulose paper yielded four distinct peaks corresponding to $M_r$ 15, 21, 32 and 52 kD. Immunocytochemical demonstration of FGF immunoreactivity with an antibody that recognizes an epitope shared by bFGF and aFGF (kindly provided by M. Sensenbrenner, Strasbourg) in both IMR 32 and C1300 cells might support the assumption of an identity of the 15 kD band with FGFs (Gospodarowicz et al. 1986b). It is apparent, therefore, that NB cells, like the closely related chromaffin cells, contain multiple NTF species. NB cell extracts and purified (chick) CNTF failed to promote IMR 32 and C1300 cell differentiation or proliferation. The function of the NTFs stored in NB cells, therefore, is still enigmatic.

## CONCLUSIONS

The results of recent studies reviewed in this report indicate that neuroectodermal cells store a multitude of NTFs, some of which may be identical to established NTFs (e.g. NGF, CNTF) and growth factors such as FGF. Localization of growth factors in neurons strengthens the concept of trophic interactions between neurons validating the view that target cell-regulated neuronal maintenance includes trophic contributions from neurons themselves. Particularly striking is the finding that NTF activities are associated with a class of molecules, the chromogranins, that have a wide-spread distribution in the PNS and CNS. The search for and characterization of novel NTF molecules as well as an extension of studies on NTFs such as CNTF and FGF to the level of regulation of their synthesis and release are research goals that will ultimately affect our understanding of CNS regeneration and suggest possibilities for its manipulation.

Acknowledgements

We thank Ch. Fiebiger, I. Ganski, M. Johannsen, W. Lorenz, H. Reichert-Preibsch and H. Schneider for technical and editorial help. Work described in this article was supported by a grant of the German Research Foundation to K.U. (Un 34/11-1).

REFERENCES

Barde YA, Lindsay RM, Monard D, Thoenen H (1978) New factor released by cultured glioma cells supporting survival and growth of sensory neurons. Nature 274:818

Lindsay RM, Barber PC, Sherwood MRC, Zimmer J, Raisman G (1982) Astrocyte cultures from adult rat brain. Derivation, characterization and neurotrophic properties of pure astroglial cells from corpus callosum. Brain Res 243:329-343

Manthorpe M, Engvall C, Ruoslahti E, Longo FM, Davis GE, Varon S (1983) Laminin promotes neuritic regeneration from cultured peripheral and central neurons. J Cell Biol 97: 1882-1890

Rudge JS, Manthorpe M, Varon S (1985) The output of neuronotrophic and neurite-promoting agents from rat brain astroglial cells. A microculture method for screening potentially regulatory molecules. Dev Brain Res 19:161-172

Varon S, Skaper StD, Facci L, Rudge JS, Manthorpe M (1987) Trophic and metabolic couplings between astroglia and neurons. In Glial-Neuronal Communication in Development and Regeneration. Althaus HH, Seifert W (eds) Springer Berlin Heidelberg New York

Guenther J, Nick H, Monard D (1985) A glial-derived neurite-promoting factor with protease inhibitory activity. EMBO J 4:1963-1966

Barbin G, Selak I, Manthorpe M, Varon S (1984) Use of central neuronal cultures for the detection of neuronotrophic agents. Neurosci 12:33-43

Varon S, Manthorpe M, Longo FM, Williams LR (1983) Growth factors in regeneration of neural tissues. In Nerve Organ and Tissue Regeneration. Res Perspectives Seil FJ (ed) Academic Press New York

Bottenstein JE, Skaper SD, Varon S, Sato GH (1980) Selective survival of neurons from chick embryo sensory ganglionic dissociates utilizing serum-free supplemented medium. Exp Cell Res 125:183-190

Westermann R, Hardung M, Meyer DK, Erhard P, Otten U, Unsicker K (1987) Neuronotrophic factors released by C6 glioma cells. J Neurochem (to be submitted)
Unsicker K, Müller ThH (1981) Purification of bovine adrenal chromaffin cells by differential plating. J Neurosci Meth 4:227-241
Livett BG (1984) Adrenal medullary chromaffin cells in vitro. Physiol Rev 64:1103-1161
Unsicker K, Lietzke R (1987) Chromaffin cells: modified neurons that are both targets and storage sites of neuronotrophic and neurite promoting factors. In Glial-Neuronal Communication in Development and Regeneration. Althaus HH, Seifert W (eds) Springer Berlin Heidelberg New York
Tatemoto K, Efendic S, Mutt V, Makk G, Feistner GJ, Bruchas JD (1986) Pancreastatin, a novel pancreatic peptide that inhibits insulin secretion. Nature 324:476-478
Eiden EE (1987) Is chromogranin a prohormone? Nature 325:301
Huttner WB, Benedum UM (1987) Chromogranin A and pancreastatin. Nature 325:305
Brenneman DE, Eiden LE, Siegel RE (1985) Neurotrophic action of VIP on spinal cord cultures. Peptide 6:35-39
Unsicker K, Reichert-Preibsch H, Schmidt R, Pettmann B, Labourdette G, Sensenbrenner M (1987) Astroglial and fibroblast growth factors have neuronotrophic functions for cultured peripheral and central nervous system neurons. Proc Natl Acad Sci USA in press
Gospodarowicz A, Baird A, Cheng J, Lui GM, Esch F, Bohlen P (1986a) Isolation of fibroblast growth factor from bovine adrenal gland: physicochemical and biological characterization. Endocrinology 118:82-90
Carnow ThB, Manthorpe M, Davis GE, Varon S (1985) Localized survival of ciliary ganglionic neurons identifies neuronotrophic factor bands on nitrocellulose blots. J Neurosci 5:1965-1971
Manthorpe M, Skaper StD, Williams LR, Varon S (1986) Purification of adult rat sciatic ciliary neuronotrophic factor. Brain Res 367:282-286
Millar TJ, Unsicker K (1981) Catecholamine-storing cells in the adrenal medulla of the pre- and postnatal rat. Cell Tissue Res 217:155-170
Moore RY (1987) Parkinson's disease - a new therapy? New England J Med 316:872-873
Heymann D, Heymanns J, Unsicker K (1986) Neuronotrophic activities in neuroblastoma cells: comparison ciliary neuronotrophic factor (CNTF). Abstr Europ Soc Neurochem Prague 351
Heymann D, Heymanns J, Unsicker K (1987) Neuroblastoma cell lines as a source for multiple neuronotrophic activities. Soc Neurosci Abstr Vol 13
Heymanns J, Unsicker K (1987, submitted) Neuroblastoma cells contain a ciliary neuronotrophic factor.
Gospodarowicz D, Neufeld G, Schweigerer L (1986b) Molecular and biological characterization of fibroblast growth factor, an angiogenic factor which also controls the proliferation and differentiation of mesoderm and neuroectoderm derived cells. Cell Diff 19:1-17

ACETYL-L-CARNITINE IN THE RAT'S HIPPOCAMPUS AGING: MORPHOLOGICAL, ENDOCRINE AND BEHAVIORAL CORRELATES

L. Angelucci, M.T. Ramacci*, F. Amenta#, G. Lorentz, F. Maccari*
Farmacologia 2a, Università di Roma "La Sapienza"
* Laboratori Biologici Sigma Tau, Pomezia
# Dipartimento Biologia Cellulare, Università di Roma "Tor Vergata"

## INTRODUCTION

The search for anti-aging agents in humans primarily aims to find substances with biological activities such as to postpone irreversible morphological damage of the brain, to sustain natural reparative processes in it, and, consequently to ameliorate behavior and autonomic, endocrine, immunitary functions, importantly governed by the CNS. In this scope we have investigated acetyl-l-carnitine (ALC), a biological substance essential, with free carnitine (FC) and carnitine acetyl-transferase, to the transport and oxidation of fatty acids, as long chain acyl-carnitine (LCAC), into mitochondrion, and to the production and incorporation into membrane phospholipids of their unsaturated forms. Also, ALC promotes utilization of ketones which can constitute an accessory energy substrate available to the neuron. ALC is present at different concentrations in various brain areas of the rat (Shug et al. 1982), at highest values during perinatal maturation of the CNS (Morris and Carey 1983), when phospholipid utilization and myelin gain are at their maximum. Apart its metabolic role, ALC, by itself, independetly from FC, possibly because shares

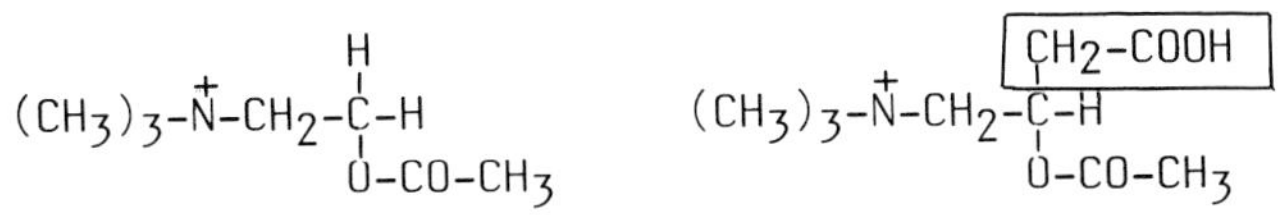

ACETYLCHOLINE ACETYL-L-CARNITINE

conformational properties with acetylcholine (Sass and Werness 1973), has

NATO ASI Series, Vol. H22
Neural Development and Regeneration
Edited by A. Gorio et al.

some cholinergic activity (Fritz 1963; Tempesta et al. 1985), and increases the high affinity choline uptake in synaptosomal preparations of cerebral cortex and hippocampus of aged rats (Curti et al. 1986). It is to remark that, as shown in table 1, concentrations of FC in the rat's blood and brain,

Table 1. Concentrations of FC, ALC and LCAC in the male Sprague-Dawley rat at various ages and following a six month treatment with ALC in the female Wistar rat.

| | 2 MONTHS (10) | 5 MONTHS (10) | 16 MONTHS (10) | 20 MONTHS (10) | ALC 20 MONTHS (12) | 30 MONTHS (10) | |
|---|---|---|---|---|---|---|---|
| Blood: nmoles/ml | | | | | | | |
| FC | 25.73 ± 1.54 | 31.90 ± 0.81$^{\#}$ | 22.71 ± 1.41$^{*}$ | | | 18.87 ± 1.12$^{*}$ | 59$^{a}$ |
| ALC | 11.63 ± 0.53 | 12.77 ± 0.70 | 9.78 ± 0.43$^{*}$ | | | 9.65 ± 0.85$^{*}$ | 75 |
| LCAC | 3.06 ± 0.17 | 2.98 ± 0.11 | 3.89 ± 0.25$^{*}$ | | | 3.05 ± 0.35 | 102 |
| Heart: nmoles/g | | | | | | | |
| FC | 682 ± 33 | 470 ± 20$^{\#}$ | 464 ± 20 | | | 353 ± 52$^{*}$ | 75 |
| ALC | 203 ± 18 | 390 ± 19$^{\#}$ | 206 ± 23$^{*}$ | | | 130 ± 9$^{*}$ | 33 |
| LCAC | 56.32 ±13.96 | 31.95 ± 3.95 | 41.06 ±11.66 | | | 62.55 ±10.10$^{*}$ | 195 |
| Brain: nmoles/g | | | | | | | |
| FC | 49.76 ± 0.96 | 55.00 ± 1.90$^{\#}$ | 49.86 ± 2.08 | 35.60 ± 1.59 | 43.72 ± 2.69$^{\&}$ | 43.47 ± 1.64$^{*}$ | 79 |
| ALC | 30.37 ± 1.27 | 30.71 ± 0.41 | 29.98 ± 0.86 | 20.64 ± 1.60 | 24.74 ± 1.14$^{\&}$ | 28.82 ± 1.16 | 94 |
| LCAC | 13.47 ± 0.64 | 13.81 ± 0.70 | 16.19 ± 1.48 | 16.44 ± 0.85 | 14.11 ± 1.29 | 16.55 ± 1.31$^{\#}$ | 120 |

In parentheses: number of animals. $^{\#}$ , $^{*}$ and $^{\&}$ : significant difference v. 2, 5 or 20 months. $^{a}$ Percent of the concentration at 5 months.

at variance with heart, reach their peak at 5 month age, when full maturation of the body should have since long been attained (around 60-70 day age), and thereafter progressively decline together with ALC. It is interesting, in view of the role of ALC in myelinization, to note the coincidence, maybe meaningful, of this phenomenon with the attaining of full maturation of some brain structures later than usually thought (see further on for the full development of the rat's hippocampal mossy fibers system whose area at 4 month is 56 per cent of that at 12 month age). It is evident, however, that brain in the aged rat attempts, successfully compared with blood and heart, to maintain its concentration of ALC. In fact, at 30 month age, there was a reduction of only 6 per cent with regard to concentration of ALC at 5 month age. This would indicate a relationship between the function of ALC in the nervous tissue, not uniquely a metabolic one, and the aging of brain. A long term treatment with exogenous ALC (71 mg/kg/day in drink water) was able, as shown in table 1, to improve the concentration of FC and ALC in the rat's brain: this could have been the basis of the effects of ALC treatment on hippocampus (HI) aging.

The marked decrease in the activity of carnitine-acetyl transferase accompanying the degeneration of cholinergic nerve terminals, in which is colocalized with choline acetyl-transferase (Sterri and Fonnum 1980), prompted us to explore the effects of long term treatments with ALC in aging rats (Angelucci et al. 1986). Here we report the results of a study of ALC on brain aging using an experimental model given by the comparison of hippocampal morphology, neurochemistry and behavioral function at various ages in the rat. Moreover, in consideration: a) of the existence of corticosterone (B) receptors in the HI (McEwen et al. 1969); b) of their role in behavioral adaptation (Bohus and De Kloet 1981); c) of their integration in a negative-feedback regulation of the hypothalamo-pituitary-adrenocortical axis (HPAA), especially in stress condition (Patacchioli et al. 1983), and d) of their progressive loss after adulthood (Angelucci et al. 1980), we have resorted, as a marker of brain senescence, to the typical disinhibition of the HPAA in the aged rat (Landfield et al. 1978; De Kosky et al. 1984; Angelucci et al. 1987), and ascertained its sensitiveness to the senescence ameliorating effect of ALC. This marker can have a pathogenetic importance with reagard to HI deterioration since permanently increased levels of plasma B can be of damage to neurons in the HI (Sapolsky et al. 1985). ALC was given to male and female Sprague-Dawley and Wistar rats, in drink water, about 70 mg/kg/day for not less than six months, starting at the age of not less than twelve months. It must be noticed that where possible neuromorphological, neuroendocrine, behavioral and immunitary evaluations were carried out on the same animals; this allowed for some qualitative correlations within each experimental group, whereas quantitative correlations would have necessitated larger numbers of animals in each group, due to unavoidable individual variability.

## FINDINGS

### Neuromorphological parameters of hippocampal aging.

Long term treatments with ALC, as shown in table 2, significantly reduced the loss of pyramidal cells in 22-24 month old rats. Compared to 4.5 month old rats, this was 26.5 percent in controls, but only 14.0 percent in treated rats. Gyrus dentatus granular cells too were protected: in treated animals they were 12.6 percent more than in controls. This finding was in good agreement with the mossy fibers - which originate from granular cells - occupying in treated rats a significantly larger area as compared to controls. Preservation of neuron number in the HI likely resulted from a healthier biochemical function in presence of ALC, as indicated by reduced lipofuscinosis, higher level of ribosomal (Nissl staining) and respiratory activity (diaforase). It is interesting that the increase in ACh-esterase activity we found in old rats, at variance with the report of a reduction in the aged male Fischer rat (Sastry et al. 1983), has been demonstrated in senile plaques in human brain (Friede 1965).

### Neuroendocrine parameters of hippocampal aging.

Long term treatment with ALC, as shown in table 3, reduced the disinhibition of the HPAA typical of the aged rat. The effect was statistically significant with regard to the response to psychic stress. Basal concentration of plasma corticosterone, and delayed negative feedback control from

Table 2. The effect of ALC (6-11 month treatment) on morphological and neurochemical parameters of the aging HI in the rat.

| | 4.5 MONTHS | 22-24 MONTHS | 22-24 MONTHS TREATED |
|---|---|---|---|
| NEURON N° per 0.21 $mm^2$ (13-14) | | | |
| CA1 | 979 ± 13 | 720 ± 8[#] | 832 ± 15* |
| G. dentatus | - | 1376 ± 14 | 1550 ± 16* |
| MOSSY FIBERS AREA (9-10) $um^2 \times 10^2$ | 38.8 ± 1.4[a] | 22.5 ± 1.2[#] | 28.6 ± 0.5* |
| LIPOFUSCIN (5-18) CA1 fluorescence units | < 1 | 68.1 ± 2.6 | 53.5 ± 1.4* |
| NISSL STAINING (5-9) arbitrary units | | | |
| CA1 | 71.9 ± 0.8 | 49.0 ± 0.7[#] | 54.4 ± 1.0* |
| G. dentatus | 85.0 ± 0.9 | 51.5 ± 0.8[#] | 54.6 ± 0.8* |
| PYR.L LAYER ENZYMES (5-9) arbitrary units | | | |
| NADH-diaforase | 94.9 ± 1.7 | 49.2 ± 1.6[#] | 74.3 ± 1.2* |
| ACh-esterase | 52.2 ± 0.8 | 72.4 ± 1.1[#] | 66.5 ± 0.9* |

In parentheses: number of animals per group. [a] At the age of 12 months; at 4 months number of fibers was not completed. [#] and * :significant difference v. 4.5 or 22-24 months.

a previous stress on a second psychic stress were similarly affected, although not at a statistically significant level due to large individual variability. On the whole, it appeared that rats treated with ALC were able to better control their adrenocortical responsiveness. This went parallel with the anatomical and functional preservation of the glucocorticoid receptor in the HI. In fact, the loss of binding capacity for $^3H$-corticosterone was about 35-40 percent in old controls, compared to young animals, whereas it was 20-25 percent in treated animals. To be noticed that the loss of binding capacity was to be attributed to the reduction in type I receptor, specifically neuronal, whereas type II receptor, also present in the glial

Table 3. The effect of long term ALC treatment on regulation of the HPAA and adrenocorticoid competence of the aging HI in the rat.

| | YOUNG | OLD | OLD + ALC |
|---|---|---|---|
| B SECRETION | | | |
| ug/100 ml plasma (6) | | | |
| Basal | 3.93 ± 0.75[a] | 12.66 ± 2.87#[b] | 7.55 ± 1.11[c] |
| Psychic stress[d] | 14.45 ± 1.57[a] | 39.35 ± 4.60#[b] | 22.39 ± 1.92#[c] |
| Stress-feedback[e] | 6.24 ± 0.46[a] | 20.50 ± 1.90#[b] | 15.05 ± 1.11[c] |
| HI $^3$H-B BINDING | | | |
| *In vitro* (4-5) | | | |
| fmoles/mg protein | | | |
| Individual maximal | 443 ± 32[a] | 262 ± 20#[b] | 357 ± 28*[c] |
| b (f.l.) total | 383(348-419)[f] | 253(185-322)#[g] | 289(233-344)#[h] |
| " " type I | 231(148-314) | 49(32-68)# | 78(53-102)# |
| " " type II[i] | 152 | 204 | 211 |
| *In vivo* (4-6) | | | |
| autoradiography | | | |
| Granules per 0.1 mm² and neuron nucleus | | | |
| CA1 | 1305 ± 45[a] | 505 ± 40#[m] | 847 ± 152*[n] |
| | 3.9 ± 0.09 | 2.6 ± 0.13# | 3.0 ± 0.09* |
| CA2 | 1278 ± 24 | 564 ± 11# | 987 ± 25* |
| | 4.4 ± 0.15 | 2.7 ± 0.13# | 3.1 ± 0.07* |
| CA3 | 1279 ± 27 | 602 ± 35# | 916 ± 98* |
| | 2.3 ± 0.10 | 1.8 ± 0.05# | 2.0 ± 0.05 |
| G. dentatus | 2423 ± 58 | 857 ± 151# | 1732 ± 285* |
| | 3.4 ± 0.09 | 2.5 ± 0.11* | 2.9 ± 0.06* |

In parentheses: number of animals. [a] 3, [b] 18, [c] 18 month old and ALC for 3 months. [d] Change of room and cage for 5 min and sampling at 15 min. [e] Negative feedback exerted by a previous 90 min cold stress on the response to a psychic stressor 45 min later. [f] 4, [g] 23, [h] 23 month old and ALC for 6 months. [i] By subtraction of $^3$H-B binding from total in presence of excess cold antiglucocorticoid RU 486. [m] 28, [n] 28 month old and ALC for 7 months. # and * : significant difference v. young or old group.

cell, tended to increase with aging. This finding contrasts with the interpretation that it is the type II receptor prevalently involved in feedback on stress-activated brain mechanisms (Reul and De Kloet 1985). The reduction in binding capacity in the CA1 - CA3 regions was partially due to a reduced number of glucocorticoid receptor per cell, but prevalently to loss of glucocorticoid competent cells. This was in agreement with findings of other authors (Sapolsky et al. 1984). Conversely, protection of binding capacity by ALC treatment was effected with preservation of the latter more than the former. The same was true for the gyrus dentatus.

Increased levels of plasma B can interfere with immunitary responsiveness; in fact, in 28 month old rats (plasma B above 7.85 ug/100 ml), splenocytes mitogenic response to P.H.A. and delayed type hypersensitivity were reduced, compared to young animals (data not shown). In old rats treated with ALC splenocyte mitogenic response to CON A and LPS appeared bigger than in their age matched controls (data not shown).

Behavioral parameters of hippocampal aging.

Long term treatment with ALC, as shown in table 4, reduced the impairment of some behavioral performances in the old rat. This was particularly evident with regard to HI-dependent behaviors, such as spatial orientation and short term memory in a temporal discrimination situation. These improvements

Table 4. The effect of long term ALC treatment on HI dependent behavioral performances in the old rat.

| | CONTROLS | TREATED |
|---|---|---|
| LEARNING[a] | | |
| 24 month old; 6 month ALC | 8 and 58<br>(24) | 50 and 33*<br>(12) |
| SPATIAL ORIENTATION[b] | | |
| 24 month old; 8 month ALC | 53.9 ± 11.2<br>(24) | 23.8 ± 8.4*<br>(6) |
| SHORT TERM MEMORY[c] | | |
| 18 month old; 6 month ALC | 142 ± 1.8 and 104 ± 21 | 136 ± 26 and 41 ± 12* |

In parentheses: number of animals. [a] Percent of rats in the high and low cluster of performance: totale number of failures in the last 5 out of 9 consecutive 20 trial daily sessions. [b] Sec to landing on the platform in a Morris water maze, in the last of 9 consecutive one trial daily sessions. [c] Number of reinforced and unreinforced responses in a DRL procedure with temporal discrimination > 6 sec for reinforcement, in the last of 10 consecutive 30 min daily sessions. * Significant difference.

were independent on possible effects of the treatment on motor activity and muscle endurance.

CONCLUSIONS

Long term treatments with ALC, in doses able to produce moderate increases in FC and ALC brain concentrations, have reduced the magnitude of anatomical and functional senescence markers in the rat, such as morphological and neurochemical changes in the HI, as well as disinhibition of the stress response and behavioral impairments. The endocrine and cognitive amelioration from exogenous ALC could be explained with the protection afforded on glucocorticoid competent neurons in the Ammon's horn and gyrus dentatus, made evident by the reduced loss in number of neurons and in number of adrenocorticoid receptors per neuron. So acting, exogenous ALC could oppose a circular pathogenetic mechanism by which increased concentrations of plasma corticosterone are resulting from deterioration of the HI, and, in turn, result in damage to the same structure. The better control of the HPAA so obtained in the old rat could also lead to preservation of cell mediated immunitary response and of neuronal trophic or reparative processes in the brain.

The pertinence of our findings to possible pharmacotherapeutic approaches in the treatment of human brain aging is indicated by the preeminent position of HI lesions in senile dementias (Hooper and Vogel 1976), and by the recent demonstration that increased concentrations of cortisol are present in the above conditions (McKeith 1984); Christie et al. 1986). Normal brain aging too in humans is characterized by loss of pyramidal neurons in the Ammon's horn (Mani et al. 1986), and a latent disinhibition of the HPAA, as signalled by reduced dexamethazone suppressibility (Rosenbaum et al. 1984). Chronic or recurrent hypercorticism from various pathologies or stress could damage the HI giving the basis of precocious brain aging, namely hindering synaptic plasticity and repair (De Kosky et al. 1984), carried on throughout the rat's (Cotman and Hoff 1983; Cotman and Nieto-Sampedro 1984) and man's life span (Geddes et al. 1985).

ACNOWLEDGEMENTS

Partially supported by C.N.R. Grant N° 86.00373.04 and M.P.I. Fund for 1986.

REFERENCES

Angelucci L, Valeri P, Grossi E, Veldhuis HD, Bohus B, De Kloet R (1980) Involvement of hippocampal corticosterone receptors in behavioral phenomena. In: Brambilla F, Racagni G, De Wied D (eds) Progress in Psychoneuroendocrinology. Elsevier/North Holland Biomedical Press, Amsterdam New York Oxford, p 177

Angelucci L, Ramacci MT (1986) Acetyl-l-carnitine: neuropharmacological potentialities in the senescent rat. Biol Psych 22:1343-1345

Angelucci L, Patacchioli FR, Scaccianoce S, Di Sciullo A, Catalani A, Taglialatela G, Ramacci MT (1987) Hypothalamo-pituitary-adrenocortical function and process of brain aging. In: Nerozzi D, Goodwin FK, Costa E (eds) Hypothalamic disfunction in neuropsychiatric disorders. Raven Press, New York,p 293

Bohus B, De Kloet ER (1981) Adrenal steroids and extinction behavior: antagonism by progesterone, deoxycorticosterone and dexamethasone of a specific effect of corticosterone. Life Sci 28:433-440

Christie JE, Whalley LJ, Bennie J, Dick H, Blackwood DHR, Fink G (1986) Neuroendocrine changes in Alzheimer's disease. In: Fink G, Harmar AJ, McKerns KW (eds) Neuroendocrine molecular biology. Plenum Press,New York, p 457

Cotman CW, Hoff SF (1983) Synapse repair in the hippocampus: the effects of aging. In: Haber B, Perez-Polo JR, Hashim GA, Giuffrida Stella AM (eds) Nervous system regeneration. Alan R Liss Inc.,New York,p 119 (Birth defects vol 19)

Cotman CW, Nieto-Sampedro M (1984) Cell biology of synaptic plasticity. Science 225:1287-1294

Curti D, Dagani F, Marzatico F, Benzi G (1986) Aging and acetyl-l-carnitine treatment: effects on some cerebral biochemical parameters. Biol Psych 22:1340-1342

DeKosky ST, Scheff SW, Cotman CW (1984) Elevated corticosterone levels. Neuroendocrinology 38:33-38

Friede RL (1965) Enzyme histochemical studies of senile plaques. J Neuropath Exp Neurol 24:477-479

Fritz JB (1963) Carnitine and its role in fatty acid metabolism. Adv Lipid Res 1:285-334

Geddes JW, Monaghan DT, Cotman CW, Lott IT, Kim RC, Chang Chui E (1985) Plasticity of hippocampal circuitry in Alzheimer's disease. Science 230: 1179-1181

Hooper MW, Vogel FS (1976) The limbic system in Alzheimer's disease. Am J Pathol 85:1-4

Landfield PW, Waymire J, Linch G (1978) Hippocampal aging and adrenocorticoid: quantitative correlations. Science 227:1580-1583

Mani RB, Lohr JB, Jeste DW (1986) Hippocampal pyramidal cells and aging in the human: a quantitative study of neuronal loss in sectors CA1 to CA4. Exp Neurol 94:29-40

McEwen BS, Weiss JM, Schwartz L (1969) Uptake of corticosterone by rat brain and its concentration by certain limbic structures. Brain Res 16:227-241

McKeith IG (1984) Clinical use of DST in a psychogeriatric population. Br J Psychiatry 145:389-393

Morris AJ, Carey EM (1983) Postnatal changes in the concentration of carnitine and acetylcarnitine in rat brain. Dev Brain Res 8:381-384

Patacchioli FR, Capasso M, Chiappini P, Chierichetti C, Scaccianoce S, Tozzi W, Angelucci L (1983) Variations of hippocampal cytosol glucocorticoid binding capacity as an after effect of physiological increase in brain and blood corticosterone concentrations. In: Endröczi E, De Wied D, Angelucci L, Scapagnini U (eds) Integrative neurohumoral mechanisms. Elsevier Biomedical Press, Amsterdam New York Oxford (Developments in Neurosciences, vol. 16) p 165

Reul JMH, De Kloet ER (1985) Two receptor systems for corticosterone in rat brain: microdistribution and differential occupation. Endocrinology 117: 2505-2511

Rosenbaum AH, Schatzberg AF, MacLaughlin RA, Snyder K, Jiang N-S, Ilstrup D, Rotschild AJ, Kliman B (1984) The dexamethasone suppression test in normal control subjects: comparison of two assays and effects of age. Am J Psychiatry 141:1550-1555

Sapolsky RM, Krey LC, McEwen BS, Rainbow TC (1984) Do vasopressin-related peptides induce hippocampal corticosterone receptors? Implications for aging. J Neurosci 4:1479-1485

Sapolsky RM, Krey LC, McEwen BS (1985) Prolonged glucocorticoid exposure reduces hippocampal neuron number: implications for aging. J Neurosci 5:1222-1227

Sass RL, Werness P (1973) Acetylcarnitine : on the relationship between structure and function. Biochem Biophys Res Comm 55:736-742

Sastri BVR, Janson VE, Jaiswal N, Tayeb OS (1983) Changes in enzymes of the cholinergic system and acetylcholine release in the cerebra of aging male Fischer rats. Pharmacology 26:61-72

Shug AL, Schmidt MJ, Golden GT, Fariello RG (1982) The distribution and role of carnitine in the mammalian brain. Life Sci 31:2869-2874

Sterri SH, Fonnum F (1980) Acetyl-1-CoA synthesizing enzymes in cholinergic nerve terminals. J Neurochem 35:249-254

Tempesta E, Janiri L, Pirrongelli C (1985) Stereospecific effects of acetylcarnitine on the spontaneous activity of brain stem neurones and their responses to acetylcholine and serotonin. Neuropharmacology 24: 43-50

# GLIA-PROMOTING FACTORS AND THE CONTROL OF OLIGODENDROGLIAL GROWTH DURING BRAIN DEVELOPMENT AND REGENERATION

Dana Giulian, M.D., Ph.D
Department of Neurology
Baylor College of Medicine
Houston, Texas 77030
USA

Joseph F. Krebs, B.A.
Program of Neuroscience
Baylor College of Medicine
Houston, Texas 77030
USA

The central nervous system (CNS) relies upon complex interactions among glial cells to regulate metabolic functions and to direct structural organization of neural networks. The contributions that astroglia, oligodendroglia, and microglia make to brain function are incompletely understood and include the support of tissue structure, production of myelin membrane, or mediation of inflammatory responses. One way to explore these cellular functions is to determine when and how glia are activated.

Each class of glia proliferates in defined regions of the CNS during development or in response to injury (Table 1). This pattern suggests local events help to regulate glial growth. Our laboratory has focused upon the study of soluble factors that stimulate the growth of astroglia, microglia, or oligodendroglia (Giulian, 1984; Giulian and Baker, 1985; Giulian et al, 1986a; Giulian, 1987).

Table 1.

Gliogenesis occurs during development or in response to injury. Under certain conditions extracts of brain tissues contain detectable levels of glial growth factors.

| Growth Periods for Brain Glia | |
|---|---|
| Astroglia | embryonic period<br>injury |
| Oligodendroglia | early postnatal period<br>regeneration (goldfish) |
| Microglia | late embryonic period<br>injury |

NATO ASI Series, Vol. H22
Neural Development and Regeneration
Edited by A. Gorio et al.

Our strategy to identify glial growth factors is a simple one. We extract soluble materials from tissues undergoing gliogenesis and test for the presence of mitogenic activity upon a particular class of glial cell in culture. Immunofluorescence techniques are used to identify oligodendroglia containing galactocerebroside (GC) or astroglia containing glial fibrillary acidic protein (GFAP). Several words of caution are in order. First, we carefully examine control or "quiescent" tissues for the presence of a putative growth factor in order to select only those substances which have elevated concentrations associated with gliogenesis. Second, we initially screen biologic activities using mixed populations of cultured glia. This approach allows us to monitor all three classes of glia simultaneously in order to determine specificity of action. Third, we test for direct action of a growth factor upon highly enriched preparations of glia. And fourth, we use *in vivo* bioassays to establish that a highly purified growth factor has a physiologic role in CNS function.

Application of our simple strategy and use of the four levels of biologic testing has proved successful and has allowed our laboratory to identify cell-specific growth factors for microglia (Giulian, 1987), astroglia (Giulian et al, 1986a), or oligodendroglia (Giulian et al, 1985). Here we describe the isolation and characterization of oligodendroglia-stimulating growth factors.

## Glia-Promoting Factors During CNS Regeneration

Transection of the goldfish optic tract initiates a remarkable regenerative process with regrowth of axons and recovery of sight. Our laboratory has found that in addition to neuronal growth, regeneration of the visual system involves proliferation of oligodendroglia (Giulian et al, 1985; Giulian and Iwanij, 1985). Surgical manipulation of the visual system suggested that soluble growth factors help to regulate oligodendroglia proliferation. Moreover, extracts of the regenerating CNS contained glial mitogens (Giulian, 1984).

The glial mitogens found in goldfish brain were peptides (< 20 kD) and were referred to as Glia-Promoting Factors (GPFs; Giulian, 1984; Giulian et al, 1985). As shown in Figure 1, goldfish tectal extracts separated by gel filtration contained 4 peaks of mitogenic activity for glia in dissociated cultures of mammalian brain. Closer examination of these mitogens showed that GPF-1 (apparent MW of 15 kD) and GPF-3 (6 kD) were growth factors for GC(+) oligodendroglia whereas GPF-2 and GPF-4 stimulated GFAP(+) astroglia.

Figure 1) Recovery of GPFs from goldfish optic tectum 10 d after transection of the optic tract. Soluble tectal protein was separated by gel filtration (P10, 100 x 0.9 cm) and assayed for growth of oligodendroglia or astroglia in culture. Data are expressed as fold increase in cell number when compared to control preparations. Molecular weight markers: a) 17.0 kD b) 14.5 kD c) 8.0 kD d) 6.4 kD e) 2.5 kD (from Giulian et al, 1986a).

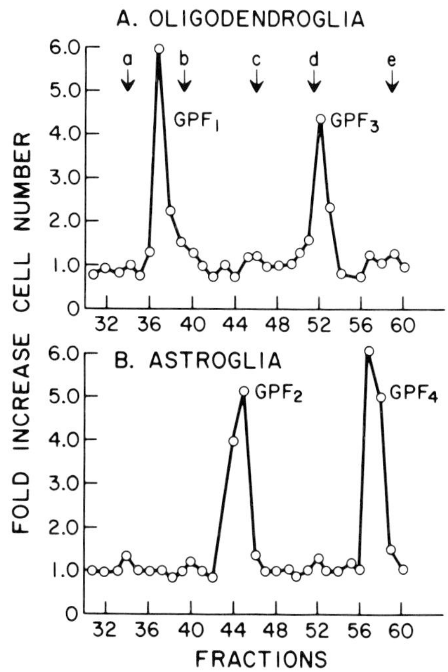


The GPFs were trypsin sensitive peptides and showed specificity of action when tested upon enriched populations of oligodendroglia or astroglia (Figure 2). Glial mitogenic activity increased during regeneration of the visual system with peak concentrations from between 7 to 14 days after axotomy (Giulian, 1984). Comparison of the different growth factors revealed GPF-1 and GPF-3, the oligodendroglia-specific factors, were produced in greater quantities than the astroglia-specific factors during regeneration (Figure 3). These observations were consistent with the fact that marked proliferation of oligodendroglia but not astroglia occurred during regeneration of the goldfish visual system (Giulian et al, 1985).

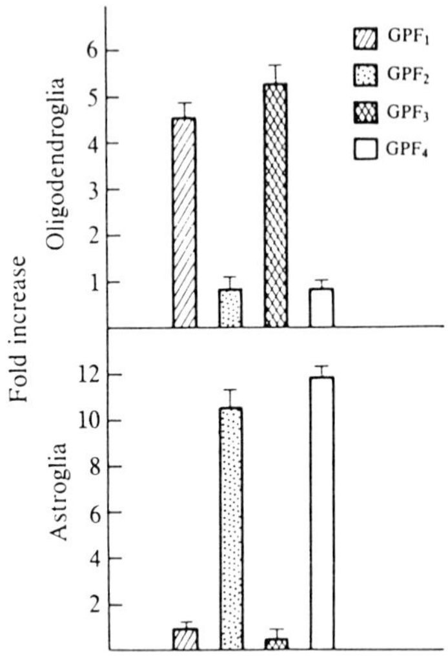


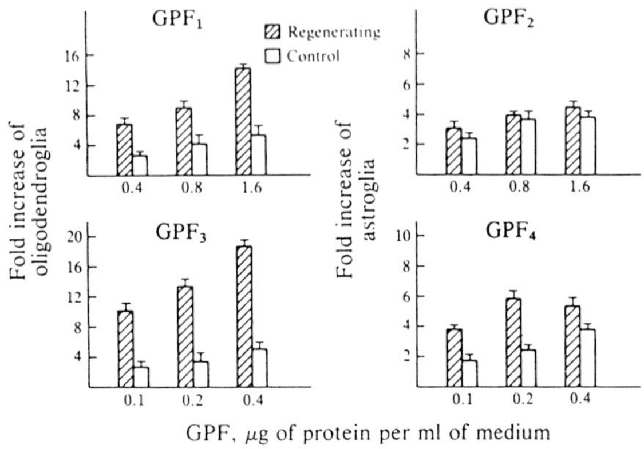


Figure 2) Action of GPFs upon enriched populations of GC(+) oligodendroglia or GFAP(+) astroglia. GPF-1 and GPF-3 show specificity as mitogens for oligodendroglia (from Giulian et al, 1985).

Figure 3) Changes in GPFs concentrations found in optic optic tectum during regeneration of the goldfish visual system. Greater concentrations of oligodendroglia-stimulating GPFs were found following axotomy of retinal ganglion cells (from Giulian et al, 1985).

In addition, GPF-1 was found to stimulate the myelin membrane-associated enzyme 2':3-'cyclic nucleotide 3'- phosphohydrolase (2':3'-CNPase) *in vitro*. Since elevations of 2':3'-CNPase occur during regeneration of the goldfish visual system (Giulian et al, 1985), it was reasonable to conclude that GPF-1 helps to stimulate oligodendroglial proliferation as well as myelin membrane formation in the goldfish visual system.

Glia-Promoting Factors and Brain Development

Oligodendroglia proliferate rapidly as myelinogenesis occurs in the postnatal brain of rat (Raff et al, 1979). Extracts of developing rat brain contain biologic activities that corresponded to the GPFs (Figure 4). In addition to GPF-1, GPF-2, GPF-3, and GPF-4, an 18 kD astroglial growth factor, the immunomodulator Interleukin-1, was also identified (Giulian et al, 1986b).

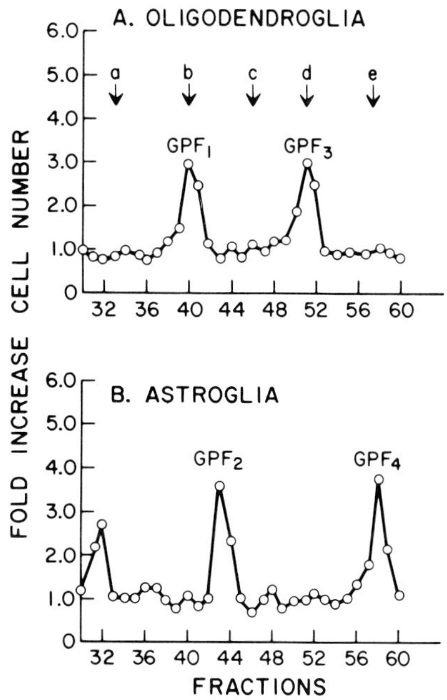


Figure 4) Presence of GPFs in the cerebral cortex of newborn rat. The two oligodendroglia-stimulating factors, GPF-1 and GPF-3, and the two astroglia-stimulating factors, GPF-2 and GPF-4, were similar to the GPFs from goldfish. In addition, the developing mammalian brain contained a 18 kD astroglia-stimulating factor which was found to be the immunomodulator Interleukin-1 (from Giulian et al, 1986a).

Examination of GPF levels during development of the cerebral cortex showed that the oligodendroglia-stimulating factors first appeared postnatally while the astroglia-stimulating factors were detected prior to birth (Figure 5). Unlike the regenerating CNS, injured mammalian brain had high levels of astroglial mitogens but low levels of oligodendroglial mitogens. The appearance of GPFs under different conditions suggested astroglia- and oligodendroglia-stimulating factors arose from different cell populations.

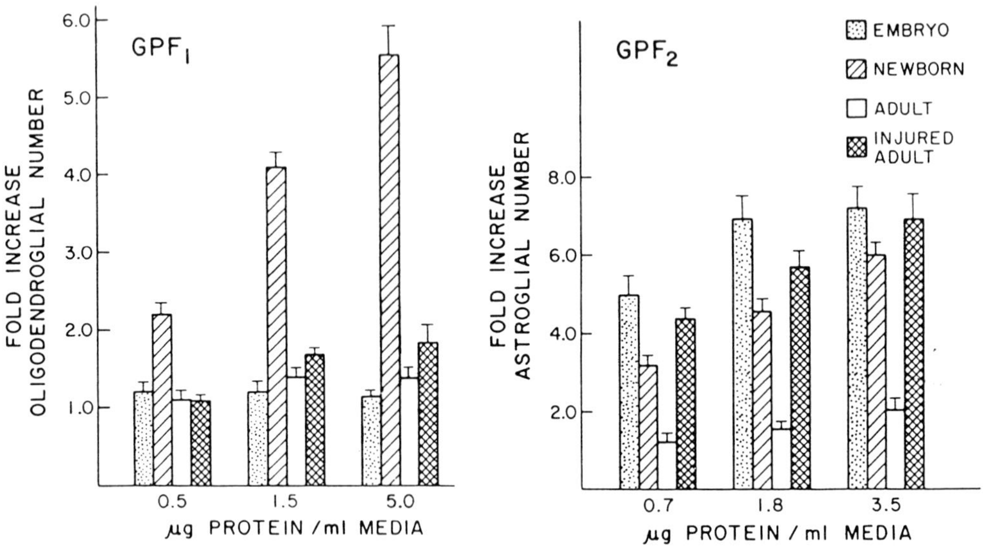


Figure 5) Recovery GPFs from the cerebral cortices of embryonic (E-16), newborn, intact adult rats, and rats receiving stab wounds (injured). The concentrations of GPF-1 was greatest during the early postnatal period and could not be elicited in the adult brain after injury (from Giulian et al, 1986).

Cellular Source of Oligodendroglia-Stimulating Growth Factors

To advance our understanding of the GPF network, we sought to determine the cellular sources of glial growth factors. Our initial study screened for the presence of GPFs in cultures of enriched glia or in neural tissue-derived cell lines. Study of conditioned medium as well as cell sonicates from various sources including astroglia and microglia, indicated that only neuroblastoma cell lines secreted oligodendroglia-stimulating GPF-1 and GPF-3 (Fibure 6). In contrast, the astroglia-stimulating GPFs were produced by ameboid microglia.

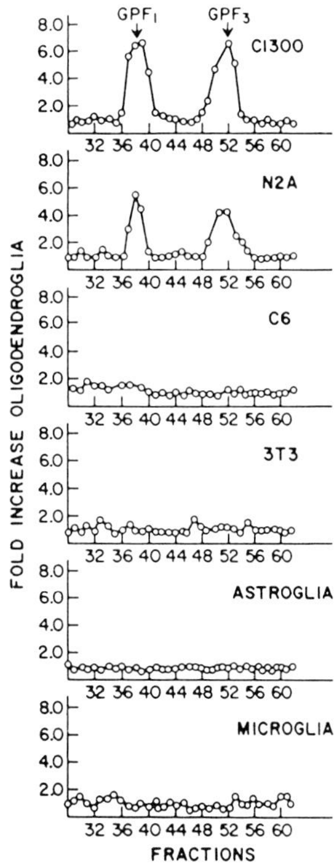


Figure 6) Secretion of oligodendroglia-stimulating GPFs by neural cell lines. Media conditioned by cells for 24 h were concentrated by ultrafiltration and separated by gel filtration. The neuronal cell lines (C1300, N2A) but not astroglia, microglia, or other non-neuronal cell lines released GPF-1 or GPF-3 (from Giulian et al, 1986a).

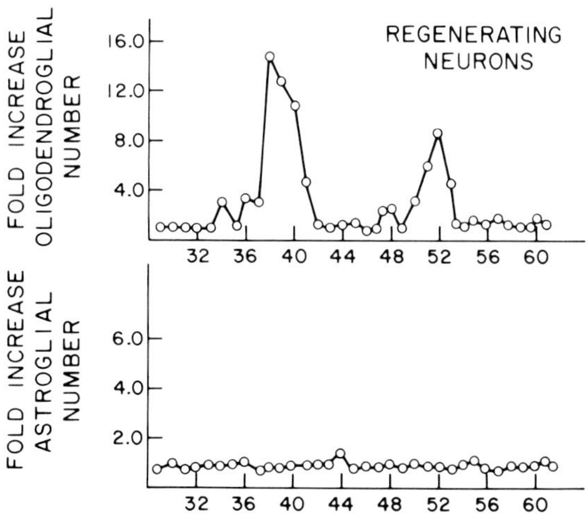


Figure 7) GPF production in goldfish neurons. Sonicates of 50 retinal ganglion cell layer dissections were separated by gel filtration. Regenerating neurons 12 d after axotomy contained GPF-1 and GPF-3 but no astroglia-stimulating growth factors (from Giulian et al, 1986).

To confirm that oligodendroglia-stimulating growth factors were produced by neurons, we isolated retinal ganglion cells from goldfish by microdissection (Giulian, 1980). This glia-free preparation showed neurons produced both GPF-1 and GPF-3 (Figure 7), but not astroglia-stimulating GPFs. The concentrations of GPF-1 and GPF-3 were greater in regenerating neurons when compared to intact control cells (Figure 8).

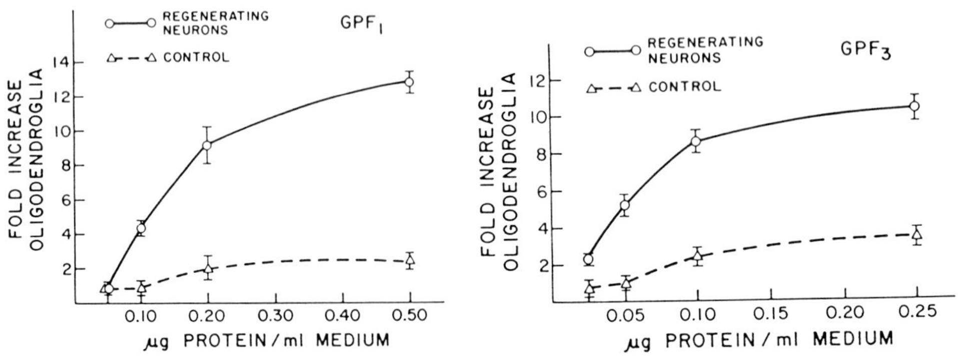


Figure 8) Comparison of GPF-1 and GPF-3 activities recovered from intact and regenerating retinal ganglion cells of goldfish. The greater specific biologic activity at 12 days after axotomy suggest that growing neurons release oligodendroglia-stimulating growth factors (from Giulian et al, 1986a).

## Purification of GPF-1

We found that GPF-1 from goldfish optic tectum, from newborn rat brain, and from the murine cell line C1300 had identical biologic properties and co-eluted by gel filtration, by anion exchange chromatrography (Figure 9), and by reverse-phase high performance liquid chromatography (Giulian and Young, 1986). Using a combination of these chromatographic techniques it was possible to recover highly purified GPF-1 from goldfish brain (Figure 10). The isolated peptide had an apparent MW of 15 kD as shown by gel filtration (Figure 11) and by SDS-PAGE (data not shown). More than 800 goldfish optic tecta were needed to yield 750 nanograms of highly purified GPF-1. Subsequent work in our laboratory has used the murine neuroblastoma as a more convenient source of GPF-1.

Figure 9) Co-purification of GPF-1 from goldfish optic tectum, newborn rat brain, and C1300 cell line using anion exchange (DEAE) chromatography (from Giulian and Young, 1986).

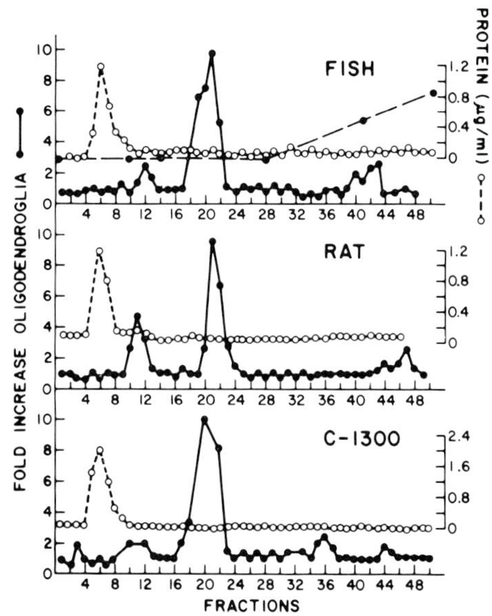


Figure 10) Highly purified GPF-1 isolated from goldfish brain or secreted by the C1300 cell line showed apparent molecular mass of 15 kD when separated by seiving HPLC. Molecular mass markers a) 68 kD b) 18 kD c) 12 kD d) 6 kD (from Giulian et al, 1986a).

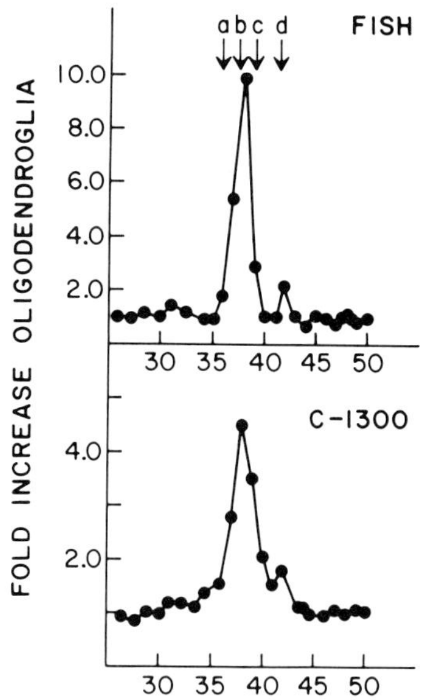


Figure 11) Dose-response curves showing purification of goldfish GPF-1. Tectal extracts were separated by gel filtraion (P-10), anion exchange chromatograophy (DEAE), reverse phase HPLC (C3) and seiving HPLC (TSK). Specific biological activity showed a 100,000-fold purification of GPF-1 when compared to tectal supernatants.

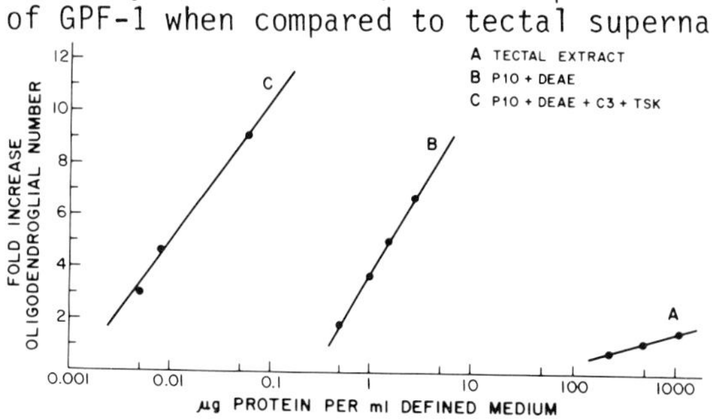

## In Vivo Effects of GPF-1

Although crude extracts from brain and other tissues will often stimulate glial growth in culture, it is unlikely that such effects are physiologically significant. To surmount the inherit artifacts of tissue culture bioassays, our laboratory has developed several methods to monitor the biologic activity of oligodendroglia-stimulating growth factors *in vivo*. Stereotaxically-placed microliter syringes allow infusion of GPFs into the cerebral cortex of adult rat in a highly reproducible fashion. Volumes of up to 2 microliters can be injected at a rate of 0.5 microliter per minute with dispersal of material to a distance of about 400 micron from the center of the needle tract. Biopsies from these injection sites are monitored for myelin protein synthesis, for 2':3'-CNPase activity, and for levels of mRNA encoding for myelin proteins.

Highly purified GPF-1 has biologic effects when injected into the cerebral cortex of adult rats. GPF-1 was found to increase enzymic activity of 2':3'-CNPase by 2 fold when compared to untreated tissue or control injection sites (Figure 12). GPF-1 had other *in vivo* effects as shown by a stimulated synthesis of myelin basic protein and elevations of mRNA encoding for phospholipoprotein (data not shown).

The observation that GPF-1 has biologic activity in the brain of the normal adult mammal is an important one for it suggests that this class of peptides has the capacity to mediate oligodendroglial growth throughout development. Secondly, it raises the possibility that growth factors infused into damaged brain would stimulate remyelination. One clinical application for GPF-1-like substances would be to accelerate regrowth of myelin membrane in patients with multiple sclerosis.

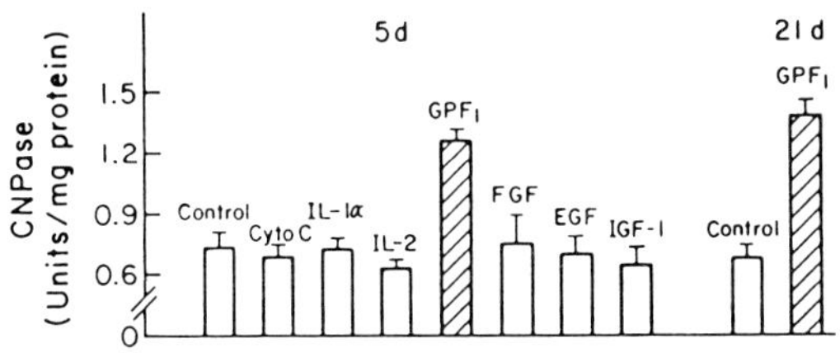


Figure 12) In vivo stimulatory effects of GPF-1 upon the oligodendroglia-marker enzyme 2':3'-CNPase. Enzymic activity was measured in biopsies obtained from sites of cerebral cortex where adult rats had been injected with growth factors 5 and 21 days earlier. Importantly, other potent growth factors have no in vivo effect, indicating the unique action of GPF-1. IL-1 - interleukin-1; IL-2 - interleukin-2; FGF - fibroblast growth factor; EGF - epidermal growth factor; IGF-1 - insulin-like growth factor-1.

## Does GPF-1 Represent a New Class of Growth Factor?

Comparisons between GPF-1 and other known growth factors show that only GPF-1 (and GPF-3) was a oligodendroglia-specific mitogen when tested in in vitro (Figure 13). Moreover, only GPF-1 stimulated myelin protein synthesis and 2':3'-CNPase activity in vivo (Figure 12). In the past year three other laboratories have reported that Fibroblast Growth Factor (FGF, Saneto et al, 1986), Interleukin 2 (IL-2, Benveniste and Merrill et al, 1986) or Insulin-Like Growth Factor-1 (IGF-1, McMorris, 1986) stimulate growth of oligodendroglia in culture. Are any of these factors related to GPF-1? FGF and IGF-1 stimulate astroglia in mixed glial cultures and have little effect upon oligodendroglia in culture medium which includes insulin (5 mg/ml). In our laboratory, IL-2 at mitogenic concentration for lymphocytes (Giulian and Lachman, 1985) had no effect upon oligodendroglial growth. At 10 to 20 fold higher concentrations, Benveniste and Merrill (1986) found a stimulatory effect of IL-2 upon oligodendroglia while Saneto et al (1986) found an inhibitory one. Importantly, we find that only GPF-1 stimulates oligodendroglia in vivo (Figure 12).

Figure 13)

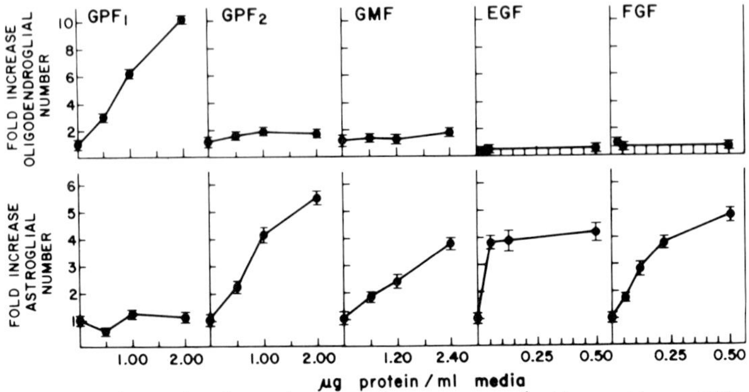


To date, no other isolated growth factor (other than GPF-3) shows the biologic effects of GPF-1 when assayed in vitro or in vivo. Our observations cannot exclude the possibilities that GPF-1 is a known growth factor not yet tested upon glial cells or that GPF-1 is structurally similar, though not identical, to a known peptide. Analysis of primary structure will be necessary in order to determine if GPF-1 in fact represents a new family of growth factors.

## CONCLUSIONS

Glia-Promoting Factors (GPFs) are brain-derived peptides which stimulate the proliferation and differentiation of oligodendroglia or astroglia in culture. Two of these factors, GPF-1 and GPF-3 are specific mitogens for oligodendroglia. These growth factors are found in highest concentrations in the regenerating visual system of goldfish and in the early postnatal brain of rat, tissues which contain rapidly proliferating oligodendroglia. Examination of isolated glial preparations, cell lines, and isolated retinal ganglion cells indicate that growing or regenerating neurons are the major source of the oligodendroglia-stimulating peptides.

Application of gel filtration, anion exchange chromatography, SDS-PAGE, and reverse phase high performance liquid chromatography has allowed purification of GPF-1 from goldfish optic tectum, rat brain, and a neuroblastoma cell line. The 15 kD growth factor is a peptide distinguished from other known growth factors by specificity of biologic activity both in vitro and in vivo.

We believe that growing neurons release peptides which regulate oligodendroglial proliferation and myelin membrane production. Manipulation of the GPF network may accelerate remyelination in lesions of the central nervous system and offer therapeutic benefit for demyelinating disorders.

REFERENCES


Benveniste EN, Merrill JE (1986) Stimulation of oligodendroglial proliferation and maturation by Interleukin-2. Nature 321:610-613

Giulian D (1980) Isolation of ganglion cells from the retina. Brain Res 189:135-155

Giulian D (1984) Peptides from the regenerating central nervous system of goldfish stimulate glia. Proc Nat Acad Sci 81:3567-3571

Giulian D, Iwanij V, Stuckenbrok H (1985) The response of optic tract glia during regeneration of the goldfish visual system I. Biosynthetic activity within different glial population after transection of retinal ganglion cell axons. Brain Res 339:87-96

Giulian D, Iwanij V (1985) The response of optic tract glia during regeneration of the goldfish visual system II. Tectal factors stimulate optic tract glia. Brain Res 339:97-104

Giulian D, Lachman LB (1985) Interleukin-1 stimulates astroglial proliferation after brain injury. Science 228:497-499

Giulian D, Baker TJ (1985) Peptides released by ameboid microglia regulate astroglial proliferation. J Cell Biol 101:2411-2415

Giulian D, Tomozawa Y, Hindman H, Allen R (1985) Peptides from the regenerating central nervous system promote specific populations of macroglia. Proc Natl Acad Sci USA 82:4287-4290

Giulian D, Baker TJ (1986) Characterization of ameboid microglia isolated from the developing mammalian brain. J Neuroscience 6:2163

Giulian D, Allen RL, Baker TJ, Tomozawa Y (1986a) Brain peptides and glial growth. 1) Glial-promoting factors as regulators of gliogenesis in the developing and injured central nervous system J Cell Biology 102:803-811

Giulian D, Young D (1986) Brain peptides and glial growth. 2) Identification of cells that secrete glial promoting factors. J Cell Biol 102:812-817

Giulian D, Baker TJ, Shih LN, Lachman LB (1986b) Interleukin-1 of the central nervous system is produced by ameboid microglia. J Exp Med 164:594-604

Giulian D (1987) Ameboid microglia as effectors of inflammation in the central nervous system. J Neurosci Res, in press

McMorris FA, Smith TM, DeSalvo S, Furlanetto RW (1986) IGF-I/Somatomedin-C: A potent inducer of oligodendrocyte development. Proc Natl Acad Sci USA 83:822-826

Raff MC, Fields KL, Hakomori S, Mirsky R, Pruss RM, Winter J (1979) Cell type specific markers for distinguishing and studying neurons and the major classes of glial cells in culture. Brain Res 174:283-308

Rio-Hortega P del (1932) Microglia. In: Cytology and Cellular Pathology of the Nervous System, (ed., W Penfield), Paul P Hocker, Inc., New York, Vol. 2, pp. 481-584

Saneto RP, Altman A, Knobler RL, Johnson HM, de Vellis J (1986) Interleukin-2 inhibition of oligodendrocyte progenitor cell proliferation depends on expression of the TAC receptor. Proc Nat Acad Sci 83:9221-9225

# CHOLINERGIC NEURONS OF THE RAT FOREBRAIN IN SLICE CULTURES; INTERACTIONS WITH TARGET TISSUE AND EFFECTS OF NERVE GROWTH FACTOR

F. Hefti and B.H. Gähwiler[1]
Department of Neurology
University of Miami
Miami, FL 33101
USA

## INTRODUCTION

The mammalian forebrain contains two distinct populations of cholinergic neurons. These populations are, first, the cholinergic neurons of the basal forebrain which are located in the medial septum, the diagonal band of Broca and the nucleus basalis of Meynert and which form an ascending and divergent projection to most cerebral cortical and limbic areas, and, second, the cholinergic interneurons of the corpus striatum (Butcher and Woolf, 1986; Mesulam et al., 1978; Wainer et al., 1983). Since their anatomy is well characterized, forebrain cholinergic neurons represent a favorite object for studying mechanisms involved in neuronal growth, targetting and regeneration. We have used the slice culture technique (Gähwiler, 1981,1984a,b) to study the interaction between axons of forebrain cholinergic neurons and their target tissues. Slices of brain tissue cultured with our technique develop into two-dimensional structures which often retain their organotypic morphology. This feature greatly facilitates tracing of fiber growth from one explant to the other. Furthermore, slice cultures can be observed and manipulated during the entire time of

[1] Institute for Brain Research, University of Zurich, 8029 Zurich, Switzerland.

NATO ASI Series, Vol. H22
Neural Development and Regeneration
Edited by A. Gorio et al.

growth.

Our first goal was to establish whether cholinergic projection neurons of the basal forebrain, when grown in culture, are capable of innervating their natural target tissues, hippocampus and cortex. Secondly, we investigated the specificity of this interaction by replacing the natural target tissues with tissues from areas not receiving a cholinergic projection in situ. Thirdly, we tested whether cholinergic interneurons of the striatum, which in situ are confined to this area, are capable of projecting to co-cultured slices of hippocampus and cortex.

We furthermore studied the effect of nerve growth factor (NGF) on the development of forebrain cholinergic neurons in slice culture. A role for NGF as a neurotrophic factor for these neurons is suggested by results from many recent studies. The evidence includes the following points. First, NGF as well as the mRNA coding for NGF are present in the rat brain and their levels correlate with the anatomical distribution of cholinergic neurons. Second, levels of NGF and its mRNA develop parallel to the growth of cholinergic neurons of the rat basal forebrain and these levels are affected by experimental lesions of the cholinergic neurons. Third, cholinergic neurons of the rat basal forebrain contain receptors for NGF. Fourth, application of NGF to rat cholinergic neurons stimulates the expression of choline acetyltransferase (ChAT), the key enzyme in the synthesis of acetylcholine and promotes survival and fiber growth of forebrain cholinergic neurons in vivo and in vitro. Finally, the notion that NGF acts as a neurotrophic factor for cholinergic neurons of the basal forebrain is supported by results from transplantation studies. These findings have been summarized in recent reviews (Hefti and Weiner, 1986: Korsching, 1986).

## METHODS

Brain tissue slices (400 µm thick) were prepared from 7 day

old rats and cultured on coverslips in roller tubes. Cultures were fed twice per week with 1 ml of medium consisting of 50% basal Eagle's medium, 25% Earle's balanced salt solution, 25% heat-inactivated horse serum, and supplemented with glucose to a final concentration of 6.5 g/l. NGF-treated cultures received 100 ng/ml NGF (2.5S NGF purified from mouse submaxillary glands) in normal medium either daily or at twice weekly intervals. Other cultures received sheep anti-NGF serum (1:1000, Suda), either daily or twice weekly. After 2-5 weeks in vitro the cultures were taken for histochemical visualization of acetylcholinesterase (AChE) or the biochemical determination of ChAT and AChE activity. Methods have been described in detail elsewhere (Gähwiler, 1981, 1984a,b; Gähwiler et al., 1987).

## SELECTIVE INNERVATION OF TARGET TISSUES BY CHOLINERGIC NEURONS OF THE BASAL FOREBRAIN

Cultures were prepared of tissue slices from the septal area and the anterior hypothalamus containing the nucleus basalis of Meynert. These slices consistently contained AChE-positive perikarya and an intricate network of fibers. The majority of these neurons had a soma diameter of approximately 30 μm and displayed two to four long dendrites. In slices cultured alone, the AChE-positive axons covered part or all of the surface area formed by the explants, but did not grow out of the explant into cell-free regions. AChE-positive neurons in these slices most probably represent cholinergic neurons, since a high degree of co-localization of AChE and ChAT has been found in these areas in situ (Eckenstein and Sofroniew, 1983; Levey et al., 1983). AChE has been shown to be a reliable marker for septal cholinergic neurons grown in cultures of dissociated cells (Hefti et al., 1985). Furthermore, findings similar to those presented in this report have recently been obtained in studies with co-cultures stained for ChAT rather than AChE (Gähwiler, unpublished observations).

Cultured slices of the cholinergic target areas, hippocampus and cortex, when kept alone, contained no AChE-positive fibers. However, AChE-positive cells were routinely encountered in the strata radiatum and oriens of the hippocampal formation and in the dentate hilar region. However, since the fibers of these cells did not stain for AChE, their presence did not interfere with the identification of cholinergic fibers derived from co-cultured slices.

In the majority of preparations containing cholinergic neurons of the septum or the nucleus basalis co-cultured together with slices of hippocampal or cortical tissue, AChE-positive fibers were seen to cross the gap between the two slices (fig. 1). The pattern of AChE-positive fibers in the hippocampal slice depended on the amount of septal tissue present. With small septal slices or slices containing few AChE-positive cells, AChE-positive fibers preferentially grew into the dentate region and area CA3 of the hippocampal formation, i.e., into hippocampal regions mainly innervated by cholinergic fibers in situ. With larger septal slices, AChE-positive fibers were present in all hippocampal subfields as well as in the fascia dentata. Ingrowth of AChE-positive fibers also depended on the distance between the two slices. In cultures with a considerable gap between the two slices, AChE-positive fibers remained restricted to the slice containing the cell bodies of these neurons. AChE-positive fibers of septal slices invaded both, hippocampal and cortical slices. The same was true for slices containing neurons of the nucleus basalis of Meynert.

To test the specificity of growth of basal forebrain cholinergic fibers into their target areas, septal slices were co-cultured with slices of various areas not innervated by forebrain cholinergic neurons in situ. These areas included the hypothalamus, the ventral mesencephalon, and the cerebellum. In the vast majority of such co-cultures, AChE-positive fibers remained confined within the septal slice. In some cultures, a few AChE-positive fibers crossed the gap between the two explants but failed to invade the adjacent culture (fig. 1).

The findings indicate that cholinergic neurons of the basal forebrain grown in slice cultures innervate co-cultured slices

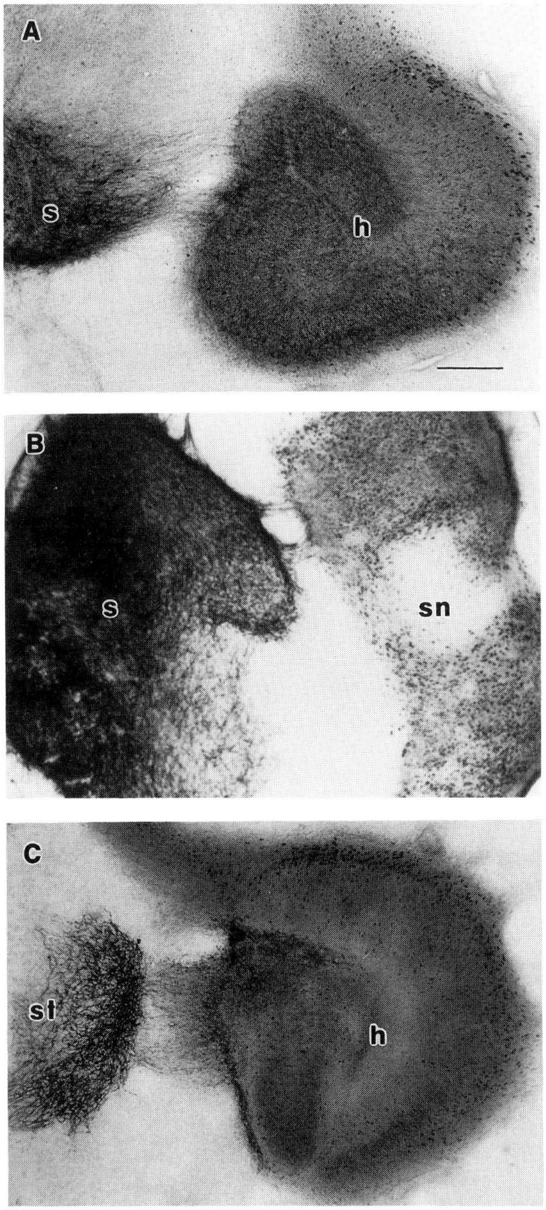


Figure 1. Growth of AChE-positive fibers in co-cultures of cholinergic tissue and other areas. (A): AChE-positive fibers originating in septal tissue invade the adjacent hippocampal slice. (B): Lack of growth of AChE-positive fibers from a septal slice into a co-cultured slice of substantia nigra tissue. (C): Invasion of a hippocampal slice by AChE-positive fibers originating in a slice of striatal tissue. Anatomical structures: c = cortex; h = hippocampus; sn = substantia nigra; st = corpus striatum. The bar represents 0.5 mm.

of their natural target tissue. As shown by electrophysiological studies, these cholinergic axons establish functional contacts with target cells (Gähwiler and Brown, 1985). The finding that cholinergic neurons of the septum and the nucleus basalis of Meynert innervate both, hippocampus and cortex, confirms the view that these neurons are part of a single population which forms a continuum of cholinergic neurons in the basal forebrain and provides a topographically organized innervation to most telencephalic areas (Butcher and Woolf, 1986; Mesulam et al, 1983; Wainer et al., 1984). Cultures of cholinergic basal forebrain neurons did not innervate slices of areas not innervated by them in situ. These findings are compatible with the notion that a selective signal from target areas is required for establishment of contacts between cholinergic neurons and their target cells.

## INNERVATION OF HIPPOCAMPAL TISSUE BY STRIATAL INTERNEURONS

Cultured slices of striatal tissue contained a variable number of AChE-positive cell bodies and a complicated network of AChE-positive fibers. When co-cultured with slices of hippocampal or cortical tissue, AChE-positive fibers originating in striatal slices invaded the hippocampal slice in the majority of the cases (fig. 1). The results demonstrate that AChE-positive fibers originating in striatal slices are capable of growing into adjacent hippocampal or cortical tissue (Gähwiler and Hefti, 1985; Gähwiler, unpublished observations). Contacts between striatal cholinergic cells and hippocampal cells were shown to be functional (Gähwiler and Hefti, 1985). These findings indicate that cholinergic neurons developing to striatal interneurons in situ (Woolf and Butcher, 1981), have the capacity to develop into projection neurons when given appropriate target tissues. Influences derived from the striatal environment therefore seem to direct the development of these cells to interneurons.

## NGF PROMOTES GROWTH OF CHOLINERGIC FIBERS IN SEPTO-HIPPOCAMPAL CO-CULTURES

Addition of NGF to the medium of cultured septal slices did not result in a diffuse, non-directed outgrowth of AChE-positive fibers as it is observed when peripheral sympathetic neurons, which respond to NGF, are cultured in the presence of NGF (for review see Thoenen and Barde, 1980). In earlier studies in which co-cultures of septal and hippocampal slices were given NGF (of other origin) once weekly, we failed to observe any stimulation of growth of AChE fibers (Gähwiler and Hefti, 1984). However, when NGF was added to the culture medium twice weekly or daily, a striking increase was observed in the number of AChE-positive fibers which grew from septum to hippocampus (fig. 2). Due to the large number of AChE-positive fibers in hippocampal slices grown in presence of NGF, the histological effect could not be quantified. The biochemically determined activities of ChAT and AChE were therefore used as indices reflecting the growth of cholinergic fibers into hippocampus. ChAT and AChE activities in co-cultured septal and hippocampal slices treated with NGF were both elevated more than 6-fold in comparison with control cultures. NGF treatment elevated ChAT activity from 0.036 ± 0.011 to 0.223 ± 0.040 and AChE activity from 5.5 ± 1.3 to 34.7 ± 5.9 pmol/min.µg protein (means ± S.E.M.; n=11). The effect of NGF was specific for cholinergic neurons, since it did not alter the protein content of the cultures.

To study the possible involvement of endogenous NGF in the establishment of the septo-hippocampal projection in vitro, co-cultured septal and hippocampal slices were grown in normal medium or in medium containing sheep anti-NGF antibodies (Suda et al., 1978). Daily addition of anti-NGF to the medium greatly reduced the incidence of hippocampal ingrowth by AChE-positive fibers (fig.2). In a few co-cultures a minimal ingrowth of AChE-positive fibers was observed. Anti-NGF produced no striking alterations in cellular or tissue morphology within the septal or hippocampal slices. No attempt however was made

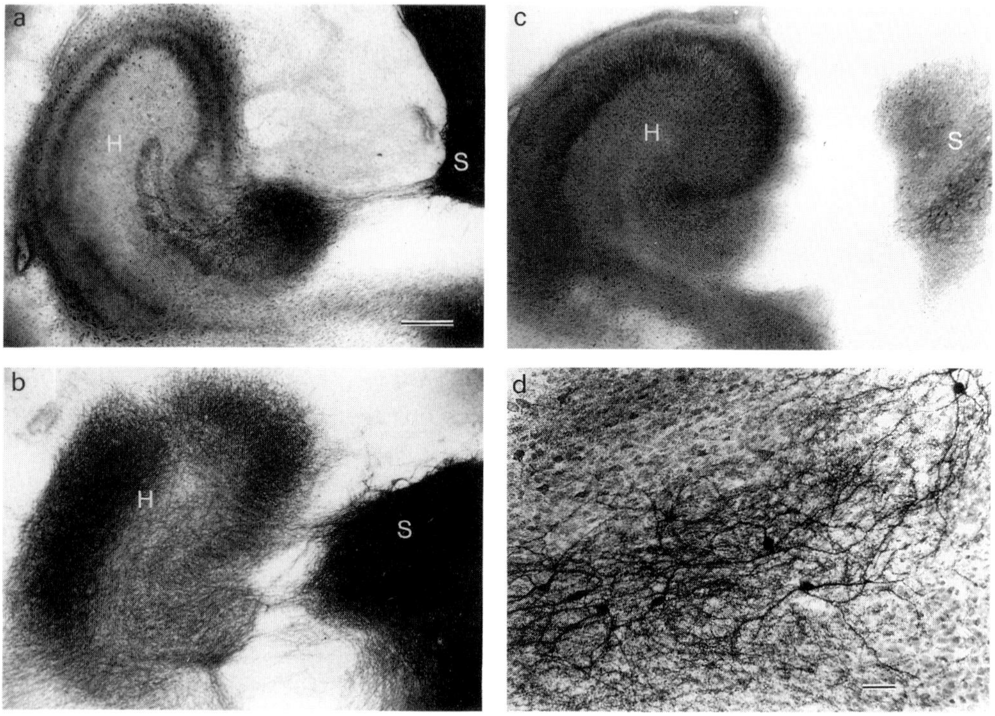


Figure 2. Effect of NGF and anti-NGF antiserum on growth of AChE-positive fibers in co-cultured slices of septal and hippocampal tissue. (a): Fiber connections as seen in a co-culture grown under control conditions. AChE-positive fibers originating in the septal explant (S) grew into the dentate gyrus and the $CA_3$ area of the hippocampal formation (H). (b): Addition of 100ng/ml of NGF induced a massive ingrowth of AChE-positive fibers into all hippocampal areas. (c): AChE staining of a septo-hippocampal co-culture grown in medium containing anti-NGF antibodies. Note the absence of fibers invading the hippocampal slice. (d): High magnification of the same culture as shown in (a) reveals a normal dendritic morphology for AChE-positive neurons in the septal slice despite daily administration of anti-NGF antiserum. Bars: (a) 1 mm, valid for a, b, c; (d) 0.1mm. Reprinted with permission (Gähwiler et al., 1987).

to quantify the number of surviving cholinergic neurons. In contrast to the anti-NGF antiserum, the administration of non-immune sheep serum failed to influence AChE-positive fiber connections between septal and hippocampal slices, excluding the possibility that the observed effects of anti-NGF reflected unspecific toxicity of the serum used.

The results indicate that NGF represents a powerful stimulus for the development of cholinergic neurons of the basal forebrain. The ability of anti-NGF antibodies to strongly attenuate the establishment of this projection in co-cultures suggests that endogenous NGF is produced and released by hippocampal target cells in control cultures and acts on the cholinergic fibers.

## CONCLUSION

The results obtained on slice cultures indicate that these cultures represent an excellent system to investigate mechanisms involved in the establishment of specific neuronal connections and, in particular, of forebrain cholinergic axonal projections. We have established that cholinergic neurons of the septum and the nucleus basalis of Meynert are capable of innervating each other's natural target area, providing further evidence that the various parts of the basal forebrain cholinergic system share most of the characteristics and can be considered part of a single population of neurons (Butcher and Woolf, 1986; Mesulam et al, 1983; Wainer et al., 1984). Striatal cholinergic interneurons were found to mimic the growth pattern of basal forebrain projection neurons when given an appropriate target tissue. This finding suggests that their development in situ reflects local environmental influences rather than an intrinsic developmental program of these neurons. It is presently not clear whether this developmental plasticity is shared by other populations of cholinergic neurons. In a limited experimental study we found that AChE-positive neurons of the spinal cord invade hippocampal tissue

(Gähwiler and Hefti, 1984). However, it remains to be established whether cholinergic neurons of the pedunculopontine area, which, besides basal forebrain neurons and striatal interneurons, represent the third population of cholinergic neurons in the brain, also respond to target tissue of forebrain cholinergic cells.

The fact that forebrain cholinergic neurons exclusively invade their natural target areas suggest that these tissues express a signal which promotes the development of their cholinergic input. Our studies with NGF strongly suggest that NGF is involved in the mechanisms establishing these pathways. The presently available data are compatible with two different mechanisms of action of NGF. First, NGF released by hippocampal target cells might diffuse to the cholinergic cells and stimulate the outgrowth of their axons. Second, NGF might be required for the stabilization of projecting cholinergic axons after they have reached their targets. This latter view is in line with findings obtained on sensory systems, which suggest that NGF-related mechanisms are involved in the stabilization rather than the guidance of axons (Davies et al., 1987). In addition, by signalling that the target has been reached, NGF might stimulate the synthesis of proteins necessary for neurotransmitter production of the cholinergic neurons.

Acknowledgements. These studies were supported in part by grants from the Alzheimer's Disease and Related Disorders Association, Chicago IL, and the National Parkinson Foundation, Miami, FL.

## REFERENCES


Butcher LL, Woolf NJ (1986). Central cholinergic systems: sypnosis of anatomy and overview of physiology and pathology. In "The Biological Substrates of Alzheimer's Disease", (eds.: Scheiber AB, Wechsler AF), New York, Academic Press, pp 73-86.

Davies AM, Bandtlow C, Heumann R, Korsching S, Rohrer H, Thoenen H (1987). Timing and site of nerve growth factor synthesis in developing skin in relation to innervation and expression of the receptor. Nature 326:353-358.

Eckenstein F, Sofroniew MW (1983). Identification of central cholinergic neurons containing both choline acetyltransferase and acetylcholinesterase and of central neurons containing only acetylcholinesterase. J Neurosci 3:2286-2291.

Gähwiler BH (1981) Organotypic monolayer cultures of nervous tissue. J Neurosci Meth 4:329-342.

Gähwiler BH (1984a) Development of the hippocampus in vitro: cell types, synapses and receptors. Neuroscience 11:751-760.

Gähwiler BH (1984b) Slice cultures of cerebellar, hippocampal and hypothalamic tissue. Experientia 40:235-243.

Gähwiler BH, Brown DA (1985). Functional innervation of cultured hippocampal neurons by cholinergic afferents from co-cultured explants. Nature 313:577-579.

Gähwiler BH, Hefti F (1984). Guidance of acetylcholinesterase-containing fibers by target tissue in co-cultured brain slices. Neuroscience 13:681-689.

Gähwiler BH, Hefti F (1985) Striatal acetylcholinesterase-containing interneurons innervate hippocampal tissue in co-cultured slices. Dev Brain Res 18:311-314.

Gähwiler BH, Enz A, Hefti F (1987). Nerve growth factor is involved in establishment of septo-hippocampal cholinergic projection. Neurosci Lett 75:6-10.

Hefti F, Weiner WJ (1986). Nerve growth factor and Alzheimer's disease. Ann Neurol 20:275-281.

Hefti F, Hartikka J, Heumann R, Eckenstein F, Schwab M (1985). Nerve growth factor (NGF) increases choline acetyltransferase but not survival or fiber growth of cultured septal cholinergic neurons. Neuroscience 14:55-68.

Korsching S (1986). The role of nerve growth factor in the CNS. Trends Neurosci 9: 570-673.

Levey AI, Wainer BH, Mufson EJ, Mesulam MM (1983). Co-localization of acetylcholinesterase and choline acetyltransferase in the rat cerebrum. Neuroscience 9:9-22.

Mesulam MM, Mufson EJ, Wainer BH, Levey AI (1983). Central cholinergic pathways in the rat: an overview based on an alternative nomenclature (Ch1-Ch6). Neuroscience 10:1185-1201.

Suda K, Barde YA, Thoenen H (1978). Nerve growth factor in

mouse and rat serum; correlation between bioassay and radioimmunoassay determination. Pro Natl Acad Sci USA 81:4042-4046.

Thoenen H, Barde YA (1980) Physiology of nerve growth factor. Physiol Revs 60:1284-1335.

Wainer BH, Levey AI, Mufson EF, Mesulam MM (1984). Cholinergic systems in mammalian brain identified with antibodies against choline acetyltransferase. Neurosci Int 6:163-182.

Woolf NJ and Butcher LL (1981). Cholinergic neurons in the caudate-putamen complex proper are intrinsically organized: a combined evans blue and acetylcholinesterase analysis. Brain Res. Bull. 7:487-507.

# NERVE GROWTH FACTOR EFFECTS ON CNS CHOLINERGIC NEURONS IN VIVO

S. Varon, F.H. Gage*, T. Hagg, H.L. Vahlsing, M. Manthorpe
Departments of Biology and Neurosciences*
University of California San Diego
La Jolla, California 92093
U.S.A.

Levi-Montalcini's discovery of Nerve Growth Factor (NGF) some 40 years ago has inspired dramatic changes in our perception of the nervous system as a highly regulated cell society. The concept that specific proteins (designated as neuronotrophic factors, or NTFs) are required for survival, growth and function of selected neuronal populations in the _peripheral_ nervous system (PNS) during its _development_ is being increasingly extended to the _central_ nervous system (CNS) as well as to _adult_ neurons in both PNS and CNS (Varon et al 1984; 1987a-d). If adult CNS neurons do depend throughout life on appropriately supplied NTFs, then it is possible to speculate that i) conditions leading to a deficient or defective NTF supply may be responsible for certain involutive or pathologic situations (Varon, 1975; Appel 1981), and/or ii) administration of exogenous NTFs could protect CNS neurons against such a deficit or alleviate their functional impairments.

The septo-hippocampal system of the adult rat has been well studied in both anatomical and functional terms (cf. Cotman 1978), and has become a favorite in vivo model for the investigation of CNS plasticity and repair processes (Bjorklund & Stenevi 1979; Gage et al 1984a; Kromer et al 1981; among others). Most of the cholinergic neurons in the medial septum and vertical diagonal band nuclei in the septum project their axons through the fimbria/fornix tract to the hippocampal formation, an important participant in the limbic system which is involved in cognitive activities of the brain. Recent investigations in several laboratories have established that _NGF_ may be a major neuronotrophic factor for most _cholinergic neurons_ of the basal forebrain including those in the Medial Septum (MS) and the Nucleus Basalis. For example: i) both NGF

NATO ASI Series, Vol. H22
Neural Development and Regeneration
Edited by A. Gorio et al.

and its messenger RNA are present in the hippocampal formation (MS innervation territory) and the cerebral cortex (NBM territory) (Korsching et al 1985); ii) cholinergic deafferentation of these territories leads to increased accumulation of NGF, presumably no longer taken up and retrogradely transported away by the innervating cholinergic axons (Korsching et al 1986); iii) NGF receptors are demonstrable on MS and NBM neurons, and co-exist with cholinergic neurons (Taniuchi et al 1986); and iv) treatment with NGF of septal neurons causes increases in their choline acetyltransferase (ChAT) activity (Hefti et al 1984, 1985). Most compellingly, intraventricular administration of exogenous NGF has been found to promote the maintenance of MS cholinergic neurons after their mechanical damage (Williams et al 1986; Hefti 1986; Kromer 1987).

We shall review here recent demonstrations, in our laboratories and/or in collaboration with Bjorklund's group in Sweden, that exogenously supplied factors can support adult rat basal forebrain cholinergic neurons in at least three respects: (1) protection against damage imposed by experimental axotomy, (2) promotion of axonal regeneration to the innervation territory, and (3) restoration of functional capabilities.

## (1) NGF prevents the numerical reduction of axotomized MS neurons

Mechanical interruption of MS cholinergic axons, via fimbria/fornix transection, should prevent the septal neurons from receiving neuronotrophic contributions from their hippocampal innervation territory and presumably lead to dysfunction, atrophy or even death of such trophically deprived nerve cells (Varon et al 1987c). Indeed, unilateral complete aspirative fimbria/fornix transection was shown to cause, within two weeks, the disappearance of most of the MS (and vertical diagonal band) cholinergic neurons, as visualized by either acetylcholinesterase histochemistry or ChAT immunoreactivity (Gage et al 1986a, Armstrong et al 1987).

We have developed a microcannula device connected to an osmotic minipump for continuous infusion of exogenous agents into the lateral ventricle (or the parenchyma) in close proximity to the septum (Williams et al 1987). By use of a minipump loaded with NGF in an appropriate vehicle, rats receiving a unilateral fimbria-fornix lesion could be immediately infused with exogenous NGF and the infusion could be continued over the 2-week period that normally leads to the disappearance of a maximal number of cholinergic MS neurons (Williams et al 1986).

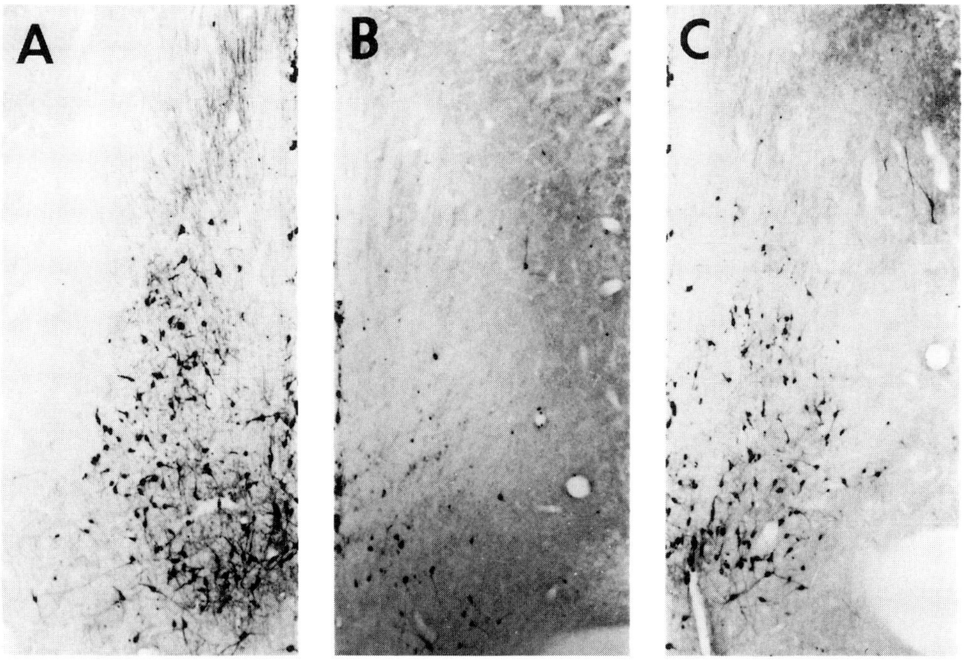


Figure 1. Coronal sections of adult rat forebrain, stained for ChAT immunoreactivity. Unilateral fimbria/fornix transection leaves largely intact the cholinergic population of the contralateral side (A), but causes the disappearance within 2 weeks of most of the ChAT-positive neurons in the ipsilateral medial septum (B). This disappearance is largely prevented by continuous intraventricular NGF infusion (C).

As shown in Figure 1, coronal sections of the rat forebrain, stained with anti-ChAT antibodies, display an extensive population of ChAT-positive neurons (Fig. 1A), which is largely lost on the fimbria/fornix-transected side of untreated animals (Fig. 1B). In dramatic contrast, the operated side of NGF-infused rats exhibits a nearly normal extent of ChAT-positive neurons (Fig. 1C). Unquestionably, then, NGF protects most of the MS cholinergic neurons from the obvious consequences of their axotomy. One must stress, however, that the available information does not prove the actual death of the cholinergic neurons rather than the reduction of their ChAT content below the levels of present detectability.

Figure 2 summarizes some numerical analyses obtained from coronal sections by counting directly either the ChAT-positive cells or cresyl-violet stained total neurons. The ChAT-positive population on the operated side was reduced to less than 20% of the initial number (or of the population measured on the contralateral, unoperated side), while in the NGF-treated

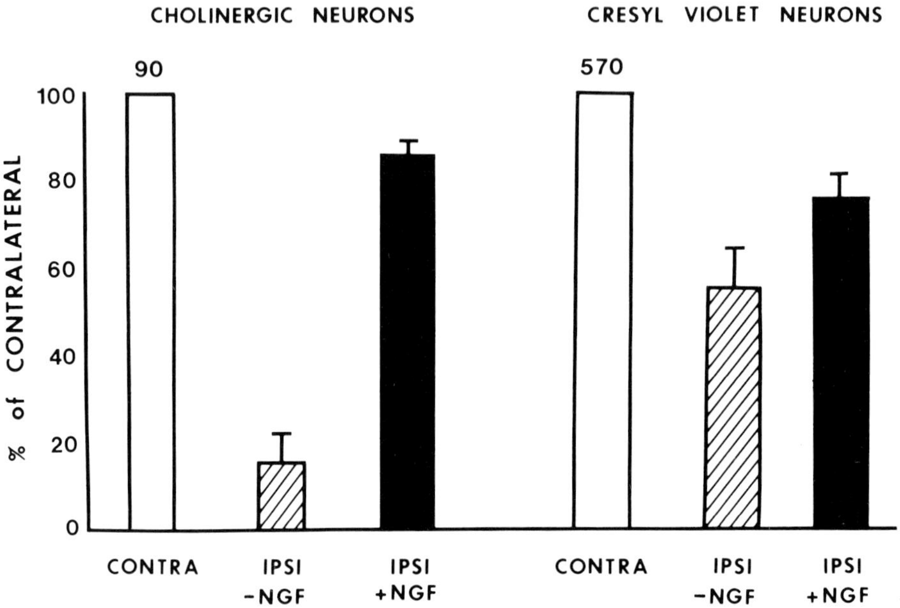


Figure 2. Numerical analyses of ChAT-positive and total (cresyl violet stained) neurons in the medial septum of adult rats following unilateral fimbria/fornix transection without or with continuous intraventricular NGF infusion.

animals nearly all (over 80%) of the normal cholinergic neurons were still counted. Total neuronal counts (i.e., cresyl violet stained neurons) were also substantially reduced on the lesion side, as noted previously (Gage et al 1986). This was to be expected since at least as many non-cholinergic as cholinergic septal neurons send their axons through the fimbria/fornix. What was more intriguing was the reduction that the NGF treatment imposed on the loss of cresyl violet stained neurons (Williams et al 1986). If the NGF-spared "cresyl violet" neurons actually correspond to the NGF-spared cholinergic ones, then the cholinergic neuronal "loss" is more likely to represent cell atrophy and/or death rather than only a loss of cholinergic enzyme contents. If, on the other hand, the cresyl violet neurons spared by the NGF treatment markedly exceed in number the cholinergic population at risk, then the question arises whether NGF addresses directly neurons that are not recognizably cholinergic or benefits these neurons only by some indirect means (Varon et al 1987d). These questions are crucial to the understanding of the role of NTFs for adult CNS neurons and are being currently addressed in our laboratory.

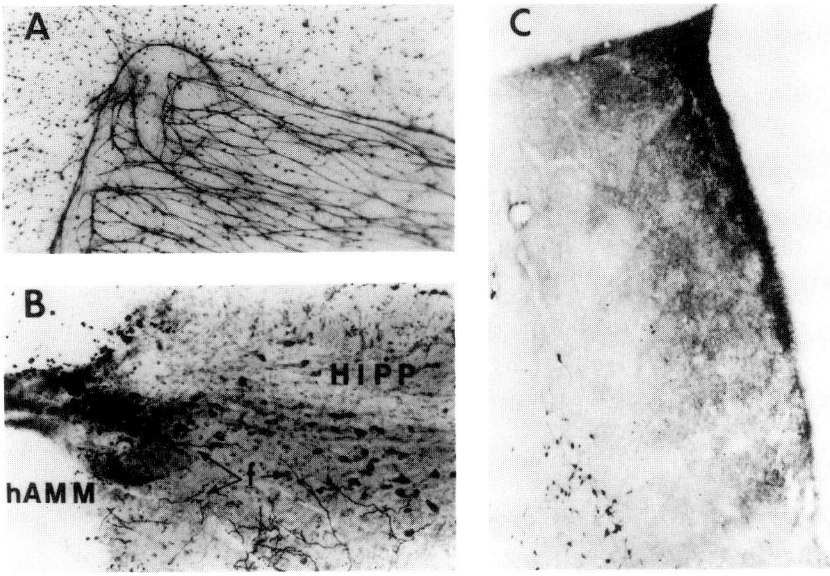


Figure 3. An approach to cholinergic axonal regeneration in the adult rat septo-hippocampal model. A: massive, oriented neurite growth is promoted in vitro by a human amnion membrane matrix (HAMM). B: a coil of HAMM, implanted into the fimbria/fornix lesion, allows some septal cholinergic axons to grow across the lesion gap into the host hippocampus. C: NGF infusion causes massive cholinergic sprouting inside the dorsal lateral region of the operated septum, suggesting that a concurrent availability of a HAMM bridge may result in substantial hippocampal reinnervation.

(2) Bridges rich in neurite promoting factors promote and guide axonal regeneration across a fimbria/fornix lesion

In vitro studies had demonstrated the existance of anchorage-dependent neurite promoting factors, released into the medium by cultured glial and other cells in the form of laminin-proteoglycan complexes (Collins 1978; Manthorpe et al 1983; Longo et al 1984; Rudge et al 1985; Lander et al 1985; Davis et al 1987c). The extracellular matrix nature of these neurite promoting molecules led us to the examination of extracellular matrix collected in its nearly native form from human amnion membranes (Davis et al 1987b). The amnion membrane is collected from discarded placenta, freed of its epithelial cell layer by treatment with ammonium hydroxide, and anchored onto a nitrocellulose strip with its basal membrane (containing the laminin) face up. Both CNS and PNS neurons, when seeded on this human amnion membrane matrix (HAMM) preparation, will attach, survive and grow a dramatic amount of neurites -- often, though not always, in a highly oriented manner, as illustrated in Figure 3A.

If an appropriate "bridge" were to be made available across a fimbria/fornix lesion gap, and if septal neurons could be encouraged to sprout, cholinergic axons might be able to regenerate across from septum to hippocampus and, possibly, invade and reinnervate the hippocampal territory. To begin exploring this possibility, HAMM material was rolled into a cylinder and a cylinder segment inserted into the fimbria/fornix lesion, taking care that the cut ends of the insert would closely abut the septal and hippocampal tissues (Davis et al 1987a). As illustrated in Fig. 3B, cholinergic fibers are seen to extend onto the HAMM bridge and leave it on the other side to regrow into their natural hippocampal territory. These preliminary results were obtained in the absence of continuous intraventricular infusion of NGF. We already know, however, that continuous NGF treatment in the fimbria/fornix transected animals also causes considerable sprouting of cholinergic axons in the dorsal lateral quadrant of the septum (Fig. 3C) (Williams et al 1986). Improvements are now being sought of the ways by which the HAMM material can be best manipulated and implanted. With NGF treatment to optimize the axonal reinnervation of the hippocampal formation, electrophysiological and behavioral consequences of such a reinnervation will be evaluated.

## (3) Long-term infusion of NGF in aged rats reduces memory impairments

The beneficial effects of exogenous neuronotrophic (and neurite promoting) factors discussed thus far have concerned the acute response of septal cholinergic neurons to a mechanical lesion imposed by the investigator. Different approaches are needed to justify the more general speculation that NTFs could provide similar benefits in chronic, non-experimental brain damage situations. In Alzheimer's Disease, memory impairments are accompanied by functional and morphologic deficits in the cholinergic neurons of basal forebrain (e.g., Terry and Davies 1980; Coyle et al 1983). Similar losses in cholinergic function accompany cognitive deficits during physiologic brain aging (e.g., Bartus et al 1982; Hepler et al 1985). If aging deficits could be alleviated by exogenous NTF administration and, specifically, cholinergic CNS deficits be reduced by exogenous NGF, a major step would have been taken to validate the hypothesis of neuronotrophic involvements in degenerative brain processes.

Promising results in this direction have been obtained in a recent study (Gage et al 1986b). Aged (over 23 months) female Sprague-Dawley rats were tested for their ability to identify and remember the location of a submerged platform in a specially constructed swimming tank. This Morris "water-maze" task had been previously used to show improved learning behaviors of aged rats before and after intra-hippocampal grafts of fetal septal tissue (Gage et al 1984b,c). Rats placed into the water are allowed to swim freely until they find the platform to escape from the water, and the time and swimming pathway required to reach the escape platform are recorded in a series of daily trials. About one third of the aged rats screened on this task showed learning and retention difficulties. These "impaired" rats were then implanted with an intraventricular cannula connected to an osmotic minipump and were infused for 4 weeks, half of these rats with NGF and half with vehicle only. One week after implantation, the rats were tested again for 5 consecutive days, then given a rest period of 11 days (while still under infusion) and tested once more for 4 days.

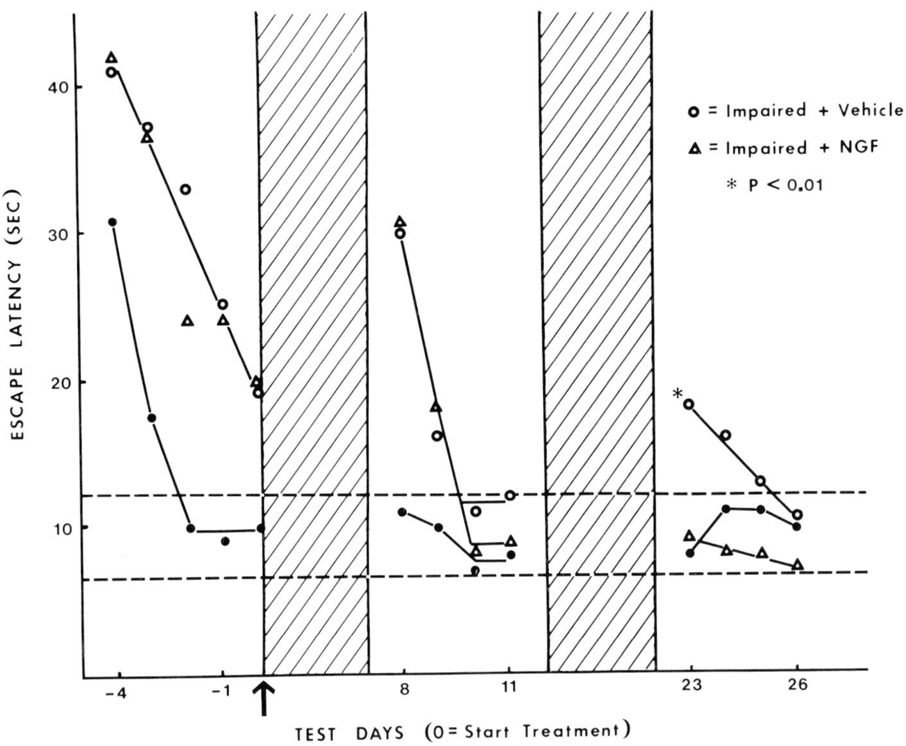


<u>Figure 4.</u> Three successive trial series of aged rats on a Morris "water-maze" task. <u>Unimpaired animals</u> (•) reached a competent performance level in the first series and retained it through the second (1 week later) and third (another 11 days later) series. <u>Impaired rats</u> (o) learned slowly and retained poorly across the three test series. <u>Continuous infusion of NGF</u> (Δ) to initially impaired rats led to significant ($p < 0.01$) retention improvements after 3 weeks of treatment.

Figure 4 illustrates some of the results. A competent performance was achieved by the non-impaired aged animals over the first 3 trial days of the screening period (Fig. 4A) and maintained from one trial series to the next (Fig. 4B,C). The "impaired" animals failed to reach this level of competence even after 5 trial days in the screening series, and had to start learning again when tested over the second week of treatment regardless of whether they received NGF or not (Fig. 4B). However, the third series of tests showed the NGF-treated rats performing optimally from the very first trial day, whereas vehicle-treated rats continued to display retention problems (Fig. 4C). Thus, 3 weeks of continuous NGF treatment brought the initially impaired rat to a performance level which was no longer distinguishable from that of unimpaired animals. Morphometric analyses on sections, taken at the end of the treatment and behavior test period and stained for acetylcholinesterase (not shown here), revealed a substantial reduction in the size of nucleus basalis cholinergic cell bodies in the impaired versus unimpaired rats, and a significant increase -- or a significantly smaller reduction -- in the size of initially impaired but NGF-treated animals. Thus, the longer-term (3-4 weeks) continuous treatment with NGF both improved cholinergic-supported functional performance and reduced function-correlated hypotrophy of certain cholinergic CNS neurons.

## Discussion and projections

The neuronotrophic hypothesis for CNS function and dysfunction has not only been inspired by the discovery and investigation of Nerve Growth Factor, it has drawn from NGF itself the supportive evidence available thus far. Other neuronotrophic factors are under investigation in several laboratories and encourage the expectation that some of them will also prove critical for non-cholinergic as well as cholinergic adult CNS neurons. For the near future, the beneficial effects of NGF administration into adult CNS are likely to be further investigated in several main directions:

(1) How much exogenous NGF is needed? Protection against the disappearance of septal cholinergic neurons in the adult rat has been obtained with as little as 2 μg of NGF per treatment, delivered at 5 ng/hr over a 2-week continuous period (Williams et al 1986). Longer treatments were needed for memory improvements in the aged rat (Gage et al 1986). Higher NGF doses may prove to be more effective on some aspects of cholinergic damage or on some temporal parameters of NGF treatment (see further on). Conversely, if NGF

doses were reduced below the threshold required for the detection of its effects by present methods, it would become possible to recognize and evaluate other agents given concurrently with NGF for their ability to potentiate the latter.

(2) How permanent are the NGF effects? The cholinergic protection currently observed over 2 weeks of continuous NGF treatment may or may not gradually dissipate after interruption of the NGF administration. On one hand, one could speculate that the fimbria/fornix lesion triggers an acute crisis which the septal neurons can weather with only a temporary administration of NGF. On the other hand, exogenous NGF may remain needed for as long as it takes for the axotomized neurons to re-acquire an adequate source of endogenous NTF. If the latter condition, in turn, requires restored connections between septal neurons and their hippocampal innervation territory, then the combined use of a neurite-promoting septal-hippocampal bridge will be needed to terminate the requirement for exogenous NGF administration.

(3) How soon after the lesion must NGF be supplied? This question has, in fact, two major aspects. One, on the practical side, relates to the disappearance of ChAT- (or acetylcholinesterase) positive MS neurons after fimbria/fornix transection, and the delay in NGF presentation which would still allow full prevention of their disappearance -- an obviously important point for clinical NTF treatments of acute trauma. The other, more biological, aspect concerns the permanence of the cholinergic neuronal losses, and specifically the possibility that disappearance of the cholinergic enzyme(s) by which the neurons are recognized need not coincide, temporally or even at all, with the actual death of the cell. Both aspects of the question can be investigated by evaluating the effects of progressive NGF delays on the persistence, disappearance and/or re-appearance of ChAT-positive MS neurons.

Acknowledgements. This work has been partially supported by NSF grants BNS-85-01766 and BNS-85-02198, NINCDS grant NS-16349, NIA grant AG-06088, and by the Office of Naval Research.

## Literature references

Appel SH (1981) A unifying hypothesis for the cause of Amyotrophic Lateral Sclerosis, Parkinsonism, and Alzheimer disease. Ann Neurol 10:499-505

Armstrong DM, Terry RD, DeTeresa RM, Bruce G, Hersh LB, Gage FH (1987) Response of septal cholinergic neurons to axotomy. J Comp Neurol, submitted

Bartus RT, Dean RL, Beer B, Lippa AS (1982) The cholinergic hypothesis of geriatric memory dysfunction. Science 217:408-417

Bjorklund A, Stenevi U (1979) Regeneration of monoaminergic and cholinergic neurons in the mammalian central nervous system. Physiol Rev 59:62-100

Collins F (1978) Induction of neuritic outgrowth by a conditioned-medium factor bound to the culture substratum. Proc Natl Acad Sci USA 75:5210-5213

Cotman CW (ed) (1978) Neuronal plasticity. Raven Press, New York

Coyle JT, Price DL, DeLong MR (1983) Alzheimer's disease: A disorder of cortical cholinergic innervation. Science 219:1184-1190

Davis GE, Blaker SN, Engvall E, Varon S, Manthorpe M, Gage FH (1987a) Human amnion membrane serves as a substratum for growing axons in vitro and in vivo. Science, in press

Davis GE, Engvall E, Varon S, Manthorpe M (1987b) Human amnion membrane as a substratum for cultured peripheral and central nervous system neurons. Dev Brain Res, in press

Davis GE, Klier, FG, Engvall E, Cornbrooks C, Varon S, Manthorpe M (1987c) Association of laminin with heparan and chondroitin sulfate-bearing proteoglycans in neurite-promoting complexes from rat Schwannoma cells. Neurochem Res, in press

Gage FH, Bjorklund A, Stenevi U (1984a) Denervation releases a neuronal survival factor in adult rat hippocampus. Nature (London) 308:637-639

Gage FH, Bjorklund A, Stenevi U, Dunnett SB, Kelly PAT (1984b) Intrahippocampal septal grafts ameliorate learning impairment in aged rats. Science 225:533-536

Gage FH, Kelly PAT, Bjorklund A (1984c) Regional changes in brain glucose metabolism reflect cognitive impairments in aged rats. J Neurosci 4(11):2856-2866

Gage FH, Wictorin K, Fischer W, Williams LR, Varon S, Bjorklund A (1986a) Retrograde cell changes in medial septum and diagonal band following fimbria-fornix transection: quantitative temporal analysis. Neurosci 19:241-255

Gage FH, Wictorin K, Fisher W, Williams LR, Varon S, Bjorklund A (1986b) Chronic intracerebral infusion of Nerve Growth Factor (NGF) improves memory performance in cognitively impaired aged rats. Soc Neurosci Abstr 12:1580

Hefti F (1986) Nerve Growth Factor promotes survival of septal cholinergic neurons after fimbrial transections. J Neurosci 6:2155-2162

Hefti F, Dravid A, Hartikka J (1984) Chronic intraventricular injections of Nerve Growth Factor elevate hippocampal choline acetyltransferase activity in adult rats with partial septo-hippocampal lesions. Brain Res 293:305-311

Hefti F, Hartikka JJ, Eckenstein F, Gnahn H, Heumann R, Schwab M (1985) Nerve Growth Factor increases choline acetyltransferase but not survival or fiber outgrowth of cultured fetal septal cholinergic neurons. Neuroscience 14:55-68

Hepler DJ, Wenk GL, Cribbs BL, Olton DS, Coyle JT (1985) Memory impairments following basal forebrain lesions. Brain Res 346:8-14

Korsching S, Auburger G, Heumann R, Scott J, Thoenen H (1985) Levels of nerve growth factor and its mRNA in the central nervous system of the rat correlate with cholinergic innervation. EMBO J 4:1389-1393

Korsching S, Heumann R, Thoenen H, Hefti F (1986) Cholinergic denervation of the rat hippocampus by fimbrial transection leads to a transient accumulation of nerve growth factor (NGF) without change in mRNA NGF content. Neurosci Lett 66:175-180

Kromer LF (1987) Nerve Growth Factor treatment after brain injury prevents neuronal death. Science 235:214-216

Kromer LF, Bjorklund A, Stenevi U (1981) Regeneration of the septo-hippocampal pathways in adult rats is promoted by utilizing embryonic hippocampal implants as bridges. Brain Res 210:173-200

Lander AD, Fujii DK, Reichardt LF (1985) Laminin is associated with the "neurite outgrowth promoting factors" found in conditioned media. Proc Natl Acad Sci USA 82:2183-2189

Longo FM, Hayman EG, Davis GE, Ruoslahti E, Engvall E, Manthorpe M, Varon S (1984) Neurite promoting factors and extracellular matrix components accumulating in vivo within nerve regeneration chambers. Brain Res 309:105-117

Manthorpe M, Engvall E, Ruoslahti E, Longo FM, Davis GE, Varon S (1983) Laminin promotes neuritic regeneration from cultured peripheral and central neurons. J Cell Biol 97:1882-1890

Rudge JS, Manthorpe M, Varon S (1985) The output of neuronotrophic and neurite-promoting agents from rat brain astroglial cells: A microculture method for screening potential regulatory molecules. Dev Brain Res 19:161-172

Taniuchi M, Schweizer JB, Johnson EM (1986) Nerve growth factor receptor molecules in rat brain. Proc Natl Acad Sci USA 83:1950-1954

Terry RD, Davies P (1980) Dementia of the Alzheimer type. Annu Rev Neurosci 3:77-95

Varon S (1975) In vitro approaches to the study of neural tissue aging. In: Maletta G (ed), Survey of the Aging Nervous System. DHEW Pub (NIH) 74-296, pp 59-76

Varon S, Manthorpe M, Williams LR (1984) Neuronotrophic and neurite promoting factors and their clinical potentials. Dev Neuroscience 6(2):73-100

Varon S, Manthorpe M, Davis GE, Williams LR, Skaper SD (1987a) Growth Factors. In: Waxman SG (ed), Physiological Basis for Functional Recovery in Neurological Disease. Raven Press, in press

Varon S, Manthorpe M, Williams LR, Gage FH (1987b) Neuronotrophic factors and their involvements in the adult CNS. In: Terry R, Klier FG, Cornbrooks C (eds), Aging and the Brain. Raven Press, New York, in press

Varon S, Williams LR, Gage FH (1987c) Exogenous administration of neuronotrophic factors in vivo protects central nervous system neurons against axotomy induced degeneration. In: Seil FJ, Herbert E, Carlson BM (eds), Neural Regeneration. Progress in Brain Research, Vol 71, Elsevier, pp 191-201

Varon S, Williams LR, Gage FH (1987d) In vivo protection by an exogenous neuronotrophic factor against neuronal death in adult rat CNS. In: Masland R, Portera-Sanchez A, Toffano G (eds), Neuroplasticity: A New Therapeutical Tool in CNS Pathology. FIDIA Research Series, Liviana Press, Padova, Italy, in press

Williams LR, Vahlsing HL, Lindamood T, Varon S, Gage FH, Manthorpe M (1987) A small gauge cannula device for continuous infusion of exogenous agents into the brain. Exp Neurol 95:743-754

Williams LR, Varon S, Peterson G, Wictorin K, Fischer W, Bjorklund A, Gage FH (1986) Continuous infusion of Nerve Growth Factor prevents basal forebrain neuronal death after fimbria-fornix transection. Proc Natl Acad Sci 83:9231-9235

# EXPRESSION OF NGF RECEPTORS DURING DEVELOPMENT OF CENTRAL SENSORY PATHWAYS IN THE RAT

Rebekah Loy and Sookyong Koh
Department of Neurobiology and Anatomy
University of Rochester Medical Center
601 Elmwood Avenue
Rochester, New York 14642

Neuronal sensitivity to nerve growth factor (NGF) is conferred by the presence of specific high affinity receptors (Stach and Perez-Polo, 1987). Based on immunocytochemical and autoradiographic studies of adult rat and human brains, NGF receptors (NGF-R) are known to be present on cholinergic neurons located in the basal forebrain and on their terminals in the neocortex and hippocampus (Schwab et al., 1979; Seiler and Schwab, 1984; Hefti et al., 1986; Richardson et al., 1986; Johnson et al., 1987; Raivich and Kreutzberg, 1987; Springer et al., 1987; Loy et al, in press). In addition, measurement of NGF-R by immunoprecipitation reveals the presence of significant quantities of NGF-R in rat cerebellum, thalamus, olfactory bulb, and particularly in the brainstem (Taniuchi et al., 1986b). Recently, NGF-R have also been identified autoradiographically on a variety of neurons in the rat brainstem, including those of the cochlear nucleus and nucleus of the lateral lemniscus, components of the auditory system, suggesting that some central sensory neurons may be sensitive to NGF (Richardson et al., 1986; Raivich and Kreutzberg, 1987).

During development there is a substantial decrease in NGF-R levels in many tissues (Raivich et al., 1985) . Brain levels of NGF-R decrease 11-fold between embryonic day 15 (ED15) and adulthood (Yan and Johnson, 1987). Such changes in the presence of NGF-R on cell bodies of neural crest-derived sensory neurons of the PNS correlate well with the temporally restricted appearance of NGF sensitivity (Rohrer and Barde, 1982). In order to determine if some CNS systems show similar developmental changes in NGF sensitivity, we have immunocytochemically examined the brains of rats between ED11 and adulthood using a monoclonal antibody to the rat NGF-R.

NATO ASI Series, Vol. H22
Neural Development and Regeneration
Edited by A. Gorio et al.

## METHODS

A total of 63 fetuses from ED13 through ED21, pups from the day of birth (postnatal day 0, PD0) through PD21, and 10 adult Long-Evans rats were used in this study. Embryonic tissues were immersion fixed for 6 hours in ice-cold 1% paraformaldehyde in 10 mM phosphate buffer, pH 7.4, followed by overnight immersion in the same fixative containing 20% sucrose. Postnatal and adult rats were perfused transcardially with buffered 4% paraformaldehyde. The brains were removed, then placed in sucrose as above. For ED13-15 embryos, 30 µm cryostat sections were cut, thaw-mounted onto slides, and stained on slides. For older animals, 50 µm freezing microtome sections were collected and every third free-floating section was processed for immunocytochemistry. Adjacent sections were stained with cresyl violet. Following preincubation with 4% normal horse serum, the sections were incubated at 4°C for 24 hours in 0.002 mg/ml 192-IgG (Taniuchi and Johnson, 1985), in 1:150 affinity purified, biotinylated horse anti-mouse secondary antibody at 4°C overnight, and in an avidin-biotin-horseradish peroxidase complex (Vector) for 3 hours. The sections were reacted with 3,3'-diaminobenzidine as chromagen, in a solution containing cobalt chloride or nickle sulfate. Control sections were run either with no primary antibody, or with monoclonal antibody to epidermal growth factor receptor.

## RESULTS

Embryonic days 13-14. NGF-R immunoreactivity (NGF-RI) is clearly present in cells of the nucleus basalis and medial septal nucleus/diagonal band, located within the ventral lateral telencephalic wall adjacent to the developing internal capsule. Also, (NGF-RI) appears in ascending somatosensory tracts within the brainstem, and in the roots and entry zones of the cranial and spinal sensory nerves (Figs. 1 and 2). In the eye cup and stalk, NGF-RI is radially-oriented and restricted to the proximal segment of the optic nerve and central retina (Fig. 3).

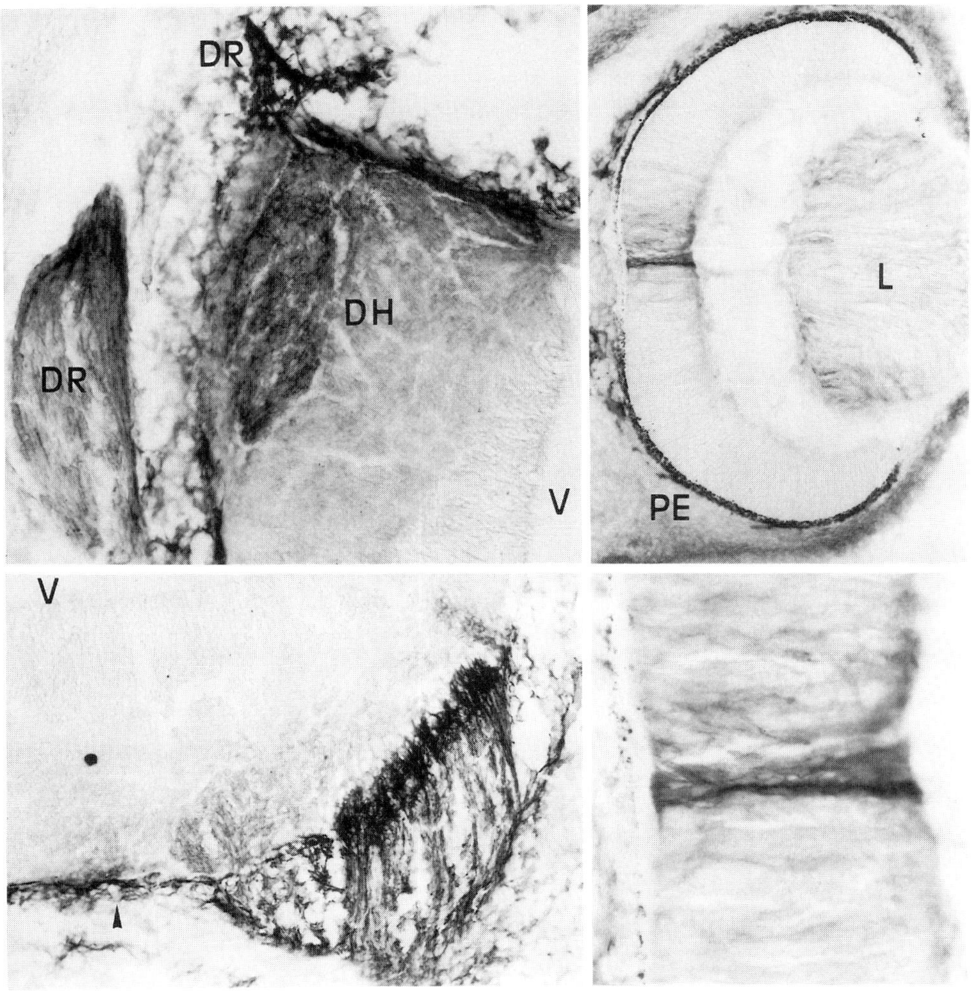


**Figure 1.** Dorsal root (DR) and horn (DH) of spinal cord, ED14; V=ventricle; in all figures, pia is indicated by arrows
**Figure 2.** VIIIth nerve entry zone in medulla oblongata, ED14
**Figure 3.** Optic cup, ED13; PE=pigmented epithelium, L=lens; inset shows NGF-RI fibers at higher magnification

*Embryonic days 15 and 16.* In subcortical regions, NGF-RI axons fill the optic tract and extend into superficial regions of the lateral geniculate nucleus (Fig. 4). NGF-RI axons from the medial septal/diagonal band nuclei begin to course dorsally and caudally into the hippocampus (Fig. 5). Axons arising from cells in the basal forebrain distribute to the intermediate

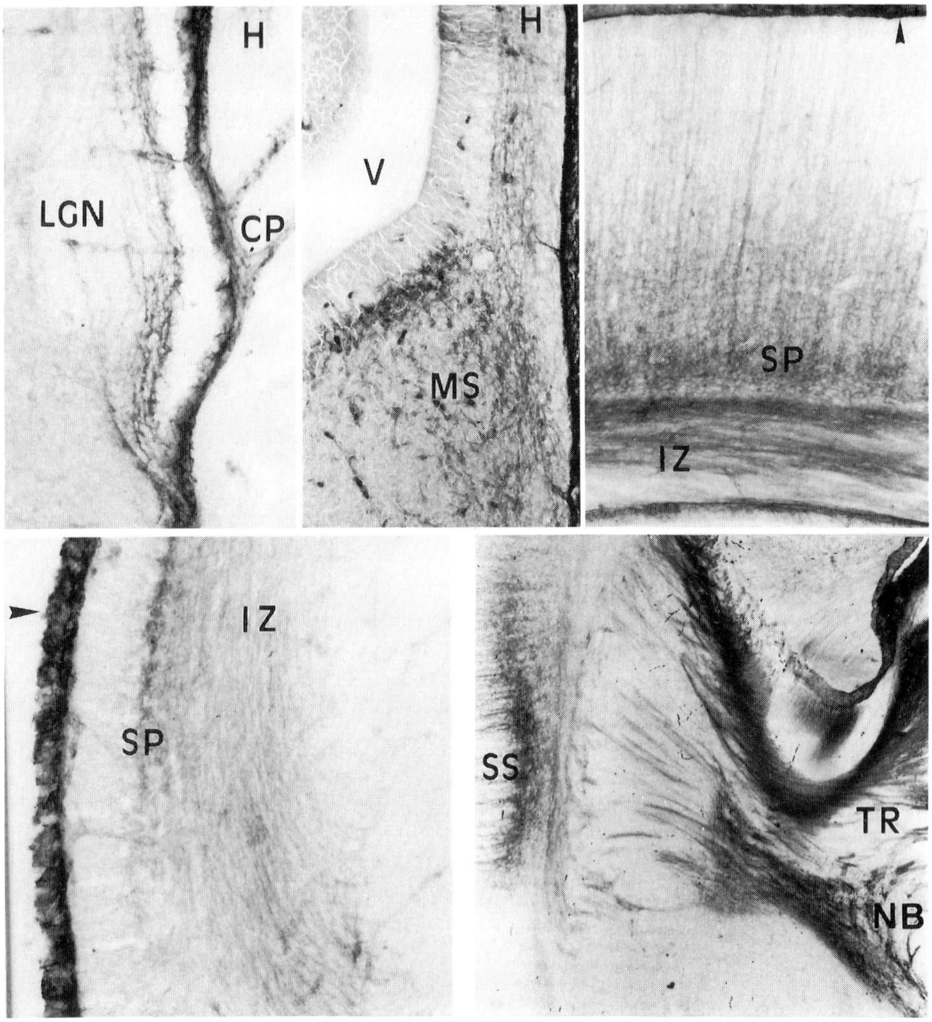


**Figure 4**. Axons entering lateral geniculate nucleus (LGN), E15; CP=choroid plexus; H=hippocampus

**Figure 5**. Axons of medial septal cells (MS) coursing dorsally through the intermediate zone towards the hippocampus, E15

**Figure 6**. Nucleus basalis axons entering the intermediate zone (IZ), subjacent to NGF-RI cells within subplate zone of the somatosensory cortex, E17

**Figure 7**. Radially-oriented NGF-R fibers extending from the cortical subplate zone (SP) to the pial surface (arrow), with tangentially-oriented axons of nucleus basalis and thalamic origin within the intermediate zone (IZ), PD1

**Figure 8**. Nucleus basalis axons (NB) and thalamic radiations (TR) within internal capsule, afferent to somatosensory cortex (SS), PD1

zone of the neocortex, and in addition NGF-RI appears within cortical cells of the subplate zone.

*Postnatal days 17 and 18.* At this age, the intermediate zone of the cortex is considerably wider and filled with NGF-RI fibers coursing tangentially to the surface (Fig. 6). This fiber-associated NGF-RI appears to collect at the deeper surface of the cortical plate, and can be traced back through the external and internal capsules to the nucleus basalis. In addition, there are radially-oriented NGF-RI fibers connecting the subplate zone with the pial surface of the cortex.

*Embryonic day 19 through Postnatal day 5.* More radially-oriented fibers are apparent throughout the superificial part of the cortical plate and the marginal zone, and NGF-RI appears to be concentrated around cells within the intermediate zone (Fig. 7). There is also NGF-RI in the thalamic radiations, which gather in the lower intermediate zone, beneath the band

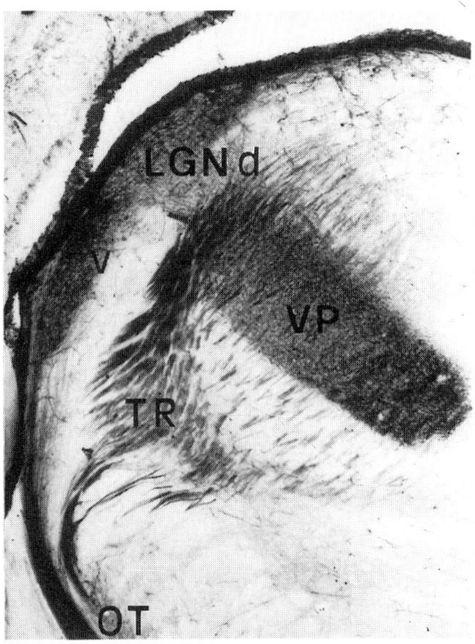


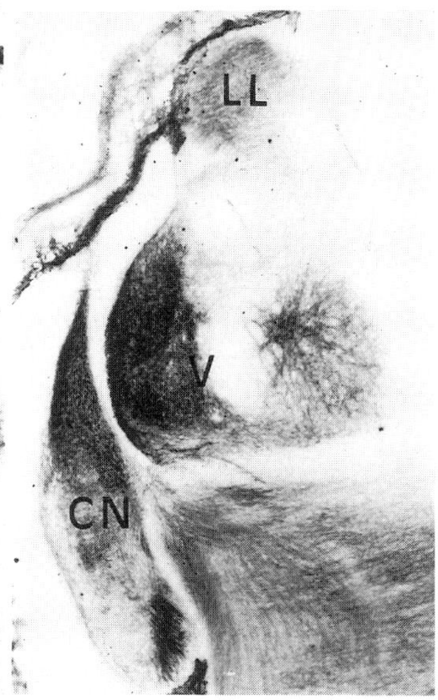


**Figure 9.** NGF-RI within the ventral posterior nucleus of the thalamus (VP), the thalamic radiations (TR), the dorsal (LGNd) and ventral (LGNv) components of the lateral geniculate nucleus, and the optic tract (OT), PD1

**Figure 10.** Horizontal brainstem section through the cochlear nucleus (CN), principal sensory nucleus of the trigeminal nerve (V) and nucleus of the lateral lemniscus (LL), PD0

of nucleus basalis-associated NGF-RI. NGF-RI is also dense within the ventral posterior nucleus of the thalamus (Figs. 8 and 9), throughout the extent of the medial lemniscus caudal to the dorsal column nuclei, and within the principal and spinal sensory nuclei of the trigeminal complex (Fig. 10). Within the auditory system, NGF-RI is also present in the medial geniculate nucleus, and in the deep layers of the inferior colliculus, the nucleus of the lateral lemniscus, the superior olive and the cochlear nucleus (Fig. 10). Within the visual system, NGF-RI is dense within the optic tract, both dorsal and ventral components of the lateral geniculate nucleus (Fig. 9), and the superficial layer of the superior colliculus. NGF-RI is present in periglomerular cells and axons deep to the granular layer of the olfactory bulb (Fig. 11), and in the islands of Calleja within the olfactory tubercle (Fig. 12).

Postnatal day 6 through 21. The radially-oriented cortical staining begins to disappear after PD5, leaving only the NGF-RI fibers of basal forebrain origin. The NGF-RI associated with subcortical sensory areas also decreases substantially after the first postnatal week. In the visual system, NGF-RI

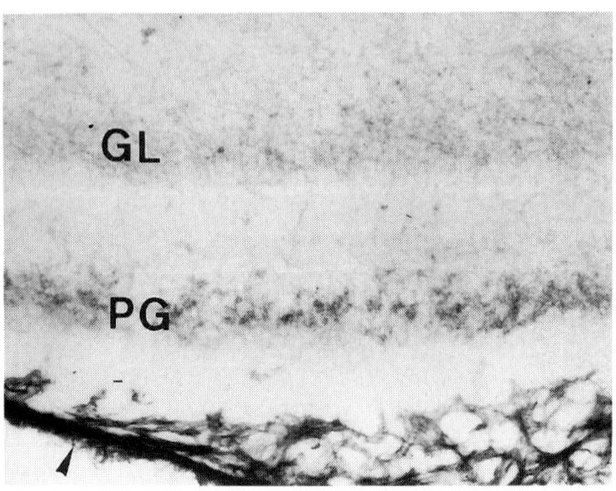


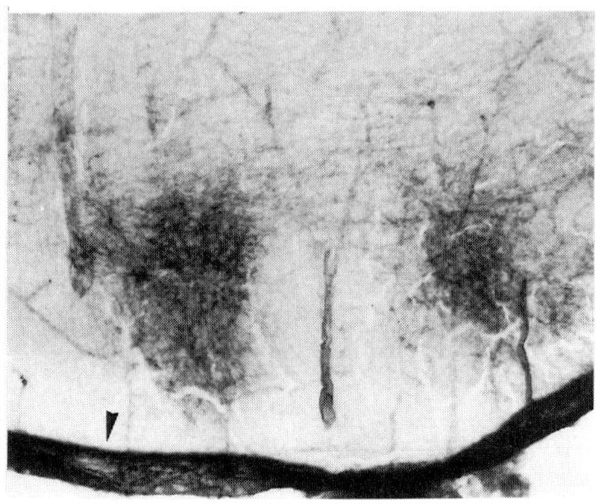

**Figure 11.** NGF-RI periglomerular cells (PG) in the olfactory bulb and within axons in the granular layer (GL), PD2
**Figure 12.** NGF-RI axons within islands of Calleja of the olfactory tubercle, PD1

remains only in small amounts in the ventral, but not the dorsal component of the lateral geniculate nucleus, and no longer appears within the optic tract after PD10. The large, pseudounipolar neurons of the mesencephalic trigeminal nucleus retain NGF-RI into adulthood, as do neurons of the cochlear nucleus, the sensory trigeminal tracts, and the glomeruli of the olfactory bulb.

## DISCUSSION

Receptors for NGF appear within the developing central nervous system in many brain areas where they are not present in appreciable numbers in the adult. Interestingly, most of these brain areas are components of central sensory pathways, some of which had been previously suggested to be NGF-sensitive. For instance, Ayer-Lelievre et al. (1983) localized NGF protein immunocytochemically within many longitudinal pathways of the spinal cord and brainstem, and within the superficial layers of the tectum, the olfactory bulb and cortex of the embryonic rat. Levi-Montalcini and Aloe (1985) also identified sites of [125I]-NGF uptake in the dorsal funiculi of the spinal cord and in dorsolateral sensory and other longitudinal fiber tracts of the tadpole brainstem. The present immunocytochemical analysis thus provides further evidence that NGF and NGF-R may play a role in regions of the central nervous system which are not associated with cholinergic neurons or their target tissues.

At the earliest developmental stages examined NGF-R are present in the entry zones of the dorsal roots and cranial sensory nerves. If NGF can be identified in these regions as well, trophic activity involving these molecules may serve the guidance function which Altman and Bayer (1982) proposed for such "boundary cap" areas in the regulation of afferent and/or efferent establishment of contacts between center and periphery, or in the determination of which groups of fibers will constitute specific cranial nerves.

The timing of appearance of NGF-R in the central visual

and somatosensory nuclei also corresponds fairly closely with the arrival of afferent fibers within the various components of the respective pathways. For instance, NGF-RI appears first in the visual system within the optic cup and proximal part of the optic stalk on ED13, then associated with optic axons within the lateral geniculate nucleus two days later. According to traditional tract-tracing techniques, the first optic axons arrive in the lateral geniculate nucleus on ED16 (Lund and Bunt, 1976), while geniculocortical axons first reach the subplate zone of the visual cortex on ED18 (Lund and Mustari, 1977). Similarly, somatosensory thalamocortical axons first invade the intermediate zone beneath the cortical plate between ED17 and ED20 in the rat (Jones, 1981), a time when NGF-RI also appears in this region.

Prior to the arrival of thalamic afferents, NGF-RI appears in the early-arriving axons of the nucleus basalis, and in association with cells of the cortical subplate zone. At this age the subplate zone contains the first-born neurons, which have become postmitotic on ED14 (Bruckner et al., 1976). At later embryonic and early postnatal ages there is a dramatic increase in NGF-RI in the cortex, primarily in radially-oriented fibers spanning the subplate zone to the pial surface. While some of this immunoreactivity is associated with cells within the intermediate zone, it is not clear without ultrastructural studies if this NGF-RI is located on neurons or glia. The radially-oriented cortical NGF-RI begins to disappear at the end of the first postnatal week, leaving only the immunoreactive fibers of basal forebrain origin.

NGF-RI within the cortex thus appears to be associated transiently with thalamic afferents at a time when these axons are actively invading their target field, establishing synaptic contacts, and segregating into zonal, laminar and columnar patterns of distribution, based in part on the sensory experience of the animal. The transient appearance of NGF-RI in the cortex and sensory relay nuclei suggests a possible role for NGF and NGF-R in the establishment of specific synaptic connections during the development of these pathways. As the relay nuclei of the olfactory, somatosensory, auditory and visual pathways, as well as the corresponding cranial nerves and spinal tracts all appear to express NGF-R, we propose that the receptor is expressed first in the "pioneer" axons or in glia at the advancing edge of the outgrowing neurites, on which it acts to increase the local concentration of NGF, effectively guiding sensory axons to their appropriate CNS targets. In support of this, NGF-R are co-expressed on chick sensory neurons and glial cells at the time when their interaction is commencing (Zimmerman and Sutter, 1983), and both NGF and NGF-R expression are induced in Schwann cells distal to a sciatic nerve crush during the time when cut axons are regenerating (Taniuchi et al., 1986a; Heumann et al., in press). Since motoneurons and skeletal muscle also transiently co-express NGF-R during the time of neuromuscular synapse formation and motoneuron cell death following synapse elimination (Raivich et al., 1985), it seems likely that NGF and its specific receptors act together to guide the development and connectivity of a seemingly wide range of neuronal-target systems in both the peripheral and central nervous systems.

## REFERENCES


Ayer-Lelievre CS, Ebendal T, Olson L, Seiger A (1983) Localization of nerve growth factor-like immunoreactivity in rat nervous tissue. Med Biol 61:296-304

Bruckner G, Mares V, Biesold M (1976) Neurogenesis in the visual system of the rat. An autoradiographic investigation. J Comp Neurol 166:245-256

Hefti F, Hartikka J, Salvatierra A, Weiner WJ, Mash DC (1986) Localization of nerve growth factor receptors in choliner gic neurons of the human basal forebrain. Neurosci Let 69:37-41

Heumann R, Korsching S, Bandtlow C, Thoenen H (to be published) Changes of nerve growth factor synthesis in nonneuron al cells in response to sciatic nerve transection. J Cell Biol

Jones EG (1981) Development of connectivity in the cerebral cortex. In:Cowan WM (ed) Studies in Developmental Neurobiology. Oxford University Press, New York Oxford, p 354

Levi-Montalcini R, Aloe L (1985) Differentiating effects of murine nerve growth factor in the peripheral and central nervous systems of Xenopus laevis tadpoles. Proc Natl Acad Sci USA 82:7111-7115

Loy R, Springer JE, Tayrien MW, Koh S (to be published) Septal and lesion-induced sympathetic afferents to the hippocampus are immunoreactive for nerve growth factor receptor. Exper Neurol

Lund RD, Bunt AH (1976) Prenatal development of central optic pathways in albino rats. J Comp Neurol 165:247-264

Lund RD, Mustari MJ (1977) Development of the geniculocortical pathway in rats. J Comp Neurol 173:289-305

Raivich G, Kreutzberg GW (1987) The localization and distribution of high affinity beta-nerve growth factor binding sites in the central nervous system of the adult rat. A light microscopic autoradiographic study using [125I]beta-nerve growth factor. Neurosci 20:23-36

Raivich G, Zimmermann A, Sutter A (1985) The spatial and temporal pattern of beta-NGF receptor expression in the developing chick embryo. EMBO J 4:637-644

Richardson PM, Verge Issa VMK, Riopelle RJ (1986) Distribution of neuronal receptors for nerve growth factor in the rat. J Neurosci 6:2312-2321

Rohrer H, Barde Y-A (1982) Presence and disappearance of nerve growth factor receptors on sensory neurons in culture. Devel Biol 89:309-315

Springer JE, Koh S, Tayrien MW, Loy R (1987) Basal forebrain magnocellular neurons stain for nerve growth factor receptor: correlation with cholinergic cell bodies and effects of axotomy. J Neurosci Res 17:111-118

Stach RW, Perez-Polo JR (1987) Binding of nerve growth factor to its receptor. J Neurosci Res 17:1-10.

Taniuchi M, Clark HB, Johnson EM Jr (1986a) Induction of nerve growth factor receptor in Schwann cells after axotomy. Proc Natl Acad Sci USA 83:4094-4098

Taniuchi M, Johnson EM Jr (1985) Characterization of the binding properties and retrograde axonal transport of a monoclonal antibody directed against the rat nerve growth factor receptor. J Cell Biol 101:1100-1106

Taniuchi M, Schweitzer JB, Johnson EM Jr (1986b) Nerve growth factor receptor molecules in rat brain. Proc Natl Acad Sci USA 83:1950-1954

Yan Q and Johnson EM Jr (1987) A quantitative study of the developmental expresssion of nerve growth factor (NGF) receptor in rats. Devel Biol 121:139-148

Zimmermann A, Sutter A (1983) Beta-nerve growth factor (beta-NGF) receptors on glial cells. Cell-cell interaction between neurons and Schwann cells in cultures of chick sensory ganglia EMBO J 2:879-885

## ACKNOWLEDGEMENTS

We thank Dorothy Heyer and Diane Alesi for their cheerful technical assistance, and Dr. E.G.Johnson, Jr. for his gift of the monoclonal antibodies and many helpful discussions. We also thank the Dysautonomia Foundation for their financial support of this work.

# RATE LIMITING EVENTS IN NEURITE OUTGROWTH

D. Monard
Friedrich Miescher Institut
P.O. Box 2543
CH-4002 Basel
Switzerland

Neurite outgrowth is one of the early cellular events leading to the differentiation of the neuronal cell. The timing and rate of neurite outgrowth is of crucial importance since the first synaptical contact established appears to have certain advantages in the process of selection during the maturation of the nervous system (Changeux and Danchin, 1976). The rate of neurite outgrowth determines the success or failure in the regeneration phenomena. Indeed, neurons of the central nervous system have the ability to regenerate neurites if provided a proper environment (Benfey and Aguayo, 1982). Therefore the identification of the biochemical events which increase the rate of neurite outgrowth could as well increase our chances to influence the regeneration of functional connections.

Neurite outgrowth is obviously a multifacet phenomenon where different interactions between the growth cone, the growing neuritic membrane and some components of the extracellular matrix all play an important role. The growth cone is not only a morphological entity. Time-lapse cinematography and careful analysis of its anatomical organisation stress its extreme motility. The rapid extension and retraction of microspikes, their instable contacts with the surrounding, indicate alternating phases of adhesion and deadhesion similar to those required for the cellular migration during development or metastasis.

## Growth cone motility and proteolytic activity

Increased amounts of plasminogen activator activity have been

NATO ASI Series, Vol. H22
Neural Development and Regeneration
Edited by A. Gorio et al.

detected at the level of the growth cone (Krystosek and Seeds, 1981). Cell-released proteases are thought to determine the transient interactions of the growth cone with its surrounding vicinity by either degrading specific components of the extracellular matrix or affecting the turnover of membrane proteins involved in cellular adhesion. Plasminogen activators (urokinase or tissue type) can initiate a cascade of proteolytic cleavages which will lead to different types of active proteases, each with a unique substrate specificity. For example, plasmin resulting from plaminogen activator activity would, in turn cleave procollagenase thus cause a localized degradation of one of the most important components of the extracellular matrix, collagen. As collagen serves as an anchor for many other ECM components, its localized degradation would by itself have drastic consequences for other adhesion promoting molecules. It has recently been shown that plasminogen activator can directly cleave fibronectin at a specific cleavage site and thus possibly alter the fibronectin mediated adhesion (Quigley et al. ,1987). It has also been shown that plasminogen activator can bind to fibronectin without loss of activity. Thus it is also possible that some proteases released by the growth cone would associate with specific components of the extracellular matrix, thus creating non permissive zones where further membranal adhesion would become unlikely as long these proteolytic enzymes remain active. Fibronectin does not seem to be an important ECM component in the nervous system. Nevertheless, these results indicate that similar degradative processes could modify the density or the properties of other ECM constituants, more relevant for the nervous tissue. As in the case of migrating cells, one can also expect that other cell-derived proteases are involved as driving forces for growth cone movement. For example, a calcium-dependent protease activity has also been localized at the level of the growth cone (Pittman, 1985). Its physiological substrates are not yet identified but it is conceivable that it could as well be one of the proteases regulating the transient interactions of the growth cone with its environment. If a number of proteases are involved, it is unlikely that all of them will have the same importance, at the same location, at the same time. Obviously, not only their activity but also the concentration of their respective substrates in the extracellular matrix or at the cell surface will determine the importance of their contribution.

## Neurite outgrowth and protease inhibition

The unexpected discovery that a neurite-promoting factor purified from the medium conditioned by glial cells is a very potent serine protease inhibitor (Monard et al.,1983; Guenther et al., 1985) has allowed one to consider a role not only for proteases but also for their respective inhibitors in the process of neurite elongation (Monard, 1985). If, as discussed above, cell-derived proteases are required for the motility of the microspikes, their inhibition could lead to the stabilization required for the elongation of neuritic zone behind the growth cone. The cDNA coding for both the human and the rat glia-derived neurite promoting factor have now been cloned (Gloor et al., 1986; Sommer et al., in press). The knowledge of the primary amino acid sequences has indicated that these glia-derived protease inhibitors belong to the serpin family (Sommer et al., in press). The aminoterminal of the human glia-derived protein is even identical with the 28 amino acid residues presently identified in protease nexin I, a serine inhibitor released by cultured human foreskin fibroblats (Scott et al., 1985). The biochemical properties of rat glia-derived protein are as well similar to those of protease nexin I (Stone et al., 1987). The glia-derived neurite promoting factor has therefore been renamed glia-derived nexin (GDN) (Sommer et al., in press). Rat GDN was shown to make SDS-resistant complexes with proteases such as tissue plasminogen activator, urokinase or thrombin (Guenther et al., 1985). This property is certainly of prime importance for its neurite promoting activity. One can consider that the presence of GDN in the vicinity of the growth cone would lead to the formation of such stable complexes with some of the growth cone associated proteases. This resulting local reduction in proteolytic activity would contribute to the stabilisation of the zone located just at the origin of the growth cone and thus allow a net increase in neurite extension. One can as well envisage that such a complex formation could exist at very specific locations in the area explored by the microspikes. Such a mechanism could then be involved in the preferential stabilisation of adhesive properties of some of the components of the growth cone. It has in fact already been proposed that such local "immobilisation" of discrete parts of microspikes could drag the growth cone forward (Bray and Chapman, 1985). Localized membrane stabilisation would lead to a reduction of the deadhesion phases caracteristic of growth cone activity and to the establishment or consolidation of the adhesion between the neuritic membrane and its environment.

**Proteases, protease inhibitors, membranal and extracellular matrix components**

The reduction in cell-associated proteolytic activity could act by increasing the density or the stability of cell adhesion molecules. Alternatively, nothing is presently known about the density and the turnover of the cell-surface associated receptors specific for extracellular matrix components. As example laminin promotes neurite outgrowth in certain neuronal cells (Baron-van Evercooren et al., 1982) and also potentiates the survival-promoting effects of neurotrophic factors (Edgar et al., 1984). This effect of laminin is thought to be mediated through an interaction with a specific membranal receptor. The regulation of the balance between protease and protease inhibitor could influence the turnover of such a type of receptor and therefore affect the sensitivity of the cell for the laminin available in its surrounding. This reasoning is as well applicable to other ECM components which could turn out to facilitate the neurite outgrowth.

Some experiments indicate that the inhibition of proteolytic activity is necessary but not sufficient to explain the neurite promoting activity of GDN. In neuroblastoma cells, hirudin and synthetic inhibitory peptides with thrombin specificity are as potent as GDN indicating that inhibition of proteolysis seems sufficient to promote neurite outgrowth (Monard et al., 1983). Recent experiments have indicated that it is not the case in cultures of primary neurons where such proteases inhibitors do not compare with the potency of GDN in promoting neurite outgrowth (Zurn et al., submitted). These data suggest that the formation of the stable high molecular weight complex with a protease is implicated in the biological activity of GDN. It is tempting to postulate that, under complex formation, GDN (or the protease) is undergoing certain conformational changes which would allow the complex to be involved in the membrane stabilisation leading to a net increase in neurite length. It is tempting to consider that the protease/protease inhibitor complex would present epitopes which could interact with some ECM components, thus contributing to a better anchorage of the neuritic membrane with its environment.

**Membrane lipids and neurite outgrowth**

The metabolism of lipids is as well expected to be involved in the increase and/or the reorganisation of membrane components required for neurite outgrowth. Incubation of neuroblastoma cells in delipidated serum can lead to a neurite outgrowth which can be prevented by the addition of certain fatty acids, especially oleic acid (Monard et al., 1977). On the other hand, sterol depletion does not influence the initial rate of neurite outgrowth but causes neurite retraction within 24 hours. Addition of low density lipoprotein was able to restore neurite outgrowth indicating that incorporation of cholesterol into the cell membrane is apparently important for long-term elongation and maintenance of neurites (Maltese et al., 1981). These observations are interesting since lesion of the rat sciatic nerve leads to an invasion of macrophages which release large quantities of apolipoprotein E (Ignatius et al., 1986; Snipes et al., 1986). The uptake of lipoprotein by neuronal growth cones has recently been demonstrated in cultured rat pheochromocytoma cells (Ignatius et al., 1987) supporting the idea that apolipoprotein E may deliver lipids necessary for the membrane biosynthesis required by the growing neurite.

Glycosphingolipids are also able to modulate neurite outgrowth (Gorio et al., 1980; Roisen et al., 1981). Different types of neuronal cells are sensitive to different molecular species of gangliosides. As example $G_{M1}$ ganglioside accelerates neurite outgrowth in rat pheochromocytoma cells (Ferrari et al., 1983), in cultured peripheral and central neurons (Skaper et al., 1985), but not in human neuroblastoma cells where the $G_{Q1b}$ form is active (Nakajima et al., 1986). In rat pheochromocytoma cells, gangliosides are not stimulatory by themselves but potentiate the neurite outgrowth triggered by Nerve Growth Factor (NGF) (Ferrari et al., 1983). In primary cultures of peripheral and central neurons, the stimulation by the $G_{M1}$ form depends on culture conditions appropriate for each type of neuronal cell. The response of ciliary ganglionic neurons requires a serum-free medium supplemented with the ciliary neurotrophic factor. Dorsal root ganglionic neurons only respond to ganglioside if the medium is supplemented by both serum and NGF. Rat central neurons have to be cultured in a serum-free pyruvate containing medium to be sensitive to $G_{M1}$ (Skaper et al., 1985). These data clearly illustrate the permissive effect of gangliosides on neurite outgrowth.

Inhibition of S-adenosylmethionine-linked methylation can lead to neurite extension in mouse neuroblastoma cells. Numerous substances known to induce neurite outgrowth are also inhibiting phospholipid methylation in those cells. However, the neuritogenesis induced by GDN does not affect phospholipid methylation (Murato and Monard, 1982). Similarly, in rat pheochromocytoma cells, NGF does not significantly influence phospholipid methylation (Ferrari and Greene, 1985). Nevertheless NGF increases the metabolism of phosphatidyl inositol and phosphatidic acid. In the same cells, a variety of agents which stimulate neurite extension increases both cyclic AMP and the metabolism of inositol (Traynor, 1984). Elevated concentrations of KCl which promote neurite outgrowth without affecting the level of cyclic AMP also modify the metabolism of inositol (Traynor, 1984). Taken together, these results support the idea that changes in the phospholipid metabolism are not absolutely required but can contribute to, or even initiate membranal modifications regulating neurite outgrowth.

**Dynamics of neurite outgrowth**

Most of the results considered above have been obtained using *in vitro* experimental models. It remains to be seen to which extent they are still valid for the *in vivo* situation. Nevertheless they indicate that many different events could initiate or sustain the target-independent neurite outgrowth which takes place when the neuroblast has reached its final location. This possibility of multiple environmental influences could explain the specific caracteristics of neurite outgrowth detected and required at distinct time and at different locations during the development of the nervous system. If a multiplicity of interactions are involved in the mechanisms regulating neurite outgrowth, it is obviously very unlikely that all the different permissive factors could simultaneously influence the rate of neuritic growth to the same extent at the same time and at the same location. One has even to consider that each of these permissive factors can be rate limiting in certain situations and have only a marginal influence in others. For example, in an environment where the quality and the density of the ECM components is adequate for a certain type of neuroblast, the balance between proteases and protease inhibitors would not have a decisive influence on the rate of neurite outgrowth. On the other hand, the same balance between proteases and protease inhbitors could become rate-limiting when the density of the neurite-promoting ECM components is not optimal. Similarly, the types of lipids provided by the environment could be crucial in certain situations but be of only secondary importance in others.

Our present knowledge also indicates that the neurite extension induced by target-derived specific neurotrophic factors such as NGF could as well be further modulated by a multiplicity of mechanisms.

**Acknowledgements.** I thank Dr. George Thomas for critical reading of the manuscript.

## References

Baron-van Evercooren A, Kleinman HK, Ohno S, Marangos P, Schwartz JP, Dubois-Dalcq ME (1982) Nerve growth factor, laminin and fibronectin promote neurite growth in human fetal sensory ganglia cultures. J. Neurosci. Res. **8**: 179-193

Benfey M, Aguayo AJ (1982) Extensive elongation of axons from rat brain into peripheral nerve grafts. Nature **296**: 150-152

Bray D, Chapman K (1985) Analysis of microspike movements on the neuronal growth cone. J. Neuroscience **5**: 3204-3213

Changeux JP, Danchin A (1976) Selective stabilization in developing synapses as a mechanism for the specification of neuronal networks. Nature **264**: 705-712

Edgar D, Timpl R, Thoenen H (1984) The heparin-binding domain of laminin is responsible for its effects on neurite outgrowth and neuronal survival. EMBO J. **3**: 1463-1468

Ferrari G, Greene LA (1985) Does phospholipid methylation play a role in the primary mechanism of action of nerve growth factor. J. Neurochem. **45**: 853-859

Ferrari G, Fabris M, Gorio A (1983) Gangliosides enhance neurite outgrowth in PC-12 cells. Dev.Brain Res. **8**: 215-221

Gloor S, Odink K, Guenther J, Nick H, Monard D (1986) A glia-derived neurite promoting factor with protease inhibitory activity belongs to the protease nexins. Cell **47**: 687-693

Gorio A, Carmignoto G, Facci L, Finesso M (1980) Motor nerve sprouting induced by ganglioside treatment. Possible implications for gangliosides on neuronal growth. Brain Res. **197**: 236-241

Guenther J, Nick H, Monard D (1985) A glia-derived neurite-promoting factor with protease inhibitory activity. EMBO J. **4**: 1963-1966

Ignatius MJ, Gebicke-Haerter PJ, Skene JHP, Schilling JW, Weisgraber KH, Mahley RW, Shooter EM (1986) Expression of apolipoprotein E during nerve degeneration and regeneration. Proc. Natl. Acad. Sci. USA **83**: 1125-1129

Ignatius MJ, Shooter EM, Pitas RE, Mahley RW (1987) Lipoprotein uptake by neuronal growth cones in vitro. Science **236**: 959-962

Krystosek A, Seeds NW (1981) Plasminogen activator release at the neuronal growth cone. Science **213**: 1532-1534

Maltese WA, Reitz BA, Volpe JJ (1981) Effects of prior sterol depletion on neurite outgrowth in neuroblastoma cells. J. Cell. Physiol. **108**: 475-482

Monard D (1985) Implications of proteases and protease inhibitors in neurite outgrowth. In Neurobiochemistry, Selected Topics, Colloquium-Mosbach 1985 Hamprecht B and Neuhoff V eds **36**: 7-12

Monard D, Rentsch M, Schuerch-Rathgeb Y, Lindsay R (1977) Morphological differentiation of neuroblastoma cells in medium supplemented with delipidated serum. Proc. Natl. Acad. Sci. (USA) **74**: 3893-3897

Monard D, Niday E, Limat A, Solomon F (1983) Inhibition of protease activity can lead to neurite extension in neuroblastoma cells. Prog. Brain Res. **58**: 359-364

Murato K, Monard D (1982) Inhibition of S-adenosylmethionine-linked methylation can lead to neurite extension in neuroblastoma cells. FEBS Letters **144**: 321-325

Nakajima J, Tsuji S, Nagai Y (1986) Bioactive gangliosides: analysis of functional structures of the tetrasialoganglioside $G_{Q1b}$ which promotes neurite outgrowth. Biochim. biophys. Acta **876**: 65-71

Pittman RN (1985) Release of plasminogen activator and a calcium-dependent metalloprotease from cultured sympathetic and sensory neurons. Dev. Biol. **110**: 91-101

Quigley JP, Gold LI, Schwimmer R, Sullivan LM (1987) Limited cleavage of cellular fibronectin by plasminogen activator purified from transformed cells. Proc. Natl. Acad. Sci. USA **84**: 2776-2780

Roisen FJ, Bartfeld H, Nagele R, Yorke G (1981) Ganglioside stimulation of axonal sprouting in vitro. Science **214**: 577-578

Scott RW, Bergman BL, Bajpai A, Hersh RT, Rodriguez H, Jones BN, Barreda C, Watts S, Baker JB (1985) Protease nexin. J. Biol. Chem. **260**: 7029-7034

Skaper SD, Katoh-Semba R, Varon S (1985) GM1 ganglioside accelerates neurite outgrowth from primary peripheral and central neurons under selected culture conditions. Dev. Brain Res. **23**: 19-26

Snipes GJ, McGuire CB, Norden JJ, Freeman JA (1986) Nerve injury stimulates the secretion of apolipoprotein E by nonneuronal cells. Proc. Natl. Acad. Sci. USA **83**: 1130-1134

Sommer J, Gloor SM, Rovelli GF, Hofsteenge J, Nick H, Meier R, Monard D (in press) cDNA sequence coding for a rat glia-derived nexin and its homology to members of the serpin superfamily. Biochemistry

Stone S, Nick H, Hofsteenge J, Monard D (1987) Glia-derived neurite promoting factor is a slow-binding inhibitor of trypsin, thrombin and urokinase Arch. Biochem. Biophys. **252**: 237-244

Traynor AE (1984) The relationship between neurite extension and phospholipid metabolism in PC12 cells. Dev. Brain Res. **14**: 205-210

Zurn A, Nick H, Monard D (submitted) A glia-derived nexin promotes neurite outgrowth in cultured chick sympathetic neurons.

# STUDIES OF THE NEUROTRANSMITTER PLASTICITY OF CULTURED RAT SYMPATHETIC NEURONS AT THE MOLECULAR LEVEL

M.J. Weber, B. Raynaud and S. Vidal
Laboratoire de Pharmacologie et
Toxicologie Fondamentales, CNRS
205, route de Narbonne
31077 Toulouse cédex
France

N. Faucon-Biguet and J. Mallet
Laboratoire de Neurobiologie
Cellulaire et Moléculaire, CNRS
91140 Gif-sur-Yvette
France

## INTRODUCTION

Cultures of sympathetic neurons from new-born rats constitute an attractive model to study the triggering and modulation of the expression of neurotransmitter phenotypic traits during neuronal differentiation. These neurons can express a variety of neurotransmitters and neuropeptides, and experiments performed *in vivo* or in cultures have led to insights on the molecular mechanisms of this phenotypic plasticity. In particular, several extracellular cues have been identified, which modify the expression of cholinergic and catecholaminergic characters in these cultured neurons (for a review, see Patterson, 1978) : conditioned medium (CM) by certain non-neuronal cells induces the biosynthesis of acetylcholine in such cultures, and depress that of catecholamines (Patterson and Chun, 1977). On the other hand, neuronal depolarization fosters the development of noradrenergic characteristics and depresses acetylcholine (ACh) biosynthesis (Walicke *et al.*, 1977 ; Walicke and Patterson, 1981). In addition, neuronal depolarization inhibits the development of substance P in rat sympathetic neurons, both *in vivo* and in culture (Kessler *et al.*, 1981 ; Adler and Black, 1984).

A number of neurotransmitter metabolic enzymes are regulated by extracellular cues in sympathetic neuron cultures : CM induces up to 100-100-fold the activity of choline acetyltransferase (CAT), and depresses the development of the three catecholamine synthesizing enzymes, tyrosine hydroxylase (TOH), dopa decarboxylase (DDC) and dopamine-β-hydroxylase (Patterson and Chun, 1977 ; Wolinski and Patterson, 1983 ;

NATO ASI Series, Vol. H22
Neural Development and Regeneration
Edited by A. Gorio et al.

Swerts *et al.*, 1983). In addition, CM impaires the development of acetylcholinesterase (AChE) and in particular, of its asymmetric $A_{12}$ form (Swerts *et al.*, 1983 ; 1984). The cholinergic factor from CM has been purified to homogeneity (Weber, 1981 ; Fukada, 1985). This factor both increases the cholinergic character of cultured sympathetic neurons and depresses the development of catecholaminergic traits (Fukada, 1985 ; Raynaud *et al.*, 1987b). On the other hand, elevated $K^+$ ions depress the development of CAT activity (Kessler, 1985 ; Raynaud *et al.*, 1987ab) and induces TOH activity (Hefti *et al*, 1982).

A new dimension was added to the study of neuronal plasticity with the use of TOH cDNA probes, which allowed to monitor variations of TOH-mRNA level by Northern blot analysis, both *in vivo* and in culture (Lamouroux *et al.*, 1982 ; Lewis *et al.*, 1983 ; Black *et al*, 1985 ; Faucon-Biguet *et al.*, 1986 ; Raynaud *et al.*, 1987a). In particular, CM, as well as the purified CM factor, decreases TOH-mRNA level in cultured sympathetic neurons, whereas elevated $K^+$ ions have an opposite effect (Raynaud *et al.*, 1987a).

In this article, we further describe the antagonistic effects of CM and $K^+$ ions on CAT and TOH development, and characterize the voltage-sensitive $Ca^{++}$ channels responsible for the modulation of the expression of neurotransmitter metabolic enzymes by neuronal depolarization. In addition, we report on the effects of Nerve Growth Factor (NGF) on TOH-mRNA level and suggest a molecular mechanism for the well-characterized TOH induction by this factor.

## MATERIALS AND METHODS

*Neuron cultures* : sympathetic neurons from newborn rat superior cervical ganglia were cultured in the virtual absence of non neuronal cells as described by Swerts *et al.* (1983). CM was collected after a 1-day contact with confluent cultures of muscle cells grown with 10 % foetal calf serum, and diluted twice with fresh medium.

*Enzymatic assays* : CAT activity was measured by the Fonnum (1975) assay in the presence of 1.6 µM [$^3$H]AcCoA (4.8 Ci/mmole), TOH and AChE activities were measured as described by Waymire *et al.* (1971) and Ellman *et al.* (1961), respectively.

*Northern blot analysis of TOH-mRNA level* : this was permormed as described in detail by Faucon-Biguet *et al.* (1986) and Raynaud *et al.*

(1987a). Briefly, total RNA extracted from neuron cultures was separated on denaturing 1 % agarose gels, transferred to nitrocellulose membranes, and hybridized with the nick-translated Pst 1 insert (742bp) of TOH cDNA clone pTH1 (Lamouroux et al., 1982). Serial dilutions of poly ($A^+$) RNA from PC12 cells were included on each gel to assess the linearity of the hybridization signal.

## RESULTS AND DISCUSSION

### Comparison of the effects of CM and $K^+$ ions on CAT and TOH development

The effects of CM and elevated $K^+$ ions on CAT and TOH development are compared on Table 1.

| Culture condition | CAT activity cpm/min/dish (x $10^{-3}$) | TOH activity pmole/min/dish |
|---|---|---|
| Control | 10.26 ± 0.22 | 62.1 ± 6.9 |
| 40 mM KCl | 1.08 ± 0.02 | 114.8 ± 14.3 |
| 50 % CM | 928 ± 78 | 19.3 ± 2.0 |
| 50 % CM + 40 mM KCl | 24.4 ± 10 | 78.0 ± 5.5 |

Table 1 : Antagonistic effects of CM and $K^+$ ions on CAT and TOH development. Neuron cultures were grown for 13 days (CAT assay) or 20 days (TOH assay) in the presence of CM and/or 40 mM KCl, as indicated. The data are means ± SEM for three cultures.

Elevated $K^+$ ions decrease by 90-97 % the development of CAT activity, both in the absence and in the presence of CM, whereas CM increases by 90-fold CAT development. Conversely CM depresses about 3-fold TOH development (Wolinski and Patterson, 1983 ; Swerts et al., 1983), whereas $K^+$ ions produce a 2-fold increase (Hefti et al., 1982 ; Raynaud et al., 1987b). The antagonism of the effects of CM and $K^+$ ions is suggested by the fact that cultures grown with CM in high $K^+$ medium display similar CAT and TOH activities than control cultures grown without CM in low $K^+$ medium. However, this antagonism does not extent to all neurotransmitter metabolism enzymes. As demonstrated by Swerts et al. (1983), CM depresses the development of dopa-decarboxylase (AADC) in sympathetic neuron cultures, but $K^+$ ions has not significant effect on the development of this enzyme. Moreover, CM depresses 2-3-fold the development of acetylcholinesterase (AChE) activity and in particular totally block the appearence of the asymmetric $A_{12}$ (or 16S) form of AChE (Swerts _et al._, 1984). Surprisingly, $K^+$ ions have similar effects, although the rate of $A_{12}$ AChE development is not blocked, but decreased about 7-fold (Verdière _et al._, 1984 ; Raynaud _et al._, 1987b). Although CM and $K^+$ ions regulate AChE in the same direction, their mode of action can be distinguished with $Ca^{++}$ antagonists (see below).

In summary, CM and $K^+$ ions have mirror-image and antagonistic effects on CAT and TOH, but this does not extend to AADC, the second enzyme in norepinephrine synthesis pathway. Moreover the regulation of AChE by these two agents is not correlated with the expression of cholinergic or catecholaminergic phenotypic traits, but may be associated with the expression of another neurotransmitter/neuropeptide.

_The effects of $K^+$ ions are mediated by $Ca^{++}$ entry through dihydropyridine-sensitive voltage-activated channels_

Although depolarization with $K^+$ ions is likely to open voltage-sensitive $Ca^{++}$ channels, conflicting data were reported on the role of $Ca^{++}$ influx in the differentiation of cultured sympathetic neurons. Walicke and Patterson (1981) showed that lowering external $Ca^{++}$ with EGTA increased the acetylcholine/catecholamine ratio of depolarized neurons, but Hefti _et al._ (1982) reported that TOH induction by $K^+$ ions was not affected in these conditions. Both groups reported that the effects of depolarization were depressed by $Ca^{++}$ channel blockers like D-600 and diphenylhydantoin, but these two drugs now appear of questionable specificity. Nethertheless, these experiments, and other using inorganic $Ca^{++}$ blockers, strongly suggested that $Ca^{++}$ entry mediated the effects of depolarization.

Since these early experiments were performed, two types of voltage-sensitive $Ca^{++}$ channels have been identified in cultured sympathetic neurons (Perney _et al._, 1986) : fast inactivating channels of the N type are insensitive to dihydropyridine drugs and are implicated in norepinephrine secretion, whereas slowly inactivating channels of the L type are blocked by dihydropyridine antagonists. These drugs do not affect norepinephrine release, except when $Ca^{++}$ entry through L channels is stimulated by a calcium agonist like BAY K 8644 or (+) 202 791 (for a review, see Miller, 1987).

The following experiments suggest that, in cultured sympathetic neurons, L channels are specifically involved in the expression of neurotransmitter metabolism enzymes. Fluspirilene is a neuroleptic drug which blocks L channels present in transverse tubule membranes of striated muscle (Galizzi _et al._, 1986). This drug has no effect of CAT induction by CM in low $K^+$ (5 mM) medium, but totally reversed the inhibition of CAT induction caused by 35 mM KCl (figure 1). Moreover, fluspirilene had no effect of TOH development in low $K^+$ medium, but

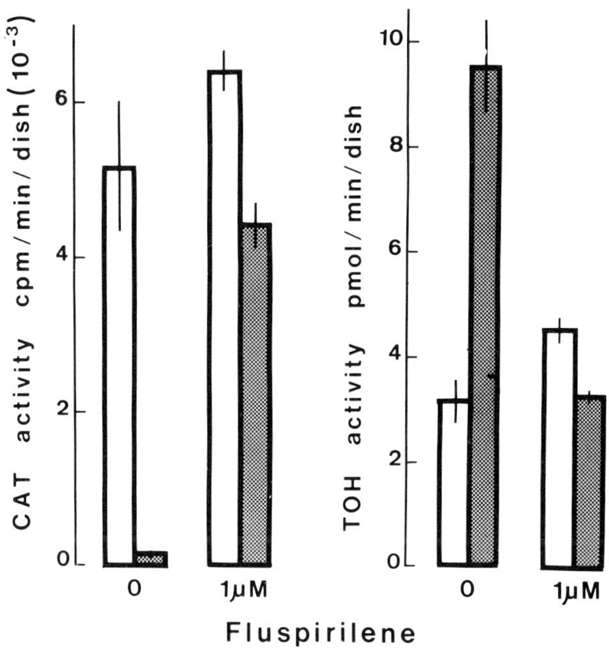


Figure 1 : Fluspirilene inhibits the effects of depolarization on CAT and TOH development. Sympathetic neurons were cultured between days 3 and 9 in the presence of 50 % CM. The medium contained either 5 (dear bars) or 35 (hatched bars) mM KCl, and fluspirilene, as indicated. The medium was renewed every 2-3 day. The data are means ± SEM for 3 cultures.

totally suppressed TOH induction by high $K^+$ medium. Similar results were obtained with 1-3 μM nitrendipine and 1 μM PN 200-110, two dihydropyridine drugs, and with the diphenylmethylpiperazine flunarizine (1 μM). Other $Ca^{++}$ antagonists only produced partial inhibitions at 1 μM : D888 (or desmethoxyverapamil), cinnarizine and lidoflazine.

On the other hand, the $Ca^{++}$ agonist (+) 202 791 (1 μM) depresses by 62 % the induction of CAT by CM in 5 mM KCl medium. This drug shifts to lower concentrations the dose-response curve of CAT inhibition by KCl (data not shown). This experiment confirms that $Ca^{++}$ entry through L channels regulates CAT expression.

As mentioned above, both CM and elevated $K^+$ ions depress the development of AChE, and in particular of the $A_{12}$ form. Again, $Ca^{++}$ antagonists (fluspirilene, nitrendipine) have no effects on AChE development in low $K^+$ medium. Also, these drugs do not antagonize the effects of CM on AChE (Figure 2). However, both drugs completely inhibited the impairment of AChE development caused by high $K^+$, and in particular reesta-

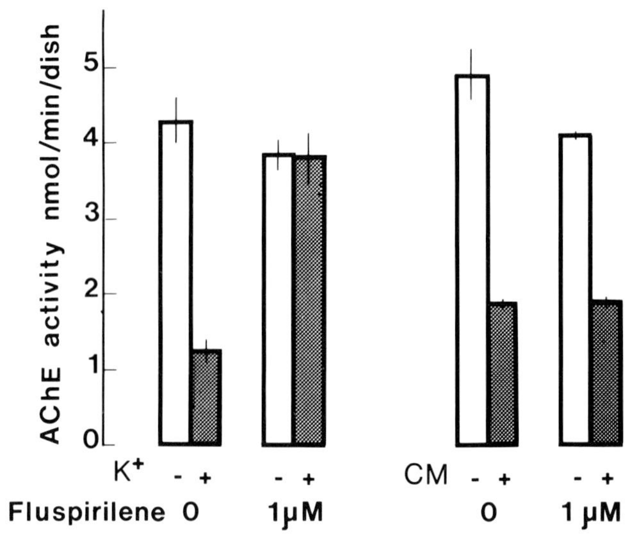


Figure 2 : Fluspirilene reverses the deficit in AChE activity caused by elevated $K^+$ ions, but not by CM. Left panel : neurons were grown for 10 days in a medium containing either 5 (clear bars) or 35 (hatched bars) mM KCl. Right panel : neurons were cultured for 12 days in 5 mM KCl medium in the absence (clear bars) or presence (hatched bars) of 50 % CM. Fluspirilene was present during the culture period, as indicated.

blished that of $A_{12}$ AChE to control values. Whereas, elevated $K^+$ ions and CM have similar effects on AChE, the former, but not the latter, acts by $Ca^{++}$ entry through L channels.

We have not measured the effects of the $Ca^{++}$ antagonists used on $^{45}Ca^{++}$ entry. However, Miller (87) reported that 1 μM nitrendipine decreased by only 50 % the $Ca^{++}$ entry caused by 70 mM KCl in cultured sympathetic neurons. Presumably, fluspirenele as well only partially inhibits $Ca^{++}$ entry in our cultures treated with 35 mM KCl. It is thus remarkable that both nitrendipine and fluspirilene totally suppress the effects of elevated $K^+$ on CAT, TOH and AChE. This suggest that $Ca^{++}$ entry through dihydropyridine insensitive N channels has no effect on the expression of neurotransmitter metabolic enzyme. This is in agreement with the notion that N channels are localized on nerve terminals near neurotransmitter release sites, whereas L channels are preferentially localized on the soma (Miller, 1987). $Ca^{++}$ entering through L, but not N channels, may thus diffuse to the nucleus and modulate gene expression.

Regulation of TOH-mRNA level in cultured sympathetic neurons

To gain more information on the molecular mechanisms of TOH regulation by various extracellular cues, TOH-mRNA level has been measured in cultured sympathetic neurons by classical Northern blot analysis using a rat TOH-cDNA probe (Lamouroux *et al.*, 1982 ; Faucon-Biguet *et al.*, 1986). This probe hybridizes with a single ARN species of the same size (1.9 kb) as the TOH-mRNA from PC12 cells. Cultures grown for 4 to 15 days in 50 % CM display a clear-cut deficit in TOH-mRNA level, as compared to sister cultures grown without CM. This deficit correlates with the deficit in TOH enzymatic activity (Raynaud *et al.*, 1987a). On the other hand, elevated $K^+$ ions (35-45 mM KCl) produce an increase in TOH-mRNA level comparable in magnitude to the increase in TOH activity. Hefti *et al.* (1982) have previously shown that TOH induction by $K^+$ ions in similar cultures is blocked by α-amanitin. These results thus clearly establish that elevated intracellular $Ca^{++}$ regulates TOH gene at the transcriptional level. On the other hand, the mechanisms by which CM depresses TOH-mRNA level are still uncertain.

In addition to promoting the survival of sympathetic neurons in culture, Nerve Growth Factor (NGF) stimulates in parallel the biosynthesis of catecholamines and acetylcholine, and thus acts as a permissive, rather than instructive signal in the neurotransmitter choice made by these neurons (Chun and Patterson, 1977). It is now well established that the increase in TOH activity caused by NGF is insensitive to inhibitors of RNA polymerase II (Rohrer *et al.*, 1978 ; Hefti *et al.*, 1982). On the other hand, TOH induction by NGF in cultured chromaffin cells is blocked by 9-β-arabinofuranosyl-adenine, an inhibitor of RNA polyadenylation (Achelson *et al.*, 1984). In cultures of rat sympathetic neurons, NGF increases in a dose-dependent manner the level of TOH-mRNA, measured by Northern analysis (Figure 3). To take into account the effects of NGF on the content of total RNA per neuron, the filters have been rehybridized with a probe specific for 18S rRNA. Again, NGF produced a clear-cut increase in the TOH/18S ratio of the hybridization signals, which correlates with the increase in TOH enzymatic specific activity (data not shown). Interestingly enough, the decline in mature TOH-mRNA observed at low NGF concentration is not accompanied by a compensatory increase in high molecular weight TOH transcripts. As NGF presumably does not affect the frequency of TOH gene transcription, this observation suggests that, at low NGF concentration, a sizeable fraction of TOH primary transcripts are rapidly degraded, and than higher NGF concentrations increase their probability of being processed into mature mRNA rather than being degraded. The regulation of TOH expression by NGF may thus be an example of a process-versus-discard control, as defined by Darnell (1982).

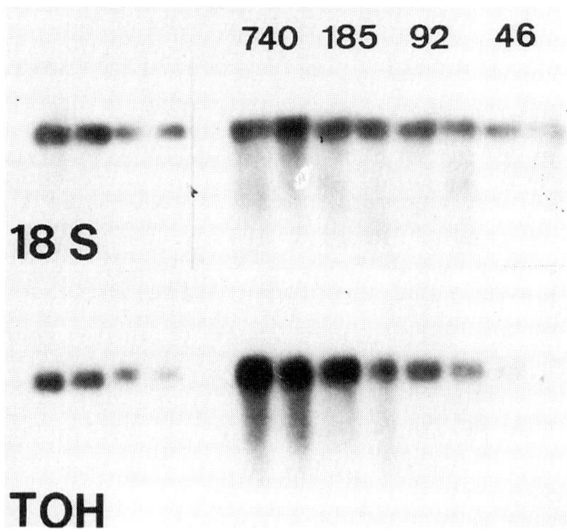


Figure 3 : Effects of NGF on TOH-mRNA level in cultured sympathetic neurons. Total RNA was extracted separately from two pools of two sister cultures grown for 15 days in the presence of 46, 92, 185 or 740 ng/ml 7S-NGF as indicated. The four lanes on the left contain 120, 60, 30 and 15 ng poly $(A^+)$RNA from PC12 cells. The blots was sequentially hybridized with a TOH, and a 18S cDNA, probe.

## REFERENCES

ACHESON A.L., NAUJOKS K., THOENEN H. (1984) Nerve growth factor-mediated enzyme induction in primary cultures of bovine adrenal chromaffin cells : specificity and level of regulation. J. Neurosci. 4 : 1771-1780.

ADLER J.E., BLACK I.B. (1984) Plasticity of substance P in mature and aged sympathetic neurons in culture. Science 225 : 1499-1500.

BLACK I.B., CHIKARAISHI D.M., LEWIS E.J. (1985) Trans-synaptic increase in RNA coding for tyrosine hydroxylase in a rat sympathetic ganglion. Brain Res. 339 : 151-153.

DARNELL J.E. Jr (1982) Variety in the level of gene control in eukaryotic cells. Nature 297 : 365-371.

ELLMAN G.L., COURTNEY K.D., ANDRES V., FEATHERSTONE R.M. (1961) A new and rapid colorimetric determination of acetylcholinesterase activity. Biochem. Pharmacol. 7 : 88-95.

FAUCON-BIGUET N., BUDA M., LAMOUROUX A., SAMOLYK D., MALLET J. (1986) Time course of the changes of TH mRNA in rat brain and adrenal medulla after a single injection of reserpine. EMBO J. 5 : 287-291.

FONNUM F. (1975) A rapid radiochemical method for the determination of choline acetyltransferase. J. Neurochem. 24 : 407-409.

FUKADA K. (1985) Purification and partial characterization of a cholinergic neuronal differentiation factor. Proc. Natl. Acad. Sci. USA 82 : 8795-8799.

GALIZZI J.P., FOSSET M., ROMEY G., LADURON P., LAZDUNSKI M. (1986) Neuroleptics of the diphenylbutylpiperidine series are potent calcium channel inhibitors. Proc. Natl. Acad. Sci. USA 83 : 7513-7517.

HEFTI F., GNAHN H., SCHWAB M.E., THOENEN H. (1982) Induction of tyrosine hydroxylase by Nerve Growth Factor and by elevated $K^+$ concentrations in cultures of dissociated sympathetic neurons. J. Neurosci. 2 : 1554-1566.

KESSLER J.A. (1985) Differential regulation of peptide and catecholamine characters in cultured sympathetic neurons.. Neuroscience. 15 : 827-839.

KESSLER J.A., ADLER J.E., BOHN M.C., BLACK I.B. (1981) Substance P in level principal sympathetic neurons : regulation by impulse activity. Science. 214 : 335-336.

LAMOUROUX A., FAUCON BIGUET N., SAMOLYK D., PRIVAT A., SALOMON J.C., PUJOL J.F., MALLET J. (1982) Identification of cDNA clones coding for rna tyrosine hydroxylase antigene. Proc. Natl. Acad. Sci. USA 79 : 3881-3885.

LEWIS E.J., TANK A.W., WEINER N., CHIKARAISHI D.M. (1983) Regulation of tyrosine hydroxylase mRNA by glucocorticoid and cyclic AMP in a rat pheochromocytoma cell line. J. Biol. Chem. 256 : 14632-14637.

MILLER R.J. (1987) Multiple calcium channels and neuronal function. Science 235 : 46-52.

PATTERSON P.H. (1978) Environmental determination of autonomic neurotransmitter functions. Ann. Rev. Neurosci. 1 : 1-17.

PATTERSON P.H., CHUN L.L.Y. (1977a) The induction of acetylcholine synthesis in primary cultures of dissociated rat sympathetic neurons. I. Effects of conditioned medium. Dev. Biol 56 : 263-280.

PERNEY T., HIRNING L.D., LEEMAN S.E., MILLER R.J. (1986) Multiple calcium channels mediate neurotransmitter release from peripheral neurons. Proc. Natl. Acad. Sci. USA 83 : 6656-6659.

RAYNAUD B., CLAROUS D., VIDAL S., FERRAND C., WEBER M.J. (1987b) Comparison of the effects of elevated $K^+$ ions and muscle-conditioned medium on the neurotransmitter phenotype of cultured sympathetic neurons. Dev. Biol. (in press).

RAYNAUD B., FAUCON-BIGUET N., VIDAL S., MALLET J., WEBER M.J. (1987a) The use of a tyrosine hydroxylase cDNA probe to study the neurotransmitter plasticity of rat sympathetic neurons in culture. Dev. Biol. 119 : 305-312.

ROHRER H., OTTEN U., THOENEN H. (1978) On the role of RNA synthesis in the selective induction of tyrosine hydroxylase by nerve growth factor. Brain Res. 159 : 436-439.

SWERTS J.P., LE VAN THAI A., VIGNY A., WEBER M.J. (1983) Regulation of enzymes responsible for neurotransmitter synthesis and degradation in cultured rat sympathetic neurons. I. Effects of muscle conditioned medium. Dev. Biol. 100 : 1-11.

SWERTS J.P., LE VAN THAI A., WEBER M.J. (1984) Regulation of enzymes responsible for neurotransmitter synthesis and degradation in cultured rat sympathetic neurons. II. Regulation of 16S acetylcholinesterase by conditioned medium. Dev. Biol. 103 : 230-234.

WALICKE P.A., CAMPENOT R.B., PATTERSON P.H. (1977) Determination of transmitter function by neuronal activity. Proc. Natl. Acad. Sci. USA 74 : 5767-5771.

WALICKE P.A., PATTERSON P.H. (1981b) On the role of $Ca^{++}$ in the transmitter choice made by cultured sympathetic neurons. J. Neurosci. 1 : 343-350 .

WAYMIRE J.C., BJUR R., WEINER N. (1971) Assay for tyrosine-hydroxylase by coupled decarboxylation of dopa formed from [1-$^{14}$C]tyrosine. Analyt. Biochem. 43 : 588-600.

WEBER M. (1981) A diffusible factor responsible for the determination of cholinergic functions in cultured sympathetic neurons. Partial purification and characterization. J. Biol. Chem. 256 : 3447-3453.

WOLINSKY E., PATTERSON P.H. (1983) Tyrosine hydroxylase activity decreases with induction of cholinergic properties in cultured sympathetic neurons. J. Neurosci. 3 : 1495-1500.

# SEROTONIN AND MORPHOGENESIS IN THE CULTURED MOUSE EMBRYO

J.M. Lauder and T.W. Sadler
Department of Anatomy 217H
Univ. of North Carolina Sch. of Med.
Chapel Hill, NC 27514, USA

## Introduction

Morphogenesis is the process whereby cell movements, changes in cell shape and cell-cell interactions result in the formation of tissues and organs in the embryo. Beginning with the work of Vogt (1929), who traced the complex movements of cells during gastrulation, and the discovery that the dorsal lip of the blastopore moving underneath the overlying ectoderm was responsible for induction of the nervous system during gastrulation (Spemann and Mangold, 1924), the importance of morphogenetic cell movements for the shaping and patterning of the embryo has become increasingly evident (see Gurdon, 1987; Gustafson and Wolpert, 1963; Holtfreter, 1968; Holtfreter and Hamburger, 1955). However, little is known concerning the forces which set in motion or control these dynamic processes, although a variety of basic cellular mechanisms have been implicated. This chapter reviews evidence that neurotransmitter substances, in particular serotoinin (5-HT) may be involved in the regulation of some morphogenetic processes in neural and non-neural tissues.

NATO ASI Series, Vol. H22
Neural Development and Regeneration
Edited by A. Gorio et al.

Neurotransmitters and morphogenesis

The hypothesis that neurotransmitters play roles in morphogenesis has its origins in the work of the Russian embryologist, G. Buznikov, who demonstrated the presence of these substances in the sea urchin embryo during cleavage and gastrulation (Buznikov et al., 1964, 1968; reviewed by Buznikov, 1980, 1984). Based on subsequent studies in which various neurochemicals were applied to sea urchin embryos, Buznikov and his co-workers suggested that dopamine, acetylcholine, 5-HT (or related substances) acting at intracellular binding sites, are important triggers for cleavage divisions and particular phases of gastrulation, such as the migration of primary mesenchyme and the onset of coelomic activity (Buznikov et al., 1970; Buznikov and Shmukler, 1981; Deeb, 1972; Gustafson and Toneby, 1970, 1971; Toneby 1977b; Manukhin et al., 1981; Markova et al., 1985; Renaud et al., 1983. See also reviews by Buznikov, 1980 and Toneby, 1977a).

Neurotransmitters such as the catecholamines and 5-HT are also present during early phases of vertebrate neuroembryogenesis (Baker and Quay, 1969; Burden and Lawrence, 1973; Ignarro and Shideman, 1968a,b), raising the possibility that they may influence early development of the nervous system and associated structures. For example, the neural tube and notochord of neurulating chick and amphibian embryos have the ability to transiently take up 5-HT or catecholamines at specific sites along the neuraxis (Allen and Newgreen, 1977; Godin, 1986; Godin and Gipouloux, 1986; Kirby and Gilmore, 1972; Lawrence and Burden,

1973; Newgreen et al., 1981; Rais et al, 1981; Sako et al., 1986; Sims, 1977; Wallace, 1982). In the caudal part of the chick embryo, 5-HT uptake sites are located in the floorplate of the neural tube and underlying notochord. As closure of the caudal neuropore proceeds, these sites progressively disappear in concert with this process (Wallace, 1982). In addition, there are indications that the notochord and even the yolk itself may be sites of 5-HT synthesis in the chick embryo (Emanuelsson, 1974; Godin, 1986; Ignarro and Shideman, 1968a; Strudel,1977a,b; Wallace, 1982; Wallace et al., 1985). Finally, neurochemicals which interfere with these and other neurotransmitters have been found to be teratogenic in the chick embryo (Landauer, 1975, 1976; Palen et al., 1979). Thus, sites of 5-HT and catecholamine localization could have functional signficance during neurulation in the chick embryo.

Until recently, little information has been available concerning the presence of sites for uptake or synthesis of 5-HT or catecholamines in mammals during early phases of embryogenesis, although Burden and Lawrence (1973) have reported that at the 4 cell stage, the blastomeres of the rat embryo have uptake mechanisms for these substances. Also, Schlumpf and Lichtensteiger (1979) have demonstrated that the visceral yolk sac of the rat embryo can synthesize catecholamines. Although little is known about sites of action of these substances, a number of pharmacologic studies have indicated that 5-HT, L-tryptophan or tricyclic antidepressants (particularly those which act through serotonergic mechanisms) can cause malformations of the skull, brain, spinal cord or vertebral column in rodents and humans

(Guram et al., 1980, 1982; Idanpaan-Heikkila and Saxen, 1973; Jurand, 1980; Van Cauteren et al., 1986). These findings suggest that the monoamine neurotransmitters may be involved in morphogenesis of the nervous system and some skeletal components in the embryo.

The developing palate represents a model system in which the possible role of neurotransmitters in the regulation of morphogenesis can be studied both in vivo and in vitro, including perturbation by appropriate pharmacologic agents. Serotonin, catecholamines and GABA have all been measured in the palate during murine palatogenesis, including changes in the levels of these transmitters during different phases of palate formation (Zimmerman et al., 1981; Pisano and Greene, 1985; Wee et al., 1986). These neurotransmitters, when added to the medium in whole embryo or tissue cultures, produce different biochemical, cellular and morphologic responses. Catecholamines and related drugs (e.g., norepinephrine, isoproterenol) stimulate adenylate cyclase (Waterman et al., 1976; Schreiner et al., 1986) apparently through a B-adrenergic receptor mechanism (Garbarino and Greene, 1984) and suppress the growth of mesenchymal cells in culture (Pisano et al., 1986). However, 5-HT stimulates cyclic GMP levels and protein carboxymethylase actvity, while inhibiting cyclic AMP levels in the same system (Zimmerman et al., 1983). In addition, evidence exists that neurotransmitters may modulate palatal morphogenesis. For example, 5-HT and acetylcholine have been shown to stimulate palatal shelf reorientation in whole embryo culture, whereas GABA exerts an inhibitory effect, and norepinephrine and dopamine have no effect at all. Moreover, the GABA-related drug diazepam also partially inhibited palatal shelf reorientation in culture and produces cleft palate in embryos when administered to pregnant mice (Wee et al., 1979, 1980; Wee and Zimmerman, 1983, 1985; Zimmerman and Wee, 1984). Since 5-HT stimulates palatal shelf reorientation in this system, its effect on motility of cells in palatal cultures has also been examined where it was found to exert a stimulatory effect on migration of mesenchymal cells from explants of palatal shelves (Venkatasubramanian and Zimmerman, 1983), and to stimulate migration of dissociated mesenchymal cells toward a chemotactic stimulus (Zimmerman et al., 1983).

As discussed below, we have undertaken studies to determine whether 5-HT may act to regulate morphogenesis in the mouse embryo during neurulation and craniofacial development (Lauder et al., 1987, 1988; Lauder and Zimmerman, 1987; Zimmerman and Lauder, 1987). For this purpose, the method of whole embryo culture (Sadler, 1979) has been employed, together with immunocytochemistry with a specific 5-HT antiserum, to analyze sites of uptake and/or synthesis of 5-HT in mouse embryos grown in the presence of 5-HT or its precursors. In addition, a specific antiserum to the purified 45 kd form of serotonin binding protein (SBP; Kirschgessner et al., 1987; Liu et al., 1985, 1987; Tamir 1983) has been used to study possible sites of 5-HT binding in these embryos. SBP binds 5-HT with high affinity (Tamir and Huang, 1974), acts as a storage protein to bind 5-HT in synaptic vesicles (Gershon et al., 1983; Tamir and Gershon, 1979), and is released along with 5-HT during exocytosis (Jonakait et al., 1979). Once in the extracellular milieu, 5-HT dissociates from SBP, an event which can be modulated by such molecules as ions and gangliosides (Tamir and Liu, 1982; Tamir et al., 1980). We have also determined the teratogenicity of 5-HT and related compounds for embryos grown in their presence during critical phases of morphogenesis.

<u>Sites of serotonin uptake in the headfold stage mouse embryo</u>

In mouse embryos at the headfold stage (embryonic day 9, E9), when the neural tube is still closing in the head and tail regions, we have observed sites of 5-HT immunoreactivity (IR) in the hindgut and heart, following incubation with 5-HT, fixation, and processing for immunocytochemistry, which was performed on tissue sections using a specific 5-HT antiserum (Wallace et al., 1982), as shown in Fig. 1. Unlike the chick (Wallace, 1982; Wallace et al., 1985), described above, no 5-HT IR has yet been found in the notochord or in the underlying floorplate of the neural tube in mouse embryos. However, a prominent site of 5-HT IR was observed in the mouse hindgut adjacent to the caudal neuropore in a similar configuration to that of the notochord in the chick (Wallace, 1982). Thus, considering the small size of the notochord in the mouse, it is possible that,with regard to 5-HT, the hindgut performs a function analogous to that of the large notochord in the chick embryo (Lauder, Thomas and Sadler, in preparation).

We have attempted to determine whether sites of 5-HT uptake in the mouse heart and hindgut are also sites of synthesis of this neurotransmitter (Lauder, Thomas and Sadler, in preparation). These studies have already demonstrated that sites of

5-HT IR are visible in both the heart and hindgut following incubation of embryos with either 5-HT or its immediate precursor 5-hydroxytryptophan (5-HTP), whereas only the heart site is visible after treatment with L-tryptophan (L-TRP), the first precursor in the 5-HT pathway. Thus, the heart represents a possible site of 5-HT synthesis in the mouse embryo, although further experiments with specific inhibitors of 5-HT uptake together with precursors of 5-HT will be required before this conclusion can be made (see below). The finding of a major site of 5-HT accumulation in the heart raises the possibility that some congenital heart malformations could have a drug-related etiology, if correlated with the use of serotonergic drugs during pregnancy. Studies are now in progress to pharmacologically characterize these sites and to follow their appearance and disappearance in early mouse embryos.

## Sites of 5-HT uptake and binding protein in the midgestation mouse embryo

The possible involvement of 5-HT in morphogenesis of the craniofacial region has been investigated using the method of whole embryo culture to expose day 11-12 (E11-12) embryos to 5-HT or related compounds, followed by fixation and processing for immunocytochemistry with antisera to 5-HT or its binding protein (Lauder et al., 1988; Lauder and Zimmerman, 1987; Zimmerman and Lauder, 1987). Sites of 5-HT IR have been found in a number of locations in tissues of the head and neck, which are either 1) epithelia derived from the non-neural ectoderm or 2) non-neuronal midline brain structures. These sites include: the surface epithelia of the head, face, nasal prominences, branchial arches, palate, oral cavity and associated nasal epithelium, the epithelium covering the eye, parts of the otic vesicle, and in the brain: the epiphysis and roof of the diencephalon (Fig. 2).

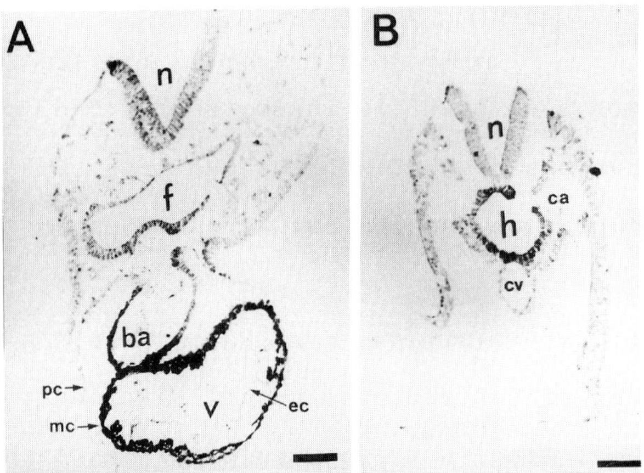


Figure 1. Sites of 5-HT uptake in the day 9 (headfold stage) mouse embryo following 3 hr incubation in medium containing 5-HT (10-5M) + nialamide and L-cysteine (10-5M each; added 1 hr prior to 5-HT). A: anterior neuropore; B: caudal neuropore. n: neural tube, f: foregut, ba: bulbus arteriosus, v: ventricle, ec: endocardium, pc: pericardium, mc: myocardium. Bars = 100 μm. (From: Lauder, Thomas and Sadler, in preparation).

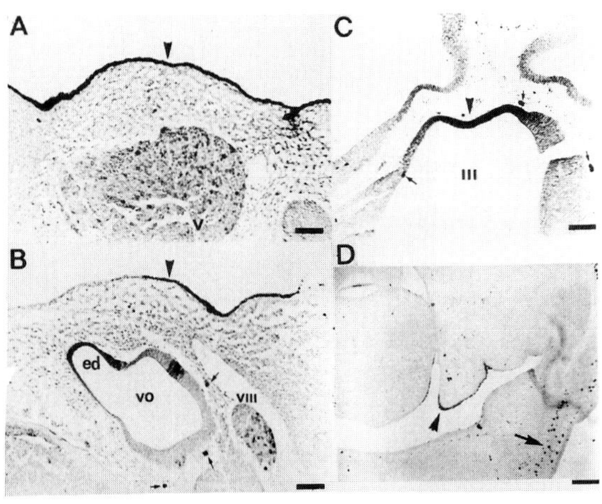


Figure 2. Sites of 5-HT uptake in the day 12 (A-C) and day 14 (D) mouse embryo following 3 hr incubation in medium containing 5-HT (10-5M) + nialamide and L-cysteine (10-5M each; added 1 hr

prior to 5-HT). A: surface epithelium of head (arrowhead); B: otocyst and surface epithelium of head (arrowhead); C: brain: epiphysis (arrowhead); D: anterior palate (arrowhead; From: Lauder and Zimmerman, 1987). v: trigeminal ganglion of 5th cranial nerve, III: 3rd ventricle, VIII: acoustic ganglion of 8th cranial nerve, small arrows: mast cells. Bars = 100 μm.

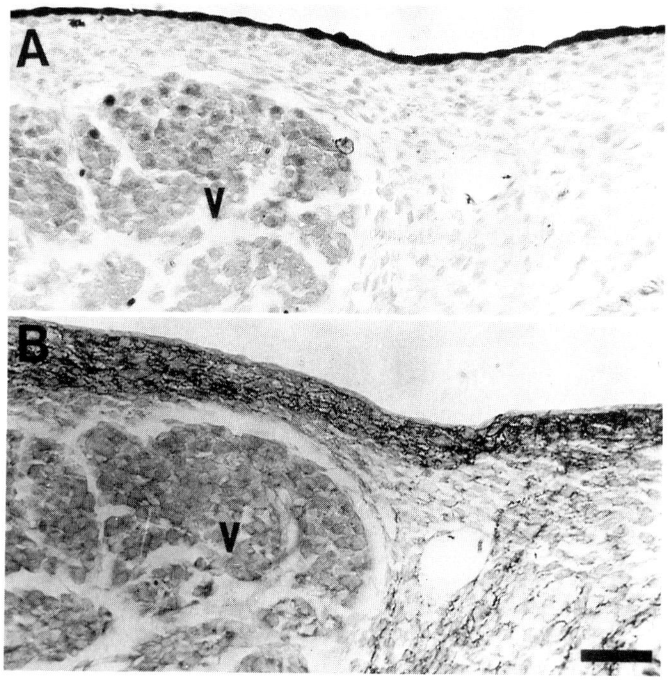


Figure 3. Sites of 5-HT uptake and serotonin binding protein (SBP) in the head of the day 12 mouse embryo. A: 5-HT immunoreactivity in the surface epithelium following incubation in 5-HT (10-5M) + nialamide and L-cysteine (10-5M each; added 1 hr prior to 5-HT); B: SBP immunoreactivity in the nearby head mesenchyme on an adjacent section. v: trigeminal ganglion of 5th nerve. Bar = 180 μm.

Regions of immunoreactivity for serotonin binding protein (SBP IR) have been identified in the mesenchyme adjacent to all of these epithelial and brain sites of 5-HT IR (e.g., Fig. 3), with the exception of the palate, oral cavity, and nasal epithelium. In addition, SBP IR has been observed in a number of other locations in the E12 mouse embryo, including the region between the surface epithelium and the somites, the perinotochordal sheath and adjacent mesenchyme, and within the meninges, especially those covering the hindbrain and fourth ventricle. The appearance of this SBP IR (see Fig. 3), suggests that this molecule is located on the outside of mesenchyme cells, filling the spaces between them. In such a location it could be associated with components of the extracellular matrix or with cell adhesion molecules. This interpretation is supported by the finding that 5-HT binding to SBP can be modulated by gangliosides (Tamir et al., 1980), as discussed above.

We have characterized the epithelial and brain sites of 5-HT IR found in E12 mouse embryos in terms of their ability to take up and/or synthesize 5-HT (Lauder et al., 1988; Lauder and Zimmerman, 1987). Embryos were exposed to 5-HT, or to its precursors (L-TRP or 5-HTP) with or without the specific 5-HT uptake inhibitor fluoxetine (Wong et al., 1979). The appearance of 5-HT IR at these sites was then examined using anti5-HT immunocytochemsitry, as described above. All of the epithelial sites of 5-HT IR could be visualized following incubation of embryos in medium containing either 5-HT precursor, whereas brain sites were only observed after treatment with 5-HT itself. This information might suggest that the epithelia contain sites of 5-HT synthesis as well as uptake. However, since the appearance of these sites after incubation with precursors was blocked by fluoxetine, we must conclude that they are only sites of uptake for 5-HT, which is normally synthesized elsewhere in the embryo. Another characteristic of these sites is their apparent ability to rapidly metabolize 5-HT, since without an inhibitor of monoamine oxidase in the medium, no detectable accumulation of 5-HT could be seen with either 5-HT or its precursors.

The sites of 5-HT uptake in epithelia and brain, and the adjacent regions of mesenchymal SBP IR are transient, such that by E14, most of them have disappeared, except in the anterior palate where a site of 5-HT uptake persists (Fig. 2D). However, new sites of SBP IR have appeared by this time, particularly in regions of chondrogenesis in the head, face and jaw (Lauder et al., 1988).

Possible functional significance of adjacent 5-HT uptake and binding sites

All of the epithelial structures where sites of 5-HT uptake have been found are derived from the non-neural ectoderm (that part of the ectoderm not induced by the chordamesoderm; Vogt 1929), whereas the mesenchyme, in which sites of SBP IR are located, is formed from the neural crest (Johnston and Hazelton, 1972; Johnston, 1974; LeLievre and LeDouarin, 1975; Nichols, 1986; Noden, 1984; Tan and Morriss-Kay, 1985) which is of neurectodermal origin (from the induced neural plate; Holtfreter and Hamburger, 1955). This mesenchyme gives rise primarily to skeletal elements and connectives tissue in the head and first two branchial arches (Ciment and Weston, 1985; Noden, 1983), as a result of reciprocal interactions (Grobstein, 1967) with adjacent epithelia of the head and face (Bee and Thorogood, 1980; Tyler and Hall, 1977), where we have found sites of 5-HT uptake. The presence of SBP IR in neural crest-derived mesenchyme in E12 embryos, and in chondrogenesis sites at later ages, suggests that SBP could be involved in the differentiation of these mesenchyme cells into skeletal elements in the craniofacial region, an event which may involve interactions with epithelia containing sites of 5-HT uptake.

## Serotonin and malformations of the craniofacial region

In current studies (Lauder, Thomas and Sadler, in preparation) we have begun to address the issue of whether 5-HT does in fact play a role in neurulation and craniofacial development in the mouse embryo. For this purpose, we have used the method of whole embryo culture to grow mouse embryos in the presence of 5-HT or agents which interfere with its uptake or metabolism. Embryos have been cultured beginning at the headfold stage (E9) for 24 or 48 hours in medium containing 5-HT (Fig. 4B,C) or the 5-HT uptake inhibitor fluoxetine (Fig. 4D). The morphological appearance of these experimental embryos has been assessed using scanning electron microscopy or 1 μm plastic sections, and compared to embryos cultured in control media. In embryos grown in the presence of 5-HT or fluoxetine, a number of defects have been observed, including deficiencies in the head mesenchyme, hypoplastic maxillary processes and mandibular arches (Fig. 4B,C), hypoplastic forebrains or open cranial neural folds (Fig. 4C,D), and abnormal eyes (Figs. 4B-D). Interestingly, the most dramatic and rapidly occurring defects have been seen with fluoxetine (Fig. 4B). Although further studies are required to assess their specificity, these effects, together with previous observations of sites of 5-HT uptake and binding protein in these same regions, discussed above, raise the possibility that

5-HT uptake by epithelia and the expression of its binding protein in adjacent mesenchyme could play an important role in morphogenesis of the craniofacial region in the mouse embryo.

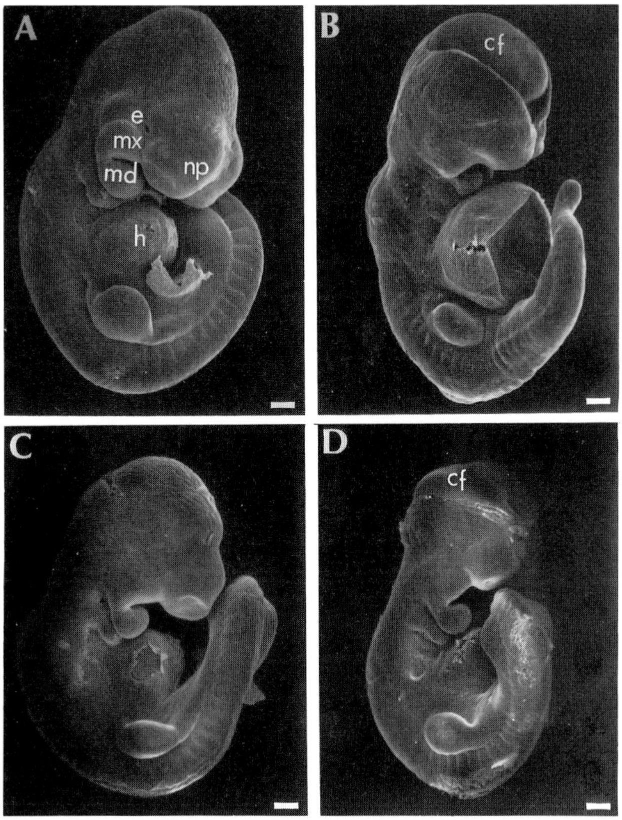


Figure 4. Malformations in mouse embryos cultured in medium containing fluoxetine (B: 10-5M) or 5-HT (C: 10-5M, D: 10-4M). Treatments were for 48 hrs beginning on embryonic day 9 in medium containing nialamide and L-cysteine (10-5M each). A: control (medium contained L-cysteine only). Nialamide + L-cysteine controls were also done. These embryos appear intermediate between those shown in A and C. Note the hypoplastic maxillary process (mx), mandibular (md; 1st branchial arch) and nasal (np) prominences in embryos treated with 5-HT (C,D), which is more pronounced with increasing dose. Note also the open cranial folds in embryos treated with fluoxetine (B) or a high concentration of 5-HT (D). An enlarged heart (h) is also apparent in the fluoxetine treated embryo (B). Eye rudiments (e) are hypoplastic or missing in all of the treated embryos (B-D). Bars = 250 µm. (From: Lauder, Thomas and Sadler, in preparation).

## References

Allen IJ, Newgreen DF (1977) Catecholamine accumulation in neural crest cells and the primary sympathetic chain. Amer. J. Anat. 149: 413-421

Baker PC, Quay WB (1969) 5-hydroxytryptamine metabolism in early embryogenesis, and the development of brain and retinal tissues. Brain Res. 12: 273-295

Bee J, Thorogood P (1980) The role of tissue interactions in the skeletogenic differentiation of avian neural crest cells. Dev. Biol. 78: 47-62

Burden RW, Lawrence IE (1973) Presence of biogenic amines in early rat development. Am. J. Anat. 136: 251-257

Buznikiv GA (1980) Biogenic monoamines and acetylcholine in protozoa and metazoan embryos. In Salanki J, Turpaev TM (eds) Neurotransmitters, Comparative Aspects. Akademiai Kiado, Budapest, pp 7-29

Buznikov GA (1984) The action of neurotransmitters and related substances on early embryogenesis. Pharmac. Ther. 25: 23-59

Buznikov GA, Chudakova IV, Zvezdina ND (1964) The role of neurohumors in early embryogenesis. I. Serotonin content of developing embryos of sea urchin and loach. J. Embryol. exp. Morph. 12: 563-573

Buznikov GA, Chudakova IV, Berdysheva LV, Vyazmina NM (1968) The role of neurohumors in early embryogenesis. II. Acetylcholine and catecholamine content in developing embryos of sea urchin. J. Embryol. exp. Morph. 20: 119-128

Buznikov GA, Kost AN, Kucherova, NF, Mndzhoyan AL, Suvorov NN, Berdysheva LV (1970) The role of neurohumours in early embryogenesis III. Pharmacological analysis of the role of neurohumours in cleavage divisions. J. Embryol. exp. Morph. 23: 549-569

Buznikov GA, Shmukler YB (1981) Possible role of "prenervous" neurotransmitters in cellular interactions of early embryogenesis. Neurochem. Res. 6: 55-68

Ciment G, Weston J (1985) Segregation of developmental abilities in neural crest-derived cells: Identification of partially restricted intermediate cell types in the branchial arches of avian embryos. Dev. Biol. 111: 73-83

Deeb SS (1972) Inhibition of cleavage and hatching of sea urchin embryos by serotonin. J. exp. Zool. 181: 79-87

Emanuelsson H (1974) Localization of serotonin in cleavage embryos of Ophryotrocha labronica La Greca and Bacci. Roux' Arch. Entw.-mech. 175: 253-271

Garbarino M, Greene R (1984) Identification of adenylate cyclase-coupled B-adrenergic receptors in the developing mammalian palate. Biochem. Biophys. Res. Commun. 119, 193-202

Gershon MD, Liu KP, Karpiak SE, Tamir H (1983) Storage of serotonin in vivo as a complex with serotonin-binding protein in central and peripheral serotonergic neurons. J. Neurosci. 3: 1901-1911

Godin I (1986) Explanted and implanted notochord of amphibian anuran embryos. Histofluorescence study on the ability to synthesize catecholamines. Anat. Embryol. 173: 393-399

Godin I, Gipouloux J-D (1985) Notochordal catecholamines in exogastrulated Xenopus embryos. Dev. Growth and Diff. 28: 137-142

Grobstein C (1967) Mechanisms of organogenetic tissue interactions. Nat. Cancer Inst. Monog. 26: 279-299

Guram MS, Gill TS, Geber WF (1980) Teratogenicity of imipramine and amitriptyline in fetal hamsters. Res. Com. Psychol.Psychiat. Behav. 5: 275-282

Guram MS, Gill TS, Geber WF (1982) Comparative teratogenicity of chlordiazepoxide, amitriptyline, and a combination of the two compounds in the fetal hamster. Neurotoxicol. 3: 83-90

Gustafson T, Toneby M (1970) On the role of serotonin and acetylcholine in sea urchin morphogenesis. Exp. Cell. Res. 62: 102-117

Gustafson T, Toneby M (1971) How genes control morphogenesis. Amer. Sci. 59: 452-462

Gurdon JB (1987) Embryonic induction - molecular aspects. Development 99: 285-306

Gustafson T, Wolpert L (1963) Cellular mechanisms in the morphogenesis of the sea urchin larva. Exp. Cell. Res. 27: 260-279

Holtfreter J, Hamburger V (1955) Amphibians. In: Willier BH, Weiss PA, Hamburger V (eds) Analysis of Development. W.B. Saunders, Philadelphia and London, pp 230-296

Holtfreter J (1968) On mesenchyme and epithelia in inductive and morphogenetic processes. In: Fleischmajer R, Billingham RE (eds) Epithelial-Mesenchymal Interactions. Williams and Wilkins, Baltimore, pp 1-30

Idanpään-Heikkila J, Saxen L (1973) Possible teratogenicity of imipramine/chloropyramine. Lancet 2: 282-284

Ignarro LJ, Shideman FE (1968a) Appearance and concentrations of catecholamines and their biosynthesis in embryonic and developing chick. J. Pharmacol. exp. Ther. 159: 38-48

Ignarro LJ, Shideman FE (1968b) Norepinephrine and epinephrine in the embryo and embryonic heart of the chick: Uptake and subcellular disribution. J. Pharmacol. exp. Ther. 159: 49-58

Johnston MC, Hazelton RD (1972) Embryonic origins of facial structures related to oral sensory and motor functions. In: Bosma JF (ed) Third Symposium on Oral Sensation and Perception. C.C. Thomas, Springfield, pp 76-97

Johnston M (1974) Facial malformation in chick embryos resulting from removal of neural crest. J. Dent. Res. (Suppl.) 43: 822

Jonakait GM, Tamir H, Gintzler AR, Gershon MD (1979) Release of [3H]serotonin and its binding protein from enteric neurons. Brain Res. 174: 55-69

Jurand A (1980) Malformations of the central nervous system induced by neurotropic drugs in mouse embryos. Dev. Growth and Diff. 22: 61-78

Kirby ML, Gilmore SA (1972) A fluorescence study on the ability of the notochord to synthesize and store catecholamines in early chick embryos. Anat. Rec. 173: 469-478

Kirschgessner AL, Liu KP, Gershon MD, Tamir H (1987) Co-localization of serotonin with specific serotonin binding proteins in serotoninergic neurons of the rat brain and spinal cord. Anat. Rec. 218: 73A

Landauer W (1975) Cholinomimetic teratogens: Studies with chicken embryos. Teratology 12: 125-146

Landauer W (1976) Cholinomimetic teratogens III. Interaction with amino acids known as neurotransmitters. Teratology 13: 41-46

Lauder JM, Zimmerman E (1987) Sites of serotonin uptake in the epithelium of the developing mouse palate, oral cavity and face: Possible role in morphogenesis? J. Craniofac. Genet. Dev. Biol. (submitted)

Lauder JM, Tamir H, Sadler TW (1987) Sites of serotonin uptake and binding protein immunoreactivity in the cultured mouse embryo: Roles in morphogenesis? Soc. Neurosci. Abst. 12: (in press)

Lauder JM, Tamir H, Sadler TW (1988) Serotonin and morphogenesis I. Sites of serotonin uptake and binding protein immunoreactivity in the midgestation mouse embryo. Development (submitted)

Lawrence IE Jr., Burden HW (1973) Catecholamines and morphogenesis of the chick neural tube and notochord. Amer. J. Anat. 137: 199-208

LeLièvre CS, LeDouarin NM (1975) Mesenchymal derivatives of the neural crest: Analysis of chimeric quail and chick embryos. J. Embryol. exp. Morph. 34: 125-154

Liu K-P, Gershon MD, Tamir H (1985) Identification, purification, and characterization of two forms of serotonin binding protein from rat brain. J. Neurochem. 44: 1289-1301

Liu K-P, Hsiung SC, Kirschgessner AL, Gershon MD, Tamir H (1987) Co-localization of serotonin with serotonin binding proteins in the rat CNS. J. Neurochem. (Suppl.) 48: 63

Manukhin BN, Volina EV, Markova LN, Rakic L, Buznikov GA (1981) Biogenic monoamines in early embryos of sea urchins. Dev. Neurosci. 4: 322-328

Markova LN, Buznikov GA, Kovačević N, Rakić L, Salimova NB, Volina EV (1985) Histochemical study if biogenic monoamines in early ("prenervous") and late embryos of sea urchins. Int. J. Dev. Neurosci. 3: 493-499

Newgreen DF, Allan IJ, Young HM, Southwell BR (1981) Accumulation of exogenous catecholamines in the neural tube and non-neural tissues of the early fowl embryo. Correlation with morphogenetic movements. W. Roux's Arch. 190: 320-333

Nichols DH (1986) Formation and distribution of neural crest mesenchyme to the first pharyngeal arch region of the mouse embryo. Am. J. Anat. 176: 221-231

Noden DM (1983) The role of the neural crest in patterning of avian cranial skeletal, connective, and muscle tissues. Dev. Biol. 96: 144-165

Noden DM (1984) Craniofacial development: New views on old problems. Anat. Rec. 208: 1-13

Palen K, Thorneby L, Emanuelsson H (1979) Effects of serotonin and serotonin antagonists on chick embryogenesis. W. Roux's Arch. 187: 89-103

Pisano MM, Greene RM (1985) Hormone and growth factor involvement in craniofacial development. IRCS Medical Science 14: 635-640

Pisano M, Schneiderman M, Greene R (1986) Catecholamine modulation of embryonic palate mesenchymal cell DNA synthesis. J. Cell. Physiol. 126: 84-92

Raïs R, Girard C, Gipouloux JD (1981) Mise en évidence de catécholamines dans la chorde dorsale des embryons d'Amphibiens anoures. Relations possibles avec l'activité adénylate cyclasique de cet organe et la migration des cellules germinales primordinales. Arch. Anat. Micr. Morphol. Exp. 70: 149-160

Renaud F, Parisi E, Capasso A, De Prisco P (1983) On the role of serotonin and 5-methoxy-tryptamine in the regulation of cell division in sea urchin eggs. Dev. Biol. 98: 37-46

Sadler TW (1979) Culture of early somite mouse embryos during organogenesis. J. Embryol. exp. Morph. 49: 17-25

Sako H, Kojima T, Okada (1986) Immunohistochemical study on the development of serotoninergic neurons in the chick: I. Distribution of cell bodies and fibers in the brain. J. Comp. Neurol. 254: 61-78

Schlumpf M, Lichtensteiger W (1979) Catecholamines in the yolk sac epithelium of the rat. Anat. Embryol. 156: 177-187

Shreiner CM, Zimmerman EF, Wee EL, Scott WJ (1986) Caffeine effects on cyclic AMP levels in the mouse embryonic limb and palate _in vitro_. Teratology 34: 21-27

Sims TJ (1977) The development of monoamine-containing neurons in the brain and spinal cord of the salamander, _Ambystoma mexicanum_. J. Comp. Neurol. 173: 319-335

Spemann H, Mangold H (1924) Uber Induktion von Embryonalanlagen durch Implantation artfremder Organisatoren. Arch. mik. Anat. EntwMech. 100: 599-638.

Strudel G, Meinel P, Gateau G (1977a) Recherches d' amines flurigènes dans les chordes d'embryons de Poulet traités par des cholinergiques. C.R. Acad. Sci. Paris 284: 1097-1100

Strudel G, Recasens M, Mandel P (1977b) Identification de catécholmines et de sérotonine dans les chordes d'embryons de Poulet. C.R. Acad. Sci. Paris 284: 967-969

Tamir H (1983) Serotonin-binding protein: Function in synaptic vesiles. Trans. N.Y. Acad. Sci. 41: 237-242

Tamir H, Brunner W, Casper D, Rapport MM (1980) Enhancement by gangiosides of the binding of serotonin to serotonin binding protein. J. Neurochem. 34: 1719-1724

Tamir H, Gershon MD (1979) Storage of serotonin and serotonin binding protein in synaptic vesicles. J. Neurochem. 33: 35-44

Tamir H, Huang, YL (1974) Binding of serotonin to soluble binding protein from synaptosomes. Life Sci. 14: 83-93

Tamir H, Liu K-P (1982) On the nature of the interaction between serotonin and serotonin binding protein: Effect of nucleotides, ions, and sulfhydryl reagents. J. Neurochem. 38: 135-141

Tan SS, Morriss-Kay, G (1985) The development and distribution of the cranial neural crest in the rat embryo. Cell Tiss. Res. 240: 403-416

Toneby M (1977a) Functional aspects of 5-hydroxytryptamine and dopaine in early embryogenesis of _Echinoidea_ and _Asteroidea_. Stockholm: Wenner-Gren Institute.

Toneby M (1977b) Functional aspects of 5-hydroxytryptamine in early embryogenesis of the sea urchin _Paracentrotus lividus_. W. Roux's Arch. 181: 247-259

Tyler MS, Hall BK (1977) Epithelial influences on skeletogenesis in the mandible of the embryonic chick. Anat. Rec. 188: 229-240

Van Cauteren H, Vandenberghe J, Marsboom R (1986) Protective activity of ketanserin against serotonin-induced embryotoxicity and teratogencity. Drug Dev. Res. 8: 179-185

Venkatasubramanian K, Zimmerman EF (1983) Palate cell motility and substrate interaction. J. Craniofacial Genet. Dev. Biol. 3: 143-157

Vogt W (1929) Gestaltungsanalyse am Amphibienkeim mit örtlicher Vitalfärbung. Roux' Arch. Entw.-Mech. 120: 384-706

Wallace JA (1982) Monoamines in the early chick embryo: Demonstration of serotonin synthesis and the regional distribution of serotoninconcentrating cells during morphogenesis. Amer. J. Anat. 165: 261-276

Wallace JA, Lilly S, Maez RR (1985) Characterization of serotonin uptake mechanisms in the region of the caudal neuropore of the early chick embryo. Soc. Neurosci. Abst. 11: 605

Wallace JA, Petrusz P, Lauder JM (1982) Serotonin immunocytochemistry in the adult and developing rat brain: Methodological and pharmacoogical considerations. Brain Res. Bull. 9: 117-129

Waterman R, Palmer G, Palmer J, Palmer S (1976) Catecholamine-sensitive adenylate cyclase in the developing golden hamster palate. Anat. Rec. 185: 125-138

Wee EL, Babiarz BS, Zimmerman S, Zimmerman EF (1979) Palate morphogenesis IV. Effects of serotonin and its antagonists on rotation in embryo culture. J. Embryol. exp. Morph. 53: 75-90

Wee EL, Norman EJ, Zimmerman EF (1986) Presence of $\gamma$-aminobutyric acid in embryonic palates of AJ and SWV mouse strains. J. Craniofacial Genet. Dev. Biol. 6: 53-61

Wee EL, Phillips NJ, Babiarz BS, Zimmerman EF (1980) Palate morphogenesis V. Effects of cholinergic agonists and antagonists on rotation in embryo culture. J. Embryol. exp. Morph. 58: 177-193

Wee EL, Zimmerman EF (1983) Involvement of GABA in palate morphogenesis and its relation to diazepam teratogenesis in two mouse strains. Teratology 28: 15-22

Wee EL, Zimmerman EF (1985) GABA uptake in embryonic palate mesenchymal cells of two mouse strains. Neurochem. Res. 10: 1673-1688

Wong DT, Horng JS, Bymaster FP, Hauser KL, Molloy BB (1974) A selective inhibitor of serotonin uptake: Lilly 11040, 3-(p-trifluoromethylphenoxyl)-N-methyl-3-phenylpropyl-amine. Life Sci. 15: 471-479

Zimmerman EF, Lauder JM (1987) Sites of serotonin uptake in the epithelium of the developing mouse palate, oral cavity and face: Possible role in morphogenesis? Teratology 35: 39A

Zimmerman EF, Wee EL (1984) Role of neurotransmitters in palate development. In: Zimmerman EF (ed) Current Topics in Developmental Biology (vol. 19: Palate Development). New York, Academic Press, pp 37-63

Zimmerman EF, Wee EL, Phillips N, Roberts N (1981) Presence of serotonin in the palate just prior to shelf elevation. J. Embryol. exp. Morphol. 64: 233-250

Zimmerman EF, Clark RL, Ganguli S, Venkatasubramanian K (1983) Serotonin regulation of palatal cell motility and metabolism. J. Craniofacial Genet. Dev. Biol. 3: 371-385

Acknowledgements

This work was supported by NIH grant HD 22052. The authors would like to thank Robin Thomas for technical assistance and Hadassah Tamir for the gift of antisera to serotonin binding protein.

# GABA AND TAURINE AS SIGNALS FOR NEURONAL DEVELOPMENT AND DIFFERENTIATION

Arne Schousboe, Gert H. Hansen, Bo Belhage, Jens H. Abraham & Eddi Meier*

Department of Biochemistry A, Panum Institute, University of Copenhagen, DK-2200 Copenhagen N, Denmark

## INTRODUCTION

During recent years evidence has been accumulating that different classical neurotransmitters such as serotonin, catecholamines and the amino acids GABA and taurine may serve as epigenetic factors during neuronal development and differentiation (Lauder,1983; Haydon *et al.*,1984; König *et al.*, 1986; Redburn & Schousboe,1987). Since a variety of macromolecular compounds, mainly peptides, are also known to act as neurotrophic factors (Manthorpe *et al.*,1986) it is clear that the extremely complex processes which govern the development and differentiation of the neuronal network and communication system in the central nerve system are subject to regulation at a number of different levels. The present review will concentrate on a summary of the recent progress in studies concerned with the possible role of GABA and taurine as agents stimulating neuronal development.

---

*Present address: Department of Pharmacology, H. Lundbeck & Co.,Ltd., DK-2500 Valby, Denmark.

NATO ASI Series, Vol. H22
Neural Development and Regeneration
Edited by A. Gorio et al.

## NEUROTROPHIC ACTIVITY OF GABA

### a. Morphological development.

Since the original observation by Wolff and coworkers (Wolff *et al.*,1978) that GABA enhances synaptogenesis in rat superior cervival ganglia, a number of studies mainly on neurons in tissue culture have been concerned with a characterization of the effects of GABA on the morphological development of neurons. In cerebellar granule cells (Hansen *et al.*, 1984) as well as in retinal neurons (Spoerri,1987) and neuroblastoma cells (Spoerri & Wolff,1981) addition of GABA to the culture media has been shown to promote neurite formation (Table 1). At the electron microscope level this effect seems to be associated with increases in the cytoplasmic densities of e.g. rough endoplasmic reticulum, Golgi apparatus and coated vesicles whereas the densities of mitochondria and smooth endoplasmic reticulum are unaffected (Table 2). These effects of GABA on the morphological differentiation of the neurons were found to be induced *via* an interaction between GABA and high affinity $GABA_A$ receptors since the action of GABA could be completely blocked (Meier *et al.*,1985) by the specific GABA receptor antagonist (Curtis *et al.*,1971) bicuculline and mimicked (Meier *et al.*,1985) by the specific GABA receptor agonist (Schousboe *et al.*,1985) 4,5,6,7-tetrahydroisoxazolo[5,4-*c*]pyridin-3-ol (THIP).

The temporal development of these GABA or GABA receptor agonist-induced morphological changes has recently been studied (Hansen *et al.*,1987b). It was found that very short exposure times (Table 3) for THIP were sufficient to induce the increase in the cytoplasmic density of the different subcellular structures.

TABLE 1. Effect of GABA or THIP on formation of neurites and neuronal colonies in granule cell cultures.

| Culture condition | | Neurite-ext. cells per mm$^2$ | Colonies per mm$^2$ |
|---|---|---|---|
| | 4-days-in culture | 7-days-in culture | 7-days-in culture |
| Control | 1804± 90 | 629±33 | 19±3 |
| + GABA (50 µM) or THIP (150 µM) | 2160±104* | 931±82** | 43±7** |

Cerebellar granule cells were cultured for 4 or 7 days in the absence or presence of 150 µM THIP (4 days) or 50 µM GABA (7 days) and phase contrast micrographs were taken randomly and scored double blind for neurite-extending cells and colonies of neuronal cell bodies. Results are averages of 6-12 micrographs taken of 2-3 cultures of each group. Asterisks indicate statistically significant differences from cells grown under standard conditions (*P<0.025, Mann-Whitney test; **P<0.01, t-test). From Hansen _et al._,(1984;1987a).

TABLE 2. Summary of effects of GABA on the ultrastructure of cerebellar granule cells.

| Organelle | Effect of GABA | |
|---|---|---|
| Mitochondria | none | - |
| Golgi apparatus | increased | p<0.0005 |
| Neurotubules | increased | p<0.025 |
| Ribosomes | none | - |
| Rough endoplasmic reticulum | increased | p<0.025 |
| Smooth endoplasmic reticulum | none | - |
| Coated vesicles | increased | p<0.05 |
| Other vesicles | increased | p<0.05 |

Cerebellar granule cells were cultured for 1-7 days in the absence or presence of 50 µM GABA and the temporal development of the cytoplasmic densities of the different organelles was followed. Electron micrographs were taken at random and the densities of the structures were determined double-blind using the point method for morphometric analysis. Summary from Hansen _et al._,(1984)

b. Biochemical development.

Two of the basic characteristics of cerebellar granule cells are that they utilize glutamate as their neurotransmitter (Young _et al._,1974; Stone,1979; Drejer _et al._,1982;1983;

TABLE 3. Temporal development of the neurotrophic effect of THIP on cerebellar granule cells

| Organelle | Cytoplasmic density (%) 1 h Control | THIP | 24 h Control | THIP |
|---|---|---|---|---|
| Rough endoplasmic reticulum | 3.60±0.44 | 5.65±0.44* | 3.57±0.44 | 5.93±0.44* |
| Smooth endoplasmic reticulum | 3.36±0.21 | 2.85±0.21* | 3.43±0.21 | 2.79±0.21* |
| Golgi apparatus | 5.35±0.77 | 6.75±0.77* | 4.97±0.77 | 6.94±0.77* |
| Vesicles | 9.04±0.74 | 12.13±0.74* | 8.32±0.74 | 11.73±0.74* |
| Coated vesicles | 1.34±0.18 | 2.14±0.18* | 1.28±0.18 | 2.28±0.18* |

Cerebellar granule cells were cultured for 4 days in plain culture media prior to the addition of 150 μM THIP. The cultures were prepared for morphometric analysis after exposure to THIP for respectively 1 and 24 hours. The results are averages + SEM of 27 independent countings calculated on the basis of a two-way analysis of variance. Asterisks indicate statistically significant differences from the controls (P<0.002). From Hansen *et al.*(1987b).

Gallo *et al.*,1982) and express a high density of GABA receptors (Palacios *et al.*,1980; Simantov *et al.*,1976; Meier & Schousboe,1982). GABA receptors in CNS normally consist of a mixture of high and low affinity entities (Wang *et al.*,1979; Falch & Krogsgaard-Larsen,1982; Meier & Schousboe, 1982). On the basis of this it was surprising that cerebellar granule cells in culture exhibiting basic characteristics of glutamatergic neurons (Drejer *et al.*,1982; Gallo *et al.*,1982) only expressed the high affinity GABA receptors (Meier & Schousboe,1982). It was subsequently shown that treatment of the cultures with GABA (50 μM) during the culture period led to induction of low affinity GABA receptors in addition to high affinity GABA receptors (Meier *et al.*,1983; 1984). Simultaneously it was reported that GABA or GABA agonists injected intraocularly induced GABA receptors in retina (Madtes & Redburn,1983a,b). It was also demonstrated that elevation of brain GABA levels by GABA-transaminase inhibitors led to an increase in GABA receptors in the brain (Sykes *et al.*,1984; Beart *et al.*,1985). All of these findings strongly indicate

TABLE 4. Effects of GABA and GABA agonists or antagonists on expression of GABA receptors on cerebellar granule cells.

| Culture condition | GABA-binding $K_D$ (nM) High | Low |
|---|---|---|
| Control | 7.0 | - |
| 50 μM GABA | 7.0 | 546 |
| 150 μM THIP | 6.8 | 476 |
| 150 μM THIP, 150 μM BIC | 14.3 | - |
| 250 μM Taurine | 10.0 | 438 |

Cells were cultured for 7-12 days in plain culture media (controls) or media to which the agonists or antagonists were added.
BIC: Bicuculline methobromide.
From Meier et al.(1984), Belhage et al.(1986) and unpublished results of J.H.Abraham and A.Schousboe.

that GABA is able to regulate the expression of its own receptors by induction of additional receptor sites which at least in some of the models studied exhibited different affinities for GABA. The mechanism by which GABA induces low affinity GABA receptors has been studied using GABA receptor agonists and antagonists. It was found (Table 4) that the ef-

TABLE 5. Kinetic constants ($K_D$ and $B_{max}$) for GABA binding to membranes prepared from 4-day-old cultures of cerebellar granule cells exposed to THIP for respectively 1, 3, 6 and 24 h.

| Time of treatment with 150 μM THIP (Hours) | $K_D$ (nM) High | Low | $B_{max}$ (pmol x $mg^{-1}$) High | Low |
|---|---|---|---|---|
| 1 | 22.3±5.8 | - | 1.00±0.06 | - |
| 3 | 6.5±2.4 | 537±376 | 0.81±0.02 | 5.31±0.39 |
| 6 | 5.7±0.9 | 500±410 | 1.79±0.09 | 5.42±0.41 |
| 24 | 7.6±1.8 | 502±265 | 1.35±0.18 | 4.69±0.27 |

Cells were cultured for 4 days in plain culture media and subsequently for 1, 3, 6 and 24 h in the presence of 150 μM THIP. Values for $K_D$ and $B_{max}$ are derived from GABA binding curves by computer analysis (Munson and Rodbard,1980; McPherson,1983) and represent the statistically significantly best fits to the curves among either one or two binding sites. Values are given as means ± S.E.M. From Hansen et al.(1987b).

fect of GABA could be mimicked by the GABA receptor agonist THIP and blocked by the receptor antagonist bicuculline (Belhage et al.,1986) or picrotoxin (Meier et al.,1987a), a blocker (Olsen,1981) of GABA gated chloride channels. These results strongly imply that the action of GABA is mediated via the preexisting high affinity GABA receptors on the cells. This appears to be the same mechanism by which GABA acts as a neurite promoting agent (cf. above).

The temporal development of the induction by GABA of low affinity GABA receptors has recently been studied. It was found (Table 5) that low affinity GABA receptors can be demonstrated in membranes prepared from cerebellar granule cells 3 h after addition of THIP to the culture media (Hansen et al., 1987b). Moreover, it appears that this induction is only possible at early developmental stages of the neurons since cultures older than 7 days did not respond to THIP treatment (Belhage et al.,1987). Similar developmental patterns have also been reported for induction of GABA receptors in retina (Madtes & Bashir-Elahi,1986).

The physiological function of the inducible low affinity GABA receptors has been studied by Meier et al.(1984). Neurotransmitter release from the cerebellar granule cells was studied under different conditions. A number of studies have shown that GABA or different GABA agonists may be able to modulate glutamate release from synaptosomes or brain slices (Potashner,1979; Johnston et al.,1980; Mitchell,1980; Levi & Gallo,1981; Kato et al.,1982). Accordingly, it was investigated if GABA could modulate evoked glutamate release from the cerebellar granule cells in culture. It was found that only when the cells had been cultured under conditions where low affinity GABA receptors are expressed, could glutamate release be inhibited by GABA or THIP (Meier et al.,1984; Belhage et al.,1986). The inhibition by GABA was shown to be blocked by bicuculline but baclofen did not have any effect on evoked glutamate release. This led to the conclusion that the inducible low affinity GABA receptors which pharmacologically are classified as $GABA_A$ receptors (cf. Hill & Bowery, 1981) mediate this inhibitory effect of GABA (Meier et al., 1984).

## NEUROTROPHIC ACTIVITY OF TAURINE

Based on the above findings, the large body of circumstantial evidence that taurine has a hyperpolarizing effect on neurons (cf. Schousboe,1982) and the reports that taurine is essential for normal development of cerebellar granule cells in the cat (Sturmann *et al.*,1985) it was investigated if taurine could mimic GABA as an inducer of low affinity GABA receptors. As seen in Table 4 treatment of cerebellar granule cells in culture with taurine led to formation of low affinity GABA receptors having kinetic characteristics indistinguisable from those observed after culture in the presence of either GABA or THIP. Moreover, these low affinity GABA receptors induced by taurine have been shown to mediate the inhibition by GABA of transmitter release from the granule cells (Schousboe & Abraham,1987) similarly to the low affinity GABA receptors induced by GABA. Altogether, these findings strongly indicate that taurine plays an important role for neuronal development and differentiation. The mechanism for its action has yet to be determined and studies pertinent to this question are now in progress. Likewise it is currently being investigated if taurine is able to mimic the effects of GABA on the morphological development of the neurons.

## CONCLUDING REMARKS

On the basis of the above findings from this and other laboratories it seems well-documented that the inhibitory neurotransmitter GABA and its sulphonic acid analogue taurine exert differentiating activity at least in certain types of neurons. In this context it may be of interest that it has recently been shown that treatment of rats during postnatal development with THIP leads to an enhanced neuronal maturation as evidenced by an enhanced development of the neuron specific markers N-CAM and glutamate decarboxylase (Meier *et al.*,1987b). This together with repeated demonstrations that also other neurotransmitters such as serotonin and catecholamines (Lauder,1983; Haydon et al.1984; König et al.,1986) affect neuronal development show that classical neurotransmitters may serve also as epigenetic factors during neurogenesis. This means that it is important to investigate the mechanism of action of these factors and compare these mechanisms with the mechanism of action of nerve growth factor and related peptides which is currently under intense investigation (see several chapters in this volume).

## REFERENCES


Beart PM, Scatton B, Lloyd K (1985) Subchronic administration of GABAergic agonists elevates [$^3$H]-GABA binding and produces tolerance in striatal dopamine catabolism. Brain Res 335:169-173

Belhage B, Meier E, Schousboe A (1986) GABA-agonists induce the formation of low affinity GABA-receptors on cultured cerebellar granule cells via preexisting high affinity GABA-receptors. Neurochem Res 11:599-606

Belhage B, Hansen GH, Schousboe A, Meier E (1987) The induction of low affinity GABA-receptors by GABA agonists on cerebellar granule cells is restricted to early development. Int J Devl Neurosci. Submitted

Curtis DA, Duggan AW, Felix O, Johnston GAR, McLennan H (1971) Antagonism between bicuculline and GABA in the rat brain. Brain Res 33:57-73

Drejer J, Larsson OM, Schousboe A (1982) Characterization of L-glutamate uptake into and release from astrocytes and neurons cultured from different brain regions. Exp Brain Res 47:259-269

Drejer J, Larsson OM, Schousboe A (1983) Characterization of uptake and release processes for D- and L-aspartate in primary cultures of astrocytes and cerebellar granule cells. Neurochem Res 8:231-243

Falch E, Krogsgaard-Larsen P (1982) The binding of the GABA agonist $^3$H-THIP to rat brain synaptic membranes. J Neurochem 38:1123-1129

Gallo V, Ciotti MT, Coletti A, Aloisi F, Levi G (1982) Selective release of glutamate from cerebellar granule cells differentiating in culture. Proc Natl Acad Sci USA 79: 7919-7923

Hansen GH, Meier E, Schousboe A (1984) GABA influences the ultrastructure composition of cerebellar granule cells during development in culture. Int J Devl Neurosci 2: 247-257

Hansen GH, Meier E, Abraham JH, Schousboe A (1987a) Trophic effects of GABA on cerebellar granule cells in culture In: Redburn DA, Schousboe A (eds.): "Neurotrophic Activity of GABA During Development", New York: Alan R. Liss, Inc., in press

Hansen GH, Belhage B, Schousboe A, Meier E (1987b) Temporal development of GABA-agonist induced alterations in ultrastructure and GABA receptor expression in cultured cerebellar granule cells. Int J Devl Neurosci 5:in press

Haydon PG, McCobb DP, Kater SB (1984) Serotonin selectively inhibits growth cone motility and synaptogenesis of specific identified neurons. Science 226:561-564

Hill DR, Bowery NG (1981) $^3$H-baclofen and $^3$H-GABA bind to bicuculline-insensitive $GABA_B$ sites in rat brain. Nature 290:149-152

Johnston GAR, Hailstone MH, Freeman CG (1980) Baclofen: Stereoselective inhibition of excitant amino acid release. J Pharm Pharmacol 32:230-231

Kato K, Goto M, Fukada H (1982) Baclofen: Inhibition of release of L-[$^3$H]glutamate and L-[$^3$H]aspartate from rat whole brain synaptosomes. Gen Pharmacol 13:445-447

Konig N, Drian M-J, Privat A, Lamande N, Pares-Herbute N, Schachner M (1986) Dissociated cells of foetal rat pallium grown in culture medium supplemented with noradrenaline: Effects of the expression of neuron-specific enolase and cell adhesion molecule L1. Neurosci Lett 66:67-72

Lauder JM (1983) Hormonal and humoral influences on brain development. Psychoneuroendocrinology 8:121-155

Levi G, Gallo V (1981) Glutamate as a putative transmitter in cerebellum: Stimulation by GABA of glutamic acid release from specific pools. J Neurochem 37:22-31

Madtes PC, Bashir-Elahi R (1986) GABA receptor binding site 'induction' in rabbit retina after nipecotic acid treatment: Changes during development. Neurochem Res 11:55-61

Madtes PC, Redburn DA (1983a) GABA as a trophic factor during development. Life Sci 33:979-984

Madtes PC, Redburn DA (1983b) Synaptic interactions in the GABA system during postnatal development in retina. Brain Res Bull 10:741-745

Manthorpe M, Rudge JS, Varon S (1986) Astroglial cell contributions to neuronal survival and neuritic growth In: Fedoroff S, Varnadakis A (eds.) Astrocytes, Vol.2, New York: Academic Press, pp. 315-376

McPherson GA (1983) A practical computer-based approach to the analysis of radioligand binding experiments. Comp Prog Biomed 17:107-114

Meier E, Schousboe A (1982) Differences between GABA receptor binding to membranes from cerebellum during postnatal development and from cultured cerebellar granule cells. Dev Neurosci 5:546-553

Meier E, Drejer J, Schousboe A (1983) Trophic actions of GABA on the development of physiologically active GABA receptors: In Mandel P, DeFeudis FV (eds): "CNS-Receptors from Molecular Pharmacology to Behaviour", New York: Raven Press, pp 47-58

Meier E, Drejer J, Schousboe A (1984) GABA induces functionally active low-affinitive GABA receptors on cultured cerebellar granule cells. J Neurochem 43:1737-1744

Meier E, Hansen GH, Schousboe A (1985) The trophic effect of GABA on cerebellar granule cells is mediated by GABA-receptors. Int J Devl Neurosci 3:401-407
Meier E, Belhage B, Drejer J, Schousboe A (1987a) The expression of GABA receptors on cultured cerebellar granule cell is influenced by GABA In: Redburn DA, Schousboe A, (eds.):"Neurotrophic Activity of GABA During Development", New York: Alan R. Liss, Inc., in press
Meier E, Jorgensen OS, Schousboe A (1987b) Effect of repeated treatment with a GABA receptor agonist on postnatal neural development in rats. J Neurochem 49:in press
Mitchell R (1980) A novel GABA receptor modulates stimulus-induced glutamate release from cortico-striatal terminals. Eur J Pharmacol 67:119-122
Munson PI, Rodbard D (1980) A versatile computerized approach for characterization of ligand binding systems. Anal Biochem 107:220-239
Olsen RW (1981) GABA-benzodiazepine-barbiturate receptor interactions. J Neurochem 37:1-13
Palacios JM, Young S, Kuhar MJ (1980) Autoradiographic localization of γ-aminobutyric acid (GABA) receptors in the rat cerebellum. Proc Natl Acad Sci USA 77:670-674
Potashner SJ (1979) Baclofen: Effects on amino acid release and metabolism in slices of guinea pig cerebral cortex. J Neurochem 32:103-109
Redburn DA, Schousboe A (Eds)(1987) Neurotrophic Activity of GABA During Development. New York: Alan R. Liss,Inc., In press
Schousboe A (1982) Metabolism and function of neurotransmitters In: Pfeiffer S (ed.):"Neuroscience Approached Through Cell Culture" Vol.1, Boca Raton: CRC Press, pp. 107-141
Schousboe A, Abraham JH (1987) Taurine induces low affinity GABA receptors on cerebellar granule cells. J Neurochem 48 Supl: S 104
Schousboe A, Larsson OM, Krogsgaard-Larsen P (1985) Lack of a high affinity uptake system for the GABA agonists THIP and isoguvacine in neurons and astrocytes cultured from mouse brain. Neurochem Int 7:505-508
Simantov R, Oster-Granite ML, Herndon RN, Snyder SH (1976) Gamma-aminobutyric acid (GABA) receptor binding selectively depleted by viral-induced granule cell loss in hamster cerebellum. Brain Res 105:365-371
Spoerri PE (1987) GABA-mediated developmental alterations in cultured neurons In: Redburn DA, Schousboe A (eds.): "Neurotrophic Activity of GABA During Development", New York: Alan R. Liss, Inc., in press
Spoerri PE, Wolff JR (1981) Effect of GABA-administration on murine neuroblastoma cells in culture. Cell Tiss Res 218:567-579
Stone TW (1979) Glutamate as the neurotransmitter of cerebellar granule cells in the rat: Electrophysiological evidence. Int J Pharmacol 66:291-296
Sturman JA, Moretz RL, French JH, Wisniewski HM (1985) Taurine deficiency in the developing cat: persistence of the cerebellar external granule layer. Prog Clin Biol Res 179:47-52

Sykes C, Prestwich S, Horton R (1984) Chronic administration of the GABA-transaminase inhibitor ethanol amine O-sulphate leads to up-regulation of GABA binding sites. Biochem Pharmacol 33:387-393

Wang Y-J, Salvaterra P, Roberts E (1979) Characterization of $^{3}$H-muscimol binding to mouse brain membranes. Biochem Pharmacol 28:1123-1128

Wolff JR, Joo F, Dames W (1978) Plasticity in dendrites shown by continuous GABA administration in superior cervical ganglion of adult rat. Nature Lond 274:72-74

Young AB, Oster-Granite ML, Herndon RM, Snyder SH (1974) Glutamic acid: Selective depletion by viral induced granule cell loss in hamster cerebellum. Brain Res 73: 1-13

# ADAPTIVE CHANGES IN AN ANIMAL MODEL OF MICRO-ENCEPHALY

F. Cattabeni, D. Cocchi*, M. Cimino, M. Di Luca, L. Mennuni, P. Zaratin and M.P. Abbracchio.

Institute of Pharmacological Sciences, School of Pharmacy, and
*Department of Pharmacology, School of Medicine
University of Milano,
Italy.

## INTRODUCTION

As a result of pre-natal or early post-natal exposure to a variety of agents (viruses, irradiation and cytotoxins) humans may develop microencephaly, characterized by reduction of brain size (Crome & Stern, 1967), with different involvement of selective brain regions depending on the type of agent and duration of exposure. Since neurons in different brain areas undergo their final division at quite distinct times during C.N.S. development, interference with neurogenesis will result in different kinds of brain lesions, strictly depending upon time of the insult, being actively dividing cells more affected than differentiated neurons. This mechanism is at the base of the neuronal lesions induced perinatally by cytotoxic agents such as hydroxy-urea, 5-azacytidine and methyl-azoxy-methanol acetate (MAM), which selectively interfere with DNA synthesis (Jonhston & Coyle, 1982). As a consequence of these lesions, the developing and maturing brain seems to undergo a series of adaptive changes not yet fully characterized, and whose consequences are totally unknown.

We describe here an animal model of microencephaly induced by

---

Reprints requests: F.C., Inst. Pharm. Sci., Via Balzaretti 9, 20133 Milano, Italy.

NATO ASI Series, Vol. H22
Neural Development and Regeneration
Edited by A. Gorio et al.

prenatal administration of MAM, and some of the neurochemical adaptive changes observed in the brain areas affected.

In our opinion, this animal model might become an interesting and useful tool to investigate the trophic relationships existing between neurons in the CNS, and to study the long term consequences of interferences with normal neuronal developmental patterns.

## I. Time and dose-dependency of MAM-induced micro-encephaly

Methyl-azoxy-methanol is the aglicone of the naturally occuring glucoside cycasin present in seeds, roots and leaves of plants belonging to the Cycadaceae family. The presence of this compound in the diet of populations indigenous to tropical islands in the Pacific area has been associated with an increased incidence of neurological disorders (amiotrophic lateral sclerosis and Parkinsonian dementia, Kurland, 1972).

Although this association has not been established with certainty, this hypothesis has lead to an intensive investigation of the neurological consequences of MAM administration to experimental animals during pregnancy. In rats, treatment on different gestational days induces reductions of brain size characterized by involvement of different brain areas, and, within the same area, of different neuronal populations.

For example, in cortex, MAM effects closely reflect the neurogenetic timetables of cortical layers (Johnston & Coyle, 1982). According to the theory of the inside-out formation of cortex, neuronal elements originating deeper layers divide in the germinal zone and migrate outwards before neurons generating more superficial layers (Angevine & Sidman, 1961). Therefore, treatment with MAM at day 13 of gestation induces hypoplasia of cortical inner layers, whereas reduction of cortex produced by administrátion of the antimitotic agent at day 14 or 15 is characterized by major neuronal losses in layers II-IV, with relative preservation of deeper neurons (Jonhston et al., 1981). Accordingly, treatment at day 17 of gestation produces significantly less pronounced neuronal losses, being almost all cortical neurons completely differentiated at this time.

This time-dependency of MAM effects is also evident for neuroblasts originating intrinsic neurons of other cerebral areas, such as n. striatum and hippocampus showing marked reductions after MAM administration at day 15 of gestation. It is therefore evident that MAM has minimal effects on neuroblasts in Go phase or on post-mitotic neuroblasts, as also shown by the absence of effects on cerebellum after administration at day 15 of gestation (Johnston & Coyle, 1982). It is instead possible to interfere with cerebellar development by administering MAM to newborn rats during the first weeks of life (a time when cerebellar interneurons undergo their final division).

The effects of MAM are dose-dependent, as shown in Fig. 1. Selective

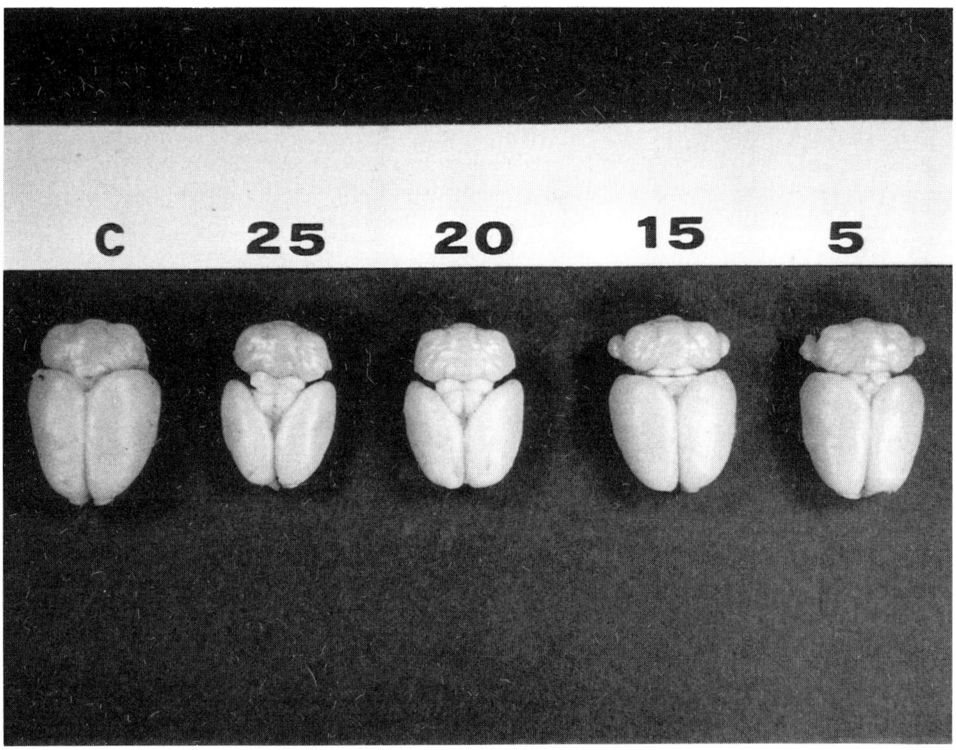


Fig. 1. Reduction in brain size induced by intraperitoneal administration of different doses (5, 15, 20 and 25 mg/Kg) of MAM at day 15 of gestation. Animals were 10 weeks old at time of sacrifice.

and significant reductions were observed in cortex, hippocampus and n. striatum for 25 and 15 mg/Kg, whereas the dose of 5 mg/Kg is not affecting the weight of these brain regions (Tab. 1).

**TABLE 1**

**WEIGHTS OF SELECTED BRAIN REGIONS OF RATS PRENATALLY EXPOSED TO MAM**

| mg | TREATMENT (at day 15 of gestation) | | | |
|---|---|---|---|---|
| | | MAM | | |
| | SALINE | 5 mg/Kg | 15 mg/Kg | 25 mg/Kg |
| Cortex | 807.0 $\pm$ 54.5 | 788.0 $\pm$ 50.8 | 545.0 $\pm$ 64.2** | 301.0 $\pm$ 77.8°° |
| Hippocampus | 87.9 $\pm$ 1.4 | 104.8 $\pm$ 12.1 | 77.7 $\pm$ 2.16** | 45.7 $\pm$ 6.87°° |
| N. striatum | 90.7 $\pm$ 0.7 | 94.0 $\pm$ 9.5 | 77.3 $\pm$ 3.7** | 49.0 $\pm$ 6.6°° |
| Cerebellum | 277.0 $\pm$ 25 | 290.0 $\pm$ 17 | 265.0 $\pm$ 18 | 255.0 $\pm$ 29 |

Values are mean $\pm$ S.E. (n= 3).
**$p < 0.05$ (Student's "t" test)
°°$p < 0.01$ (Student's "t" test).

In MAM treated rats, cerebral areas which should not be affected by administration of the antimitotic agent at gestational day 15 (e.g., pons-medulla and cerebellum) did not show any significant weight difference with respect to controls (Tab. 1). It must be also noted that the treated animals do not show any body weight decrease with respect to controls at 2 months of age.

In order to analyze the functional trophic relationships existing between neurons and between neurons and glia, morphological, neurochemical and behavioural parameters should be studied longitudinally.

## II. Adaptive changes in MAM rats.

MAM-induced micro-encephaly in adult animals is not only due to differences in brain size at birth, but also results from an earlier growth arrest of the brain (Fig. 2). This is probably also due to the fact that

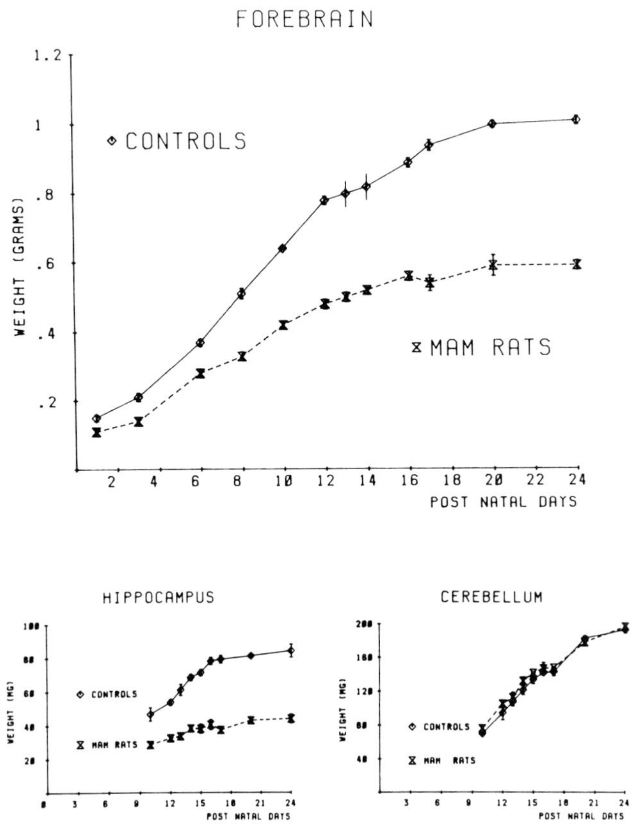


**Fig. 2.** Postnatal growth curves of forebrain, hippocampus and cerebellum in control rats and in the offspring of dams treated at gestational day 15 with 25 mg/Kg MAM. Results represent the mean $\pm$ S.E. of 5 animals for each time point.

the astrocytic development adjusts in response to the changed neuronal environment. Indeed, the density of astrocytic structures is similar to controls in MAM rats, and their morphology is normal in all the structures affected (Eriksdotter-Nilsson et al., 1986), suggesting that the number of astrocytes is not predetermined, but is probably dependent upon the size of the intrinsic neuronal population. No detailed studies are available on the degree of myelination in MAM rats. Matsutani et al. (1980) have reported that in these animals the activity of 2',3'-cyclic nucleotide 3'-phosphohydrolase, a marker for cerebral myelination, is not changed in the affected areas, when results are expressed as Units/mg protein. This of course indicates a decrease of total activity proportional to the reduction of brain weight. Such a result therefore suggests that a lower number of oligodendroglia is formed during post-natal myelination in MAM rats, probably due to the reduced amount of neuronal processes to envelop in hypoplastic brain regions, and accounting for the observed growth arrest in the affected areas (Fig. 2).

Another consequence of the reduced number of intrinsic neurons is the local hyperinnervation occurring in hypoplastic brain regions receiving axonal projections from other non-affected cerebral areas. This is particularly evident for aminergic afferents to cerebral cortex in rats treated with MAM at day 15 of gestation (Johnston & Coyle, 1982). In fact, at this time, noradrenergic neuroblasts in locus coeruleous have already undergone their final division and they originate a normal quantity of axonal arbors to the hypoplastic cortex, with a consequent local hyper-innervation. In rats prenatally treated with MAM, a similar condition is observed in the hypoplastic n. striatum receiving intact afferents from perikarya of nigral dopaminergic neurons (Beaulieu & Coyle, 1981). These findings are rather interesting, since they demonstrate that the quantitative aspects of axonal development are not influenced by loss of neurons in the target field, suggesting a growth independency of afferent fibers from the integrity of the innervated area. This is strikingly different from what is observed in periphery, where axons appear to adjust their terminal projections to fit the innervated field, and would suggest that in the CNS the quantitative aspects of terminal development are rather rigidly pre-programmed.

This local hyperinnervation induces a number of adaptive changes both on morphological, neurochemical and functional parameters. Morphometric analysis of neurons in cortical sections of rats prenatally treated with different doses of MAM showed that the observed dose-dependent reduction of cell number per section is accompanied by a proportional increase of mean

TABLE 2

**MORPHOMETRIC ANALYSIS OF NEURONAL CELLS IN CORTICAL SECTIONS OF RATS RECEIVING DIFFERENT DOSES (MG/KG) OF MAM AT DAY 15 OF EMBRYONIC LIFE**

| | n. of cells/section | cell surface increase (%) |
|---|---|---|
| Controls | 1157 ± 12 | 0 |
| MAM 20 | 735 ± 11[1] | + 31 |
| MAM 25 | 579 ± 9[1,2] | + 66 |

[1] $p < 0.001$ with respect to controls

[2] $p < 0.01$ with respect to MAM 20

Morphometric analysis was performed on a TAS-Leitz apparatus

cell surface (Tab. II). This probably reflects an adaptation of surviving neurons to the local increase of afferent terminals.

Also from a biochemical point of view, there are evidences supporting the occurence of adaptive changes in cortical neurons of MAM-rats. Due to MAM-induced noradrenergic hyperinnervation, cortical beta-adrenoreceptors are down-regulated, and are not subject to additional down-regulation with chronic antidepressant treatment, whereas they normally respond to situations inducing up-regulation, such as treatment with 6-hydroxy-dopamine (Beaulieu & Coyle, 1982).

Compensatory mechanisms also develop in hypoplastic corpus striatum of MAM rats receiving intact afferents from DAergic nigral neurons.

Studies conducted in our laboratory (Balduini et al., 1984) showed a reduction of dopamine-dependent adenylate cyclase activity in n. striatum of micro-encephalic MAM rats. Michaelis-Menten kinetic analysis of the decreased response to dopamine (DA) did not reveal any significant difference in either the apparent affinity of the enzyme for its substrate (km), or the maximal velocity of adenylate cyclase activity (Vmax), suggesting that this effect was not due to alterations in the properties of the enzyme, but probably to a reduction of the total amount of the enzyme itself. Measurement of $^{3}$H-Spiroperidol binding showed a 30% reduction of DAergic receptors in hypoplastic striata of MAM rats; this reduction was not due to decreases of DAergic $D_2$ receptors present on cortico-striatal glutamatergic fibers, since kainic acid, monolaterally injected in c. striatum, retained its neurotoxic activity. Since $^{3}$H-Spiroperidol in striatum labels both $D_1$ and $D_2$ receptors, on the bases of the DA-dependent cyclase reduction and of the retention of kainic acid neurotoxic effect, we concluded that only neurons intrisic to striatum and bearing DAergic $D_1$ -cyclase-linked receptors were affected by gestational MAM administration (Balduini et al., 1984). These conclusions later found a pharmacological counterpart in subsequent studies performed by other authors. Sanberg et al. (1985) demonstrated that the increased activity of striatal tyrosine hydroxylase (consistent with a relative increase in the density of DAergic terminals) is accompanied by a reduced response to DA agonists and antagonists. In fact, the administration of the DA receptor agonist apomorphine or of the receptor antagonist haloperidol produced less stereotypy and catalepsy, respectively, suggesting a loss of striatal perikarya induced by gestational MAM.

It therefore seems that, similarly to ß-receptor down-regulation in hyperinnervated cortex of MAM rats, also DAergic receptors in c. striatum are reduced in response to the increased local nigro-striatal input. We have later confirmed the reduced activity of striatal $D_1$ receptors from a functional point of view with behavioural data (Balduini et al., 1986). We showed that MAM rats display a reduced response to pharmacological agents known to increase locomotor activity, either through an agonistic activity on DAergic striatal receptors (apomorphine), or through an indirect action mediated by the release of DA from its terminals (amphetamine). We also showed that subsensitivity of DAergic receptors in adult MAM rats develops as an adaptive mechanism which takes place in the neuronal circuitry in the striatum of these animals (Balduini et al., 1986). A few day after the onset of DAergic activity in the striatum (21 days of age) MAM rats show an increase of spontaneous motility which is paralleled by increments of striatal levels of DOPAC (3,4-dihydroxy-phenyl-acetic-acid), the DA metabolite reflecting DAergic functional activity. This initial hyperactivity, which is a likely consequence of striatal hyperinnervation, is no longer present in adult MAM rats (60 days of age), when DOPAC levels in striatum are back to control values and $D_1$ receptors are downregulated.

Despite the above described compensatory mechanisms, MAM rats show deficits in behavioural tests normally taken as measures of learning and memory such as passive avoidance (Cannon-Spoor and Freed, 1984; Vorhees et al., 1984) and several kinds of mazes (Haddad et al., 1969; Lee et al., 1982; Banfi et al., 1984; Mohammed et al., 1986). The effects induced by MAM on learning and memory are dose-dependent, as shown by results obtained by us on the adult offspring (2 months of age) of dams treated at gestational day 15 with 5, 15 and 25 mg/Kg MAM and subjected to evaluation of passive avoidance and to a water-maze test.

In the passive avoidance test, rats have been tested for avoidance latencies 1 and 24 h after the session where the unescapable foot-shock was given, and the number of amnestic animals has been recorded. Performances of animals 1 h after the training session are generally taken as an index of learning abilities, whereas results at 24 h are thought to mainly reflect memorization. As shown in fig. 3, a dose-dependent effect of MAM was observed. At 1 h, only 25 mg/Kg MAM rats behaved differently from controls in a statistically significant manner; at 24 h, statistically significant differences were observed also in rats treated with the intermediate dose of antimitotic, suggesting that MAM affects memorization more than learning processes.

The different behaviour of MAM rats when compared to controls in this test cannot be due to modifications of spontaneous motor activity (see this chapter) or to alterations of the pain threshold in these animals. In fact,

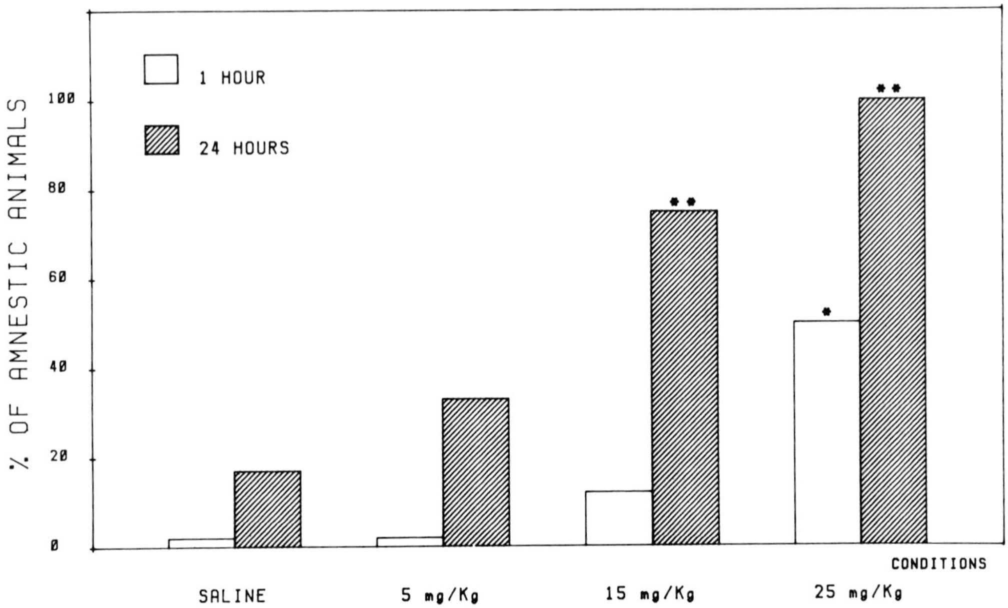


**Fig. 3.** Passive avoidance test in control animals and in rats prenatally treated with graded doses of MAM. The test was performed according to Lo Conte et al., 1982. Data are expressed as percent of amnestic animals. Rats (n= 12) were trained in one trial passive avoidance task. The retest was carried out 1 h or 24 h after the training (*$p < 0.05$; **$p < 0.01$, $\chi^2$ test versus controls).

performances of MAM rats in two tests classically used to measure pain sensitivity (tail flick and hot plate tests) were practically identical to those of control animals (Panerai, Personal Communication).

In the water-maze test, rats treated with the two higher doses of MAM performed significantly worse than control animals (Tab. 3), as shown by the higher number of errors during learning sessions.

## III. Future perspectives

On the bases of the above reviewed results, several interesting issues can be addressed for future research investigations on MAM-induced micro-encephaly. One first important point concerns the adaptive mechanisms taking place in the brains of micro-encephalic animals, as a consequence of the lesion induced during CNS development. We have shown how this

TABLE 3

WATER MAZE TEST IN RATS PRENATALLY EXPOSED TO MAM ACETATE

| TREATMENT | SESSION NUMBER | | | | | | | |
|---|---|---|---|---|---|---|---|---|
| | 1 | 2 | 3 | 4 | 5 | 6 | 7 | 8 |
| | NUMBER OF ERRORS DURING THE LEARNING SESSION | | | | | | | |
| Saline | 15.6 ± 1.7 | 8.9 ± 2.2 | 2.6 ± 0.7 | 2.0 ± 0.4 | 2.2 ± 0.4 | 3.0 ± 0.8 | 0.6 ± 0.2 | 1.9 ± 0.6 |
| MAM | | | | | | | | |
| 5 mg/Kg | 15.7 ± 1.2 | 4.6 ± 1.1 | 6.7 ± 1.7 | 3.2 ± 1.1 | 2.2 ± 0.8 | 1.7 ± 0.6 | 2.5 ± 1.5 | 1.5 ± 0.6 |
| 15 mg/Kg | 15.5 ± 1.7 | 11.2 ± 2.5 | 7.8 ± 1.3** | 5.9 ± 1.6* | 4.6 ± 2.2 | 2.6 ± 0.8 | 3.3 ± 1.7* | 1.4 ± 0.4 |
| 25 mg/Kg | 18.7 ± 2.4 | 18.8 ± 3.5* | 14.0 ± 3.6*** | 7.7 ± 2.0** | 4.5 ± 1.1 | 8.5 ± 2.5 | 5.1 ± 1.5*** | 2.9 ± 0.4 |

The test was performed according to Giurgea and Mouravieff-Lesuisse (1972). Each animal was given 2 trials/day for 4 consecutive days. Errors and time/trial were recorded. Values are mean ± S.E. (n= 12).

*$p < 0.05$ versus saline treated rats (Mann-Whitney test)
**$p < 0.02$ versus saline treated rats (Mann-Whitney test)
***$p < 0.002$ versus saline treated rats (Mann-Whitney test).

micro-encephaly also results from a growth arrest occuring during the very first weeks of postnatal life, when myelination and astroglia formation occur, suggesting that the number of glial cells in brain is not predetermined but is strictly dependent upon the intrinsic neuronal population (Eriksdotter-Nilsson et al., 1986, Matsutani et al., 1980). Also, we have here reviewed the morphological and neurochemical adaptive changes occurring in surviving neurons, as a consequence of the local hyperinnervation at the level of hypoplastic areas. Therefore, as anticipated in the Introduction, MAM animals might represent a valuable model to study the relationships existing between different cell types in the CNS, and to investigate how the developing brain responds to exogenous factors disrupting the normal establishment of neuron-neuron and neuron-glia interactions. In this respect, it is interesting to mention a preliminary result, recently obtained in our laboratory, when measuring somatostatin levels in the hypoplastic cortex of MAM rats. At 2 months of age, the levels of this peptide are reduced after gestational administration of the antimitotic agent (25 mg/Kg), and such a reduction is evident not only when results are expressed as total amount of neuropeptide, but also in terms of peptide concentration. This is a quite unusual situation in the hypoplastic cortex of MAM rats, since, for all the other systems of interneurons, neurotransmitter decreases are proportional to the reduction of cortical mass. In fact, as schematized in Fig. 4, two different types of neurotransmitter situations have been so far described in the cortex of MAM rats. For projections from subcortical unaffected areas (e.g., monoaminergic terminals originating from locus coeruleus), being the quantity of afferent fibers independent from the number of neurons in the target region, the total amount of neurotransmitter in the hypoplastic cortex of MAM rats is not decreased it compared to age-matched controls and therefore its concentration is increased. On the contrary, for intrinsic neurons differentiating at the time of antimitotic administration (e.g., GABAergic interneurons), the number of neuronal cells is reduced in parallel to the reduction of cortex size, so that the total amount of neurotransmitter is decreased but its concentration remains comparable to that of control cortex (Fig. 4). Somatostatin levels, instead, are reduced not only as total amount of peptide, but also in terms of peptide concentration (Fig.

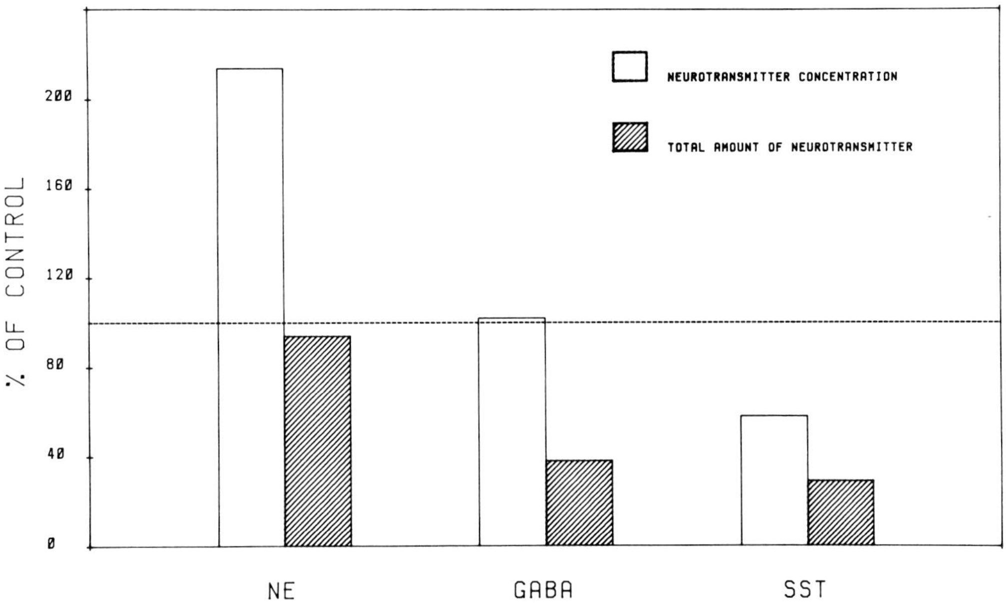


**Fig. 4.** Cortical levels of norepinephrine (NE), $\gamma$ -amino-butyric acid (GABA) and somatostatin (SST) in rats prenatally treated with MAM (25 mg/Kg). Measurements of NE and GABA levels have been performed according to Koslow et al. 1972 and to Cattabeni et al. 1976, respectively. SST levels have been measured with radio-immuno-assay according to Petraglia et al. 1983.

4), suggesting that this decrease cannot be exclusively attributed to a loss of somatostatinergic neurons parallel to the reduction of the cortical mass, but that some other functional modification is occuring at the level of this interneuron population. Experiments are now in progress in our laboratory to ascertain whether this reduction is due to modifications in the synthesis of this peptide, also in view of the hypothesized interrelationships between cortical somatostatinergic neurons and cholinergic afferents to the cortex. It has been indeed postulated that in dementias of the Alzheimer type, the degeneration of cholinergic neurons located to n. basalis of Meynert could be the result of alterations of some kind of "trophic" interactions between their cortical afferents and somatostatinergic interneurons in the target area. Recent findings suggest that the primary defect in Alzheimer patients could be a functional modification of somatostatinergic cortical neurons eventually leading to a retrograde degeneration of cholinergic afferents (Roberts et al., 1985; Morrison et. al., 1985).

Being somatostatin levels reduced in the cortex of MAM rats, it would be very interesting to assess whether, in the long run, these animals show precocius degeneration of cholinergic neurons in n. basalis of Meynert, and whether this can be related to the reduced learning and memory abilities of these animals. The answer to this question also concerns a second important issue in future investigations on MAM-induced micro-encephaly, that is the evaluation of the long-term consequences of MAM interference with neuronal developmental patterns. In other words, will the adaptive changes occurring in the brain of micro-encephalic animals compensate for the neuronal damage for the rest of the life of these animals? Will the undamaged afferent fibers to cortex be kept in place by a sustained release of trophic factors produced by the surviving cells in the target area? And, if this is so, will these target cortical neurons be always able to produce a sufficient amount of these factors? We do not have the answers yet, but some preliminary data indicate that, after the second month of life, the compensatory mechanisms in MAM-rats start failing. For example, for cortical monoaminergic fibers, in preliminary experiments we have observed a decrease of norepinephrine markers at 4 months of age, indicating perhaps that noradrenergic afferents start to degenerate, maybe due to "exhaustion" of trophic factors. Delucidation of these points in the near future will help to verify whether MAM-rats can represent an useful model for neuro-degenerative disorders and could shed light inside the complex and fascinating mechanisms regulating neuronal aging and plasticity.

## AKNOWLEDGEMENTS

This work was partially supported by the National Research Council (CNR), Target Project "Preventive Medicine and Riabilitation", Sub-project "Toxicological Risk", Contract No. 86.01715.56, and by the Regione Lombardia, Progetti di Ricerca Finalizzati nel Settore Sanitario (Project.

n. 397).

Authors are grateful to Miss S. Giovannazzi and R. Pacchioni for technical help, and to Miss S. Scattolon and M. Zamati for typing the manuscript.

## REFERENCES

Angevine JB, Sidman RL (1961) Autoradiographic study of cell migration during histogenesis of cerebral cortex in the mouse. Nature 192: 766-768

Balduini W, Abbracchio MP, Lombardelli G, Cattabeni F (1984). Loss of intrinsic striatal neurons after methyl-azoxy-methanol acetate treatment in pregnant rats. Dev Brain Res 15: 133-136

Balduini W, Cimino M, Lombardelli G, Abbracchio MP, Peruzzi G, Cecchini T, Gazzanelli GC, Cattabeni F (1986) Micro-encephalic rats as a model for cognitive disorders. Clin Neuropharmacol 9(3): S8-18

Banfi S, Dorigotti L, Abbracchio MP, Balduini W, Coen E, Ragusa C, Cattabeni F (1984) Methyl-azoxy-methanol micro-encephaly in rats: neurochemical characterization and behavioral studies with the nootropic oxiracetam. Pharmacol Res Comm 16(1): 67-83

Beaulieu M, Coyle JT (1981) Effects of fetal methyl-azoxy-methanol acetate lesion on the synaptic neurochemistry of the adult rat striatum. J Neurochem 37(4): 878-887

Beaulieu M, Coyle JT (1982) Fetally-induced noradrenergic hyperinnervation of cerebral cortex results in persistent down-regulation of beta-receptors. Dev Brain Res 4: 491-494

Cannon-Spoor EH, Freed WJ (1984) Hyperactivity induced by prenatal administration of methyl-azoxy-methanol: association with altered performance on conditioning tasks in rats. Pharmacol Biochem and Behavior 20: 189-193

Cattabeni F, Galli CL, Eros T (1976) A simple and highly sensitive mass-fragmentographic procedure for $\gamma$ -aminobutyricacid determinations. Anal Biochem 72: 1-7

Crome L, Stern J (1967) The pathology of mental retardation, Churchill, London

Eriksdotter-Nilsson M, Jonsson G, Dahl D, Bjorklund H (1986) Stroglial development in microencephalic rat brain after fetal methyl-azoxy-methanol treatment. J Devl Neurosci 4(4); 353-362

Giurgea C, Mouravieff-LeSuisse F (1972) Effect facilitateur du piracetam sur un apprentissage repetitif chez le rat. J. Pharmacol 3(1): 17-30

Haddad RK, Rabe A, Laquer GL, Spatz M, Valsamis MP (1969) Intellectual deficit associated with transplacentally induced microcephaly in the rat. Science 163: 88-90

Johnston MV, Carman AB, Coyle JT (1981) Effects of fetal treatment with methyl-azoxy-methanol acetate at various gestational dates on the neurochemistry of the adult neocortex of the rat. J Neurochem 36(1): 124-128

Johnston MV, Coyle JT (1982) Cytotoxic lesion and the development of transmitter systems. TINS May: 153-156

Koslow SH, Cattabeni F, Costa E (1972) Norepinephrine and dopamine: assay by mass-fragmentography in the picomole range. Science 176: 177-180

Kurland LT (1972) An appraisal of the neurotoxicity of cycad and the etiology of amiotrophic lateral sclerosis on Guam. Fed Proc 31(5): 1540-1542

Lee MH, Haddad R, Rabe A (1982) Impaired learning of the Lasheley II maze by rats with chemically induced micrencephaly. Teratol 25: 58-59

Lo Conte G, Bartolini L, Casamenti F, Marconcini-Pepeu I, Pepeu G (1982) Lesions of cholinergic forebrain nuclei: changes in avoidance behaviour and scopolamine actions. Pharmacol Biochem & Behavior 17: 933-937

Matsutani T, Nagayoshi M, Tamaru M, Tsukada Y (1980) Elevated monoamine levels in the cerebral hemispheres of microencephalic rats treated prenatally with methyl-azoxy-methanol or cytosine arabinoside. J Neurochem 34(4): 950-956

Mohammed AK, Jonsson G, Sundstrom E, Minor BG, Soderberg U, Archer T (1986) Selective attention and place navigation in rats treated prenatally with methyl-azoxy-methanol. Dev Brain Res 30: 145-155

Morrison JH, Rogers J, Scherr S, Benoit R, Bloom FE (1985) Somatostatin immunoreactivity in neuritic plaques of Alzheimer's patients. Nature 314: 90-92

Petraglia F, Locatelli V, Peñalva A, Cocchi D, Genazzani AR, Müller EE (1984) Gonadal steroid modulation of naloxone-induced LH secretion in the rat. J Endocr 101: 33-39

Roberts GW, Crow TJ, Polak JM (1985) Location of neuronal tangles in somatostatin neurons in Alzheimer's disease. Nature 314: 92-94

Sanberg PR, Pevsner J, Antuono PG, Coyle JT (1985) Fetal methyl-azoxy-methanol acetate-induced lesions cause reductions in dopamine receptor-mediated catalepsy and stereotypy. Neuropharmacol 24(11): 1057-1062

Vorhees CV, Fernandez K, Dumas RM, Haddad RK (1984) Pervasive hyperactivity and long-term learning impairments in rats with induced micrencephaly from prenatal exposure to methyl-azoxy-methanol. Dev Brain Res 15: 1-10

# T H E M E   II

# MECHANISMS OF GENE EXPRESSION

## Theme II - INTRODUCTION

The now routine application of recombinant DNA techniques to developmental neurobiology has allowed for the precise determination of the molecular participants and processes involved in the regulation of gene expression in the nervous system. From xenobiotic responses to oncogene products and cell lineage expression, it has become possible to use appropriate DNA probes in order to dissect events on chromosomes as well as demonstrate direct interactions between regulator molecules and specific genomic sites that determine gene expression. The significance of these findings to neuropathology and regeneration is just beginning to emerge as the regulation of the expression of myelin protein or of nerve growth factor receptors has become amenable to direct chemical manipulation at the genomic level. This is particularly true for Alzheimer's and other neurodegenerative diseases where genetic components were already suspected. More active intervensions are likely to become possible in other aspects of trauma and disease of the nervous system.

# CELL FATE AND GENE EXPRESSION IN THE DEVELOPING NEURAL CREST

D. J. Anderson
Division of Biology, 216-76
California Institute of Technology
Pasadena, CA 91125 USA

Our laboratory has been interested in the cellular and molecular mechanisms that govern the way cells choose their developmental fates during embryonic neurogenesis. We have focused on the differentiation of a subset of neural crest derivatives: the endocrine (chromaffin) cells of the adrenal medulla, and the principal noradrenergic neurons of the sympathetic ganglia (LeDouarin, 1982). Previous studies have suggested that environmental signals, such as Nerve Growth Factor (NGF) and glucocorticoids (GC), may play an important role in the development of these two cell types (Aloe and Levi-Montalcini, 1979). In particular, apparently mature chromaffin cells are able to convert into cells phenotypically indistinguishable from sympathetic neurons, when cultured in the presence of NGF and absence of GC (Unsicker et al., 1978; Ogawa et al., 1984; Lillien and Claude, 1985; Doupe et al., 1985a,b). We now wish to account for this plasticity in terms of the developmental history of these cells. Do sympathetic neurons and chromaffin cells in fact share a common embryonic progenitor? What is the phenotype of this progenitor? How much of this progenitor's ultimate fate is controlled by its earlier history, and how much by its immediate environment? What environmental factors control this decision, and how do they work?

In order to begin to address these questions, we have used antibodies and specific cloned sequences as molecular markers to identify developing cells in embryo sections and in primary cultures. In particular, we have used a differential screening strategy to isolate cDNA clones complementary to mRNAs expressed by sympathetic neurons but not chromaffin cells (Anderson and Axel, 1985). Using these markers, we first asked at what stage in the development of this lineage

NATO ASI Series, Vol. H22
Neural Development and Regeneration.
Edited by A. Gorio et al.

these genes first become expressed. Northern blot and *in situ* hybridization analysis indicated that none of our markers is specifically expressed by premigratory, or even migrating, neural crest cells. Rather, these genes first become expressed at the time cells begin to coalesce into the sympathetic ganglion primordia (Anderson and Axel, 1985). A similar pattern of expression has been observed previously for other phenotypic markers, such as tyrosine hydroxylase (TH) (Cochard et al., 1979) and neurofilament (Cochard and Paulin, 1984).

**A Transient Population of Neuronal Precursors in the Embryonic Adrenal Gland**

Some of the cells which initially populate the developing sympathetic ganglia (on or about E12 in the rat) undergo a secondary migration over the next 48 hr, and invade the mesodermally-derived adrenocortical primordium (Fig. 1). If the chromaffin cells of the adrenal derive from the same precursor as sympathetic neurons, we might expect that the population of crest cells invading the adrenal early in embryogenesis would initially express neural-specific genes.

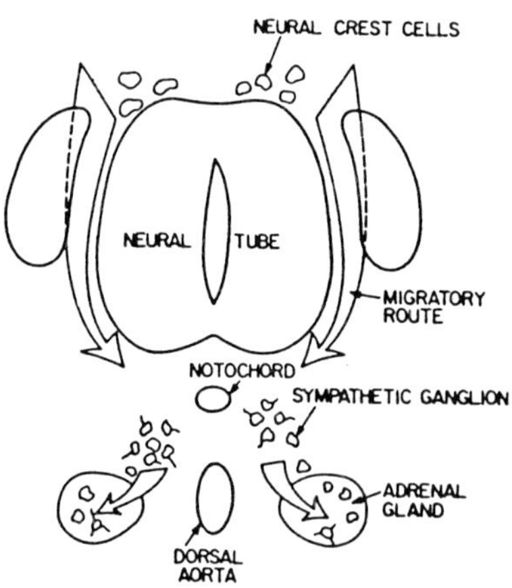


Fig. 1. Schematic indicating the migratory route taken by cells in the sympathoadrenal lineage.

We found that the embryonic adrenal gland is in fact transiently populated by cells expressing two independent neural-specific markers: SCG10 and NF68. Expression of both markers follows a similar spatial pattern, whether detected by immunohistochemistry or by *in situ* hybridization. Expression is most intense at the medio-dorsal region of the gland, near the site where migrating progenitor cells first invade the adreno-cortical primordium (Fig. 2B,D; Anderson and Axel, 1986). SCG10 and NF68 both appear to label a subpopulation of the cells labeled with anti-TH (Fig. 2A,C), and this subpopulation appears to be distributed in a steep medial-lateral gradient within the gland.

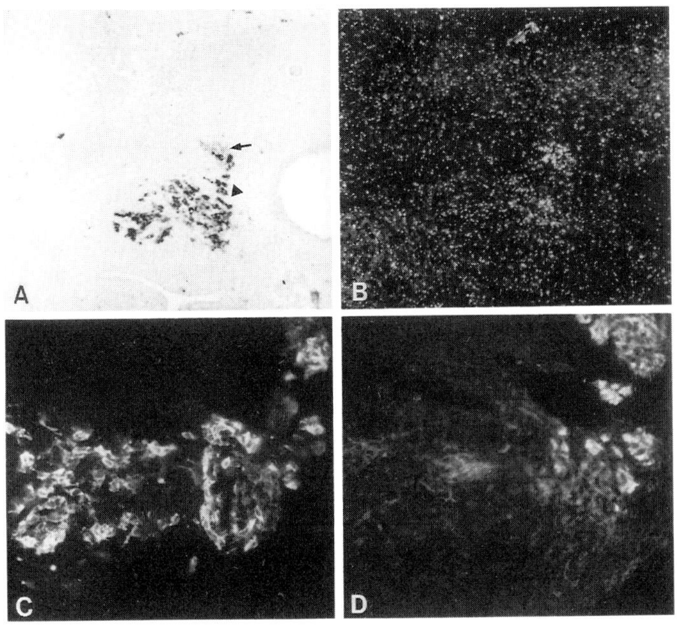


Fig. 2. Expression of SCG10 mRNA (B) and protein (D) in the E14.5 adrenal gland. Adjacent serial sections are stained for TH by immunoperoxidase (A) or immunofluorescence (C). Arrow: sympathetic ganglion; arrowhead: point of entry of invading precursors (A).

Double-labeling of freshly-dissociated suspensions of embryonic adrenal cells confirmed that the neural-specific markers are indeed expressed by a subset of the $TH^+$ cells: at E14.5, fully 50% of the $TH^+$ cells are $NF68^+$. By performing this single-cell assay at different stages of development, we established that both the proportion and absolute number of $TH^+NF^+$ cells declines over the last two weeks of gestation. In a six week-old rat, expression of the neurofilament proteins in adrenal chromaffin cells _in situ_ is essentially below the level of detection of immunohistochemistry (Anderson and Axel, 1986; Trojanowski _et al._, 1986).

The observation that catecholaminergic cells expressing neural-specific markers transiently populate the embryonic adrenal medulla, raises the question of the developmental fate of these cells. Do these cells die, or do they develop into mature chromaffin cells? A series of in vitro experiments suggests the answer is both (Anderson and Axel, 1986). When E14.5 adrenal glands are placed in dissociated cell culture at moderate density, in the presence of the synthetic glucocorticoid dexamethasone (DEX), the $TH^+NF^+$ cells decline to a minority population within a few days (30%). In contrast, if DEX is omitted from the culture medium, the $TH^+NF^+$ cells rapidly become the predominant population (85%). Morphologic examination of these cultures indicates that the $TH^+NF^+$ cells have a neuron-like morphology, extending long processes (Fig. 3A,C). In contrast, the $TH^+NF^-$ cells that predominate in DEX-treated cultures have no neurites, and a rounded or flattened chromaffin-like morphology (Fig. 3B,D).

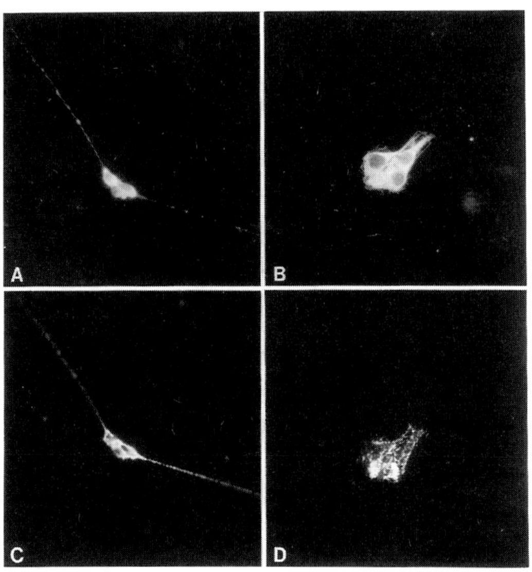


Fig. 3. Two types of $TH^+$ (A,B) cells develop in control medium (A,C) or in medium containing DEX (B,D). Both types are HNK-$1^+$ (C,D). Cells as in (B,D) were $NF^-$ (not shown).

Quantitative analysis of these cultures, as well as single-cell tracking experiments, suggest that some $TH^+NF^+$ cells can convert to $TH^+NF^-$ cells, under the influence of DEX. However, a significant fraction appear refractory to the influence of DEX. This finding was confirmed using cells isolated from the embryonic adrenal gland by fluorescence-activated cell sorting. We found that a cell-surface monoclonal antibody, B2 (J. Dodd, unpublished), exhibited a pattern of staining *in situ* virtually identical to that obtained using SCG10 and NF68 (Anderson and Axel, 1986). This antibody thus allowed us to isolate a subpopulation of $TH^+$ cells, of which 100% were expressing NF68 at high levels. When this population was cultured in the presence of DEX, a significant proportion of the cells (~30%) lost NF immunoreactivity, developed a rounded, chromaffin-like morphology and expressed the chromaffin-specific marker, PNMT. Since 100% of these cells expressed NF68 at the time of plating, it follows that many of these cells are able to extinguish the expression of this neural-specific marker under the influence of DEX, and convert to chromaffin cells.

The remainder of $B2^+$ cells appear refractory to the influence of DEX: despite the presence of steroid, they continue to extend neurites and then eventually die. We infer that these cells have developed further along the neuronal pathway than their DEX-responsive counterparts, to a point where they are unresponsive to glucocorticoids. Since at least some of these cells are NGF-dependent, this result suggests that, *in vivo*, those neuronal precursors that escape the action of steroid hormone should not survive in an adrenal environment lacking NGF. In this way, the presence of one hormone (GC) and the absence of another (NGF) control the phenotype of the emerging adrenal medullary population, through two distinct cellular mechanisms.

**Origin of $B2^+$ Cells: Necessary Precursors or Plastic Intermediate?**

The data described above suggest that both selection and phenotypic conversion underlie the gradual disappearance of neuronal precursors from the embryonic adrenal gland. This explanation, however, raises the question of what these cells were doing in the adrenal gland in the first place. Do all chromaffin cells necessarily pass through a $B2^+$ precursor state? Or are B2$^+$ cells a more developmentally restricted subpopulation, which still retains some plasticity?

At the earliest time we are able to dissect the adrenal gland (E14.5), B2$^+$ cells constitute about 30% of the total TH$^+$ adrenal population. Although the *in vitro* data unequivocally indicate that some of the B2$^+$ cells can be converted to TH$^+$NF$^-$ cells by DEX, this does not mean that *all* TH$^+$NF$^-$ cells obligatorily derive from B2$^+$ precursors. If this were the case, we would only expect to observe TH$^+$NF$^-$ cells within the adrenal gland, where the local GC concentration is high enough to convert B2$^+$ precursors. In fact, however, at early times, TH$^+$NF$^-$ cells can also be observed in the developing sympathetic ganglia (Fig. 4, E14.5). With ensuing development, the number of these cells declines dramatically in the ganglia while it increases steadily in the adrenal (D. Anderson and A. Michelsohn, unpublished observations). This population of cells can be distinguished by its intense immunoreactivity for TH, compared to B2$^+$ cells (Fig. 4), its lack of staining with B2, and its intense reactivity with a series of monoclonal antibodies that stain postnatal adrenal chromaffin cells, but not sympathetic neurons (J. Carnahan and P. H. Patterson, personal communication). Therefore, *in vivo*,

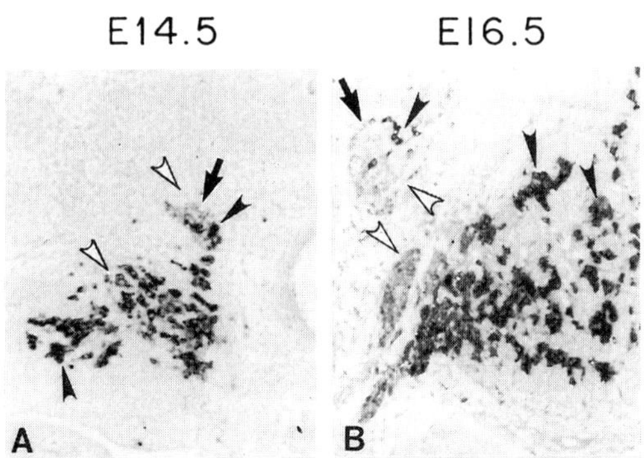


Fig. 4. TH$^+$NF$^-$ cells develop in early sympathetic ganglia. (A) Dark TH$^+$ cells (black arrow head) are clearly distinguishable from light TH$^+$ cells (white arrow head), in both the ganglia (arrow) and the adrenal, at E14.5. The dark TH$^+$ cells are usually NF$^-$ or only weakly NF$^+$. By E16.5 (B), only a few dark TH$^+$ cells remain in the ganglion (black arrow), while in the adrenal they predominate.

these $TH^+NF^-B2^-$ cells can apparently develop outside of the adrenal gland. Since _in vitro_ these cells can only be derived from $B2^+$ cells under the influence of DEX, it is difficult to imagine how _in vivo_ they could develop exclusively from such $B2^+$ precursors in the (presumably) steroid-poor sympathetic ganglia.

We therefore feel that _in vivo_, the $TH^+NF^-$ cells do not obligatorily develop from $B2^+$ precursors, but can be generated without passing through this transient state. If the $B2^+$ cell is not the fully bipotential progenitor, what is the phenotype of this cell? Recently, we have been able to isolate $B2^-$ precursors from the embryonic adrenal by sorting with the monoclonal antibody, HNK-1 (Abo and Balch, 1981). In contrast to $B2^+$ cells, most of which extend long neurites rapidly after plating (Fig. 5C,D), $B2^-HNK-1^+$ cells predominantly have short

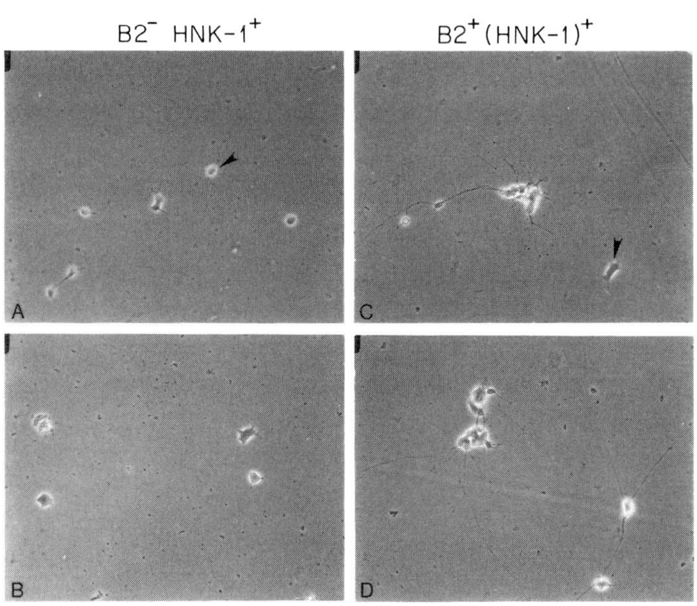


Fig. 5. Two types of precursor isolated by cell sorting. Cells isolated with B2 have extended long processes 24 hrs after plating (C,D); those isolated with HNK-1 from the $B2^-$ fraction are less developed (A,B), although with time these cells begin to extend processes as well (arrow, A). The $B2^+$ fraction contains a subpopulation which is less mature and still responsive to DEX (arrow, C).

processes or are round (Fig. 5A,B), although a small proportion do extend neurites (Fig. 5A, arrow). In the presence of DEX, virtually all of these cells survive and develop into chromaffin cells expressing PNMT (data not shown); therefore, these cells appear less committed to the neuronal pathway than their $B2^+$ counterparts. Consistent with this, only 35% of these $B2^-HNK\text{-}1^+$ cells are $NF^+$, and the NF68 staining is weak and diffuse. In the presence of NGF, however, virtually all of these cells develop into neurons (not shown). Therefore, this population of cells appears to be fully bipotential, and probably represents an earlier developmental stage than the $B2^+$ population.

If the $HNK\text{-}1^+$ $B2^-$ cells are indeed the true progenitors to both neurons and chromaffin cells (Fig. 6, $P_{CN}$), their appearance <u>in vivo</u> should developmentally precede the appearance of $B2^+$ cells. Experiments to address this prediction are now in progress. If this model proves to be correct, it suggests that the origin of $B2^+$ cells inside the E14.5 adrenal is in a subpopulation of migrating progenitors, which have begun to differentiate along the neuronal pathway prior to invading the adrenal primordium. The process of neuronal differentiation is sufficiently gradual, however, that some $B2^+$ cells (Fig. 6, $P_N$) are able to switch back to

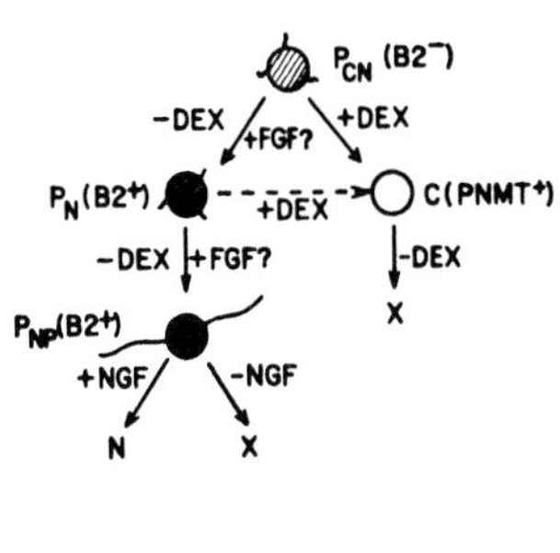


| Cell type | TH | B2 | HNK-1 | NF68 | SCG10 | PNMT | neurites | mitotic |
|---|---|---|---|---|---|---|---|---|
| $P_{CN}$ | ++ | − | + | +/− | +/− | − | − | + |
| $P_N$ | + | + | + | + | + | − | − | + |
| $P_{NP}$ | + | + | + | + | + | − | + | + |
| N | + | − | + | ++ | ++ | − | ++ | − |
| C | ++ | − | + | − | − | + | − | − (+) |

Fig. 6. Multiple stages of neuronal development defined by cell morphology and antigenic properties. "FGF?" indicates that recent data suggest the neuronal pathway may require FGF, or an FGF-like inducer. N = sympathetic neuron; C = chromaffin cell; X = cell death. $P_{NP}$ are committed neuronal precursors. Shading indicates level of SCG10/NF68 expression.

the chromaffin pathway under the influence of glucocorticoids, after they have entered the adrenal gland. The remainder (Fig. 6, $P_{NP}$) are committed neuronal precursors, most of which probably degenerate due to the absence of local NGF. If a small number of cells escaped this selection, they could provide the source of the subpopulation of ganglionic neurons which persist in the adult medulla. These neurons could not develop from $B2^-$ progenitors due to the inhibitory influence of GC. $B2^+$ cells, however, being committed neuronal precursors, would be insensitive to this GC inhibition. Thus, a relatively late lineal restriction would permit the development of phenotypic diversity in the face of a strong environmental influence. In this way, the asynchronous development of the migrating progenitor population may be exploited to generate cellular heterogeneity in the adrenal medulla.

**The Relationship of Chromaffin Cell Plasticity to Development**

Chromaffin cell plasticity is an unusual phenomenon, and raises the question of whether this process is fundamentally different from normal development, or simply a protracted extension thereof. The answer depends upon the way one views the chromaffin-neuron "decision." If, for example, one views it as a traditional "binary choice" (Raff _et al_., 1983) made by a bipotential progenitor, then the process of phenotypic conversion would necessarily involve a reversal of a developmental progression (Fig. 7A). If, on the other hand, one views the decision as the choice of whether or not to proceed along a linear pathway, where chromaffin cells are actually metastable neuronal "precursors," then the process of phenotypic conversion would not involve the recapitulation of an earlier developmental process, but simply the activation of the "next step" in a developmental program otherwise held in abeyance. An analogous dichotomy has faced those investigators studying limb regeneration (Kintner and Brockes, 1984). The branch model would be supported if chromaffin cells during their conversion could be shown to transiently express a marker normally present on embryonic precursors, but

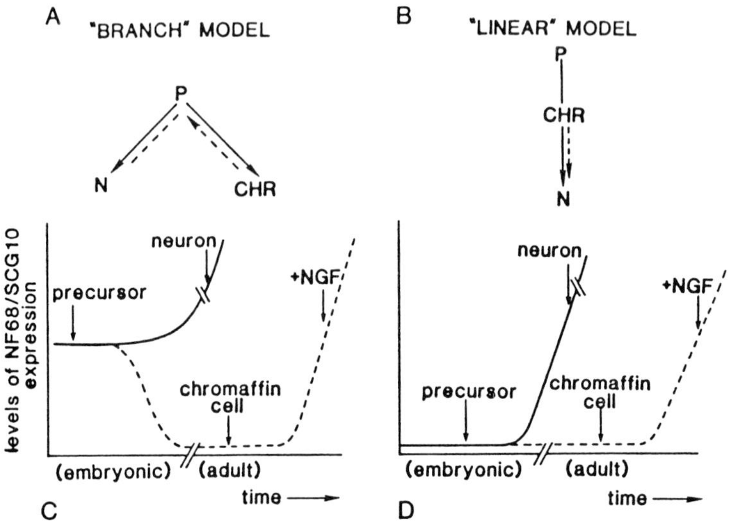


Fig. 7. "Branch" (A) and "linear" (B) models of the chromaffin-neuron decision. Solid arrows indicate developmental events; broken arrows indicate later phenotypic conversion (C,D): Mature chromaffin cells may suppress neural-specific gene expression from initially high levels (C), or simply maintain basal levels (D).

not on either chromaffin cells or sympathetic neurons. Such a marker, unfortunately, does not yet exist. Although the linear model is more consistent with the view of the related adrenergic-cholinergic conversion (Landis and Patterson, 1981; Landis and Keefe, 1983), the exclusive expression of the marker PNMT by mature chromaffin cells and not by sympathetic neurons or, apparently, their embryonic precursors, tends in our current view to support the branch model.

**The Molecular Basis of Chromaffin Cell Plasticity**

Chromaffin cells express a stable, endocrine phenotype, but are able to activate a program of neural-specific gene expression in response to an altered environment. We have shown that the developmental origin of this plasticity lies in the fact that chromaffin cells develop from a bipotential progenitor which begins to express neural-specific genes very early on, before choosing between the neuronal and endocrine pathways. Thus, the embryonic adrenal gland is transiently populated by cells expressing high levels of several neuronal markers. While many of these cells probably die, some of these neuronal precursors are sufficiently plastic to be diverted to the chromaffin pathway. We originally suggested that chromaffin cell plasticity might be due to a "memory" of this transient embryonic expression of neural-specific genes (Fig. 7C). However, it now seems possible that many chromaffin cells may develop without necessarily passing through a stage of high neural-specific gene expression (Fig. 6). In that case, plasticity could reflect simply the persistent, low-level expression of neural-specific genes which are initially activated at these basal levels in uncommitted progenitor cells (Fig. 7D). In support of this, we have recently found, by nuclear run-on experiments, that adult chromaffin cells maintain a basal level of neural-specific gene transcription. Thus, the persistence of the potential to express the neuronal phenotype, in chromaffin cells, lies in the maintenance of neural-specific genes in a transcriptionally competent, but highly suppressed state. This raises the question of whether this state is achieved through GC-mediated active repression, or through the absence of NGF-dependent inducers. The recent isolation of genomic sequences for SCG10, and the identification of potential regulatory elements therein (Stein _et al_., in preparation), now permits us to address this question. The answers to this and related issues may yield insights not only into fundamental mechanisms of development, but also of regeneration and plasticity in the adult nervous system.

## Acknowledgements

We thank R. Axel for his contributions to and support for the development of this project. Supported by NIH grant NS23476-01 and an NSF Presidental Young Investigator Award. We thank P. Patterson, J. Brockes, D. Stemple, and A. Michelsohn for helpful discussions.

## References

Abo T, Balch CM (1981) A differentiation antigen of human NK and K cells identified by a monoclonal antibody (HNK-1). J Immunol 127:1024-1029

Aloe L, Levi-Montalcini R (1979) Nerve growth factor-induced transformation of immature chromaffin cells in vivo into sympathetic neurons: effect of antiserum to nerve growth factor. Proc Natl Acad Sci USA 76:1246-1250

Anderson DJ, Axel R (1985) Molecular probes for the development and plasticity of neural crest derivatives. Cell 42:649-662

Anderson DJ, Axel R (1986) A bipotential neuroendocrine precursor whose choice of cell fate is determined by NGF and glucocorticoids. Cell 47:1079-1090

Cochard P, Goldstein M, Black I (1979) Initial development of the noradrenergic phenotype in automatic neuroblasts of the rat embryo in vivo. Dev Biol 71:100-114

Cochard P, Paulin D (1984) Initial expression of neurofilaments and vimentin in the central and peripheral nervous system of the mouse embryo in vivo. J Neurosci 4:2080-2094

Doupe AJ, Patterson PH, Landis SC (1985a) Environmental influences in the development of neural crest derivatives: glucocorticoids, growth factors and chromaffin cell plasticity. J Neurosci 5:2119-2142

Doupe AJ, Patterson PH, Landis SC (1985b) Small intensely fluorescent (SIF) cells in culture: role of glucocorticoids and growth factors in their development and phenotypic interconversions with other neural crest derivatives. J Neurosci 5:2143-2160

Kintner C, Brockes JP (1984) Monoclonal antibodies identify blastemal cells derived from de-differentiating muscle in limb regeneration. Nature 308:67-69

Landis SC, Keefe D (1983) Evidence for neurotransmitter plasticity in vivo: Developmental changes in properties of cholinergic sympathetic neurons. Dev Biol 98:349-372

Landis SC, Patterson PH (1981) Neural crest cell lineages. Trends Neurosci 4:172-175

LeDouarin NM (1982) The Neural Crest. Cambridge University Press, Cambridge

Lillien L, Claude P (1985) Nerve growth factor is a mitogen for cultured chromaffin cells. Nature 317:632-634

Ogawa M, Ishikawa T, Irimajiri A (1984) Adrenal chromaffin cells form functional cholinergic synapses in culture. Nature 307:66-68

Raff MC, MIller, RH, Noble M (1983) A glial progenitor cell that develops in vitro into an astrocyte or an oligodendrocyte depending on culture medium. Nature 303:390-396

Trojanowski JQ, Walkenstein N, Lee VM-Y (1986) Expression of neurofilament subunits in neurons of the central and peripheral nervous system: an immunohistorchemical study with monoclonal antibodies. J Neurosci 6:650-660

Unsicker K, Krisch B, Otten J, Thoenen H (1978) Nerve growth factor-induced fiber outgrowth from isolated rat adrenal chromaffin cells: impairment by glucocorticoids. Proc Natl Acad Sci USA 75:3498-3502

# TRANSIENTLY INDUCED SEQUENCES AS POTENTIAL MEDIATORS OF CELLULAR PROLIFERATION AND DIFFERENTIATION

H.R. Herschman, R.W. Lim, B.C. Varnum, and D.A. Kujubu
Department of Biological Chemistry,
and Laboratory of Biomedical and Environmental Sciences
School of Medicine
University of California, Los Angeles
Los Angeles, California 90024 (USA)

Our laboratory has, for a number of years, been interested in the causal biochemical, molecular, and physiological alterations that accompany mitogen-induced transitions from quiescent, non-dividing cells to cells committed to reenter the cell cycle. We have used the clonal murine embryo cell line Swiss 3T3 as a model system to study this transition. In this chapter we will first describe this mitogen-response system, present background data from our laboratory that led to the results to be reported here, summarize our recent studies on the isolation of a family of mitogen response genes, and then describe the expression of these genes in a developmental neurobiology context. We will conclude with a brief description of our plans for the future.

## Swiss 3T3 Cells as a Model for the Study of Mitogenesis:

Although some cells in the body are post-mitotic (e.g. platelets, erythrocytes, CNS neurons), many cells are in a growth-arrested, Go, state but can respond to specific mitogens by reentering the cell cycle and dividing. Thus, non-dividing hepatocytes are stimulated to proliferate and repopulate the liver following hepatectomy, antigen-responsive precursor cells undergo a clonal expansion after antigen challenge, mammary cells experience both hypertrophy and hyperplasia in the course of hormonally induced responses during pregnancy, etc. The study of the mitogen response *in vivo* is hampered, however, by a large number of factors. These include cellular heterogeneity within target tissues, lack of synchrony in target cell populations, problems in interpretation of data due to the potential

NATO ASI Series, Vol. H22
Neural Development and Regeneration
Edited by A. Gorio et al.

involvement of intervening endocrine systems, and the large quantities of mitogen required for in vivo studies. The vast majority of studies on the mechanisms of mitogenic responsiveness have, for these reasons, been carried out with cultured cells.

Swiss 3T3 cells are a clonal population of murine embryo cells that grow in culture as a monolayer in serum-supplemented medium. The cells will reach a saturation density proportional to the amount of serum in the medium, exit the cell cycle and enter a quiescent, non-dividing state. If 3T3 cells are cultured in media containing differing levels of serum supplement, the number of cells present when cell division ceases will be proportional to the amount of serum in the growth medium. The growth arrest is reversible. If additional serum is added to growth arrested 3T3 cells the cells will reenter the cell cycle, and divide.

A wide variety of studies have shown that growth arrested 3T3 cells are synchronized in the "Go" phase of the cell cycle. After addition of serum there is a 12-14 hour lag. The cells then enter S phase and duplicate their DNA content prior to mitosis and cell division. A variety of agents other than additional serum can stimulate growth arrested 3T3 cells to divide. These include the polypeptide mitogens epidermal growth factor (EGF), platelet derived growth factor (PDGF), and fibroblast growth factor (FGF), fatty acid derivatives such as prostaglandin F2$\alpha$, and the potent tumor promoters tetradecanoyl phorbol acetate (TPA) and teleocidin.

## Mitogen-specific Nonproliferative Mutants of Swiss 3T3 Cells:

A wide variety of biological responses accompany the mitogenic response. These include alterations in transport of small molecules and ions, a wide range of phosphorylation events, induction of new gene expression, changes in cytoskeletal arrangement, etc. It is difficult to sort out causal, necessary steps in the mitogen-response from correlative events that accompany, but are not essential for, the commitment to proliferation. A number of years ago we initiated a somatic cell genetic approach to this problem. We developed a procedure, recently described in detail (Herschman, 1987a), for the isolation of mitogen-specific nonproliferative variants of 3T3 cells. We reasoned that, should we be able to isolate cells blocked in specific steps in the mitogenic response to single agents (e.g. EGF nonproliferative variants that are unable to respond to this growth factor but can still respond to FGF, TPA, etc.), these cells were likely to be lesioned in a step causal in the response to that mitogen.

Identification of the molecular defects in such variants would be instructive in our understanding of the mitogenic pathway.

We utilized our selective procedure to isolate both EGF nonproliferative variants (Pruss and Herschman, 1977; Terwilliger and Herschman, 1984) and TPA nonproliferative variants (Butler-Gralla and Herschman, 1981). To our surprise, the EGF-nonproliferative variants all failed to bind EGF; they were functionally EGF receptorless. When antisera for the EGF receptor and molecular probes for the EGF receptor message became available we discovered that the EGF nonresponsive 3T3 variants were unable to produce EGF receptor-related proteins or message; the EGF receptor gene was silent (Schneider et al., 1986).

In recent years TPA has been shown to exert the bulk of its biological activities by binding to and activating the serine threonine protein kinase known as protein kinase C. In contrast to our results with EGF nonproliferative variants, our TPA nonproliferative variants retained TPA binding activity (Blumberg et al., 1981), and had levels of c-kinase equivalent to those found in the parental 3T3 cells (Bishop et al., 1985). Moreover, the TPA nonproliferative variant 3T3-TNR9, when treated with TPA, demonstrated induced phosphorylation of protein kinase C substrates similar in nature and extent to that observed with 3T3 cells (Bishop et al., 1985). We concluded from these data that 3T3-TNR9 cells are lesioned in the TPA-stimulated mitogenic pathway at a point distal to activation of protein kinase C; i.e., at a "post-receptor" locus.

One simple potential explanation for the TPA nonresponsive phenotype of the 3T3-TNR9 variant suggests that stimulation of all transcriptional activity in response to TPA is blocked in this cell line; the TPA specific mitogenic defect is due to an inability of a c-kinase mediated pathway to stimulate new gene expression. One of our initial studies suggested this might be the case. Competent mitogens for 3T3 cells, such as serum, TPA or EGF, stimulate transient elevation in the levels of ornithine decarboxylase (ODC) activity. While serum induced a similar increase in ODC levels in 3T3-TNR9 cells, no increase in ODC levels occured when the variant was treated with TPA. The ODC gene is apparently fine; it responds appropriately to serum. Some aspect, specific to ODC, of the transcription or translation of this gene must be defective in this variant. We are current examining the transcriptional status of the ODC gene in 3T3 and 3T3-TNR9 cells. To determine if TPA-mediated transcription is, in general, shut down in these TPA nonproliferative variants we turned to a gene whose induction by TPA had been well characterized in 3T3 cells. Major excreted protein (MEP) had previously been shown to be inducible by TPA (Gottesman and Sobel, 1980). Using a cDNA probe and antisera provided by Dr. Michael Gottesman, we demonstrated that TPA is able to induce the accumulation of MEP mRNA (Herschman, 1987b) and synthesis of MEP protein (Herschman, unpublished) in TPA mitogenically nonresponsive 3T3-TNR9 cells in a manner indistinguishable from that observed in TPA mitogenically responsive 3T3 cells. While the TPA induction of some functions (e.g. ODC) is blocked in the 3T3-TNR9 variant, induction of expression of other genes (e.g. MEP) is not impaired. The block in TPA-induced cell division in 3T3-TNR9 cells is not due to a generalized defect in TPA-mediated gene expression.

Rationale for the Isolation of TPA-induced mRNAs:

We have recently taken a new (for our laboratory) approach to the question of the causal steps in TPA-induced proliferation of quiescent cells. We reasoned that new gene expression is required for the transition from resting to proliferating cells. Our plan was to clone cDNAs for genes induced by TPA in 3T3 cells, and search for those genes whose transcriptional activation in response to TPA is defective in 3T3-TNR9 cells. Yamamoto and Alberts (1976) have divided gene expression in response to exogenous agents into "primary" and "secondary" responses. Primary response genes are genes whose transcriptional activation can occur in the absence of any new protein synthesis; all the components necessary for their transcription in response to an exogenous agent (hormone, growth factor, tumor promoter) are present in the cell and simply require activation by the extracellular ligand. Secondary response genes require the synthesis of an intervening protein in response to the effector before their transcription can be activated. Primary and secondary response to an extracellular agent can be distinguished experimentally. Increased transcription of primary response genes will occur in the presence of effector and an inhibitor of protein synthesis. In contrast, protein synthesis inhibitors will block effector-mediated transcription of secondary response genes.

We decided to restrict out attention to primary response genes, and to look for genes whose transcription was induced by TPA in quiescent, non-dividing 3T3 cells. We would then examine the expression of these genes in TPA nonproliferative 3T3-TNR9 cells in response to TPA.

## Cloning of cDNAs for TPA-induced Primary Response Genes in 3T3 Cells:

3T3 cells were grown to density arrest in medium containing 5% serum. Cells were then treated with TPA and the protein synthesis inhibitor cycloheximide (CHX). After three hours RNA was isolated, enriched for poly $A^+$ mRNA, and copied into double stranded cDNA. The cDNA preparation was then cloned into a bacteriophage cloning vector (λgt10) via Eco $R_1$ linkers. We obtained a cDNA library of approximately 150,000 phage (Lim et al., 1987). Our next task was to identify those cDNA clones representing TPA-induced sequences. Duplicate transfers to nitrocellulose supports were made for 50,000 phage plaques. Each plaque was then screened for hybridization with two cDNA probes. The single-stranded $^{32}P$-labeled "plus" probe was prepared from quiescent 3T3 cells treated with TPA plus CHX. A similarly labeled "minus" probe was prepared from quiescent 3T3 cells treated only with CHX. Plaques that showed more extensive hybridization with "plus" than "minus" probe are candidates for cDNA clones of messages induced by TPA. Candidate plaques were picked and rescreened; 50 plaques that consistently demonstrated greater hybridization with "plus" cDNA were isolated. Cross-hybridization data and comparison of mRNA sizes by northern analyses using the phage DNA as probes reduced a sub-population of these initial 50 clones to a collection of seven new cDNA clones that represent distinct mRNAs, from different genes, induced as primary responses to TPA (Lim et al., 1987). We initially referred to these genes as TPA induced sequences, or TIS genes.

## One of the TIS Genes Is the c-fos Protooncogene:

We examined the expression of the various TIS genes in response to CHX and to TPA + CHX, to be certain that CHX alone did not induce an inordinately large level of expression. We also examined the time course of expression of the TIS genes in response to TPA alone. A representative experiment is shown in Figure 1.

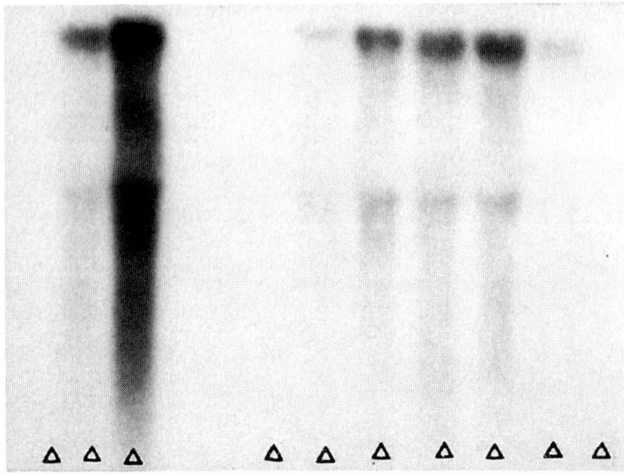

Figure 1. TPA induction of TIS 8. The left three panels show RNA from control cells, cells treated with CHX for three hours, and cells treated with TPA plus CHX for three hours. On the right are RNA samples from control cells and cells treated for 15, 30, 60, 120, 180, and 300 minutes.

From this data we note that (i) little or no mRNA is present in untreated cells, (ii) CHX alone causes an elevation in mRNA level, (iii) TPA alone induces a rapid, transient increase in mRNA levels; mRNA levels for the various TIS genes peaked at 30-90 minutes and returned to baseline by three to four hours (Lim et al., 1987), and (iv) the level of mRNA was greatly superinduced by the combined presence of TPA plus CHX. These characteristics were shared by all seven TIS mRNAS.

The c-fos protooncogene is the cellular homologue of the v-fos oncogene, the oncogene of two murine osteosarcoma viruses. Several laboratories have shown that c-fos expression shares with the TIS genes the characteristics of rapid, transient induction in 3T3 cells by mitogens and an extraordinary superinducibility by cycloheximide. To determine whether any of our TIS cDNAs were related to c-fos (or to other genes known to be induced by TPA) we screened our λ clones with probes for fos, myc, metallothionein, and ODC. One clone, TIS28, cross-reacted with a v-fos probe. When RNA sizes and inducibility were compared using TIS 28 and v-fos probes the results appeared identical. When genomic restriction digests of 3T3 DNA were analyzed with v-fos and TIS28 probes, similar restriction fragments occured (Lim et al., 1987). We conclude that the TIS28 clone is a partial cDNA for the c-fos message. Our screening procedure was able to identify this low abundance message. It is of interest and importance to note that we observed TIS 28 -- and several other TIS genes -- only once in our screen. Had we not obtained superinduction of these genes through the use of CHX, the abundance of these rare messages would probably not have been sufficient to allow their isolation in the 50,000 plaques screened.

Induction of TIS Genes by Polypeptide Mitogens:

Although TPA is a potent mitogen for 3T3 cells, it also has biological activities (e.g., tumor promotion, inhibition of cellular communication) that are not shared with other mitogens. A subset of the TIS genes might, therefore, be restricted to TPA responsiveness, and not be induced by other 3T3 mitogens. However, all the TIS genes were rapidly and transiently induced in 3T3 cells by mitogenic levels of serum, EGF, or FGF. Moreover, superinduction by CHX occured with each of these mitogens (Lim et al. 1987). Induction of the entire collection of TIS genes appears to be a common qualitative response in 3T3 cells to all mitogens, although quantitative differences may occur in response to the various mitogens. The name TPA induced sequence appears, therefore, to be a misnomer. Happily, however, the TIS acronym remains quite useful, as these are transiently induced sequences in all the mitogen responses.

Induction of the TIS Genes in the TPA Nonproliferative 3T3-TNR Variant:

One rationale for the isolation of TIS gene cDNAs was the possibility that the defect in the TPA nonproliferative variants might be the consequence of a lack of TPA-induced expression of one or more of the TIS genes. To examine this possibility, density arrested 3T3-TNR9 (TPA nonproliferative) cells were exposed to serum, TPA, EGF or FGF in the presence of CHX. All the mitogens, including TPA, stimulated accumulation of each TIS mRNA. When 3T3 cells were exposed to TPA or serum in the absence of CHX rapid, transient induction of all the TIS genes occured (Lim et al., 1987). In summary, none of the TIS genes was qualitatively "shut-down" in TPA response potential in the TPA nonproliferative variant. Although quantitative differences might exist in the TPA induction of various TIS messages between 3T3 and 3T3-TNR9 cells, we did not pursue such differences. We reasoned that, since we have no idea of the roles of the TIS gene products and, consequently, no knowledge of the threshold values of TIS mRNAs or proteins required for their function, we would be unable to place any meaning on quantitative differences in their expression in 3T3 vs. 3T3-TNR9 cells.

## The c-fos Protooncogene Is Expressed in Differentiation As Well As Mitogenic Responses:

The tumorigenic nature of the v-fos oncogene led to speculation that the product of its cellular homologue, the c-fos protooncogene, is likely to be involved in mediating cellular proliferation. The demonstrations of rapid, transient induction of c-fos expression by a variety of mitogens further enhanced the popularity of this hypothesis. More recently, however, a variety of laboratories have shown that expression of c-fos mRNA is rapidly and transiently induced in biological systems in which proliferation is, in fact, inhibited and differentiation pathways are initiated. The include (but are not limited to) induced differentiation of HL-60 cells (Muller et al., 1985), and nerve growth factor (NGF) treated PC12 cells (Kruijer et al., 1985).

PC12 cells are derived from a rat pheochromocytoma. When exposed to NGF, PC12 cells stop dividing and extend long neurite processes. One also observes increased electrical excitability, altered cellular adhesion and changes in neurotransmitter synthesis. When PC12 cells are exposed to NGF, c-fos mRNA is rapidly and transiently induced.

## Induction of a Subset of TIS Genes by NGF in PC12 Cells:

The TIS genes are induced in 3T3 cells by agents that induce c-fos expression. Indeed, c-fos can be considered a member of the TIS gene "family". To analyze the expression of the TIS genes in a differentiating, rather than a mitogenic, system we analyzed the expression of the TIS genes in NGF-treated PC12 cells (Kujubu et al., 1987).

We first examined the levels of TIS mRNA's in cells exposed to TPA + CHX or NGF + CHX, to both enhance potential induction via superinduction, and to avoid the problems of different kinetics of induction and de-induction for the various TIS genes. Five of the six TIS genes tested (TIS1, TIS7, TIS8, TIS11, TIS21) were induced by either NGF or TPA in the presence of CHX. A representative induction is shown in Figure 2.

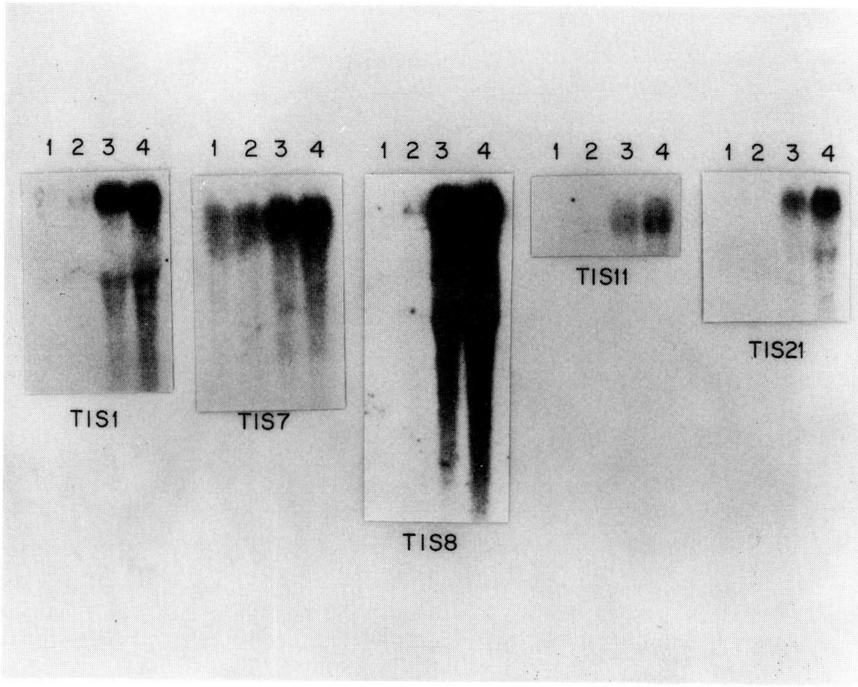


Figure 2. NGF induces accumulation of some TIS messages in PC12 cells. RNA was isolated from control PC12 cells (lane 1), cells exposed to CHX for 3 hours (lane 2), cells exposed to TPA + CHX for 3 hours (lane 3), or cells exposed to NGF + CHX for 3 hours (lane 4). Data are from Kujubu et al., 1987.

<u>In contrast, TIS10 was not induced by NGF or TPA in PC12 cells</u>. Not all the TPA-induced TIS genes are responsive in PC12 cells. TIS10 probe was able to detect mRNA in TPA-treated 3T3 cells; the probe used in this experiment was capable of hybridization.

We thought it possible that the TIS10 probe might not be sufficiently homologous to PC12 message, since PC12 cells are derived from rat, and the probes are from murine cells. However, TIS10 was able to detect a unique restriction fragment in a Southern blot of total rat genomic DNA (Kujubu et al., 1977), suggesting that lack of homology is not the basis for our inability to detect TIS10 mRNA in NGF-treated PC12 cells.

When PC12 cells were exposed to NGF without CHX, the levels of TIS1, TIS7 TIS8, TIS11, TIS21 and c-fos mRNA all rose rapidly, and peaked within 30-90 minutes. The levels of TIS1, TIS8, TIS11 and TIS21 then dropped toward baseline over the next 90 minutes (Fig. 3).

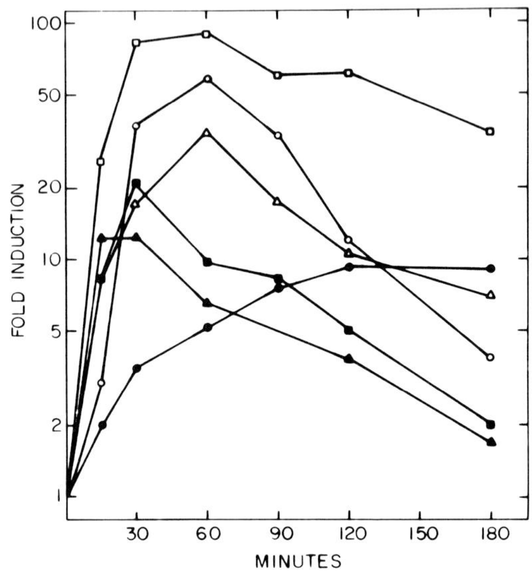


Figure 3. Kinetics of the induction by NGF of the TIS genes in PC12 cells. PC12 cells were treated with NGF (50 ng/ml) and RNA was harvested at the times shown. Data are derived from densitometry of autoradiographs. The various symbols represent different TIS probes. Data are from Kujubu et al., 1987.

TIS7 mRNA, in contrast both to its own behavior in 3T3 cells and to that of the other TIS genes in PC12 cells, remained elevated for the 180 minutes tested in these experiments, and did not return rapidly to uninduced levels. Thus, although in general terms the TIS genes were, like c-fos, rapidly and transiently induced in PC12 cells by NGF, significant qualitative and quantitative variations could be observed in the responses of 3T3 and PC12 cells.

## Induction of TIS Genes in PC12 Cells by EGF and by Depolarizing Agents:

Induction of c-fos in PC12 cells is not restricted to NGF; other polypeptide growth factors (e.g. EGF) and activation of a voltage dependent calcium channel also led to transient increases in c-fos mRNA (Morgan and Curren, 1986). These treatments also lead to the induction of expression of the TIS genes. Once again, TIS10 was the sole exception; neither EGF nor elevated $K^+$ induced expression of TIS 10. In contrast, these two agents stimulated expression of the other TIS genes, including c-fos (Kujubu et al., 1987).

Benzodiazepines Superinduce the TIS Gene NGF Response:

The benzodiazepine RO-3351 is not, by itself, able to substantially induce c-fos expression. However, if RO-3351 is administered concomitantly with NGF, substantial superinduction of the NGF mediated increase in c-fos message occurs (Curran and Morgan, 1985). RO-3351 mediated superinduction of c-fos differs from that observed with CHX. The benzodiazepine does not alter the transient nature of the response; fos mRNA levels peak at the same time for NGF + RO-3351 and NGF alone. The levels of c-fos mRNA are, however, much greater with NGF + RO-3351 than with either agent alone. In contrast, CHX blocks the rapid decrease in c-fos mRNA induced by NGF, and mRNA levels remain elevated for a much longer period.

We found that RO-3351 was also able to superinduce the NGF-responsive TIS genes. Like c-fos, these mRNAs were substantially elevated in the presence of NGF + RO-3351, but were not responsive to the benzodiazepine alone. The times required to reach peak levels of expression were not altered, but RO-3351 + NGF induced levels of the TIS mRNAs were much greater than the sum of the mRNAs induced in response to either agent alone. Representative data are shown in Figure 4.

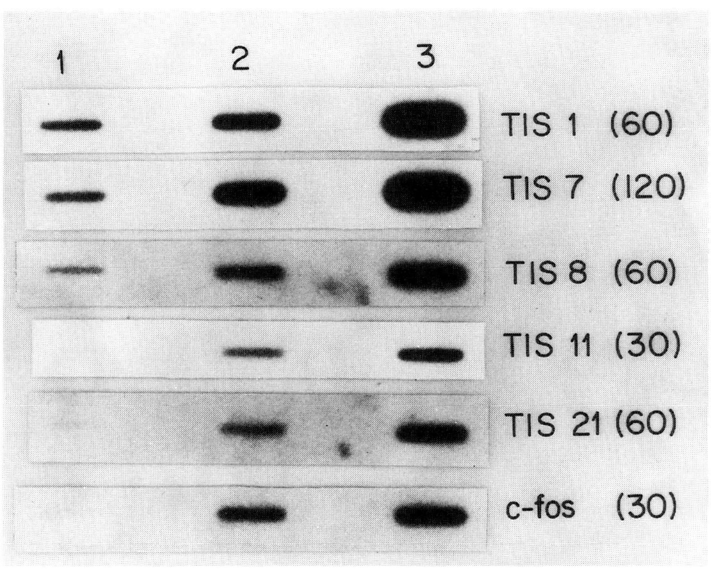


Figure 4. Benzodiazepines superinduce the TIS gene NGF response. Slot 1 has RNA from RO-3351 treated cells, slot 2 has RNA from NGF treated cells, slot 3 has RNA from cells treated both with NGF and RO-3351-treated cells. The numbers in parentheses are the times (in minutes) when RNA was collected. These are the times to peak expression for the various TIS clones. Data are from Kujubu et al., 1987.

Speculations on the Roles of the TIS Genes:

The two best characterized TIS genes, c-fos and c-myc, code for nuclear DNA binding proteins. The TIS genes are induced by a variety of biological agents, in a number of systems in which the effectors greatly alter cellular physiology. Cells are shifted from quiescence to proliferation, proliferation to differentiation, etc. We propose that the TIS gene products may be involved in the restructuring of chromatin necessary for cells to make these major transitions in physiological function. There may exist a hierarchy of such genes; some may be generally required; for physiological responses to a wide variety of extracellular effectors. One could think of them as "promiscuous" TIS genes, in the sense that they are induced in a variety of cellular responses. Other TIS genes might be necessary for alterations in cellular physiology unique to cell type, physiological response, or species. TIS10 may be an example of this "monogamous" class of TIS genes.

If this hypothesis were correct, one would predict that TIS-type cDNA clones should be isolatable that are restricted to specific differentiation pathways. NGF induction of differentiation is among the most restrictive of the easily accessible cellular models of ligand-induced differentiation. Relatively few cell types have NGF receptors, and the NGF response is unique to a small subset of neurons. We are currently screening for TIS-type cDNAs that are restricted to the NGF response in PC12 cells.

Future Directions:

A great deal of interest and speculation exists about the roles of the c-fos and c-myc gene products. We view these genes as the "tip of an iceberg", representing a family of genes -- the TIS genes. We are currently isolating cDNAs containing complete coding regions, and sequencing these clones to determine the primary structure of the TIS gene products. Antisera will be produced to appropriate peptides and used for localization of the TIS proteins, characterization of their synthesis and degradation, etc. Developmental studies of murine organs are underway, to determine the normal tissue specificity and time of expression of these genes. We are also isolating TIS genes from genomic libraries, to study the nature of their induction by exogenous agents. We are also examining TIS gene expression in several other biological contexts (e.g.

teratocarcinoma cells, induced B-cell differentiation, primary cultures of astrocytes, oligodendrocytes and neurons from the CNS). We will over-express the TIS genes in a variety of biological systems, using appropriate expression vectors, and examine the consequences. Recently, two laboratories have used inducible antisense vectors to examine, in 3T3 cells, the consequences of shutting down c-fos production. We are currently preparing similar TIS gene antisense constructs, to examine the causal role of TIS genes in various biological responses. We anticipate that these, and related, studies should occupy our laboratory for some time to come.

Acknowledgements:

Supported by grants to HRH from the NIH (GM 24797) and the University of California Cancer Research Coordinating Committee, and by Contract DE AC03 76 SF00012 between the Regents of the University of California and the Department of Energy. BCV is an NIH predoctoral trainee (2T32 GM07104); DAK is supported by a NIDDKD training program (2T32 DK 07270-06A2).

## REFERENCES


Bishop R, Martinez R, Weber MJ, Blackshear PJ, Beatty S, Lim R, Herschman HR (1985) Protein phosphorylation in a tetradecanoyl phorbol acetate-nonproliferative variant of 3T3 cells. Mol Cell Biol 5:2231-2237.

Blumberg PM, Butler-Gralla E, Herschman, H.R. (1981) Analysis of phorbol ester receptors in phorbol ester unresponsive 3T3 cells variants. Biochem Biophys Res Commun 102:818-823.

Butler-Gralla E, Herschman HR (1981) Variants of 3T3 cells lacking mitogenic resonse to the tumor promoter tetradecanoyl-phorbol-acetate. J Cell Physiol 107:59-67.

Curran T, Morgan J (1985) Superinduction of c-fos by nerve growth factor in the presence of peripherally active benzodiazepine. Science 229:1265-1268.

Gottesman MM (1978) Transformation-dependent secretion of a low molecular weight protein by murine fibroblast. Proc Natl Acad Sci USA 75:2767-2771.

Herschman HR (1987a) Isolation of mitogen-specific nonproliferative variant cell lines. In: Barnes D, Sirbasqu D (eds) Peptide growth factors: Methods in enzymology. Academic Press, New York. (In Press)

Herschman HR (1987b) Mitogen-specific nonresponsive mutants and the initiation of cellular proliferation. BioEssays. (In Press)

Kruijer W, Schubert D, Verma I (1985) Induction of the proto-oncogene fos by nerve growth factor. Proc Natl Acad Sci USA 82:7330-7334.

Kujubu DA, Lim RW, Varnum BC, Herschman HR (1987) Induction of transiently expressed genes in PC-12 pheochromocytoma cells. Oncogene. (In Press)

Lim RW, Varnum BC, Herschman HR (1987) Cloning of tetradecanoyl phorbol ester induced "primary response" sequences and their expression in density-arrested Swiss 3T3 cells and a TPA nonproliferative variant. Oncogene. (In Press)

Morgan J, Curran T (1986) Role of ion flux in the control of c-fos expression. Nature 322:552-555.

Muller R, Curran T, Muller D, Guilbert L (1985) Induction of c-fos during myelomonocytic differentiation and macrophage proliferation. Nature 314:546-548.

Pruss RM, Herschman HR (1977) Variants of 3T3 cells lacking mitogenic response to epidermal growth factor. Proc Natl Acad Sci USA 74:3918-3921.

Schneider CA, Lim RW, Terwilliger E, Herschman HR (1986) Epidermal growth factor nonresponsive 3T3 variants do not contain epidermal growth factor receptor-related antigens or messenger RNA. Proc Natl Acad Sci USA 83:333-336.

Terwilliger E, Herschman HR (1984) 3T3 variants unable to bind epidermal growth factor cannot complement in co-culture. Biochem Biophys Res Commun 118:60-64.

Yamamoto K, Alberts B (1976) Steroid receptors: Elements for modulation of eukaryotic transcription. Ann Rev Biochem 45:721.

# EXPRESSION OF THE C-SRC PROTO-ONCOGENE PRODUCT IN NEURAL CELLS

Joan S. Brugge
Department of Microbiology
State University of New York
Stony Brook, New York 11794
United States of America

## INTRODUCTION

Investigations of retroviral oncogenes has led to the identification of many cellular genes (termed proto-oncogenes) that appear to play crucial roles in regulating cellular responses to extracellular signals. Many of these genes are directly involved in the regulation of cellular growth control, either serving as growth factors themselves (such as the c-*sis* gene product which is one of the two chains of platelet-derived-growth-factor) or as growth factor receptors, (such as the c-*erb*-b or c-*fms* gene products which are the receptors for epidermal growth factor and colony stimulating factor I). However, the protein products of proto-oncogenes have also been implicated in the induction of other aspects of signal transduction in a variety of cell types, including neural cells [i.e.the induction of neurite outgrowth in PC12 cells (Bar-Sagi and Feramisco, 1985; Hagag et al., 1986; Alema et al., 1985) and the response to the convulsant drug Metrazole (Morgan et al., 1987)]. Studies of one such proto-oncogene, c-*src*, have provided strong evidence that the c-*src* gene product, which functions as a tyrosine-specific protein kinase, may serve a specialized function in neurons.

The *src* gene product was initially identified as the transforming protein encoded by Rous sarcoma virus (Brugge and Erikson, 1977; Purchio et al., 1978). This gene is both necessary and sufficient for oncogenic transformation by Rous sarcoma virus. The viral *src* gene is closely related to a cellular gene, denoted c-*src*, which has been highly conserved through metazoan evolution (review, Bishop, 1983). Investigations of the nucleotide sequence of the viral and cellular *src*

NATO ASI Series, Vol. H22
Neural Development and Regeneration
Edited by A. Gorio et al.

genes have provided evidence that the viral gene was acquired by recombination between host cell DNA and the viral genome (review, Bishop, 1983; Bishop and Varmus, 1982).

Both the viral and cellular src gene products, pp60$^{v\text{-}src}$ and pp60$^{c\text{-}src}$, possess tyrosine-specific protein kinase activity. However, the specific activity of pp60$^{v\text{-}src}$ is 20- to 100-fold greater than that of pp60$^{c\text{-}src}$ (Iba et al., 1985; Coussens, et al., 1985). Expression of the viral src gene product in fibroblasts induces many changes in cell physiology, including alterations in growth behavior, morphology and cytoskeletal arrangements, hexose uptake, and metabolism (Hanafusa, 1977). However, these phenotypic changes have not been detected in cells that express the c-src gene product at levels comparable to the levels of pp60$^{v\text{-}src}$ in RSV-transformed cells (Iba et al., 1984, 1985; Parker et al., 1984; Johnson et al., 1985). It is of interest that mutational alterations throughout the src gene can activate the oncogenic potential of this gene, suggesting that the c-src gene product is very sensitive to alterations in conformation that affect its functional activity (reviews, Hanafusa, 1987; Hunter, 1987). Oncogenic variants of pp60$^{c\text{-}src}$ possess an activated tyrosine kinase activity, suggesting a correlation between oncogenicity and activation of pp60$^{c\text{-}src}$ protein kinase activity.

The c-src gene product is one member of a large family of cellular tyrosine kinases. These proteins can be distinguished into two groups based on the nature of their association with the plasma membrane (review, Hunter and Cooper, 1985). One group consists of the transmembrane tyrosine kinases such as the receptors for epidermal growth factor, insulin, and platelet-derived-growth-factor. The other group consists of proteins such as pp60$^{c\text{-}src}$, which are exclusively associated with the cytoplasmic face of the plasma membrane. It is clear that the membrane receptors are involved in transducing signals from peptide hormones to elicit cellular responses, including induction of DNA synthesis and cell proliferation, stimulation of phosphatidylinositol turnover, activation of the Na-H$^+$ pump, stimulation of cell proliferation, changes in cell morphology, increased transport of glucose, etc. The recent identification of the sev gene from Drosophila melanogaster as a tyrosine protein kinase membrane receptor (based on the close relationship between its amino acid sequence and that of animal cell tyrosine kinase receptors) also implicates tyrosine kinases in the regulation of critical developmental decisions. Mutations in the _sev_ gene cause a shift in the differentiation program of the R7 cells from the ommatidia of the eye such that cone cells develop in place of photoreceptor cells (Banergee et al., 1987; Hafen et al, 1987).

The function of the _src_ family of tyrosine kinases is not known. Since these proteins do not possess an extracellular domain, one cannot postulate a direct involvement for these tyrosine kinases in hormone signal transduction. In order to provide a clue to possible functions of the c-_src_ gene product in normal cells, we examined the expression of the c-_src_ protein in tissues from developing chicken embryos (Cotton and Brugge, 1983). All neural tissues, including brain, neural retina and dorsal root ganglia, expressed high levels of $pp60^{c-src}$. It was of interest that the major population of $pp60^{c-src}$ precipitated from neural tissues with monoclonal antibodies to $pp60^{c-src}$ displayed a slower electrophoretic mobility than the protein precipitated from other tissues (Brugge et al. 1987a). This protein, designated $pp60^{c-src(+)}$, contains a 6-amino acid insertion within the amino-terminal region of the molecule (described below). These studies indicated that the expression of c-_src_ gene in neural tissues could be distinguished qualitatively and quantitatively from c-_src_ expression in other tissues.

Other investigators have also found high levels of $pp60^{c-src}$ in neural tissues (Shartl and Barnekov, 1982; Levy et al., 1984; Sorge et al., 1984; Jacobs and Rubsamen, 1983). Indeed, high levels of c-_src_-related gene products have been detected in neural tissues from lower eukaryotic species such as Drosophila (Simon et al., 1985), cockroaches, fish (Shartl and Barnekov, 1984) and hydra, as well as in humans (Levy et al., 1984; Jacobs and Rubsamen, 1985) and other mammalian species. These results suggest that $pp60^{c-src}$ may play a role in events that take place in neural tissues.

## IDENTIFICATION OF THE TYPE OF NEURAL CELL THAT EXPRESSES HIGH LEVELS OF THE ALTERED FORM OF $pp60^{c-src}$.

There are many lines of evidence which indicate that neuronal cells express the majority (if not all) of the $pp60^{c-src(+)}$ detected in neural tissues.

1. **Analyses of the expression of $pp60^{c-src(+)}$ in cultured cells:**
   a) $pp60^{c-src}$ represents the majority (greater thatn 80%) of the population of $pp60^{c-src}$ expressed in cultured neurons (Brugge et al.,

1985; Cartwright et al., 1987). pp60$^{c\text{-}src(+)}$ was not detected in astrocytic cultures, other types of cultured cells, or in any non-neural tissues.

b) pp60$^{c\text{-}src(+)}$ was detected at high levels in neuron-like cells that differentiate from p19 teratocarcinoma cells after treatment with retinoic acid (Lynch et al., 1985). The appearance of high levels of pp60$^{c\text{-}src(+)}$ correlated with neurite outgrowth in the cultures.

c) Several different cell lines derived from human neuroblastoma tumors express pp60$^{c\text{-}src(+)}$ (Bolen et al, 1985; Mellstrom and Pahlman, personal communication; Yang and Walter, personal communication).

2. Analyses of pp60$^{c\text{-}src}$ in neural tissues.

Since reagents are not yet available that distinguish between the neural and non-neural forms of pp60$^{c\text{-}src}$, it has not been possible to examine the localization of these two different forms of pp60$^{c\text{-}src}$ by immunohistochemical techniques. Maness and coworkers reported that neuronal cells from the chicken neural retina (Sorge et al., 1984) and the molecular layer from the developing cerebellum (Fults et al., 1985) displayed the highest levels of pp60$^{c\text{-}src}$ immunoreactivity. Since the majority of the c-*src* gene product expressed in neural retina is pp60$^{c\text{-}src(+)}$ (Brugge et al., 1987a), these results suggested that pp60$^{src(+)}$ is expressed in neural cells *in vivo*. We have obtained the following indirect evidence that supports this conclusion through the biochemical analysis of the two c-*src* gene products separated by polyacrylamide gels.

a) We have examined the expression of pp60$^{c\text{-}src(+)}$ in developing cerebella from wild-type mice and mutant mice that display progressive degeneration of specific classes of cerebellar neurons (Brugge et al., 1987b). The loss of pp60$^{c\text{-}src(+)}$ generally correlated with the loss of granule and Purkinje cells from the cerebella of mice carrying the staggerer (*sg*/*sg*) and Lurcher (*Lc*/+) mutations, with the most pronounced changes observed in cerebella from the more severly affected *sg*/*sg* mice. There was no loss of the lower, non-neural form of pp60$^{c\text{-}src}$ in any of the mutant mice. These results indicate a correlation between the loss of cerebellar neurons and the loss of pp60$^{c\text{-}src(+)}$.

b) Lesions induced by injection of quinolinic acid in the caudate nucleus from adult rats caused a loss of pp60$^{c\text{-}src(+)}$ in both the caudate nucleus and the substantia nigra. The most feasible explanation for this finding is that pp60$^{c-\underline{src}(+)}$ is localized in both the neuronal cell bodies and the nerve termini (Walaas, Lustig, Greengard, and Brugge, unpublished results).

Thus, while one cannot rule out the possibility that a minor proportion of pp60$^{c-\underline{src}(+)}$ is expressed in non-neuronal cells in neural tissues, it is likely that neurons account for the majority of pp60$^{c-\underline{src}(+)}$ expressed in neural tissues. In collaboration with I. Walaas and P. Greengard, we have also examined the expression of pp60$^{c-\underline{src}}$ in a variety of different regions of the central nervous system. These studies indicate that pp60$^{c-\underline{src}(+)}$ is expressed in most regions of the central nervous system (unpublished results). In addition, in collaboration with R. Keane and R.J. Barrett, we have examined cultured neurons from the met- and telencephalon, striatum, and spinal cord from 14-day rat embryos. The majority of the c-*src* gene product from both cell types migrated as pp60$^{c-\underline{src}(+)}$ (Brugge et al., 1985 and unpublished results). These results indicate that the expression of this protein is not limited to a small subclass of neuronal cells. However, identification of the precise type of neuronal cells that express pp60$^{c-\underline{src}(+)}$ awaits *in situ* studies of the expression of pp60$^{c-\underline{src}(+)}$.

## NATURE OF THE STRUCTURAL DIFFERENCE BETWEEN pp60$^{c-\underline{src}}$ AND pp60$^{c-\underline{src}(+)}$

In order to determine the functional significance of the variant form of pp60$^{c-\underline{src}}$ detected in neurons , it was essential to determine the nature of the structural difference between pp60$^{c-\underline{src}(+)}$ and pp60$^{c-\underline{src}}$.

### 1. Localization of the position of the alteration in pp60$^{c-\underline{src}(+)}$.

We have performed a series of experiments using a variety of chemical and enzymatic methods to cleave pp60$^{c-\underline{src}}$ at specific amino acids. This allowed us to tentatiely map the location of the modification in pp60$^{c-\underline{src}(+)}$ to a position between amino acids 60 and 118 (Brugge et al., 1985; and Lustig, Cotton,and Brugge, unpublished results).

### 2. Analysis of the phosphorylation of pp60$^{c-\underline{src}(+)}$.

Since phosphorylation of pp60$^{c-\underline{src}}$ is known to cause a retardation of its electrophoretic mobility, we examined the phosphorylation of pp60$^{c-\underline{src}(+)}$ to determine whether the shift in electrophoretic mobility of neuronal pp60$^{c-\underline{src}(+)}$ was due to a difference in the phosphorylation of this protein in neurons. pp60$^{c\text{-}\underline{src}(+)}$ from neuronal cultures was found to contain an additional site of serine phosphorylation that was located in the amino-terminal 16,000 daltons of the molecule. However, this modification is not responsible for the slower electrophoretic mobility of pp60$^{c\text{-}\underline{src}(+)}$ since enzymatic dephosphorylation of pp60$^{c\text{-}\underline{src}(+)}$ does not alter its electrophoretic mobility (Brugge et al., 1987a).

**3. Analysis of post-translational alterations in the mobility of pp60$^{c\text{-}\underline{src}}$ in neurons.**

To follow the synthesis of pp60$^{c\text{-}\underline{src}}$, we labeled neuronal cells for varying periods of time with $^{35}$S-methionine, or pulse-labeled with $^{35}$S-methionine and then chased with unlabled methionine. These studies did not provide any evidence for a post-translational alteration in pp60$^{c\text{-}\underline{src}}$ in neurons. The same proportion of the slower and faster migrating forms of pp60$^{c\text{-}\underline{src}}$ was detected under all labeling conditions, even for periods as short as 5 min. (Brugge et al., 1987a; Brugge, Coussens, Lustig, and Keane, unpublished results).

**4. Analysis of the mobility of the c-*src* gene product translated *in vitro*.**

Since all of the protein data suggested that the modification in pp60$^{c\text{-}\underline{src}(+)}$ did not result from post-translational alterations in the c-*src* gene product, we examined the initial c-*src* translation product in lysates programmed with RNA isolated from neural (cerebral cortex) and non-neural (limb) tissues from 10-day chicken embryos (Brugge et al., 1987a). The *in vitro* translation product from RNA brain displayed a slower electrophoretic mobility than the protein translated in reactions programmed with limb RNA. These results strongly suggested that the mRNA from brain tissues encoded pp60$^{c\text{-}\underline{src}(+)}$, and that this RNA was subjected to an altered pattern of splicing in neural cells.

**5. Isolation of a c-*src* cDNA from embryonic brain mRNA.**

To investigate the possiblity of whether c-*src* mRNA is uniquely processed in neural tissues, we prepared a cDNA library from chicken brain mRNA and isolated a full-length cDNA clone encoding the c-*src* gene product (Levy et al., 1987) A similar c-*src* cDNA was also isolated from a mouse brain cDNA library by Martinez and coworkers (Martinez et al., 1987). The c-*src* cDNA from both species contains an 18-nucleotide insert located at the junction between the sequences that represent the genomic c-*src* exons 3 and 4 (see figure 1). This insertion encodes a highly charged 6-amino acid peptide located between amino acids 117 and 118. Although there are 4 nucleotide differences between the insert found in the chicken and mouse cDNAs, the amino acids encoded by these two genes are identical. Martinez and coworkers have located this 18-nucleotide sequence within the intron between exons 3 and 4 of the mouse genomic c-*src* gene (R. Martinez and D. Baltimore, unpublished results). This result indicates that the 18-nucleotide insertion represents a mini-exon which is exclusively used in neural tissues (presumably in neurons) to generate $pp60^{c\text{-}src(+)}$. Both the mouse and chicken neural cDNAs have been inserted into retroviral vectors and expressed in cultured cells (Martinez et al., 1987; Levy et al., 1987). The protein products of each cDNA displayed a retarded electrophoretic mobility compared to the fibroblast c-*src* gene product, and the peptide maps of the neural cDNA products were simlar to that of $pp60^{c\text{-}src(+)}$ from neurons. These results provide strong evidence that the c-*src* mRNA is subject to a unique form of processing in neurons to generate a novel form of $pp60^{c\text{-}src}$ which contains a 6-amino acid insertion located 117 amino acids from the amino terminus of $pp60^{c\text{-}src}$. The evidence that the amino acid sequence of the insert is identical in the mouse and chicken cDNAs suggest a functional importance for this insertion. It is possible that this highly charged insert may be important in conferring specificity to the interaction of $pp60^{c\text{-}src}$ with neural cell proteins that either regulate the functional activity of $pp60^{c\text{-}src}$, or that are substrates of tyrosine phosphorylation by $pp60^{c\text{-}src}$.

## ANALYSIS OF THE FUNCTIONAL ACTIVITY OF $pp60^{c\text{-}src(+)}$.

The $pp60^{c\text{-}src(+)}$ protein extracted from cultured neuronal cells displayed an elevated kinase activity compared to $pp60^{c\text{-}src}$ from astrocytes or fibroblasts. The assay employed to compare the kinase activity of these different forms of $pp60^{c\text{-}src}$ was performed within an immunocomplex following immunoprecipitation with a monoclonal antibody that does not interfere with the kinase activity of $pp60^{c\text{-}src}$ (Lipsich et al., 1983). Enolase was used an exogenous substrate of tyrosine phosphorylation (Cooper et al., 1984). Since the $pp60^{c\text{-}src(+)}$ expressed in neurons differs from $pp60^{c\text{-}src}$ from astrocytes by the presence of both the 6-amino acid insert and the additional site of serine phosphorylation, it is difficult to distinguish which structural difference is responsible for the elevated specific activity of pp60$^{c\text{-}src(+)}$ from neurons. However, we have recently found that the pp60$^{c\text{-}src(+)}$ protein expressed in fibroblasts following transfection with a retrovirus that carries the neural c-*src* cDNA is not phosphorylated on the novel serine residue which is detected in neurons (J. Levy, M. DeMarco, J. Brugge, unpublished results). Comparison of the kinase activity of pp60$^{c\text{-}src(+)}$ and pp60$^{c\text{-}src}$ expressed in these cells indicated that pp60$^{c\text{-}src(+)}$ possesses a higher specific activity in this assay. This result indicates that the 6-amino acid insert is responsible for the elevated specific activity of pp60$^{c\text{-}src(+)}$.

It is difficult to assess the functional significance of this structural difference between pp60$^{c\text{-}src(+)}$ and pp60$^{c\text{-}src}$. We have not detected any dramatic differences between the growth behavior of fibroblasts that express high levels of pp60$^{c\text{-}src(+)}$ (J. Levy and J. Brugge, unpublished results). In addition, we do not detect an increase in the phosphorylation of any cellular proteins on tyrosine in these pp60$^{c\text{-}src(+)}$ expressor cells (J. Levy, M. De Marco and J. Brugge, unpublished results). Mutant variants of pp60$^{c\text{-}src}$ that display activities similar to those of pp60$^{c\text{-}src(+)}$ in *in vitro* assays cause elevated phosphorylation of cellular proteins *in vivo* and dramatic phenotypic changes in cell growth and physiology (Iba et al., 1984; Levy et al., 1986; Cartwright et al., 1987; Kmiecik et al., 1987; Piwnica-Worms et al., 1987). It is possible that the 6-amino acid insert in pp60$^{c\text{-}src(+)}$ affects the stability of pp60$^{c\text{-}src(+)}$ in the *in vitro* kinase assay and does not necessarily affect the specific activity *in vivo*. Alternatively, it is possible that the specific substrate(s) of pp60$^{c\text{-}src(+)}$ phosphorylation are absent in fibroblasts and, thus, differences in activity are not detectable in fibroblasts.

## SUMMARY

The c-*src* gene product expressed in neurons can be distinguished both qualitatively and quantitatively from the c-*src* gene product expressed in other cell types. Neurons express high levels of a structurally distinct form of pp60$^{c\text{-}src}$ that is generated by an altered processing of the c-*src* mRNA. In neurons, a unique sequence of 18 nucleotides that is located within the intron between c-*src* exons 3 & 4 is inserted into the c-*src* mRNA, resulting in the production of a c-*src* mRNA that encodes a novel form of pp60$^{c-\underline{src}}$ which contains a 6-amino acid insertion. This variant form of pp60$^{c-\underline{src}}$ has not been observed in any other cell types, and the same 6-amino acid insertion is found in pp60$^{c-\underline{src}}$ from both mouse and chicken neural cells, suggesting that this variation specifically affects the function of pp60$^{c-\underline{src}}$ in neuronal cells. In the absence of information on the functional role of pp60$^{c-\underline{src}}$ in any cell type, it is difficult to predict how this modification affects pp60$^{c-\underline{src}}$ function.

One possibility is that the _src_ family of tyrosine kinases, which are localized exclusively on the cytoplasmic face of the plasma membrane, communicate directly with transmembrane receptor proteins by non-covalent protein-protein interactions (as the beta-adrenergic receptor interact with its GTP-binding protein). According to this scenario, the _src_ gene could represent one portion of an ancestral receptor kinase gene which has been truncated during evolution such that the kinase domain has become dissociated from the transmembrane signal-binding domain. This would represent one evolutionary mechanism to generate diversity in the type of signals that are transduced by different tyrosine kinases. The question is then raised whether this truncated kinase still interacts functionally with a transmembrane protein, or whether this kinase has evolved to serve a different type of function in the membrane. In either case, it is possible that the 6-amino acid insert may confer specificity to the interaction of pp60$^{c-\underline{src}}$ with protein(s) that affect its functional activity.

It is difficult to distinguish from available information whether the pp60$^{c-\underline{src}(+)}$ is involved in events that take place in mature neurons (i.e. neuronal survival, signal transduction), or events involved in neuronal differentiation (as the _sev_ gene product from Drosophila). Examination of the kinetics of expression of pp60$^{c-\underline{src}(+)}$ in neuron-like cells that differentiate in cultured p19 teratocarcinoma cells following treatment with retinoic acid indicate that a shift from the production of low levels of pp60$^{c-\underline{src}}$ to high levels of pp60$^{c-\underline{src}(+)}$ occurs either just prior to, or coincidentally with neurite extension (Lynch et al., 1986). Ideally, it would be informative to interfere with the production of pp60$^{c-\underline{src}(+)}$ during this differentiation process to evaluate the role of pp60$^{c-\underline{src}(+)}$ in the process of differentiation. Since this approach is currently not technically feasible, we plan to introduce the neural c-_src_ cDNA expression vectors into immature neuroblasts to examine whether constitutive high levels of expression of pp60$^{c\text{-}src(+)}$ affect the differentitation program of neural cells.

It would also be very useful to examine the precise localization of pp60$^{c\text{-}src(+)}$ in developing central nervous system tissues and in adults. This is now feasible with the identification of the structural difference between pp60$^{c\text{-}src}$ and pp60$^{c\text{-}src(+)}$. We have prepared antibodies to a synthetic peptide containing the 6-amino acids from the neuron-specific insert (J. Brugge and D. Marshak, unpublished results). This antibody specifically recognizes pp60$^{c\text{-}src(+)}$, thus allowing localization of this protein by _in situ_ immunohistochemical techniques.

It is difficult to reconcile the oncogenic activity of the viral _src_ gene product with a role for pp60$^{c\text{-}src}$ in either promoting the differentiation of neurons, or an event that takes place in mature neurons. Perhaps the mutational changes in the v-_src_ gene deregulate and activate the tyrosine kinase activity of the v-_src_ gene product, thus allowing it to phosphorylate the substrates of other cellular tyrosine kinases. This could lead to pleitropic alterations in cell physiology that would include a constitutive stimulation of cell proliferation as a result of the phosphorylation of growth hormone receptor substrates. The evidence that the substrates of the v-_src_ gene product overlap with those of the the epidermal and platelet-derived-growth factor receptors supports this possibility (review, Hunter and Cooper, 1984). Many of these questions will be addressed by the identification of physiologically relevant substrates of tyrosine kinases, clearly one of the most important and difficult challenges to investigators in this field.

ACKNOWLEDGMENTS

The research from J. Brugge's laboratory described in this report was supported by grants CA28146 and CA27951 from the National Cancer Institute. JSB receives partial salary support from the American Cancer Society. The author acknowledges Kathleen Donnelly for excellent secretarial assistance.

Neuronal c-src mRNA contains an additional 18 bases between exons 3 and 4.

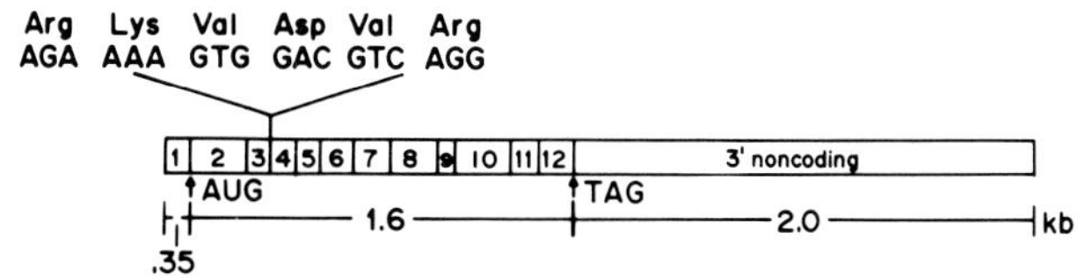


Splicing Mechanism to Generate Neuronal c-src mRNA

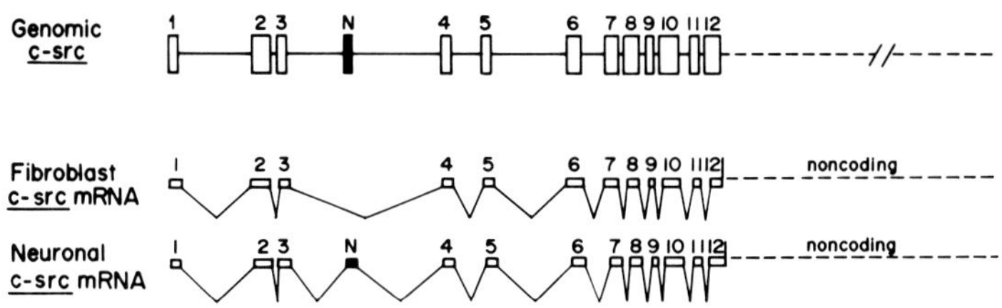


Figure Legend

Figure 1. This figure shows the structure of the cDNA isolated from a chicken brain cDNA library (Levy et al., 1987) and a proposed mechanism for the alternate splicing of c-*src* mRNA in neurons. The numbered panels refer to the corresponding exons of the c-*src* gene.

## References

Alema S, Casalbore P, Agostini E, Tato F (1985) Differentiation of pc12 phaeochromocytoma cells induced by v-*src* oncogene. Nature 316:557-559

Banerjee U, Renfranz PJ, Pollock JA, Benzer S (1987) Molecular characterization and expression of *Sevenless*, a gene involved in neuronal pattern formation in the Drosophila eye. Cell 49:281-291.

Bar-Sagi D, Feramisco J (1985) Microinjection of the *ras* oncogene protein into PC12 cells induces morphological differentiation. Cell 42:841-848

Bishop J, Varmus H (1982) Functions and origins of retroviral transforming genes. In: Weiss, Teich, Varmus, Coffin (eds) RNA tumor viruses. Cold Spring Harbor Press, Cold Spring Harbor, New York, p 999

Bishop JM (1983) Cellular oncogenes and retroviruses. Ann Rev Biochem 52:301-354.

Brugge JS, Erikson RL (1977) Identification of a transformation-specific antigen induced by an avian sarcoma virus. Nature 269:346-348

Brugge JS, Cotton PC, Queral AE, Barrett, JN, Nonner D, Keane RW (1985) Neurones express high levels of a structurally modified, activated form of $pp60^{c-src}$. Nature 316:554-557

Brugge JS, Cotton PC, Lustig A, Yonemoto W, Lipsich, L, Coussens, PM, Barrett, JN, Nonner D, Keane RW (1987a) Characterization of the altered form of the c-src gene product in neuronal cells. Genes & Development 1:287-296

Brugge JS, Lustig A, Messer A (to be published) Changes in the pattern of expression of $pp60^{c-src}$ in cerebellar mutants of mice. J Neurosci Res

Cartwright CA, Simantov R, Kaplan PL, Hunter T, Eckhart W (1987) Alterations in $pp60^{c-src}$ accompany differentiation. Mol Cell Biol 7:1830-1840

Cartwright CA, Eckhart W, Simon S, Kaplan PL (1987) Cell transformation by $pp60^{c-src}$ mutated in the carboxy-terminal regulatory domain. Cell 49:83-91

Cooper JA, Esch FS, Taylor SS, Hunter T (1984) Phosphorylation sites on enolase and dehydrogenease utilized by tyrosine protein kinases in vivo and in vitro. J Biol Chem 259:7835-7841

Cotton PC and Brugge JS (1983) Neural tissues express high levels of the cellular src gene product, $pp60^{c-src}$. Mol Cell Biol 3:1157-1162

Coussens PM, Cooper J, Hunter T, Shalloway D (1985) Restriction of the in vitro and in vivo tyrosine protein kinase activities of $pp60^{c-src}$ relative to $pp60^{c-src}$. Mol Cell Biol 10:2753-2763

Fults DW, Towle AC, Lauder JM, Maness PF (1985) $pp60^{c-src}$ in the developing cerebellum. Mol Cell Biol 5:27-32

Hafen E, Basler K, Stroem E, Rubin J-C, Rubin GM (1987) Sevenless, a cell-specific homeotic gene of Drosophila, encodes a putative transmembrane receptor with a tyrosine kinase domain. Science 236:55-63

Hanafusa H (1977) Cell transformation by RNA tumor viruses. In: Fraenkel-Conrat, Wagner R (eds) Comprehensive virology. Plenum Press, New York, p 401

Hanafusa H (1987) Activation of the c-src gene. In: P. Kahn, T. Graf (eds) Oncogenes and Growth Control. Springer-Verlag, Heidelberg, p100

Hagag M, Halegoua S, Viola M (1986) Inhibition of growth factor-induced differentiation of pc12 cells by microinjection of antibody to ras p21. Nature 319:680-682

Hunter T, Cooper JA (1984) Tyrosine protein kinases and their substrates: an overview. Adv Cyclic Nucleotide Protein Phosphorylation Res 17:443-455

Hunter T and Cooper JA (1985) Protein tyrosine kinases. Ann Rev Biochem 54:897-930

Hunter T (1987) A tail of two src's: Mutatis Mutandis. Cell 49:1-4

Iba H, Jove R, Hanafusa (1985) Lack of induction of neuroretinal cell proliferation by Rous sarcoma virus variants that carry the c-src gene. Mol Cell Biol 5:2856-2859

Iba H, Cross FR, Garber EA, Hanafusa H (1985) Low level of cellular protein phosphorylation by non-transforming over produced p60$^{c-src}$. Mol Cell Biol 5:1058-1066

Jacobs C and Rubsamen H (1983) Expression of pp60$^{c-src}$ protein kinase in adult and fetal human tissue: high activities in some sarcomas and mammalian carcinomas. Cancer Res 43:1696-1702

Johnson P, Coussens P, Danko A, Shalloway D (1985) Overexpressed pp60$^{c-src}$ can induce focus formation without complete transformation of NIH 3T3 cells. Mol Cell Biol 5:1073-1083

Kmiecik T, Shalloway D (1987) Activation and suppression of pp60$^{c-src}$ transforming ability by mutation of its primary sites of tyrosine phosphorylation. Cell 49:65-73

Levy BT, Sorge LK, Meymandi A, Maness P (1984) pp60$^{c-src}$ kinase is in chick and human embryonic tissues. Devel Biol 104:9-17

Levy JB, Iba H, Hanafusa H (1986) Activation of the transforming potential of pp60$^{c-src}$ by a single amino acid change. Proc Natl Acad Sci USA 83:4228-4232

Levy JB, Dorai T, Wang L-H, Brugge JS (to be published) The structurally distinct form of pp60$^{c-src}$ detected in neuronal cells is encoded by a unique c-src mRNA. Mol Cell Biol

Lynch SA, Brugge JS, Levine JM (1986) Induction of altered c-src product during neuronal differentiation of embryonal carcinoma cells. Science 234:873-876

Lipsich LA, Cutt JC, Brugge JS (1982) Association of the transforming proteins of Rous, Fujinami and Y73 avian sarcoma viruses with the same two cellular proteins. Mol Cell Biol 2:875-880

Morgan JI, Cohen DR, Hempstead JL, Curran T (1987) Mapping patterns of c-fos expression in the central nervous system after seizure. Science 237:192-196

Parker R, Varmus HE, Bishop JM (1984) Expression of v-src and chicken c-src in rat cells demonstrates qualitative differences between pp60$^{v-src}$ and pp60$^{c-src}$. Cell 37:131-139

Parker R, Varmus HE, Bishop JM (1984) Expression of v-src and c-src in rat cells demonstrates qualitative differences between pp60$^{v-src}$ and pp60$^{c-src}$. Cell 37:131-139

Piwnica-Worms H, Saunders KB, Roberts TM, Smith AE, Cheng SH (1987) Tyrosine phosphorylation regulates the biochemical and biological properties of pp60$^{c-src}$. Cell 49:75-82

Purchio AF, Erikson E, Brugge JS and Erikson RL (1978) Identification of a polypeptide encoded by the avian sarcoma virus src gene. Proc Natl Acad Sci USA 75:1567-1571

Schartl M, Barnekow A (1982) The expression in eukaryotes of a tyrosine kinase which is reactive with pp60$^{v-src}$ antibodies. Differentiation 23:109-114

Schartl M, Barnekow A (1984) Differential expression of the cellular src gene during vertebrate development. Devel Biol 105:415-422

Simon M, Drees B, Kornberg T, Bishop PM (1985) The nucleotide sequence and the tissue-specific expression of Drosophila c-src. Cell 42:831-840

Sorge LK, Levy BT, Maness PF (1984) pp60$^{c-src}$ is developmentally regulated in the neural retina. Cell 36:249-256

Takeya T, Hanafusa H (1983) Nucleotide sequence of c-src. Cell 32:881-890

# INDUCTION OF THE 68/72 kDa HEAT-SHOCK PROTEIN DURING HYDROGEN PEROXIDE TOXICITY

R.N. Nishimura [1,2], B.E. Dwyer [1,2], R. Cole [3], J. de Vellis [3]
Department of Neurology [1]
Veterans Administration Hospital
Sepulveda, California 91343
USA

## INTRODUCTION

The heat-shock or stress proteins (HSPs) are families of proteins synthesized in response to heat stress and other noxious stimuli in bacteria, fungi, Drosophila melanogaster, and mammalian cells (Subjeck and Shyy 1986). The function of the proteins is unknown but because they are thought to protect the stressed cell they have raised much interest. In the mammalian central nervous system induction and synthesis of these proteins has been noted after trauma (White 1980), during recovery from hypoxia-ischemia (Dienel et al 1986, Nowak 1985) and after heat shock (Clark and Brown 1985). Among those cell types which are capable of synthesizing HSPs in the brain are endothelial cells (White 1980), isolated rat glial (Nishimura et al 1986) and neuronal cells (Nishimura et al 1986a) and retinal neurons (Clark and Brown 1985). The primary HSPs synthesized in central nervous system astrocytes are 68/72, 70/74, 89, and 97 kDa (Nishimura et al 1986). The 68/72 kDa protein is not synthesized constitutively (Welch and Feramisco 1982). It is shown here that the 68/72 kDa HSP can be synthesized by purified rat astrocytes in response to an oxidative stress induced by hydrogen peroxide.

## MATERIALS AND METHODS

Purified astrocytes were prepared by the method of McCarthy and de Vellis

----------------

Departments of Neurology [2] and Anatomy [3]
UCLA
Los Angeles, California 90024-1769
USA

NATO ASI Series, Vol. H22
Neural Development and Regeneration
Edited by A. Gorio et al.

(1980), except that a mechanical rather than a trypsin dissociation of primary tissue was performed. Oligodendrocytes were separated from the astrocytes by shaking and secondary astrocyte cultures were prepared by trypsin dissociation of the primary cultures. After two weeks in-vitro, cultures were changed from the normal feeding medium (10% fetal calf serum in Dulbecco's modified essential medium/Ham's F-12, 1:1) to DMEM/F-12 alone at 37°C. Hydrogen peroxide (2, 4, and 6 μM final concentrations) was added to each culture. Controls were untreated. These results were compared with heat-stress response in astrocytes heated to 45°C ± 0.3°C for 10 or 20 minutes.

After $H_2O_2$ or heat stress treatment cultures were incubated at 37°C the remainder of the experiment except for removal of medium from $H_2O_2$ treated cultures at 1 hour and replacement with fresh DMEM/F-12 at 37°C. Radioactive labeling with $^{35}S$-methionine was performed in methionine deficient medium (30 uCi/ml) for 1 or 2 hours. After labeling the cultures were processed by successive washes of ice-cold phosphate buffered saline, 0.1M, pH 7.4, then treated with 10% TCA supplemented with 0.1% methionine and then washed again with PBS. Cells were then scraped from the flasks and homogenized in 0.1% SDS and heated 3 minutes at 100°C.

Samples were then examined by SDS protein electrophoresis, in 12.5% polyacrylamide gels as per Laemmli (1970). Two-dimensional gels were processed as per O'Farrell (1975). Western blot analysis was performed as per Towbin et al (1979). Immunostaining was performed using the avidin-biotin procedure by Vector Laboratories, Burlingame, California. A specific mouse monoclonal antibody for the 68/72 kDa HSP was provided by Dr. W. Welch, Cold Spring Harbor Laboratories, Cold Spring Harbor, New York (Welch and Feramisco 1982).

## RESULTS

Astrocytes exposed to micromolar amounts of $H_2O_2$ synthesized the 68/72 kDa heat-shock protein in a dose-dependent and time-dependent manner (figure 1).

The 68/72 kDa heat-shock protein made by astrocytes in response to H2O2 migrates to the same region after two dimensional gel electrophoresis when compared to that made by heat-stressed astrocytes (Nishimura et al 1986). This protein is negligibly present in control astrocytes. Relative increases and decreases in radioactivity were associated with many protein spots. Three of these protein spots with prominent increased radioactivity are shown (horizontal arrows, figure 2).

Immunoblot staining was performed utilizing a specific monoclonal antibody for the 68/72 kDa HSP . The faint band confirms the presence of the 68/72 kDa HSP after $H_2O_2$ exposure (figure 3).

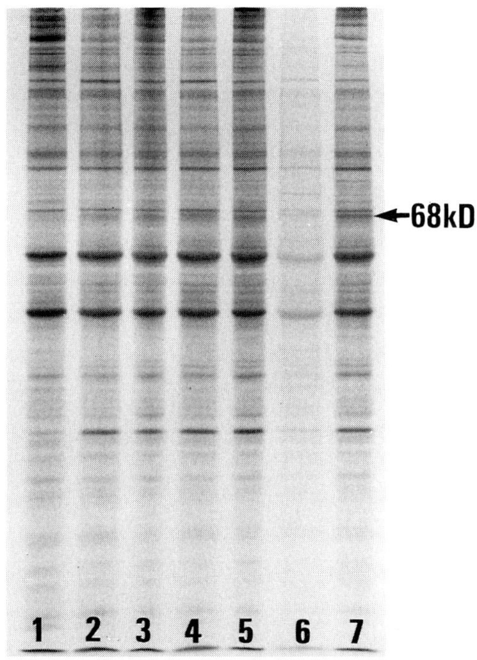


Figure 1
Polyacrylamide gel of astrocytes after one hour treatment of $H_2O_2$. Equal cpms/minute were added to each column except for lane 6 which has one-half as many cpms. The arrow denotes the 68/72 kDa protein. Lane 1-control; lanes 2,3-2 µM $H_2O_2$, labeled at 2-4 and 4-6 hours after exposure respectively; lanes 4,5-4 µM, labeled at 2-4 and 4-6 hours respectively and lanes 6,7-6 µM labeled at 2-4 and 4-6 hours respectively (Nishimura et al 1987b).

DISCUSSION

In contrast to Burdon (1986) who did not find synthesis of HSPs in mammalian cells after $H_2O_2$ exposure, this study shows that the synthesis of the 68/72 kDa HSP is induced by $H_2O_2$ in purified rat astrocytes. Love et al (1986) found that large concentrations, 50 mM, or pretreatment with 1 mM then 50 mM $H_2O_2$ induced HSP mRNA transcription in Drosophila melanogaster. The present results indicate that rat astrocytes synthesize limited amounts of the 68/72 kDa HSP and several other

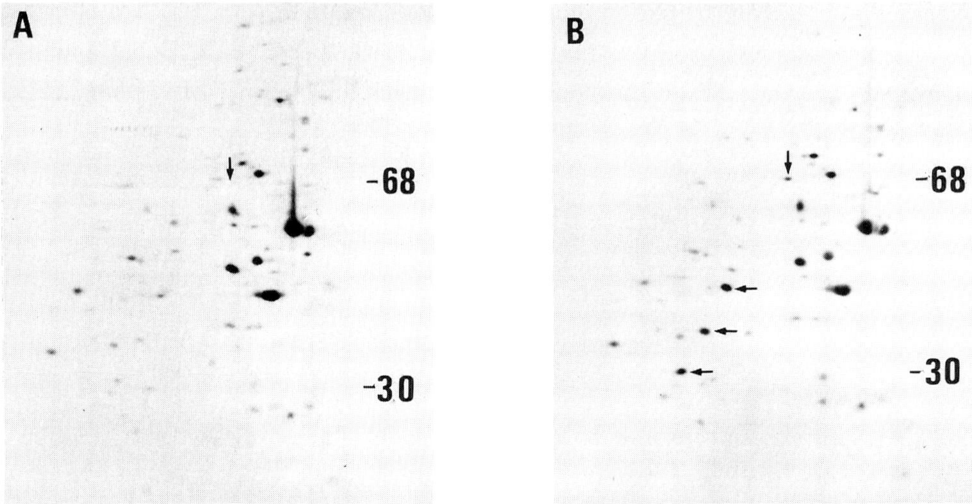


Figure 2
Two dimensional gels of control (A) and $H_2O_2$ (4 µM) treated astrocytes (B). Approximately 100,000 cpms were added to each gel. The vertical arrows show the region for the 68/72 kDa HSP. The horizontal arrows show synthesis of three protein also induced by $H_2O_2$. Molecular weights are noted in the margin (Nishimura et al 1987b).

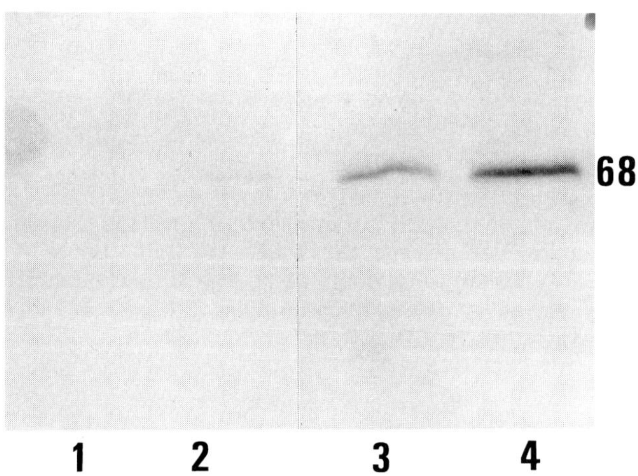


Figure 3
Immunoblot analysis of astrocytes treated with $H_2O_2$ (6 µM) compared with heat-stress of 10 and 20 minutes. Immunostaining for the 68/72 kDa HSP is much more prominent in heat-stressed astrocytes than $H_2O_2$ stressed astrocytes. All samples were harvested 6 hours after respective treatments. Lane 1-control; lane 2- $H_2O_2$ (6 µM for one hour); lane 3-10 minute heat-stress; and lane 4-20 minute heat-stress. Each lane contained 100 µg protein prior to transfer to nitrocellulose membrane (Nishimura et al 1987b).

unidentified low molecular weight proteins after $H_2O_2$ exposure. How this response benefits the cell remains unknown. It is interesting to speculate that the cellular response to $H_2O_2$ may be mediated through free radical formation (Siesjo 1981). Free radical formation is postulated to play a major role in the pathophysiology of tissue damage in trauma and hypoxia-ischemia. This relationship makes the pursuit of the function of these HSP proteins clinically relevant.

## REFERENCES

Burdon RH (1986) Heat shock and the heat shock proteins. Biochem J 240:313-324

Clark BD, Brown IR (1985) Axonal transport of a heat shock protein in the rabbit visual system. Proc Natl Acad Sci 82:1281-1285

Dienel, GA, Keissling M, Jacewicz M, Pulsinelli WA (1986) Synthesis of heat shock proteins in rat brain after transient ischemia. J Cerebral Blood Flow Metab 6:505-510.

Laemmli UK (1970) Cleavage of structural proteins during the assembly of the heat of bacteriophage T4. Nature 227:680-685

Love JD, Vivino AA, Minton KW (1986) Hydrogen peroxide toxicity may be enhanced by heat shock gene induction in Drosophila. J Cell Physiol 26:60-68

McCarthy KD, de Vellis J (1980) Preparation of separate astroglial and oligodendroglial cell cultures from rat cerebral tissue. J Cell Biol 85:890-902

Nishimura, RN, Dwyer BE, Liotta K, Cole R, de Vellis J (1986) Induction of stress proteins in astrocytes. Trans Am Soc Neurochem 17:325

Nishimura, RN, Dwyer BE, Liotta K, Cole R, de Vellis J (1987) Heat stress response in primary rat neuronal and glial cultures. Neurology 37:S370

Nishimura, RN, Dwyer BE, Cole R, de Vellis J (1987) Induction of the 68/72 kDa heat stress protein by hydrogen peroxide toxicity. submitted for publication

Nowak TS (1985) Synthesis of a stress protein following transient ischemia in the gerbil. J Neurochem 45:1635-1641

O'Farrell PH (1975) High resolution of two-dimensional electrophoresis proteins. J Biol Chem 250:4007-4021

Siesjo BK (1981) Cell damage in the brain: A speculative review. J Cerebral Blood Flow Metab 1:155-185

Subjeck JR, Shyy T-T (1986) Stress protein systems of mammalian cells. Am J Physiol 250:C1-C17

Towbin H, Staehelin T, Gordon J (1979) Electrophoretic transfer of proteins from polyacrylamide gels to nitrocellulose sheets: procedure and some applications. Proc Natl Acad Sci 76:4350-4354

Welch WJ, Feramisco JR (1982) Purification of the major mammalian heat shock proteins. J Biol Chem 257:14949-14959

White FP (1980) Differences in protein synthesized in-vivo and in-vitro in cells associated with the cerebral microvasculature. A protein synthesized in response to trauma? Neurosci 5:1793-1799

## ACKNOWLEDGEMENTS

Supported by the medical research service of the Veterans Administration and the United Cerebral Palsy Research and Educational Foundation.

# DEVELOPMENTAL EXPRESSION OF NERVE GROWTH FACTOR

Ted Ebendal[1] and Håkan Persson[2]

[1]Department of Zoology, Uppsala University,
Box 561, S-751 22 Uppsala, Sweden.

[2]Department of Medical Genetics,
Uppsala University Biomedical Center,
Box 589, S-751 23 Uppsala, Sweden.

## INTRODUCTION

Nerve growth factor supports sympathetic and sensory innervation of peripheral tissues (Levi-Montalcini & Angeletti, 1968; Thoenen & Barde, 1980). Recently NGF has also been found in the brain (Shelton and Reichardt, 1984, 1986; Korsching *et al.*, 1985; Whittemore *et al.* 1986) and attributed a trophic function for cholinergic neurons situated in the basal forebrain (Gnahn *et al.*, 1983; Large *et al.*, 1986). Although the classical biological assay for NGF (Cohen *et al.*, 1954) is based on stimulation of neurite formation in embryonic chicken ganglia, little is known about the developmental appearance and possible embryonic function of NGF. The recent isolation of the gene for chicken βNGF (Ebendal *et al.*, 1986; Meier *et al.*, 1986; Wion *et al.*, 1986) has made it possible to address the question of developmental appearance and regulation of NGF the chicken embryo.

NATO ASI Series, Vol. H22
Neural Development and Regeneration
Edited by A. Gorio et al.

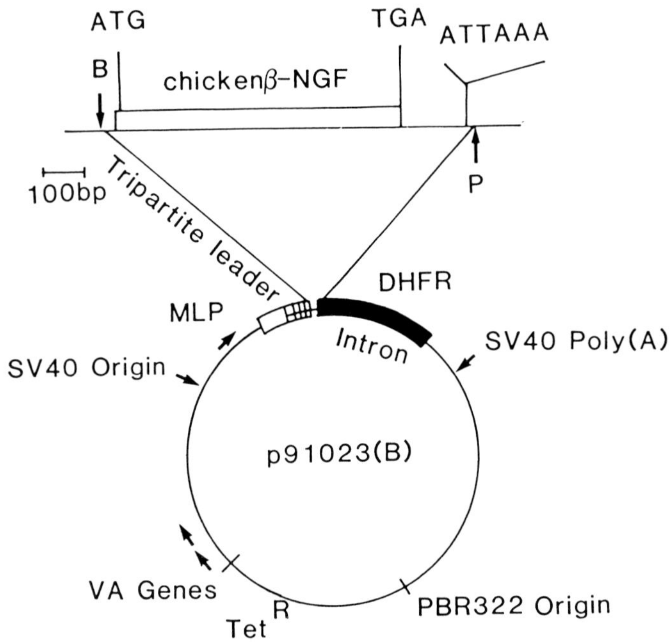


Fig. 1. Chimaeric plasmid construct for expression of recombinant chicken βNGF. A genomic chick NGF clone (Ebendal *et al.*, 1986) was restricted with BglI (B) and PvuII (P), and a 960 bp fragment containing the entire 3'-exon of the chicken NGF gene was isolated. The fragment was ligated to EcoRI linkers and inserted into the EcoRI site of the expression vector p91023(B) using standard recombinant DNA techniques (Maniatis *et al.*, 1982). The features of the vector making it suitable for transient expression in COS cells (Gluzman, 1981) have been detailed elsewhere (Wong *et al.*, 1985). ATG refers to the in-frame initiation codon at position -121 (numbering from the amino-terminus of the mature NGF protein), and TGA refers to the termination codon used for the synthesis of prepro-NGF. ATTAAA refers to the hexanucleotide sequence specifying polyadenylation of the NGF mRNA. For transfection, 5 μg of DNA was mixed with DEAE-dextran (Pharmacia) and applied for 30 min. to a 10 cm culture dish with COS cells at half confluence. The cells were treated with 0.1 mM chloroquine in Dulbecco's modified Eagle's medium containing 10% fetal calf serum for 5 hours before the medium was changed. The cells were allowed to grow for another 3 days before medium was collected for analysis.

PRODUCTION OF BIOLOGICALLY ACTIVE RECOMBINANT NGF

A recombinant NGF protein was produced using the recently cloned chicken NGF gene (Ebendal *et al.*, 1986). A 960 bp BglI-PvuII fragment including the entire 3'-exon of the chick NGF gene (Fig. 1) was inserted in the proper orientation for translation into the expression vector p91023(B) (Wong *et al.*, 1985), and the chimaeric plasmid was used for transfection of COS cells (Gluzman, 1981). Blot analysis of RNA from the transfected cells using a 900 bp PstI fragment from the chicken NGF gene (Ebendal *et al.*, 1986) showed two abundant transcripts with approximate sizes of 1.1 kb and 2.1 kb, respectively (Fig. 2 a). The smaller transcript represented 70% of the total hybridizing RNA and had a size consistent with polyadenylation at a consensus hexanucleotide sequence (ATTAAA) present 140 bp downstream of the translational termination codon (Fig. 1). The size of the larger transcript (2.1 kb) is consistent with polyadenylation occurring at the SV40 polyadenylation signal present in the vector (SV40 Poly(A)). RNA blots of COS cells transfected with p91023(B) without insert did not give any hybridization signal with the chicken NGF probe (not shown).

Conditioned medium collected three days after transfection was tested for NGF activity in a bioassay measuring fibre outgrowth from sympathetic ganglia. Medium from control COS cells transfected with the plasmid carrying the chicken NGF insert in the reverse orientation showed no NGF activity at the dilution tested (Fig. 2 b). Conditioned medium at the same

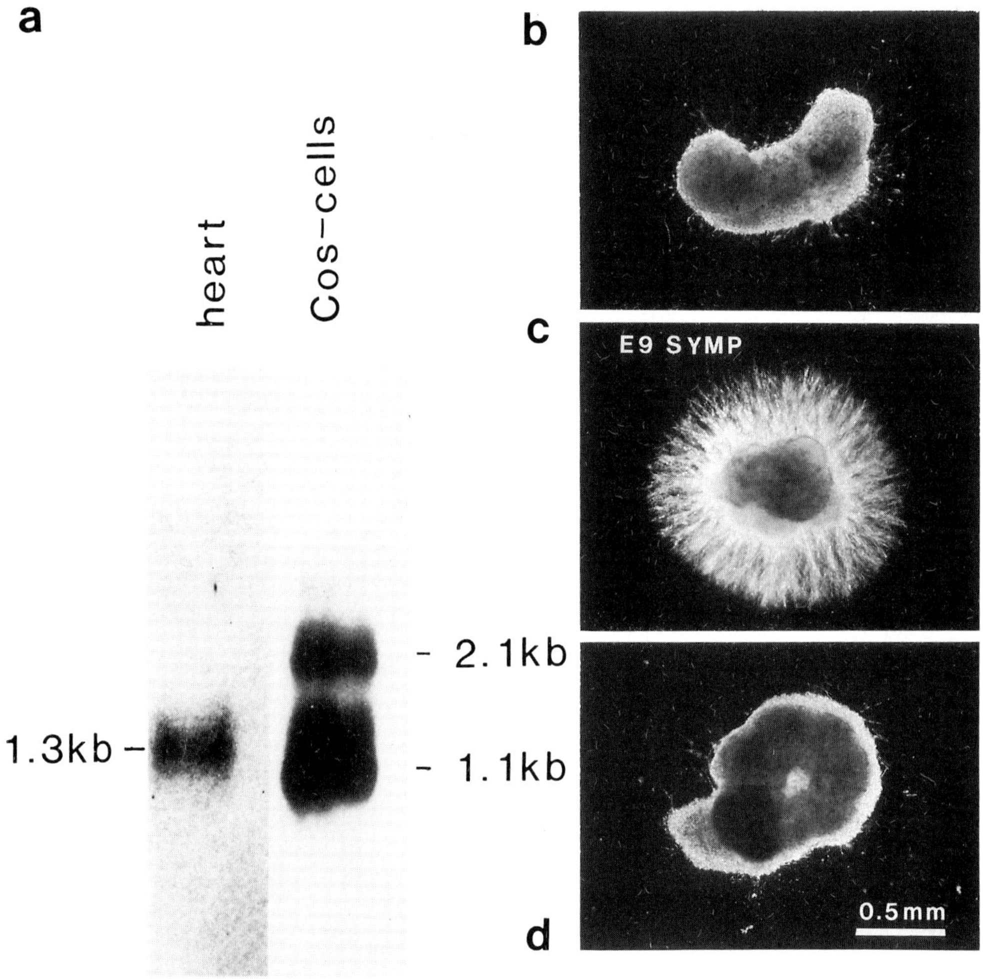


Fig. 2. a. The transfected COS cells were disrupted in 4 M guanidine isothiocyanate for preparation of RNA (Chirgwin *et al.*, 1979), and 10 μg of total cellular RNA was electrophoresed in a formaldehyde-containing agarose gel and transferred to nitrocellulose for hybridization to a nick-translated chicken NGF PstI fragment (900 bp). For comparison, 10 μg of polyadenylated (polyA+) RNA prepared from the heart of an adult chicken were analyzed in a parallel lane (heart). The lane with RNA from transfected cells (COS cells) was exposed to film for 2 hours, while the lane from the adult heart was exposed for 2 days.
b, Biological assay of NGF activity using explanted sympathetic ganglia from the 9-day (E9) chick embryo (Ebendal, 1979). The ganglia are shown by dark-field microscopy after

one day in culture. The photograph shows lack of response (no fibre outgrowth) in ganglia receiving conditioned COS-medium after transfection with a plasmid containing the chicken NGF insert in the reverse orientation. The medium was diluted 4-fold in this and subsequent experiments.
c, One day after addition of the conditioned medium from transfection with the plasmid carrying the chick NGF insert in the correct orientation for translation of chicken NGF protein. A dense outgrowth of nerve fibres has formed. By comparison with the activity of purified mouse βNGF, the concentration of NGF in the COS-medium is estimated to be around 20 ng/ml.
d, The same as in c, but with biological activity blocked by addition of 2 μg/ml of affinity-purified antibodies to mouse NGF (Ebendal *et al.*, 1984).

dilution from cells transfected with the plasmid having the chicken βNGF insert in the proper orientation for translation showed the presence of biologically active NGF (Fig. 2c). The fibre outgrowth was blocked by antibodies to mouse βNGF (Fig. 2d). These results show that the cloned chicken NGF gene (Ebendal *et al.*, 1986) contains all the information necessary for the synthesis and secretion of biologically active NGF protein. The 3'-exon of the cloned chicken NGF gene contains two ATG-codons (positions -121 and -119 relative to the amino-terminus of the mature NGF protein). A translational start at one of these two positions results in a prepro-NGF protein containing either an 18- or 16-amino-acid-long hydrophobic signal peptide. The mouse NGF gene, in addition, has a third in-frame ATG-codon located in a separate short 5'-exon at position -183 (Ullrich *et al.*, 1983, Scott *et al.*, 1983). Differential RNA splicing generates two mRNA species, with the smaller transcript lacking the ATG-codon at position -183 (Edwards *et al.*, 1986). In a cell-free system, the two

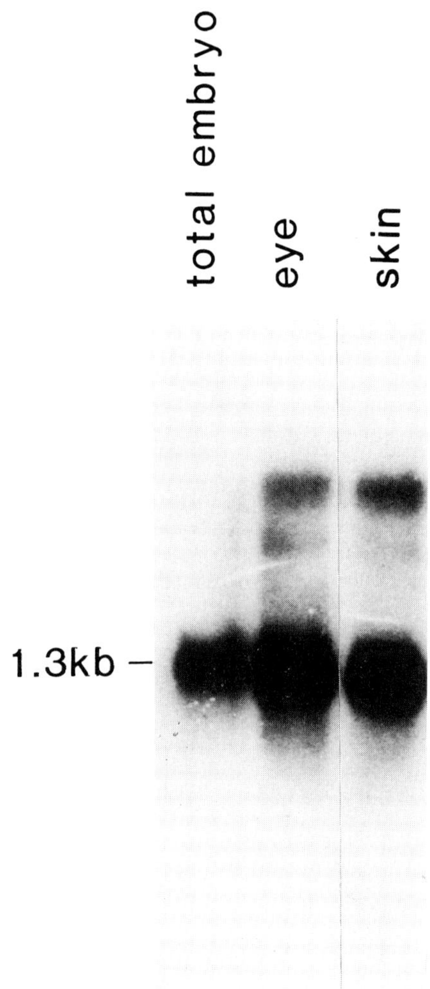


Fig. 3. Levels of NGF mRNA during chick development. Total RNA was prepared from entire embryos (embryonic day 8), or organs from E8 embryos as previously described (Ebendal *et al.*, 1986). Poly(A)$^+$ RNA was purified by oligo(dT)-cellulose chromatography (Aviv & Leder, 1972) and used for RNA blots. Ten $\mu$g of poly(A)$^+$ RNA from each sample were electrophoresed in 1% agarose gels containing 0.7% formaldehyde, then transferred to nitrocellulose filters and hybridized to a nick-translated (5 x $10^8$ cpm/$\mu$g) 900 bp Pst I fragment encoding the mature chicken NGF protein. Filters were washed at high stringency (15 mM NaCl, 1.5 mM sodium citrate, pH 7.0, 0.1% SDS, 54$^o$C) and exposed to Kodak XAR-5 film at -80$^o$C using Du Pont intensifying screens. Filters were washed and rehybridized with a probe for mouse $\alpha$-actin as a control.

transcripts have been shown to direct the synthesis of prepro-NGF proteins with molecular weights of 34kD and 27kD, respectively (Edwards *et al.*, 1986). The 27kD prepro-NGF protein most likely corresponds to initiation of protein synthesis occurring *in vitro* at the ATG-codon at positions -121 or -119. The chicken NGF construct used for transfection of COS cells in this study shows that the ATG-codons in the 3'-exon (positions -121 and -119) are functional initiation sites for synthesis of prepro-NGF in an *in vivo* system. A full report on these findings will be published elsewhere (F. Hallböök, T. Ebendal & H. Persson, submitted).

RESPONSE TO RECOMBINANT CHICKEN NGF

The conditioned medium from transfected COS cells made it also possible to study the effect of chicken NGF on the fibre outgrowth response in a number of chick ganglia at different stages of development. The spinal ganglia (neural crest origin) became responsive to recombinant NGF at day 5 (stage 26 according to Hamburger & Hamilton, 1951). Weak fibre outgrowth responses were also seen at the same stage in the trigeminal ganglion, with neurons derived both from the neural crest and from epidermal placodes (Noden, 1978). A weak, transient, response to NGF in the nodose ganglion was observed at day 5 with a much less response at day 8 or 9. In contrast, the fibre outgrowth increased in the trigeminal ganglion during this period, probably due to progressive maturation of the neural crest-derived neurons. The parasympathetic ciliary ganglion did not respond to the recombinant NGF at any stage. The paravertebral sympathetic ganglia became responsive at day 6 and then dramatically increased their density of fibre outgrowth with age.

NGF mRNA DURING DEVELOPMENT

The onset of fibre outgrowth responses to recombinant chicken NGF in several ganglia at embryonic day 5 to 8 prompted us to study the synthesis of NGF during different stages of development. We therefore used part of the genomic chicken NGF clone as a probe for determining the levels of NGF mRNA in the chicken embryo. Blots of RNA prepared from different developmental stages showed that the NGF mRNA was present already at embryonic day 3.5 (stage 20), the earliest stage examined. The size of the embryonic NGF transcript was the same as in the adult (1.3 kb). The NGF mRNA in the total embryo preparation increased slightly at day 4.5 (stage 25), showed peak levels at days 8 and 12, and was then present at distinctly lower levels during late embryonic development (day 18). The sharp rise in NGF mRNA expression in the total embryo between day 4.5 and 8 thus coincided with the time period of increasing responsiveness to the recombinant chicken NGF among several different types of neurons in the chick embryo. At day 8, particularly high levels of NGF mRNA were expressed in skin and eye (Fig. 3).

For comparison, levels of NGF mRNA were studied also in heart and brain from embryonic day 8 until one week after hatch. These two organs were previously found to be rich in NGF mRNA in the adult chicken (Ebendal *et al.*, 1986). During the entire embryonic period, the heart contained low levels of NGF mRNA, which reached adult levels one week after hatch. The brain also showed low levels of NGF mRNA throughout the embryonic period with a marked increase around hatching. As a control for the developmental changes in levels of NGF mRNA, and to ensure similar amounts of mRNA in each lane, the same blots were stripped of the NGF probe and rehybridized with a probe for α-actin. Both the entire embryo and the brain contained similar levels of α-actin mRNA at all stages analyzed. Although direct evidence is still lacking for the presence of the NGF protein in the chicken embryo until late in development (day 18, Belew & Ebendal, 1986), the presence of the NGF mRNA at day 3.5 (stage 20) is a strong indication for an early synthesis of the NGF protein.

The peak of NGF mRNA levels (days 8-12) coincides with the maximum number of NGF receptors on the spinal chick ganglia (Herrup & Shooter, 1975) and with maximal fibre outgrowth from explanted sympathetic, trigeminal, and spinal ganglia in response to mouse NGF (Ebendal, 1979). At around day 8 maximal neuronal death in spinal ganglia was also observed (Hamburger *et al.*, 1981) and suggested to be the result of competition between neurons for a limited supply of a trophic factor. The high levels of NGF mRNA found at day 8 in the skin and eye of the embryo (Fig. 3), may indicate that the early peak in NGF expression serves a function in sensory innervation.

The peak was not seen in heart and brain showing high levels of NGF mRNA in adults, suggesting a transient developmental expression of NGF in tissues that are at later stages less active in NGF production.

ACKNOWLEDGEMENTS

We are grateful to Dr. Randal J. Kaufman, the Genetics Institute, Boston, Massachusetts, for providing the expression vector p91023(B), to Dr. Dan Larhammar for suggestions on chimaeric plasmid construction and to Dr. Katherine McIntyre for reading the manuscript. Technical assistance was given by Mrs. Annika Kylberg, Mrs. Stine Söderström and Mrs. Vibeke Nilsson. Support was obtained from the Swedish Medical and Natural Science Research Councils and the Bank of Sweden Tercentenary Foundation.

REFERENCES

Aviv H, Leder P (1972) Purification of biologically active globin messenger RNA by chromatography on oligothymidylic acid-cellulose. Proc Natl Acad Sci USA 69: 1408-1412

Belew M, Ebendal T (1986) Chick embryo nerve growth factor. Fractionation and Biological Activity. Exp Cell Res 167: 550-558

Chirgwin J, Aeyble A, McDonald R, Rutter W (1979) Isolation of biologically active ribonucleic acid from sources enriched in ribonuclease. Biochemistry 18: 5294-5299

Cohen S, Levi-Montalcini R, Hamburger V (1954) A nerve growth-stimulating factor isolated from sarcomas 37 and 180. Proc Natl Acad Sci USA 40: 1014-1018

Ebendal T (1979) Stage-dependent stimulation of neurite outgrowth exerted by nerve growth factor and chick heart in cultured embryonic ganglia. Dev Biol 72: 276-290

Ebendal T, Olson L, Seiger Å, Belew M (1984) Nerve growth factors in chick and rat tissues. In: Cellular and Molecular Biology of Neuronal Development (Plenum, N.Y.) pp. 231-242

Ebendal T, Larhammar D, Persson H (1986) Structure and expression of the chicken β nerve growth factor. EMBO J 5: 1483-1487

Edwards RH, Selby MJ, Rutter WJ (1986) Differential RNA splicing predicts two distinct nerve growth factor precursors. Nature 319: 784-787

Gluzman Y (1981) SV40-transformed simian cells support the replication of early SV40 mutants. Cell 23: 175-182

Gnahn H, Hefti F, Heumann R, Schwab ME, Thoenen H (1983) NGF-mediated increase of choline acetyltransferase (ChAT) in the neonatal rat forebrain: Evidence for a Physiological role of NGF in the brain. Dev Brain Res 9: 45-52

Hamburger V, Hamilton HL. A series of nromal stages in the development of the chick embryo. J Morphol 88: 49-92

Hamburger V, Brunso-Bechtold JK, Yip JW (1981) Neuronal death in the spinal ganglia of the chick embryo and its reduction by nerve growth factor. J Neurosci 1: 60-71

Herrup K, Shooter EM (1975) Properties of the β-nerve growth factor receptor in development. J Cell Biol 67: 118-125

Korsching S, Auburger G, Heumann R, Scott J, Thoenen H (1985) Levels of nerve growth factor and its mRNA in the central nervous system of the rat correlate with cholinergic innervation. EMBO J 4: 1389-1393

Large T H, Bodary SC, Clegg DO, Weskamp G, Otten U, Reichardt LF (1986) Nerve growth factor gene expression in the developing rat brain. Science 234: 352-355

Levi-Montalcini R, Angeletti PU (1968) Nerve growth factor. Physiol Rev 48: 534-569

Maniatis T, Fritsch EF, Sambrook J (1982) Molecular Cloning. A Laboratory Manual, (Cold Spring Harbor) 545 pp.

Meier R, Becker-Andre M, Götz R, Heumann R, Shaw A, Thoenen H (1986) Molecular cloning of bovine and chick nerve growth factor (NGF): delineation of conserved and unconserved domains and their relationship to the biological activity and antigenicity of NGF. EMBO J 5: 1489-1493

Noden D (1978) The control of avian cephalic neural crest cytodifferentiation. II. Neural tissues. Dev Biol 67: 313-329

Scott J, Selby M, Urdea M, Quiroga M, Bell GI, Rutter WJ (1983) Isolation and nucleotide sequence of a cDNA encoding the precursor of mouse nerve growth factor. Nature 302: 538-540

Shelton DL, Reichardt LF (1984) Expression of the β-nerve growth factor gene correlates with the density of sympathetic innervation in effector organs. Proc Natl Acad Sci USA 81: 7951-7955

Shelton DL, Reichardt LF (1986) Studies on the expression of the β nerve growth factor (NGF) gene in the central nervous system: Level and regional distribution of NGF mRNA suggest that NGF functions as a trophic factor for several distinct populations of neurons. Proc Natl Acad Sci USA 83: 2741-2781

Thoenen H, Barde Y-A (1980) Physiology of nerve growth factor. Physiol Rev 60: 1284-1335

Ullrich A, Gray A, Berman C, Dull TJ (1983) Human β-nerve growth factor gene sequence highly homologous to that of mouse. Nature 303: 821-825

Whittemore SR, Ebendal T, Lärkfors L, Olson L, Seiger Å, Strömberg I, Persson H (1986) Developmental and regional expression of β nerve growth factor messenger RNA and protein in the rat central nervous system. Proc Natl Acad Sci USA 83: 817-821

Wion D, Perret C, Frechin N, Keller A, Behar G, Brachet P, Auffray C (1986) Molecular cloning of the avian β-nerve growth factor gene: transcription in brain. FEBS Lett. 203: 82-86

Wong GG, Witek JJS, Temple PA, Wilkens KM, Leary AC, Luxenberg DP, Jones SS, Brown EL, Kay RM, Orr EC, Shoemaker C, Golde DW, Kaufman RJ, Hewick RM, Wang EA, Clark SC (1985) Human GM-CSF: Molecular cloning of the complementary DNA and purification of the natural and recombinant proteins. Science 228: 810-815

# STRUCTURE AND EXPRESSION OF ß-NERVE GROWTH FACTOR IN THE RAT CENTRAL NERVOUS SYSTEM

Scott R. Whittemore[1], Håkan Persson, Ted Ebendal[2], Lena Lärkfors[2], Dan Larhammar and Anders Ericsson
Department of Medical Genetics
Biomedical Center Box 589
Uppsala University
S-751 23 Uppsala
Sweden

[1] Present address and correspondence: Dr. S.R. Whittemore, Department of Neurological Surgery, University of Miami School of Medicine, 1600 NW 10th Avenue - R48, Miami, FL 33136.

[2] Department of Zoology, Uppsala University, S-751 23 Uppsala, Sweden

NATO ASI Series, Vol. H22
Neural Development and Regeneration
Edited by A. Gorio et al.

## INTRODUCTION

Target-derived neuronal trophic factors have been implicated in the maturation and maintainance of both the central (CNS) and peripheral (PNS) nervous systems[1-3]. The most well characterized of these is β-nerve growth factor (NGF). The effects of NGF on PNS sensory and sympathetic neurons are well documented[4,5]. Present evidence suggests a physiological role for NGF also in the CNS. These data include the detection of molecules in the CNS with "NGF-like" physiological activity[6-10] or immunological cross-reactivity[9,11-15], as well as measurements of altered biological responses subsequent to injection of NGF or anti-NGF antibodies into the CNS[16-25]. Recent advances in recombinant DNA technology have allowed determination of NGF mRNA levels in the brain[9,11,12,15,26-28]. Finally, both the detection of specific NGF receptors in the CNS[29-33] and the observed effects of NGF on cultured CNS neurons[34-40] have supported a possible role of NGF in the CNS.

Present data strongly implies that NGF is a neuronal trophic factor for the basal forebrain cholinergic neurons. However, NGF does not have generalized effects on all CNS cholinergic cell groups. Additionally, NGF and NGF mRNA are found in CNS regions devoid of cholinergic neurons, suggesting effects on other as yet unknown central neuronal populations. Here, the structure of rat NGF is presented and the regional and developmental expression of NGF in the rat CNS documented.

## METHODS

Isolation and DNA sequence analysis of the rat NGF gene. A genomic rat Sprague-Dawley library was prepared in the EcoRI site of phage Charon 4A after partial digestion of genomic DNA with Hae III and addition of EcoRI linkers. The library was screened with a [$^{32}$-P]-labelled 900bp Pst I fragment from a mouse cDNA clone[41] using conventional procedures under high stringency conditions. One phage clone was isolated and a hybridizing 1.7kb Pvu II-Bgl II fragment was subcloned into the plasmid pUC9. The nucleotide sequence was determined with the Maxam and Gilbert procedure[42].

RNA isolation and blot hybridization. Tissues were removed and immediately frozen in liquid nitrogen. Total cellular RNA was prepared[43] and poly ($A^+$) RNA, isolated by oligo(dT) cellulose chromatography[44], separated on 1% agarose gels containing 0.7% formaldehyde and transferred to nitrocellulose filters. A 900bp Pst I fragment from a mouse cDNA clone[41] and a 1.5kb Pst I fragment from an α-actin cDNA clone[45] were nick translated, hybridized to the nitrocellulose filters, exposed on Kodak XAR-5 X-ray film and quantitated as previously described[9].

Enzyme immunoassay (EIA) for NGF. Endogenous NGF levels were determined by a two-site fluorometric EIA, as described in detail previously[14].

Surgical procedures. One week old Sprague-Dawley rats (Alab, Stockholm) were anesthetized with ether. Fimbria transection and entorhinal cortex lesions were performed as described[46]. Sham operated animals served as controls, and received a bilateral superficial knife cut through cortex which did not damage underlying structures.

## RESULTS

Nucleotide sequence of the rat prepro-NGF gene. One positive genomic clone was isolated and its hybridizing region subcloned in plasmid pUC9 (Fig. 1A). The sequenced region contains the 3' exon of the rat NGF gene and encodes the carboxyterminal 245 amino acids of prepro-NGF, including the mature protein, as well as the 3'-untranslated region of the NGF mRNA (Fig. 1B). The 894 nucleotides of this exon are 96% homologous with the corresponding part of the mouse NGF gene. Ten of the 36 nucleotide substitutions result in amino acid substitutions which are equally distributed between the propeptide and the mature NGF protein. Six of these 10 replacements are conservative.

A single polyadenylation signal is present 136 nucleotides 3' to the translation termination codon. No additional polyadenylation signal occurs in the following 533 nucleotides.

Expression of NGF in the adult rat CNS. A 1.3kb poly $(A)^+$ NGF mRNA was detected in both the mouse submaxillary gland and the rat CNS using the 900bp Pst I fragment from the mouse cDNA as a probe. An additional band which comprised 20-25% of the hybridization signal was seen only in the rat brain (Fig. 2). An identical hybridization pattern was seen when a homologous rat genomic probe was used (data not shown).

NGF mRNA was heterogeneously distributed (Fig.2), with cortex and hippocampus having roughly two-fold higher levels than total brain, which contains 2.8 pg NGF mRNA/μg poly $(A)^+$ RNA[27]. Significant levels were observed in olfactory bulb and pons/medulla, low levels in cerebellum and thalamus, while NGF mRNA was below detection limits in hypothalamus, septum and striatum. Actin mRNA levels were identical in all regions of the CNS.

A

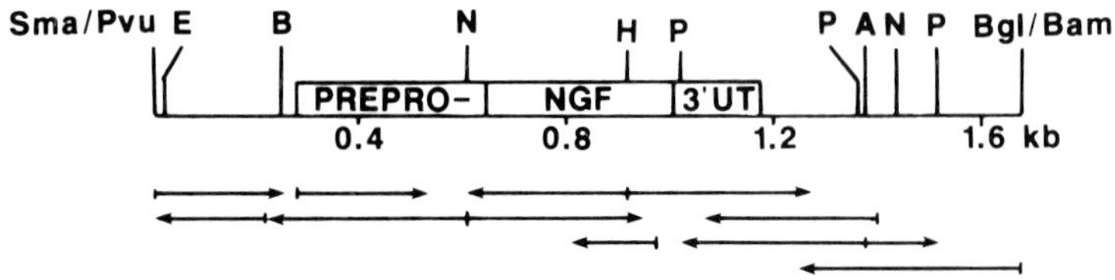


B

CAGCTGGGTTGGAATTCAAGGGCCCCATTGCTTCCCGGAACAGAACGACCACACAGCCTGCTCTGATTA 69

ATGCCAGTGATCCCAATGTGATTGCTGCCCACGCCCCTTCTCCTCTCACAAGTGTTCTACTTTGGGTGA 138

TGATTCTGGGCTCTCTTCCCATAGCCTCCTGGCATCTTCTTGGAAGAACCCTGTGAGGGGGCCTGACAC 207

CATCCCGATAATGCTTAGCACGGCTCCCCAGCGTTTAACTTAGGTAACCTCTCGGTCTTTGTCTTTCCAG▼ 277

GTG CAT AGC GTA ATG TCC ATG TTG TTC TAC ACT CTG ATC ACA GCG TTT TTG 328

Val His Ser Val Met Ser Met Leu Phe Tyr Thr Leu Ile Thr Ala Phe Leu

ATC GGC GTA CAG GCA GAA CCG TAC ACA GAT AGC AAT GTC CCA GAG GGA GAC 379

Ile Gly Val Gln Ala Glu Pro Tyr Thr Asp Ser Asn Val Pro Glu Gly Asp

TCT GTC CCT GAA GCC CAC TGG ACT AAA CTT CAG CAT TCC CTT GAC ACA GCC 430

Ser Val Pro Glu Ala His Trp Thr Lys Leu Gln His Ser Leu Asp Thr Ala

CTC CGC AGA GCC CGC AGT GCC CCT GCT GAA CCA ATA GCT GCC CGT GTG ACA 481

Leu Arg Arg Ala Arg Ser Ala Pro Ala Glu Pro Ile Ala Ala Arg Val Thr

GGG CAG ACC CGC AAC ATC ACT GTG GAC CCC AAA CTG TTT AAG AAA CGG AGA 532

Gly Gln Thr Arg Asn Ile Thr Val Asp Pro Lys Leu Phe Lys Lys Arg Arg

CTC CGT TCA CCC CGC GTG CTG TTT AGC ACC CAG CCT CCA CCC ACC TCT TCG 583

Leu Arg Ser Pro Arg Val Leu Phe Ser Thr Gln Pro Pro Pro Thr Ser Ser

GAC ACT CTG GAT TTA GAC TTC CAG GCC CAT GGT ACA ATC TCC TTC AAC AGG 634

Asp Thr Leu Asp Leu Asp Phe Gln Ala His Gly Thr Ile Ser Phe Asn Arg

ACT CAC AGG AGC AAG CGC TCA TCC ACC CAC CCA GTC TTC CAC ATG GGG GAG 685

Thr His Arg Ser Lys Arg Ser Ser Thr His Pro Val Phe His Met Gly Glu

TTT TCA GTG TGT GAC AGT GTC AGT GTG TGG GTT GGA GAT AAG ACC ACA GCC 736

Phe Ser Val Cys Asp Ser Val Ser Val Trp Val Gly Asp Lys Thr Thr Ala

ACG GAC ATC AAG GGC AAG GAG GTG ACA GTG CTG GGC GAG GTG AAC ATT AAC 787

Thr Asp Ile Lys Gly Lys Glu Val Thr Val Leu Gly Glu Val Asn Ile Asn

AAC AGT GTA TTC AAA CAG TAT TTT TTT GAG ACC AAG TGC CGA GCC CCA AAT 838

Asn Ser Val Phe Lys Gln Tyr Phe Phe Glu Thr Lys Cys Arg Ala Pro Asn

CCT GTA GAG AGT GGA TGC CGG GGC ATT GAC TCC AAG CAC TGG AAC TCA TAC 889

Pro Val Glu Ser Gly Cys Arg Gly Ile Asp Ser Lys His Trp Asn Ser Tyr

TGC ACC ACG ACT CAC ACC TTT GTC AAG GCG TTG ACA ACA GAC GAC AAA CAG 940

Cys Thr Thr Thr His Thr Phe Val Lys Ala Leu Thr Thr Asp Asp Lys Gln

GCT GCC TGG AGG TTC ATC AGG ATA GAT ACA GCC TGC GTG TGT GTG CTC AGC 991

Ala Ala Trp Arg Phe Ile Arg Ile Asp Thr Ala Cys Val Cys Val Leu Ser

AGG AAG GCT GCA AGA AGA GGC TGA CTTGCCTGCAGCCCCCTTCCCCACCTGCCCCCTCCA 1051

Arg Lys Ala Ala Arg Arg Gly **STOP**

CACTCTCCTGGGCCCCTCCCTACCTCAGCCTGTAAATTATTTTAAATTATAAGGACTGCATGATAATTT 1120

ATCGTTTATACAATTTTAAAGTCATTATTT**ATTAAA**TTTTCAAAGCATCCTG▼TGTACCCACACTTGAG 1188

TCATTTCTCTCAATAAGAGTACCCACAAAGTTTAGGAGAGTGCAGAATGAACTGTCCCCCAGCCACTCC 1287

TGGCAACACGGCCCATCTGTAACCTTCATTCCCAGCCAGAGCTGCTCCAGGGCTGGCTAACTAGTTTCA 1326

GACACTGCTCAGCACCCAGCATGATTAGCAAGGGAAGTCAGCCTGCAGGCTCTGGTCTACATTCCGGAG 1395

CCAACTCTACCAAATCCTTGGATTATCTGCTGCACAGCATGCCTCCATGGGTTTTGATTGCCTCACTTG 1464

AGGAGGGAAGAGTAGTTAAGACTGGTCAGAAAGCAGGATGCTATGTACACTGGCTGCAGTCTCCCACCT 1533

CTGAGAGACCCAGGCTGGTCCTCGGAGGATATTGGGAACTCCCTGGGTGGATAAGTAGAGGCTTCCAGG 1602

TCTTCTGGCTTCAGTCAGTTGGAAGAGCAGTCTGAAGGAGCTGTAACAAAATCATCTCCTGAGGCCTGT 1671

CATGGCAGATCT 1683

Fig 1. Restiction map (A) and nucleotide sequence (B) of chromosomal segment containing 3' exon of the rat NGF gene. In (A), exon is boxed and arrows show sequencing strategy. In (B), mature NGF is boxed, as are potential proteolytic processing sites. Arrows indicate exon boundaries and the polyadenylation site is underlined. Abbreviations: E-Eco RI; B-BstE II; N-Nco I; P-Pst I; A-Acc I.

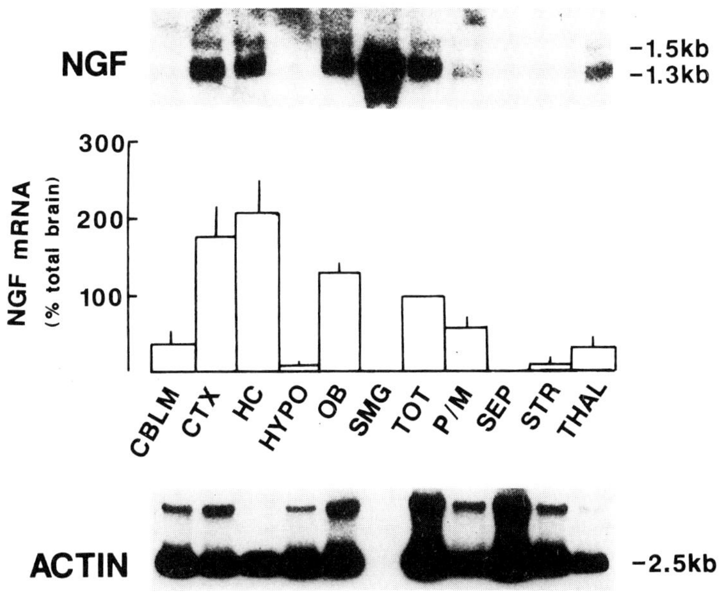


Fig. 2. Regional expression of NGF mRNA in the rat CNS. Northern blot (upper panel) and quantitation (middle panel) of NGF mRNA (15ug/lane) expression in the rat brain. Actin mRNA levels are shown in the lower panel. Abbreviations: CBLM-cerebellum; CTX-cerebral cortex; HC-hippocampus; OB-olfactory bulb; SMG-mouse submaxillary gland (80ng/lane); TOT-total brain; P/M-pons/medulla; SEP-septum; STR-corpus striatum; THAL-thalamus. Data redrawn from ref. 9.

Developmental expression of NGF mRNA and protein. NGF mRNA was undetectable prenatally in total brain. On postnatal day 1 (P1), 5% of adult levels were observed, which were reached by 3 weeks postnatal. Half-maximal levels occurred between 1 and 2 weeks. Forty seven and 84 week old total brain contained 90% and 80% respectively of the NGF mRNA found in adult brain (Fig. 3, open bars). Actin mRNA levels were constant at all developmental stages (data not shown).

In contrast, NGF protein was found at nearly adult levels in prenatal total brain, reaching peak expression (160% adult levels) at 3 weeks postnatal (Fig. 3, filled circles). A slight decrease in NGF protein levels was seen between adult and 1 year old total brain.

Lesion-induced changes in hippocampal NGF expression. Ten days after fimbrial transection in three week old rats, which removes the cholinergic afferent fibers coming from the basal forebrain[47], hippocampal NGF mRNA and protein levels were increased 60% and 50% respectively, compared to age-matched controls (Fig. 4). By 30 days post-lesion, neither NGF mRNA nor protein were different from controls (data not shown). In contrast,

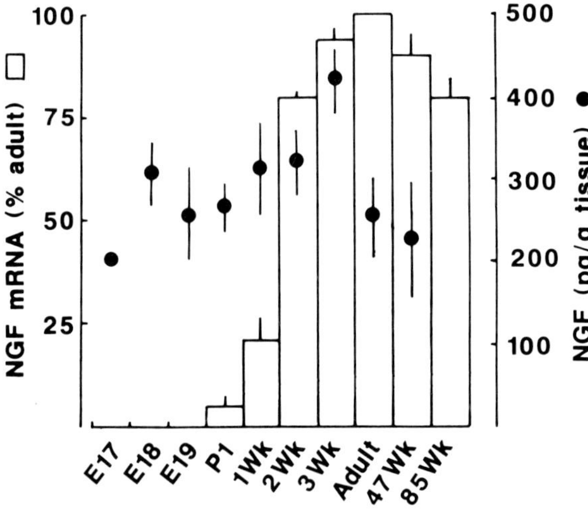


Fig. 3. Developmental expression of NGF mRNA and protein. Open bars: Poly (A)+ RNA (15μg) from total brain of the ages indicated were probed for NGF mRNA and the results (mean ± SEM, 4-6 experiments) were normalized to adult levels. Closed circles: NGF protein levels detected by EIA (Mean ± SEM, 2-15 experiments). Abbreviations: E17-19, embryonic day 17-19; P1, postnatal day 1; 1-85 Wk, 1-85 weeks. Adult, 12 weeks. Data redrawn from ref. 9.

NGF mRNA and protein levels were unaltered in either the ipsilateral or contralateral hippocampus 10 days after unilateral entorhinal cortex ablation, which removes the major excitatory amino acid afferents to the hippocampus[47]. Cortical NGF mRNA and hippocampal actin mRNA levels were unchanged following either fimbrial transection or entorhinal cortex ablation (data not shown).

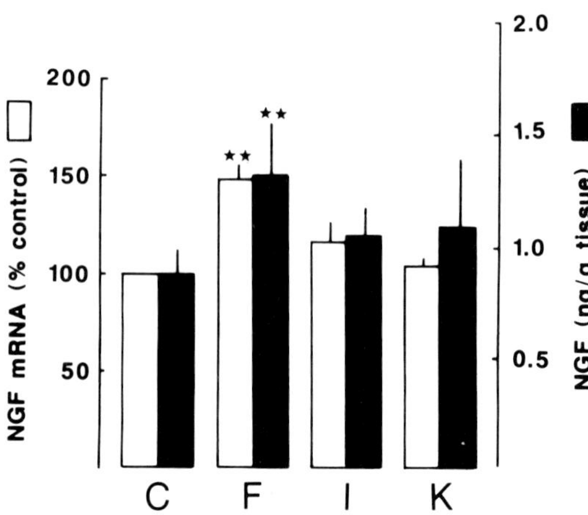


Fig. 4. Lesion-induced alterations in hippocamal NGF mRNA and protein expression. Levels of NGF mRNA (open bars) represent Mean ± SEM of densitometric scans of 4-5 Northern blots from 2 independent preparations of RNA, 10 days after lesion. NGF protein levels (filled bars) are Mean ± SEM of 2-5 experiments, each of which was assayed 5-10 times. **$p<0.05$ as compared to controls. Abbreviations: C, control; F, fimbrial transection; I and K, ipsi- and contra-lateral to unilateral entorhinal cortex lesion. Data redrawn from ref. 15.

Discussion. The 3' exon of the rat NGF gene is highly homologous (96%) to that of the mouse. Interestingly, the predicted prepropeptide is as conserved as the mature protein. Similar high homologies are seen between the murine and the human[48], chicken[49-51] and bovine[51] sequences. This high species conservation of NGF is not surprising in view of its essential role in the development of the mammalian nervous system[4,5]. The 3' untranslated region of the rat and mouse mRNA is also highly conserved, with only 1 difference in 160 nucleotides. This region has a very high AT content with a consensus ATTTA sequence, both of which have been shown to confer mRNA instability to lymphokine, cytokine and proto-oncogene mRNA[52].

Two NGF mRNAs, 1.3 and 1.5kb, were detected in the rat CNS. These could not be accounted for by an additional poly $(A)^+$ site as only one was found. Alternative splicing of NGF mRNA has been described[53], although it resulted in a shorter transcript. It remains to be determined if differential splicing or perhaps a larger size for one of the four 5' exons[53] could account for the 2 mRNA species found in the rat.

NGF mRNA is differentially distributed in the CNS, consistent with previous results[9,11,12,27,28]. The regions with the highest levels, cortex and hippocampus, contain the terminal fields of the basal forebrain cholinergic neurons. NGF is retrogradely transported from hippocampus and cortex to the basal forebrain[16,17] and intraventricularly infused NGF can prevent the death of septal cholinergic neurons induced by fimbrial transection[22-24]. These data suggest that NGF functions as a trophic factor for the septal cholinergic neurons. However, in the brain stem, where moderate levels of NGF mRNA and protein[11] are seen, NGF does not alter cholinergic metabolism[38,54,55] nor are NGF receptors associated with the main cholinergic cell groups[29]. Additionally, both NGF mRNA and protein[11,12] are found in the cerebellum, where cholinergic cell groups have not been described[56]. This would imply both that NGF does not affect all cholinergic CNS neurons and that other non-NGF factors can influence cholinergic function.

Total brain NGF mRNA expression appears postnatal. Similar developmental NGF mRNA profiles were described for hippocampus and cortex[12,71]. This time course closely parallels the maturation of synapses in cortex[57] and hippocampus[58], as well as hippocampal ChAT expression[12,71]. The detection of NGF prenatally, in the absence of NGF mRNA may reflect a rapid turnover of message and thus very low steady state levels. Auburger et al.[71] also saw similarly high levels of NGF in E17 hippocampus, in the absence of detectable NGF mRNA. In contrast, Large et al.[12] detected only low levels of NGF on P1 in cortex or hippocampus. As all three studies found identical adult levels of NGF, this discrepency is difficult to reconcile. Recently, Davies et al.[59] elegantly demonstrated that NGF mRNA, protein and receptor expression in the PNS was initiated only after afferent sensory fibers reached their targets. Hippocampal cholinergic synaptogenesis occurs primarily postnatally[58,60], but septal afferents reach the hippocampus by at least E20[61,62]. Together with the detection of NGF receptors[63,64] and NGF immunoreactivity[65] as early as E15 in the rat CNS, these data suggest that NGF is synthesized prenatally.

In aged animals, slight reductions in total brain NGF mRNA were observed. These decreases may reflect large deficits in trophic support within specific populations of neurons. Indeed, significant decreases in hippocampal NGF mRNA and protein were seen in aged Fischer rats[66]. Deficits in septal cholinergic neurons have also been reported at these ages[67,68], and these systems have been suggested to be strongly involved in memory[69]. It is conceivable that decreases in neurotrophic support during aging may result in impaired neuronal function.

NGF synthesis in the neonatal hippocampus appears to be specifically regulated by the degree of afferent cholinergic input. Fimbrial transection, but not entorhinal cortex ablation, results in a transient increase in NGF mRNA and protein levels. These data suggest either lesion-induced transcriptional control or an increase in NGF mRNA stability. Either mechanism implies an initial compensatory increase in NGF mRNA specifically in response to cholinergic denervation. The return to control levels 30 days post-lesion suggests a subsequent down-regulation, possibly in response to reinnvervation by non-cholinergic fibers which sprout to fill the vacant synaptic sites[47].

In the adult hippocampus, NGF mRNA expression is not induced by fimbrial transection[9,28,70]. The transient increase in hippocampal NGF protein seen after fimbriaectomy[13,70] is most likely secondary to the removal of the retrograde transport system. This difference in responsivity between adult and neonate may be a fundamental age-related effect, with the neonatal neurons having a greater capacity to differentially respond to an altered cellular environment.

The differential distribution and developmental regulation is consistent with the hypothesis that NGF does function as a neurotrophic factor in the mammalian CNS. The strongest evidence for central NGF function is seen for basal forebrain cholinergic neurons. High levels of NGF mRNA and protein were detected in the target zones of these neurons. Additionally, the specific induction of hippocampal NGF expression only in response to cholinergic denervations further supports this suggestion. The temporal appearance of NGF suggests a role as a maintainance factor, rather than a chemotactic one, as in the periphery[59]. However, it is apparent also that NGF does not support all cholinergic neurons in the CNS, nor is NGF the only central cholinergic growth factor[38]. Finally, the distribution of NGF mRNA suggests that NGF may also have effects on other, as yet undefined, non-cholinergic central neurons.

Acknowledgements. We thank Dr. James Bonner, Cal Tech, Pasedena, CA for providing the rat genomic library.

REFERENCES

1. Cowan WM, Fawcett JW, O'Leary DDM, Stanfield B. (1984) Regressive events in neurogenesis. Science 227:1258-1265
2. Nieto-Sampedro M, Cotman CW (1985) Growth factor induction and temporal order in central nervous system repair. In: Cotman CW (ed) Synaptic Plasticity. Guilford, New York, p 407
3. Easter SS, Purves D, Rakic P, Spitzer NC (1985) The changing view of neural specificity. Science 230:507-511
4. Levi-Montalcini R, Angeletti PU (1968) Nerve growth factor. Physiol Rev 48:534-569
5. Thoenen H, Barde Y-A (1980) Physiology of nerve growth factor. Physiol Rev 60:1285-1335
6. Crutcher KA, Brothers L, Davis JN (1979) Sprouting of sympathetic nerves in the absence of afferent input. Exp Neurol 66:778-783
7. Crutcher KA, Collins F (1982) In vitro evidence for two distinct hippocampal growth factors: basis of neuronal plasticity? Science 217:67-68
8. Collins F, Crutcher KA (1985) Neurotrophic activity in the adult rat hippocampal formation: regional distribution and increase after septal lesion. J Neurosci 5:2809-2814
9. Whittemore SR, Ebendal T, Lärkfors L, Olson L, Seiger Å, Strömberg I, Persson H (1986) Developmental and regional expression of nerve growth factor messenger RNA and protein in the rat central nervous system. Proc Nat Acad Sci USA 83:817-821
10. Gage FH, Björklund A, Stenevi U (1984) Denervation releases a neuronal survival factor in adult rat hippocampus. Nature 308:637-639
11. Korsching S, Auburger G, Heumann R, Scott J, Thoenen H (1985) Levels of nerve growth factor and its mRNA in the central nervous system of the rat correlate with cholinergic innervation. EMBO J 4:1389-1393
12. Large TH, Bodary SC, Clegg DO, Weskamp G, Otten U, Reichardt LF (1986) Nerve growth factor gene expression in the developing rat brain. Science 234:352-355
13. Gasser UE, Weskamp G, Otten U, Dravid AR (1986) Time course of the elevation of nerve growth factor (NGF) content in the hippocmapus and septum following lesions of the septohippocampal pathway in rats. Brain Res 376:351-356
14. Lärkfors L, Ebendal T (1987) Highly sensitive enzyme immunoassays for β-nerve growth factor. J Immunol Meth 97:41-47
15. Whittemore SR, Lärkfors L, Ebendal T, Holets VR, Ericsson A, Persson H (1987) Increased β-nerve growth factor messenger RNA and protein levels in neonatal rat hippocampus following specific cholinergic lesions. J Neurosci 7:244-251
16. Schwab ME, Otten U, Agid Y, Thoenen H (1979) Nerve growth factor (NGF) in the rat CNS: absence of specific retrograde axonal transport and tyrosine hydroxylase induction in locus coeruleus and substantia nigra. Brain Res 168:473-483
17. Seiler M, Schwab ME (1984) Specific retrograde transport of nerve growth factor (NGF) from neocortex to nucleus basalis in the rat. Brain Res 300:33-39
18. Gnahn H, Hefti F, Heumann R, Schwab ME, Thoenen H (1983) NGF-mediated increase of choline acetyltransferase (ChAT) in the neonatal rat forebrain: evidence for a physiological role of NGF in the brain? Dev Brain Res 9:45-52
19. Mobley WC, Rutkowski JL, Tennekoon GI, Buchanan K, Johnston MV (1985) Choline acetyltransferase activity in striatum of neonatal rats increased by nerve growth factor. Science 229:284-287
20. Mobley WC, Rutkowski JL, Tennekoon GI, Gemski J, Buchanan K, Johnston MV (1986) Nerve growth factor increases choline acetyltransferase activity in developing basal forebrain neurons. Mol Brain Res 1:53-62
21. Hefti F, Dravid A, Hartikka J (1984) Chronic intraventricular injections of nerve growth factor elevate hippocampal choline acetyltransferase activity in adult rats with partial septo hippo-

campal lesions. Brain Res 293:305-311
22. Hefti F (1986) Nerve growth factor promotes survival of septal cholinergic neurons after fimbrial transection. J Neurosci 6:2155-2162
23. Williams LR, Varon S, Peterson GM, Wictorin K, Fischer W, Björklund A, Gage FH (1986) Infusion of nerve growth factor prevents basal forebrain neuronal death after fimbria fornix transection. Proc Nat Acad Sci USA 83:9231-9235
24. Kromer LF (1987) Nerve growth factor treatment after brain injury prevents neuronal death. Science 235:214-216
25. Springer JE, Loy R (1985) Intrahippocampal injections of antiserum to nerve growth factor inhibit sympathohippocampal sprouting. Brain Res Bull 15:629-634
26. Shelton DL, Reichardt LF (1984) Expression of the β-nerve growth factor gene correlates with the density of sympathetic innervaton in effector organs. Proc Nat Acad Sci USA 81:7951-7955
27. Shelton DL, Reichardt LF (1986) Studies on the expression of the nerve growth factor (NGF) gene in the central nervous system: level and regional distribution of NGF mRNA suggest that NGF functions as a trophic factor for several distinct populations of neurons. Proc Nat Acad Sci USA 83:2714-2718
28. Goedert M, Fine A, Hunt SP, Ullrich U (1986) Nerve growth factor mRNA in peripheral and central rat tissues and in the human central nervous system: lesion effects in the rat brain and levels in Alzheimer's disease. Mol Brain Res 1:85-92
29. Richardson PM, Verge Issa VMK, Riopelle RJ (1986) Distribution of neuronal receptors for nerve growth factor in the rat. J Neurosci 6:2312-2321
30. Taniuchi M, Schweitzer JB, Johnson EM (1984) Nerve growth factor receptor molecules in rat brain. Proc Nat Acad Sci USA 83:1950-1954
31. Hefti F, Hartikka J, Salvatierra A, Weiner WJ, Mash DC (1986) Localization of nerve growth factor receptors in cholinergic neurons of the human basal forebrain. Neurosci Lett 69:37-41
32. Springer JE, Koh S, Tayrien MW, Loy R (1987) Basal forebrain magnocellular neurons stain for nerve growth factor: correlation with cholinergic cell bodies and effects of axotomy. J Neurosci Res (in press)
33. Johnson EM, Taniuchi M, Clark HB, Springer JE, Koh S, Tayrien MW, Loy R (1987) Demonstration of the retrograde transport of nerve growth factor (NGF) receptor in the peripheral and central nervous system. J Neurosci 7:923-929
34. Honegger P, Lenoir D (1982) Nerve growth factor (NGF) stimulation of cholinergic telencephalic neurons in aggregation cell cultures. Dev Brain Res 3:229-238
35. Honegger P (1983) Nerve growth factor-sensitive brain neurons in culture. Monogr neural Sci 9:36-42
36. Hefti F, Hartikka J, Eckenstein F, Gnahn H, Heumann R, Schwab M (1985) Nerve growth factor increases choline acetyltransferase but not survival or fiber outgrowth of cultured fetal septal cholinergic neurons. Neurosci 14:55-68
37. Hefti F, Hartikka J, Bolger MB (1986) Effect of thyroid hormone analogs on the activity of choline acetyltransferase in cultures of dissociated septal cells. Brain Res 375:413-416
38. Hatanaka H, Tsukui H (1986) Differential effects of nerve-growth factor and glioma-conditioned medium on neurons cultured from various regions of fetal rat central nervous system, Dev Brain Res 30:47-56
39. Gähwiler BH, Enz A, Hefti F (1987) Nerve growth factor promotes development of the rat septohippocampal cholinergic projection in vitro. Neurosci Lett 75:6-10
40. Martínez HJ, Dreyfus CF, Miller Jonakait G, Black IB (1985) Nerve growth factor promotes cholinergic development in brain striatal cultures. Proc Nat Acad Sci USA 82:7777-7781
41. Scott J, Selby M, Urdea M, Quiroga M, Bell GI, Rutter WJ (1983) Isolation and nucleotide sequence of a cDNA clone encoding the precursor of mouse nerve growth factor. Nature 302:538-540
42. Maxam AM, Gilbert W (1977) A new method for sequencing DNA. Proc Nat Acad Sci USA 74:560-564
43. Chirgwin JM, Przybyla AE, MacDonald RJ, Rutter WJ (1979) Isolation of biologically active ribonucleic acid from sources enriched in ribonuclease. Biochem 18:5294-5299
44. Aviv H, Leder P (1972) Purification of biologically active globin messenger RNA by chromatography on oligo-thymidylic acid-cellulose. Proc Nat Acad Sci USA 69:1408-1412
45. Minty AJ, Caravatti M, Benoit K, Cohen A, Daubas P, Weydert A, Gros R,

Buckingham ME (1981) Mouse actin messenger RNAs. Construction and characterization of a recombinant plasmid molecule containing a compementary transcript of mouse α-actin mRNA, J. Biol Chem 286:1008-1014

46. Lewis ER, Cotman CW (1980) Mechanisms of septal lamination in the developing hippocampus revealed by outgrowth of fibers from septal implants. Positional and temporal factors. Brain Res 196:307-330

47. Cotman CW, Nadler JV (1978) Reactive synaptogenesis in the hippocampus. In: Cotman CW (ed), Neuronal Plasticity, Raven, New York, p 227

48. Ullrich A, Gray A, Berman C, Dull TJ (1983) Human -nerve growth factor gene sequence highly homologous to that of mouse. Nature 303:821-825

49. Ebendal T, Larhammar D, Persson H (1986) Structure and expression of the chicken nerve growth factor gene. EMBO J 5:1483-1487

50. Wion D, Perret C, Fréchin N, Keller A, Béhar G, Brachet P, Auffray C (1986) Molecular cloning of the avian β-nerve growth factor gene: transcription in brain. FEBS Lett 203:82-86

51. Meier R, Becker-André M, Götz R, Heumann R, Shaw A, Thoenen H (1986) Molecular cloning of bovine and chick nerve growth factor (NGF): delineation of conserved and unconserved domains and their relationship to the biological activity and antigenicity of NGF. EMBO J 5:1489-1493

52. Shaw G, Kamen R (1986) A conserved AU sequence from the 3' untranslated region of GM-CSF mRNA mediates selective mRNA degredation. Cell 46:559-667

53. Edwards RH, Selby MJ, Rutter WJ (1986) Differential RNA splicing predicts two distinct nerve growth factor precursors. Nature 319:784-787.

54. Konkol RJ, Mailman R, Bendeich EG, Garrison AM, Mueller RA, Breese GR (1978) Evaluation of the effects of nerve growth factor and anti-nerve growth factor on the development of central catecholamine-containing neurons. Brain Res 144:277-285

55. Dreyfus CF, Peterson ER, Crain SM (1980) Failure of nerve growth factor to affect fetal mouse brain stem catecholaminergic neurons in culture. Brain Res 194:540-547

56. Mesulam M-M, Mufson EJ, Wainer BH, Levey AI (1983) Central cholinergic pathways in the rat: an overview based on an alternative nomenclature (Ch1-Ch6). Neurosci 10:1185-1201

57. Aghajanian GK, Bloom FE (1967) The formation of synaptic junctions in developing rat brai: a quantitative electron microscopic study. Brain Res 6:716-727

58. Crain B, Cotman C, Taylor D, Lynch G (1973) A quantitative electron microscopic study of synaptogenesis in the dentate gyrus of the rat. Brain Res 63:195-204

59. Davies AM, Bandtlow C, Heumann R, Korsching S, Rohrer H, Thoenen H (1987) Timing and site of nerve growth factor synthesis in developing skin in relation to innervation and expression of the receptor. Nature 326:353-358

60. Matthews DA, Nadler JV, Lynch GS, Cotman CW (1974) Development of cholinergic innervation in the hippocampal formation of the rat. I. Histochemical demonstration of acetylcholinesterase activity. Dev Biol 36:130-141

61. Milner TA, Loy R, Amaral DG (1983) An anatomical study of the development of the septo-hippocampal projection in the rat. Dev Brain Res 8:343-371

62. Crutcher KA (1982) Development of the rat septohippocampal projection: a retrograde fluorescent tracer study. Dev Brain Res 3:145-150

63. Koh S, Notter MD, Loy R (1986) Nerve growth factor (NGF) promotes cell survival and neurite outgrowth of rat CNS neurons in culture. Correlation with ontogenesis of NGF receptor immunoreactivity. Neurosci Absts 12:1093

64. Yan Q, Johnson EM (1986) NGF receptor density in developing rats Neurosci Absts 12:1093

65. Ayer-LeLievre CS, Ebendal T, Olson L, Seiger Å (1983) Localization of nerve growth factor-like immunoreactivity in rat nervous tissue. Med Biol 61:296-304

66. Lärkfors L, Ebendal T, Whittemore SR, Persson H, Hoffer B, Olson L Decreased levels of nerve growth factor and its messenger RNA in the aged rat brain. Mol Brain Res (submitted)

67. Bondareff W (1979) Synaptic atrophy in the senescent hippocampus. Mech Aging Dev 9:163-171

68. Hornberger JC, Buell SJ, Flood DG, McNeill TH, Coleman PD (1985) Stability of numbers but not size of mouse forebrain cholinergic

neurons to 53 months. Neurobiol Aging 6:269-275
69. Collerton D (1986) Cholinergic function and intellectual decline in Alzheimer's disease. Neurosci 19:1-28
70. Korsching S, Heumann R, Thoenen H, Hefti F (1986) Cholinergic denervation of the rat hippocampus by fimbrial transection leads to a transient accumulation of nerve growth factor (NGF) without change in $mRNA^{NGF}$ content. Neurosci Lett 66:175-180
71. Auburger G, Heumann R, Hellweg R, Korsching S, Thoenen H (1987) Developmental changes of nerve growth factor and its mRNA in the rat hippocampus: comparison with choline acetyltransferase. Dev Biol 120:322-328

# MOLECULAR ASPECTS OF THE RAT NERVE GROWTH FACTOR RECEPTOR.

T.P. Misko, M.J. Radeke and E.M. Shooter
Department of Neurobiology
Stanford University School of Medicine
Stanford
California 94305.

## INTRODUCTION

The role of nerve growth factor (NGF) in the development, maintenance, and regrowth (after injury) of sympathetic and some sensory neurons is well documented (Vale and Shooter 1987, Oppenheim 1981, Levi-Montalcini and Angeletti 1968). Perhaps this is most strikingly demonstrated by the ability of NGF antibodies to prevent the development of sympathetic neurons when injected into newborn rats (Levi-Montalcini and Angeletti, 1966) or of some sensory neurons when introduced into the fetus (Johnson et al. 1980). More recently, the discovery of NGF in certain cholinergic systems in the brain suggests a similar role for NGF in specific CNS neurons (Korsching et al. 1985).

Figure 1 depicts the pathway NGF follows. Synthesis of NGF occurs in the target organs of NGF-dependent neurons (Korsching and Thoenen 1983, Shelton and Reichardt 1984). Following synthesis, the mature NGF peptide chains are cleaved from the precursor (Edwards et al. 1986, Darling et al. 1983) and associate into stable noncovalent dimers (Bothwell and Shooter 1977) which are secreted by the target tissue near the nerve terminal. NGF then binds to NGF receptors (NGFR) and is subsequently internalized via receptor mediated endocytosis. Although the NGF is delivered intact and biologically active to the cell body it is quite rapidly degraded in the lysosomes (Korsching and Thoenen 1983, Korsching and Thoenen

NATO ASI Series, Vol. H22
Neural Development and Regeneration
Edited by A. Gorio et al.

1985). It is, as yet, unclear where in this pathway the intracellular signals are generated to mediate the action of NGF (Heumann et al. 1981).

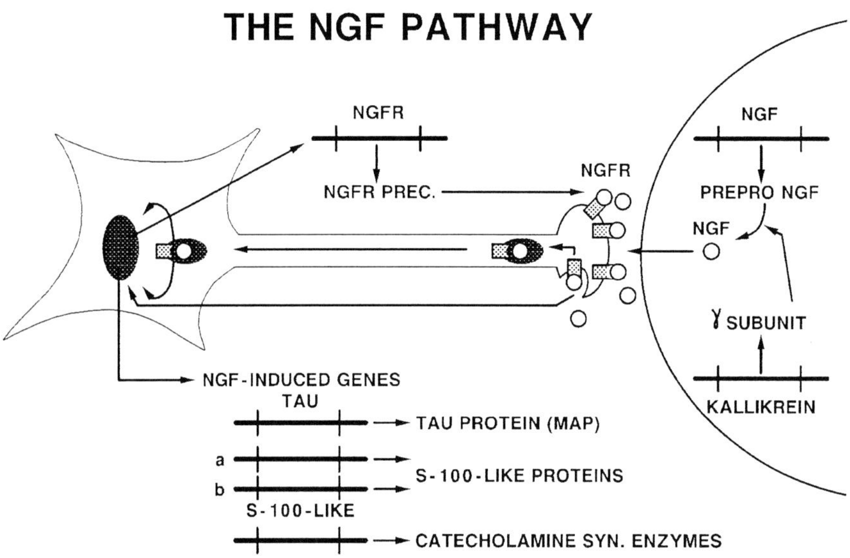


Figure 1 The NGF pathway.

NGF, synthesized under the control of a single gene and processed from two precursor proteins, is secreted by the several cell types in the target tissue into the vicinity of the nerve terminal. Binding to the NGF receptors on the nerve terminal initiates signal transduction and internalization. The internalized vesicles carrying NGF bound to the NGF receptor are transported along microtubules to the neuronal cell body. After the pH of the vesicles (endosomes) is lowered by the action of proton pumps, their fluid phase, including free NGF, is transferred to lysosomes and the proteins in it degraded. The receptors are free to recycle to the nerve terminal after anterograde transport along the microtubules although there is no evidence, as yet, for this process. The arrows emanating from the NGF-NGF receptor complex indicate locations at which intracellular signals might arise. These are (i) at the nerve terminal membrane, (ii) after internalization and/or retrograde flow up the axon and (iii) in the neuronal cell body. The cascade of reactions started by one or more of these signals leads finally to modulation of gene expression and several of the genes whose transcription is increased by the action of NGF are listed in the diagram.

Signals are neither produced by the release of NGF inside the cell nor by the generation of fragments of NGF from either vesicles or lysosomes. Moreover, inhibition of lysosomal degradation by a variety of agents does not abolish NGF-mediated induction of neurite outgrowth or the enzyme choline acetyltransferase (Seeley et al. 1983, Layer and Shooter 1983, Heumann et al. 1984). On the other hand, expression of the ras or src gene products in PC12 cells after infection with ras or src containing viruses or after microinjection of ras oncogene p21, mimics the action of NGF by inducing neurite outgrowth (Noda et al. 1985, Alema et al. 1985, Bar-Sagi and Feramisco 1985). Conversely, microinjection of the antibody to p21 into PC12 cells obviates NGF-induced neurite extension (Hagag et al. 1986). These results suggest that either gene product may be near the beginning of the pathway activated by the binding of NGF to its receptor.

Thus, at sympathetic and sensory nerve terminals and on PC12 cells, NGF first acts with its receptors and it is in this interaction that the possibility for generating second messengers or intracellular signals arises. Two types of receptors are found on primary sensory and sympathetic neurons and PC12 cells (Vale et al. 1983) (Table I). They differ in their affinities for NGF (approx. $10^{-11}$ and $10^{-9}$ M respectively), their numbers (approx. 10-times as many of the lower compared to the higher affinity receptor) and their dissociation kinetics (dissociation from the lower affinity receptor is approximately 100-fold faster than from the higher affinity receptor). In addition, NGF-occupied high affinity or slow receptors (a term suggested by Schechter and Bothwell (1981) based on dissociation rates) are trypsin resistant and insoluble in Triton X-100 while occupied low affinity or fast receptors are trypsin labile and Triton X-100 soluble (Shooter et al. 1981).

Several lines of evidence suggest a relationship between the two types of NGFR. Wheat germ agglutinin or antibodies to NGF have been used to convert NGFR exhibiting fast dissociation kinetics to a slow dissociating form (Vale and Shooter 1982, Vale and Shooter 1983, Grob and Bothwell 1983). Also NGFR clustered by the above agents become

Triton X-100 insoluble (implying cytoskeletal association), a characteristic of the high affinity NGFR. In addition, $^{125}$I-NGF bound to PC12 cells and then crosslinked to NGFR using N-hydroxysuccinimidyl-4-azido-benzoate (HSAB) produces complexes of 158,000 and 100,000 apparent molecular weight, which have been shown to correspond to the slow and fast NGFR respectively (Hosang and Shooter 1985). The 58,000 dalton difference in apparent molecular weight may represent an effector protein necessary for NGF-mediated signal transduction. Finally, internalization of NGF in PC12 cells involves only the slow NGFR, while both forms of NGFR seem to be utilized in sympathetic neurons *in vivo* (Bernd and Greene 1984, Hosang and Shooter 1987, Dumas et al. 1979).

It is clear that an understanding of the relationship between the two receptors and of their capacity to generate intracellular signals will only come from a detailed molecular characterization of the two NGFR. Therefore, the cDNA for the fast NGFR from the rat PC12 cells has been cloned and its amino acid sequence determined (Radeke et al. 1987). Briefly, a two-step approach was used involving (1) the production by genomic DNA-mediated gene transfer of a set of mouse cell lines expressing the rat fast NGFR and (2) a cDNA clone coding for the rat fast NGFR was identified by utilizing a subtractive probe, whose efficacy relied on the difference in gene expression in the newly created NGFR$^{+}$ cell lines and the original mouse cell line.

TABLE 1

**PROPERTIES OF THE TWO NGF RECEPTORS**

| PROPERTY | S-NGFR (H-NGFR) | F-NGFR (L-NGFR) |
|---|---|---|
| $K_d$ ($^{125}$I-NGF binding) | $10^{-11}$ M | $10^{-9}$ M |
| DISSOCIATION ($t_{1/2}$) ($^{125}$I-NGF release) | ∽10 min SLOW | ∽3 sec FAST |
| TRYPSIN (occupied receptor) | STABLE | LABILE |
| TRITON X-100 (occupied receptor) | INSOLUBLE | SOLUBLE |
| MOL. WT. COMPLEX | 158 K | 100 K |
| RECEPTOR | 140 K | 80 K |

## RESULTS

### Isolation and Analysis of $NGFR^+$ Transfectants

Because the rat pheochromocytoma cell line (PC12) expresses both forms of NGFR and is physiologically responsive to exogenous NGF, it was used as a source of high molecular weight genomic DNA (100-200 kb in length). 20 micrograms of PC12 genomic DNA was cotransfected along with 1 microgram of a plasmid containing the chicken thymidine kinase gene (pCHTK) into mouse $LTK^-$ cells using a modified protocol of Wigler et al (1979). Cells that integrated and expressed chicken thymidine kinase as well as the cotransfected cellular genes were then selected by growth in HAT (hypoxanthine, aminopterin, thymidine) medium. Survivors of HAT selection were then screened for those transfectants expressing the rat fast NGFR. This was accomplished by staining the $LTK^+$ transfectants with MC192, a mouse monoclonal antibody directed against the rat fast NGFR, followed by fluorescein-conjugated goat anti-mouse IgG. Positively stained cells were then isolated by sorting on a fluorescence activated cell sorter or FACS (Fig.2). Of the 8 independent transfections, 6 positively staining cell lines were obtained, and one of these, after 10 rounds of sorting and regrowth, produced a stable cell line (PCNA) that stained approximately 500 times above background.

To insure that the transfectants were, in fact, expressing PC12 NGFR and not some other antigen to which MC192 might crossreact, and to determine the form of the receptor being expressed, the transfectants were analyzed using several different criteria. Each of the positively staining transfectants specifically bound $^{125}$I-NGF. In fact, Scatchard analysis of $^{125}$I-NGF bound to the PCNA cell line showed that it expressed only the fast NGFR with a $K_D$ of 2.3 nM, and this line had over $2.3 \times 10^6$ molecules per cell. The other transfectants bound from 3-10 x $10^4$ molecules of NGF per cell with $K_D$'s of 1-6 nM; therefore also expressing only the rat fast NGFR.

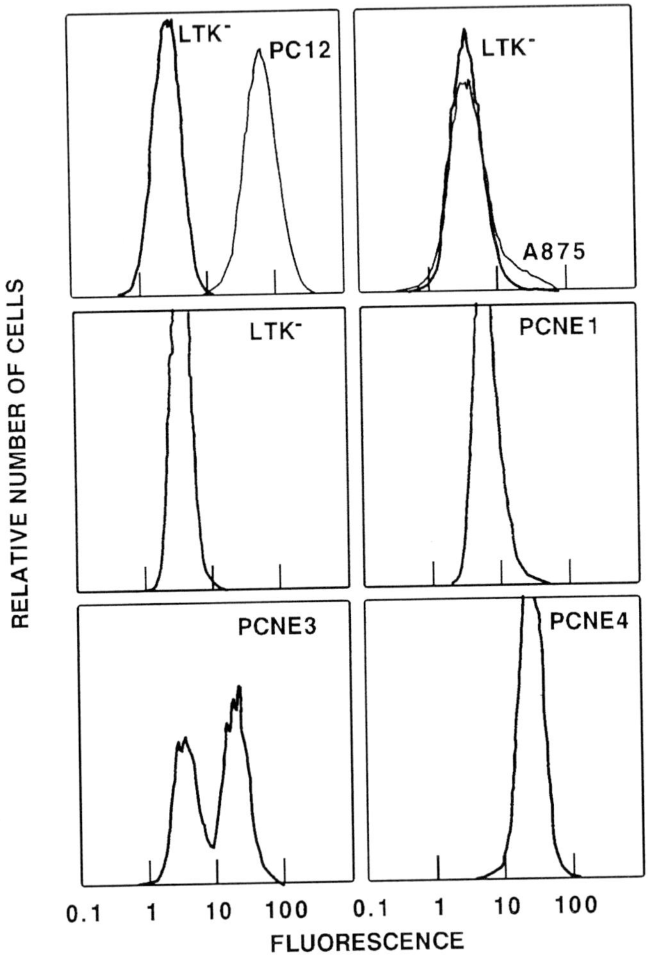


Figure 2 FACS Analysis of $NGFR^+$ Cell lines

The upper left panel shows the FACS analysis of $LTK^-$ cells and PC12 cells stained with MC192 followed by goat anti-mouse IgG-FITC. PC12 cells are clearly positive for NGFR expression while $LTK^-$ cells are negative, an observation confirmed by $^{125}$I-NGF binding studies (data not shown). The upper right panel indicates the specificity of MC192 for the rat NGFR since the FACS profile for A875, a human melanoma cell line possessing 10-20 fold more receptors per cell when compared to PC12 cells, is coincident with the $NGFR^-$ $LTK^-$ cell line. The remaining four panels show the isolation of the PCNE cell line through successive rounds of cell sorting after transfection with PC12 genomic DNA. The number following the cell line name indicates the number of times the cells had been sorted.

The second criterion compared the rates of dissociation of $^{125}$I-NGF from PC12 cells and the transfectant cell lines. All of the primary mouse cell transfectants exhibited fast dissociation kinetics indicative of the low affinity form of the NGFR. In addition, the molecular weight of the NGFR in the PCNA cell line was determined after either immunoprecipitation of radioiodinated cell surface membrane proteins with MC192 or by crosslinking NGFR to $^{125}$I-NGF with the photoreactive heterobifunctional reagent, HSAB. Both methods generated the same answer following SDS PAGE under reducing conditions: the apparent $M_r$ of the NGFR on PCNA cells was 85,000 in agreement with the size of the fast NGFR on PC12 cells. It should be noted, however, that crosslinking produces an approximately 100 kilodalton species because of the presence of NGF monomers and dimers in the complex. The preceding data shows that the transfer of the rat fast NGFR gene into the mouse L cells was successful.

## Cloning of the rat fast NGFR cDNA

To rescue the rat fast NGFR gene, advantage was taken of the fact that the NGFR$^+$ L cell transfectants express NGFR mRNA while the original host L cells do not. Therefore, cDNA was made from PCNA poly A$^+$ RNA, inserted into the PstI site of pUC9 using G·C tailing and then transformed into HB101 to give rise to a PCNA pUC9 cDNA library. A NGFR enriched probe was then made by subtracting $^{32}$P-labelled cDNA made from 3 micrograms of PCNA poly A$^+$ RNA with a 20-fold excess of LTK$^+$ poly A$^+$ RNA (the LTK$^+$ cell line was made by transfecting LTK$^-$ cells with pCHTK) in order to remove constitutive LTK$^+$ cDNA (Hedrick et al., 1984). This subtraction resulted in the removal of 90% of the PCNA cDNA. The remaining 10% of the $^{32}$P-labelled cDNA was then used to screen approximately 60,000 colonies of the PCNA pUC9 library.

Of the 30 most intensely hybridizing colonies picked during primary screening, only 19 remained positive after rescreening. Cross-hybridizational analysis of the inserts in these 19 clones identified a family of 6 clones, the longest insert in this group measuring 3.4 kb. By hybridization of this clone to total RNA from PC12, PCNA, rat dorsal root ganglia, and PCNC cells (all of which express NGFR) a 3.7 kb message was detected. In contrast, no message was detected in RNA from $LTK^+$ or rat liver which lack the NGFR. The same size message was observed in poly $A^+$ RNA from all of the other transfectants as well as in the human melanoma cell line A875 which also expresses the fast NGFR. This Northern analysis (Fig. 3) suggested that the 3.4 kb clone did contain a NGFR cDNA. Southern analysis (Fig. 4) of genomic DNA from PC12, PCNA, $LTK^+$ and the 4 remaining transfectants further supported this notion because the clone hybridized with a common rat specific gene in all of these cells, but not the $LTK^+$ cells. It is interesting to note that the NGFR gene dosage in PC12 and PCNA cells seems to be roughly equivalent whereas the hybridization signals from the remaining primary transfectants are considerably less.

This fast NGFR pUC9 clone was named pNGFR.1. To test the ability of this 3.4 kb clone to code for a full length NGFR, the entire insert was excised by digestion with Eco R1 and Hind III, blunt ended, and inserted in either orientation into the blunt ended Eco R1 site of the eukaryotic, SV40 based expression vector, pcDL1. The two resulting subclones $pcNGFR^+$ and $pcNGFR^-$ were then independently cotransfected with pCHTK and human genomic carrier DNA into $LTK^-$ cells as previously described. After HAT selection the stable transformants were reacted with MC192 and FITC coupled goat anti-mouse IgG and analyzed on the FACS.

The transformants carrying $pcNGFR^+$ with the sense orientation of the NGFR cDNA stained positively. The brightest cells of these transfectants (approx. 1%) were collected, grown in HAT medium and further analyzed using the same criteria that were applied to the genomic DNA transfectants. $pcNGFR^+$ cells have fast NGFR with a $K_D$ of 3.5 nM, similar to the fast NGFR on PC12 cells and the PCNA cells from which the clone was derived. Each cell expressed approximately 17,000 receptors having a dissociation rate for $^{125}$I-NGF similar to the PC12 fast NGFR. Furthermore, the size of the NGFR in these cells was the same as that obtained after immunoprecipitation of $^{125}$I-labelled surface PCNA cell proteins.

The nucleotide sequence of the fast NGFR cDNA indicates that the first start codon is 114 bases from the 5' end. The open reading frame continues for 1275 bases resulting in a predicted fast NGF receptor precursor of 425 amino acid residues in length. A preliminary N-terminal sequence for the purified receptor shows that 29 N-terminal amino acid residues are removed leaving a receptor peptide with 396 residues and a molecular weight of 42,478. Given the molecular weight of the mature receptor (83,000) it is probable that the fast NGF receptor is rich in carbohydrate, which is presumably attached to one or both putative N-linked glycosylation sites or a number of possible O-linked glycosylation sites in the extracellular domain.

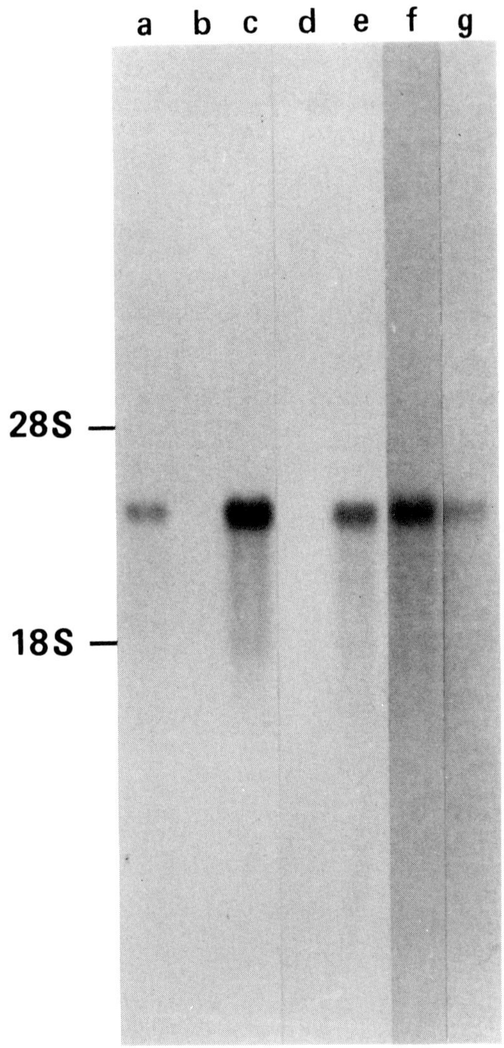


Figure 3 Northern analysis using the putative fast NGFR cDNA clone

10 μg of total RNA from each source was screened with $^{32}$P-labeled cDNA made from the 3.4-kb insert of the fast NGFR cDNA clone (pNGFR.1). Lane a) PC12 cells, b) $LTK^{+}$ cells, c) PCNA cells d) rat liver, e) newborn rat dorsal root ganglia, f) PCNC cells, g) human melanoma cell line, A875. Lanes a-e were exposed overnight, while lanes f-g were exposed for three days.

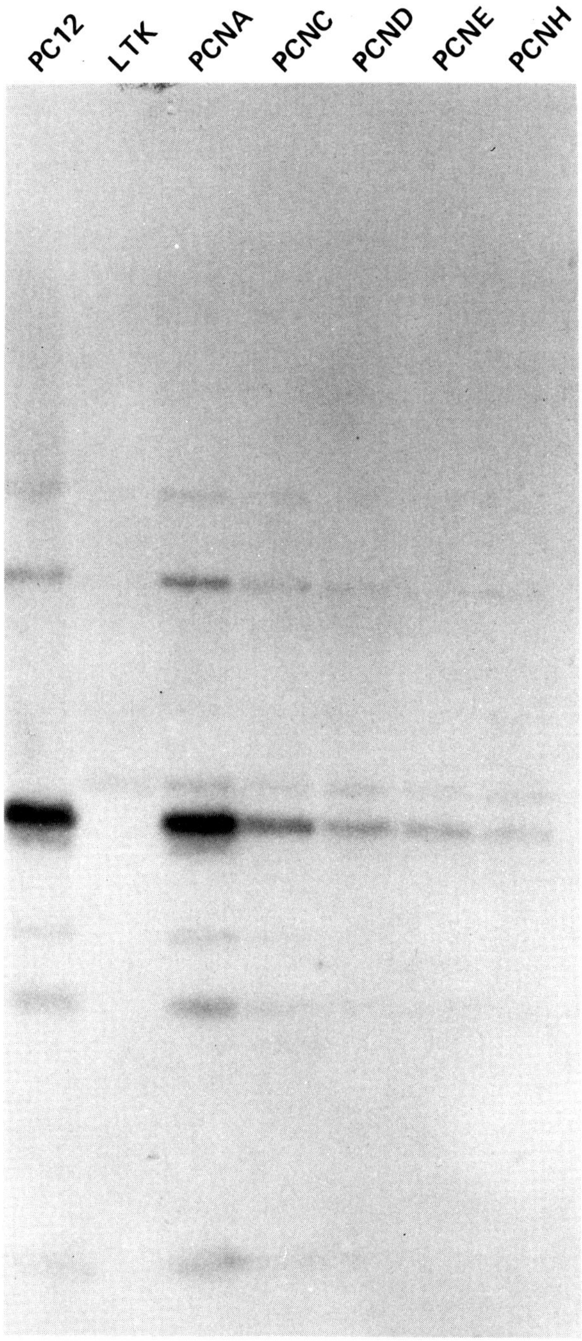


Figure 4 Southern (DNA) Analysis of Stable Transfected Cell Lines

Pstl digested DNA's using $^{32}$P-pNGFR.1 as probe.

## DISCUSSION

The NGFR appears to be unique at both nucleotide and amino acid sequence levels. It has one membrane spanning domain of 22 residues dividing the receptor into a 222 residue long extracellular domain and a 151 residue long cytoplasmic domain. The extracellular domain comprises four repeating elements rich in cysteine residues, similar to structures found in other growth factor (mitogen) receptors. The intracellular domain is too short to encode an endogenous tyrosine kinase activity and, in keeping with this, lacks the consensus sequence for an ATP binding site.

The cloning of the gene for the human NGFR has also been accomplished (Chao et al. 1986, Johnson et al. 1986). Figure 5 is a comparison of the amino acid sequence for the rat and human fast NGFR. The two forms are greater than 90% homologous, and in keeping with this, do not exhibit any major differences, except perhaps, in putative N-linked glycosylation sites. The rat NGFR has two of these sites in its extracellular domain while the human NGFR has but one.

Of considerable interest is the fact that the cDNA for the fast NGF receptor hybridizes to a single mRNA species even in cells (PC12 and sensory neurons) which express both types of receptor. This suggests that the two receptors share the protein coded for by the fast NGF receptor gene as a common NGF binding subunit. This suggestion is further strengthened by the finding of Green et al (1986) that the slow NGFR-NGF protein complex comigrates with the fast form on SDS-PAGE after crosslinking $^{125}$I-NGF bound to the NGFR on PC12 cells when the crosslinker EDAC is used. Also, by using the human NGFR anti-sense RNA as a probe, Buck et al. (1986) identified a 3.7kb message for NGFR in SY5Y neuroblastoma cells, a line which expresses only the high affinity or slow NGFR. In addition, crosslinking studies by Hosang and Shooter (1985) were able to identify a 158,000 $M_r$ form corresponding to the slow NGFR and a 100,000 $M_r$ form corresponding to the low affinity or fast receptor.

It follows that the slow NGF receptor might then contain a second subunit, the effector protein, of approximately 60,000 molecular weight whose identity is as yet unknown. As mentioned in the Introduction, c-src or ras or a GTP-binding protein may be strong candidates for such an effector protein. However, it should be noted that the 158,000 $M_r$ form produced by crosslinking $^{125}$I-NGF bound to NGFR on PC12 cells does not preclude the possibility that the second subunit is a protein of 145,000 daltons or that the high affinity or slow NGFR is a separate protein altogether. Thus, the key to the signal transduction mechanism mediated by NGF lies in understanding the difference between the structures of the fast and slow receptors, i.e. the nature of the effector protein.

# Comparison of the Rat and Human NGFR

```
HUMAN  1    MGAGATGRAMDGPRLLLLLLLGVSLGGAKEACPTGLYTHSGECCKACNLGEGVAQPCGA
               :::. .:::  :::::.:::: :::::.:.::::::::::::::::::::::::::
RAT    1   MRRAGAACSAMDRLRLLLLLILGVSSGGAKETCSTGLYTHSGECCKACNLGEGVAQPCGA

                      *
      60   NQTVCEPCLDSVTFSDVVSATEPCKPCTECVGLQSMSAPCVEADDAVCRCAYGYYQDETT
           ::::::::::.:::::::::::::::::::::.:::::::::::::::::::::::::.:
      61   NQTVCEPCLDNVTFSDVVSATEPCKPCTECLGLQSMSAPCVEADDAVCRCAYGYYQDEET

     120   GRCEACRVCEAGSGLVFSCQDKQNTVCEECPDGTYSDEANHVDPCLPCTVCEDTERQLRE
           :.::::.:::.:::::::::::::::::::::.:::::::::::::::::::::::::::
     121   GHCEACSVCEVGSGLVFSCQDKQNTVCEECPEGTYSDEANHVDPCLPCTVCEDTERQLRE

     180   CTRWADAECEEIPGRWITRSTPPEGSDSTAPSTQEPEAPPEQDLIASTVAGVVTTVMGSS
           ::.::::::::::::::::.:::::::::::::::::::.::::::..::::..::::::
     181   CTPWADAECEEIPGRWIPRSTPPEGSDSTAPSTQEPEVPPEQDLVPSTVADMVTTVMGSS

     240   QPVVTRGTTDNLIPVYCSILAAVVVGLVAYIAFKRWNSCKQNKQGANSRPVNQTPPPEGE
           ::::::::::::::::::::::::::::::::::::::::::::::::::::::::::::
     241   QPVVTRGTTDNLIPVYCSILAAVVVGLVAYIAFKRWNSCKQNKQGANSRPVNQTPPPEGE

     300   KLHSDSGISVDSQSLHDQQPHTQTASGQALKGDGGLYSSLPPAKREEVEKLLNGSAGDTW
           :::::::::::::::::::.::::::::::::::::.::::::: .::::::::::   ::::
     301   KLHSDSGISVDSQSLHDQQTHTQTASGQALKGDGNLYSSLPLTKREEVEKLLN---GDTW

     360   RHLAGELGYQPEHIDSFTHEACPVRALLASWATQDSATLDALLAALRRIQRADLVESLCS
           ::::::::::::::::::::::::::::::::..:::::::::::::::::::::.::::::
     358   RHLAGELGYQPEHIDSFTHEACPVRALLASWGAQDSATLDALLAALRRIQRADIVESLCS

     420   ESTATSPV
           ::::::::
     418   ESTATSPV
```

Figure 5 Comparison of the Rat and Human NGFR Amino Acid Sequence

Direct matches are signified by (:) while conservative substitution is represented by (.). The cysteine rich domains are underscored and the 22 amino acid transmembrane domain is boxed. The absence of a second putative N-glycosylation site in the extracellular domain of the human NGFR is noted by a star (*). There is greater than a 90% homology in amino acid sequence between the two receptors.

## REFERENCES


Alema S, Casalbore P, Agostini E, Tato F (1985) Differentiation of PC12 pheochromocytoma cells induced by v-src oncogene. Nature 316: 557-559.

Bar-Sagi D, Feramisco JR (1985) Microinjection of the ras oncogene into PC12 cells induces morphological differentiation. Cell 42: 841-848.

Bernd P, Greene LA (1984) Association of $^{125}$I-nerve growth factor with PC12 pheochromocytoma cells. J Biol Chem 259: 15509-15516.

Bothwell MA, Shooter EM (1977) Dissociation equilibrium constant of β-nerve growth factor. J Biol Chem 252: 8532-8536.

Buck CR, Chao MV, Martinez HJ, Black IB (1986) Selective expression of the nerve growth factor receptor gene *in vivo*. Neuroscience Abst 111.2:391.

Chao MV, Bothwell MA, Ross AH, Koprowski H, Lanahan AA, Buck CR, Sehgal A (1986) Gene transfer and molecular cloning of the human NGF receptor. Science 232: 518-521.

Darling TL, Petrides PE, Beguin E, Frey P, Shooter EM (1983) The biosynthesis and processing of proteins in the mouse 7S nerve growth factor complex. Cold Spring Harbor Symp. Quant. Biol 48: 427-434.

Dumas M, Schwab ME, Thoenen H (1979) Retrograde axonal transport of specific macromolecules as a tool for characterizing nerve terminal membranes. J Neurobiology 10: 179-197.

Edwards RH, Selby MJ, Rutter WJ (1986) Differential RNA splicing predicts two distinct nerve growth factor precursors. Nature 319: 784-786.

Green SH, Greene LA (1986) A single Mr 103,000 $^{125}$I-β-Nerve Growth Factor-affinity-labeled species represents both the low and high affinity forms of the nerve growth factor receptor. J. Biol. Chem. 261: 15316-15326.

Grob PM and Bothwell MA (1983) Modification of nerve growth factor receptor properties by wheat germ agglutinin. J Biol Chem 258: 14136-14143.

Hagag N, Halegoua S, Viola M (1986) Inhibition of growth factor-induced differentiation of PC12 cells by microinjection of antibody to p21. Nature 319: 680-682.

Hedrick, SM, Cohen, DI, Nielsen, EA, Davis, MM (1984) Isolation of cDNA clones encoding T cell-specific membrane associated proteins. Nature 308: 149-153.

Heumann R, Schwab M, Thoenen H (1981) A second messenger required for nerve growth factor biological activity? Nature 292: 838-840.

Heumann R, Schwab M, Merkl R, Thoenen H (1984) Nerve growth factor - mediated induction of choline acetyltransferase in PC12 cells: Evaluation of the site of action of nerve growth factor and the involvement of lysosomal degradation products of nerve growth factor. J. Neuroscience 4: 3039-3050.

Hosang M, Shooter EM (1985) Molecular characteristics of nerve growth factor receptors on PC12 cells. J Biol Chem 260: 655-662.

Hosang M, Shooter EM (1987) The internalization of nerve growth factor by high-affinity receptors on pheochromocytoma PC12 cells. EMBO J 6: 1197-1202.

Johnson D, Lanahan A, Buck CR, Sehgal A, Morgan C, Mercer E, Bothwell M, Chao M, (1986) Expression and structure of the human NGF receptor. Cell 47: 545-554.

Johnson EM Jr, Gorin PD, Brandeis LD, Pearson J (1980) Dorsal root ganglion neurons are destroyed by exposure _in utero_ to maternal antibody to nerve growth factor. Science 210: 916-918.

Korsching S, Thoenen H (1983) Quantitative demonstration of the retrograde axonal transport of endogenous nerve growth factor. Neuroscience Letter 39: 1-4.

Korsching S, Thoenen H. (1983) Nerve growth factor in sympathetic ganglia and corresponding target organs of the rat correlates with density of sympathetic innervation. Proc. Natl. Acad. Sci. U.S.A. 80: 3513-3516

Korsching S, Thoenen H (1985) Treatment with 6-hydroxydopamine and colchicine decreases nerve growth factor levels in sympathetic ganglia and increases them in corresponding target tissues. J. Neuroscience 5: 1058-1061.

Korsching S, Auburger G, Heumann R, Scott J, Thoenen H (1985) Levels of nerve growth factor and its mRNA in the central nervous system of the rat correlate with cholinergic innervation. EMBO J 4: 1389-1393.

Layer PG, Shooter EM (1973) Binding and degradation of nerve growth factor by PC12 pheochromocytoma cells. J Biol Chem 258: 3012-3018.

Levi-Montalcini R, Angeletti P.U. (1966) Immunosympathectomy. Pharmacol Rev 18, 619-628.

Levi-Montalcini R, Angeletti P.U. (1968) Nerve Growth Factor. Physiol Rev 48, 534-569.

Noda M, Ko M, Ogura A, Lin D-G, Amano T, Takano T, Ikawa Y (1985) Sarcoma viruses carrying ras oncogenes induce differentiation associated properties in a neuronal cell line. Nature 318: 73-75.

Oppenheim RW (1981) Neuronal cell death and some related phenomena during neurogenesis: A selective historical review and progress report. In Studies In Developmental Biology (ed WM Cowan) New York, Oxford: Oxford University Press, pp. 74-133.

Radeke MJ, Misko TP, Hsu C, Herzenberg LA, Shooter EM (1987) Gene transfer and molecular cloning of the rat nerve growth factor receptor: a new class of receptors. Nature 325: 593-597.

Schechter AL, Bothwell MA (1981) Nerve growth factor receptors on PC12 cells: Evidence for two receptor classes with differing cytoskeletal association. Cell 24: 867-874.

Seeley PJ, Keith CH, Shelanski ML, Greene LA (1983) Pressure microinjection of nerve growth factor and anti-nerve growth factor into the nucleus and cytoplasm: Lack of effects on neurite outgrowth from pheochromocytoma cells. J. Neuroscience 3: 1488-1494.

Shelton DL, Reichardt LF (1984) Expression of the β-nerve growth factor gene correlates with the density of sympathetic innervation in effector organs. Proc Natl Acad Sci USA 81: 7951-7955.

Shooter EM, Yankner BA, Landreth GE, Sutter A (1981) Recent Prog Hormone Res. Biosynthesis and Mechanism of action of nerve growth factor. 37: 417-446.

Vale RD, Chandler CE, Sutter A, Shooter EM (1983) The binding and internalization of nerve growth factor. In Receptors and Recognition, edited by P Cuatrecasas and MF Greaves, London: Chapman and Hall, pp. 83-119.

Vale RD, Shooter EM (1982) Alteration of binding properties and cytoskeletal attachment of nerve growth factor receptors in PC12 cells by wheat germ agglutinin. J.Cell Biol 94: 710-717.

Vale RD, Shooter EM (1983) Conversion of nerve growth factor receptor complexes to a slowly dissociating, Triton X-100 insoluble state by anti-nerve growth factor antibodies. Biochemistry 22: 5022-5028.

Vale RD, Shooter EM (1987) Nerve Growth Factor. In Cowan WM (ed) Handbook of Physiology. Baltimore Waverly Press, in press.

Wigler M, Silverstein S, Lee L-S, Pelicer A, Cheng Y-C, Axel R (1979) Transfer of purified herpes virus thymidine kinase gene to cultured mouse cells. Cell 11: 223-232.

# REGULATION OF THE SYNTHESIS OF NERVE GROWTH FACTOR AND NERVE GROWTH FACTOR RECEPTOR.

R. Heumann, D. Lindholm, C.E. Bandtlow, M. Meyer, M. Radeke[1], Th. Misko[1], E. Shooter[1] and H. Thoenen

Max-Planck-Institute for Psychiatry,
Department of Neurochemistry,
Am Klopferspitz 18a,
D-8033 Planegg-Martinsried, F.R.G.

## INTRODUCTION

The importance of Nerve Growth Factor (NGF) for the development and the maintenance of differentiated properties of peripheral sympathetic and neural crest-derived sensory neurons as well as for basal forebrain cholinergic neurons is well established (cf Levi-Montalcini & Angeletti, 1968; Greene & Shooter, 1980; Thoenen & Barde, 1980; Thoenen et al. 1987). NGF interacts with specific neuronal receptors, is internalized and is subsequently retrogradely transported to the perikaryon. During the last few years new methodological approaches allowed the direct analysis of the retrograde messenger function of NGF between target organs and corresponding NGF-responsive neurons. In the adult animal it was demonstrated that the density of sympathetic innervation is correlated with the levels of NGF (Korsching & Thoenen 1983) and $mRNA^{NGF}$ (Heumann et al. 1984, Shelton & Reichardt 1984). Thus, the ratio between NGF and $mRNA^{NGF}$ in various target tissues of sympathetic or sensory neurons is relatively constant. However, in sympathetic and sensory ganglia containing the cell bodies of NGF-responsive neurons the levels of NGF are (relatively) very high whereas the $mRNA^{NGF}$ levels are at the detection limit (Heumann et al. 1984, Davies et al. 1987a). Similarly, in the sciatic nerve (Heumann et al. 1987a) the ratio between NGF

1) Stanford University School of Medicine, Department of Neurobiology, Stanford, CA 94305, USA

NATO ASI Series, Vol. H22
Neural Development and Regeneration
Edited by A. Gorio et al.

and $mRNA^{NGF}$ is up to 100-fold higher than in peripheral target tissues of sympathetic and sensory neurons, reflecting the very low contribution of local synthesis to the sciatic NGF content. This is in agreement with the observation that after ligation of the sciatic nerve NGF accumulates distally to the ligature whereas proximally NGF levels are reduced to the detection limit of the NGF assay (Korsching and Thoenen, 1983b). The importance of the NGF supply from the peripheral target tissues is also demonstrated by the fact that destruction of sympathetic nerve terminals by 6-OH-dopamine results in a rapid decay of NGF levels in the sympathetic ganglia ($t_{1/2}$ = 4-5 hours) (Korsching and Thoenen, 1985) with a concomitant increase of NGF in the corresponding peripheral target organs.

The spectrum of NGF actions on responsive neurons (regulation of neuronal survival during critical periods of development, regulation of neurotransmitter-synthesizing enzymes, neuro-peptides and fiber-outgrowth) is well delineated. However, investigations on the regulation of NGF synthesis during embryonic development and adulthood are in a early stage.

## I) SYNTHESIS OF NGF DURING SENSORY INNERVATION OF THE WHISKER PAD

The relationship between the time course of innervation by trigeminal nerve fibers and the initiation of NGF synthesis was investigated in the mouse whisker pad (Davies et al., 1987). It was of particular interest to evaluate whether NGF synthesis precedes, coincides or follows the arrival of the sensory nerve fibers. NGF was not found in the whisker pad between E9.5 and E10.5, a stage at which nerve fibers emerge from the trigeminal ganglion to grow towards the whisker pad. At E11 the first fibers contact their target organ: at this stage NGF is first detectable. Subsequently, NGF levels increase in correlation with the increasing density of sensory innervation reaching maximum levels at E12.5. The $mRNA^{NGF}$ is detectable 12 hours before NGF protein is found in the maxillary process (E10.5) and also reaches a maximum at E12.5. After E12.5, NGF protein in the whisker pad decreases to 10-fold lower levels reflecting the removal of NGF by uptake and retrograde transport by trigeminal fibers. The counterpart to the decrease of NGF levels in the whisker pad is the increase in the trigeminal ganglion where $mRNA^{NGF}$ levels do not reach the detection limit. This indicates that the increased levels of NGF in the ganglion result from uptake and retrograde transport rather than from local synthesis in satellite cells. Previously, a molecule different from NGF has been proposed to be responsible for the initial fiber outgrowth from trigeminal ganglion (Lumsden & Davies, 1983). The observation that NGF synthesis does not precede the advent of the first trigeminal nerves fibers in the target area together with the fact that these fibers do not yet express NGF receptors is unambiguous evidence that NGF does not act as a chemotactic agent guiding the initial sensory fibers to their targets. On the other hand the coincidence of the commencement of target field innervation and the onset of NGF synthesis raises the question whether NGF synthesis is initiated by the advent of these fibers. This issue is presently under investigation in chick embryos in which it is possible to prevent the innervation of the legs by removal of the neural crest (sensory and sympathetic innervation) and neural tube (motoneurons).

In situ hybridization experiments and quantitative Northern blots demonstrated that even within a given target organ there are regional differences in the levels of $mRNA^{NGF}$ reflecting the density of innervation. In the epithelium the $mRNA^{NGF}$ levels were 10 times higher than those in the (less densely innervated) mesenchyme (Davies et al., 1987). Similar observations were made in the rat iris (Bandtlow et al., 1987).

## III) REGULATION OF NGF SYNTHESIS IN THE SCIATIC NERVE AFTER TRANSECTION

We used the rat sciatic nerve as a model to investigate possible changes in NGF synthesis during experimental conditions of degeneration and subsequent regeneration. These experiments were initiated with the hope that by analysing changes in NGF synthesis under these experimental conditions we could obtain informations on the physiological regulatory mechanisms. Moreover, the analysis of NGF synthesis regulation in the context of regeneration is of interest in its own right.

### 1) Changes in $mRNA^{NGF}$ levels after chronic denervation.

#### a) *Proximal nerve stump*

After transection, the NGF supply from the periphery is interrupted. This leads to a rapid drop in NGF levels within 6 hours to 15% of control (i.e. intact contralateral nerve) in the most proximal region of the stump. However, the situation is distinctly different at the site of lesion at the tip of the proximal stump.

In situ hybridization experiments in conjunction with quantitative $mRNA^{NGF}$ determinations identified a newly-induced source of NGF which is confined to the neuroma structure at the tip of the proximal stump and the adjacent 2 mm, which undergo retrograde Wallerian degeneration. There, the NGF concentrations correspond to those of densely innervated target organs, but the volume of the tissue is by far too small to compensate for the interrupted NGF supply from the peripheries.

That the NGF newly synthesized by this "substitute target organ" is fully available for uptake and retrograde axonal transport is demonstrated by experiments showing that in the most proximal segments NGF levels recover to about 40% of control and remain elevated while $mRNA^{NGF}$ levels in the most proximal segments persist at the very low control levels. That the local synthesis of NGF cannot fully compensate for the interrupted supply from the periphery evolves also from the observation by Rich et al. 1987 showing that sciatic nerve transection results in degeneration of 20% of sensory neurons which can be rescued by local administration of NGF.

In situ hybridization experiments on dissociated sciatic nerve indicate that all the non-neuronal cells have the capacity to synthesize NGF. Thus, Schwann cells ensheathing NGF-unresponsive motoneuron axons are also involved in the reactive synthesis of NGF (Heumann et al. 1987a). It is tempting to speculate that after nerve transection all Schwann cells (and fibroblast-like cells) attain a "rescue-function" by producing, in addition to NGF, a series of other neurotrophic molecules which may contribute to reduce neuronal cell death resulting from the interrupted trophic support from the periphery and thus promote regeneration, which however is sub-optimal even in the peripheral nervous system.

b) *Distal nerve stump*

Unlike the proximal stump, where the changes in NGF synthesis are confined to the region immediately adjacent to the transection site, in the distal stump the whole nerve is affected. The very rapid, large increase of NGF immediately adjacent to the transection site (Heumann et al. 1987a) results from accumulation of target-derived NGF by the initially still intact retrograde axonal transport. As Wallerian degeneration proceeds and the peripheral axon degenerates (Hallpike et al., 1970), NGF levels decrease again, but remain 5 -fold elevated over control levels for several weeks. This long-term increase, but not the initial rapid accumulation of NGF was also found in further distally located regions of the nerve. Consistently, 10 to 15-fold increased levels of $mRNA^{NGF}$ were found in the distal segments and persisted for at least 3 weeks. These observations demonstrate a persistent augmented NGF synthesis in the distal degenerated nerve. The increases of $mRNA^{NGF}$ were biphasic, the peak of the initial rapid phase (I) being reached already after 6 hours while the second phase (II) reached maximal levels at 3-7 days (Fig 1).

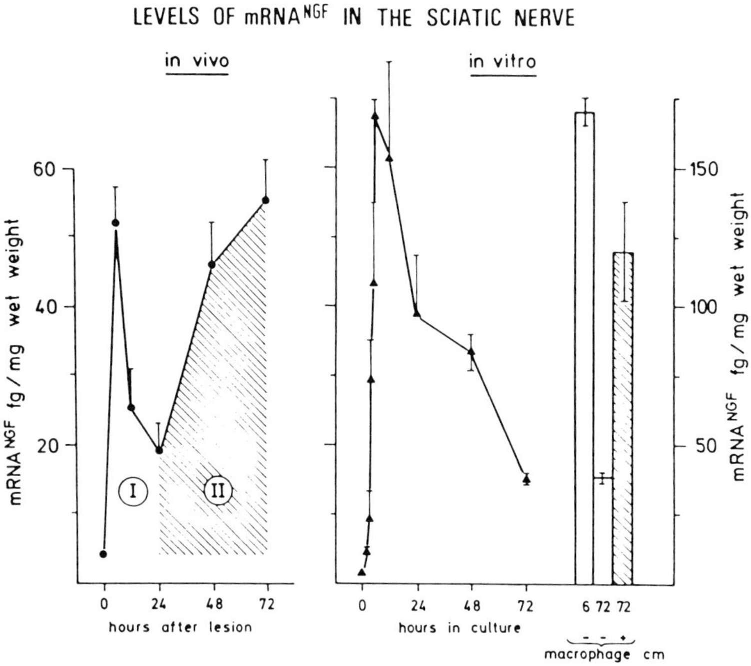


FIG. 1. Levels of mRNA$^{NGF}$ in a distal segment immediately adjacent to the cut (left panel) and in nerves kept in culture (right panel). In the left panel the initial rapid peak ("phase I") and the later increase of mRNA$^{NGF}$ ("phase II", hatched) are indicated. In the right panel the effect of macrophages on mRNA$^{NGF}$ levels (hatched column) is compared with untreated controls (open columns).(According to Heumann et al. 1987b).

II) Changes of mRNA$^{NGF}$ levels during development and under conditions that allow regeneration.

The idea that the events taking place during regeneration may be considered in part as a regression into earlier developmental stages has already been suggested by Cajal, 1928. During the first postnatal week the number of axons in the sciatic is still increasing, this net increase being due to a balance between axonal growth (Webster, 1973) and some simultaneously-occurring developmentally regulated neuronal death (see Purves & Lichtman, 1985). Possibly as a consequence of axonal degeneration of neurons a relatively large number of cells carrying the macrophage-specific marker ED1 have been detected in the newborn sciatic (Stoll & Müller, 1986). As the nerve matures during the first 3 postnatal weeks, the very low number of macrophages characteristic of the situation in the adult nerve is reached (Stoll & Müller, 1986). After lesion of the adult nerve a large number of macrophages invade the sciatic nerve. It is these macrophages which seem to be responsible for at least part of the events known as Wallerian degeneration (Abercrombie & Johnson, 1946, Scheidt et al., 1986; Beuche & Friede, 1986).

Similarly to the aforementioned changes in the numbers of macrophages, the levels of $mRNA^{NGF}$ are relatively high during the first postnatal week of normal development. In the first postnatal week $mRNA^{NGF}$ levels remain nearly constant, they then decrease relatively rapidly during the second postnatal week to approach adult levels by the third postnatal week. A level of $mRNA^{NGF}$ comparable to that of the first postnatal week was reached in adult distal sciatic nerve segments after transection precluding regeneration (Fig 2).

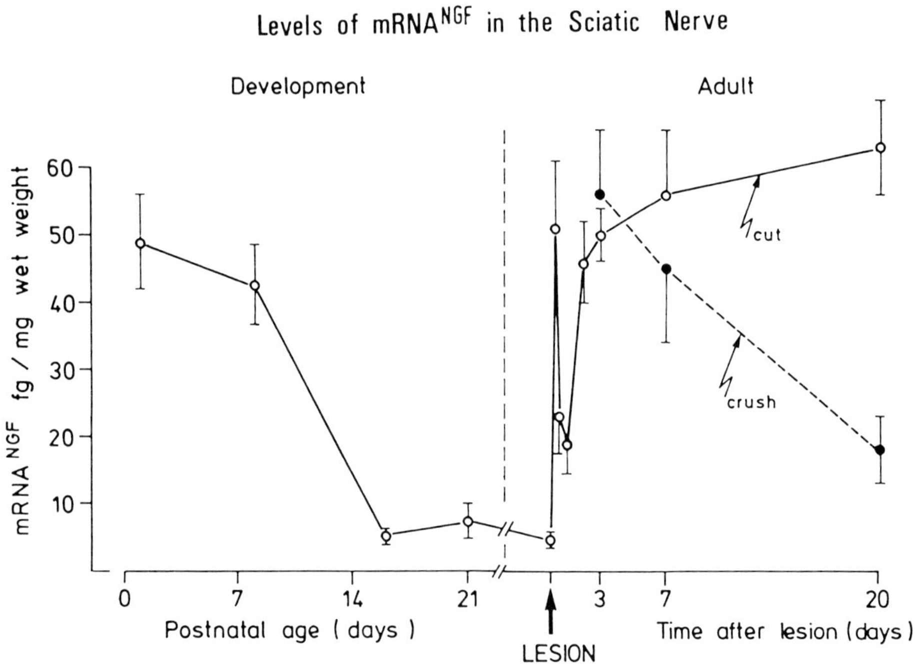


FIG. 2. Levels of $mRNA^{NGF}$ during development (left panel) and in the adult animal (right panel). The sciatic nerve was lesioned (arrow) under conditions leading either to chronic denervation (cut) or regeneration of fibers into the distal stump (crush).

In order to establish an in vitro assay allowing a detailed study of the changes of $mRNA^{NGF}$ levels we cultured isolated segments of the sciatic nerve. There was a transient rapid increase of $mRNA^{NGF}$ (Fig. 1, right panel) but in comparison to the in vivo situation (Fig. 1, left panel), a "second" phase of increase in $mRNA^{NGF}$ was not observed. The time course of the $mRNA^{NGF}$ increase during the "second" phase in vivo correlated well with that of the macrophage invasion (Perry et al., 1987). Addition of activated macrophages or of macrophage-conditioned medium to the cultured nerve segments resulted in an increase in the levels of $mRNA^{NGF}$. The activated macrophages themselves did not contain detectable levels of $mRNA^{NGF}$ indicating that they must produce signal(s) which regulate $mRNA^{NGF}$ levels in non-neuronal cells (Heumann et al., 1987b). Because the non-lesioned sciatic nerve is synthesizing very low levels of NGF locally it remained to be investigated whether NGF synthesis could also be regulated by macrophages in those non-neuronal cells which are located in sympathetic or sensory target tissues.

We found previously that after bringing iris into culture there was a rapid 35-fold increase of $mRNA^{NGF}$ which reached its maximum after 12 hours, thereafter decreasing to only 3 to 4-fold elevated levels at 48 to 72 hours (Heumann et al. 1986). The rapid and transient increase of NGF in the cultured iris was very similar to that of the cultured nerve and of the first phase of increase after sciatic nerve transection in vivo opening the possibility of a common mechanism of regulation of $mRNA^{NGF}$ in these systems. Consistently, in both sciatic and iris cultures cycloheximide blocked the increase of $mRNA^{NGF}$ when added at the beginning of the incubation period (Heumann et al. 1986, and D. Lindholm, unpublished observation), indicating that the initiation of the transient first phase of $mRNA^{NGF}$ changes is dependent on protein synthesis. A parallel regulation of $mRNA^{NGF}$ in cultured nerve segments and iris is also observed with respect to the response to activated macrophages. Addition of activated macrophages or of macrophage conditioned medium leads to a 8-fold increase of $mRNA^{NGF}$ in the cultured iris (R.Heumann, unpublished observation), which is comparable to the changes found in the cultured nerve segments (see above). In situ hybridization experiments performed on dissociated iris cell cultures (Bandtlow et al., 1987) demonstrated that all cell types, i.e. smooth muscle cells, fibroblasts, epithelial cells and Schwann cells showed $mRNA^{NGF}$ specific labelling. It remains to be investigated whether all these cell types are susceptible to the macrophage-mediated regulation of NGF synthesis.

There are a number of functions associated with activated macrophages: they present antigens, stimulate T-cell proliferation and antigen production (Unanue & Allen, 1987). In the lesioned sciatic nerve macrophages are apparently also involved in the degradation of cell debris and myelin as well as in the regulation of Schwann cell mitosis (Beuche & Friede, 1986). We now present evidence that they are also crucially involved in the regulation of NGF synthesis after nerve lesion.

We then considered the possible role of regenerating fibers in the regulation of NGF synthesis. After nerve crush the axons are destroyed, but the epineurium remains intact. This allows the regenerating nerve fibers to easily progress into the distal nerve stump along the bands of Büngner. Some days after the axons have passed through the tubes the levels of $mRNA^{NGF}$ decrease. Again, there is a correlation between the disappearance of macrophages as monitored by the synthesis of apo-lipoprotein E (Müller et al., 1985) and the decrease of $mRNA^{NGF}$ levels in the regenerating nerve. It remains to be established which of the many secretory products of macrophages is responsible for the regulation of $mRNA^{NGF}$.

## IV) REGULATION OF NGF RECEPTOR SYNTHESIS DURING DEVELOPMENT AND UNDER CONDITIONS OF DEGENERATION AND REGENERATION IN THE SCIATIC NERVE.

Expression of NGF receptors on Schwann cells during development (Zimmermann & Sutter, 1985; Rohrer, 1985) and a re-expression after sciatic nerve lesion in the adult animal have been described previously (Taniuchi et al. 1986; Heumann et al., 1987a). Correspondingly, the $mRNA^{rec}$ (see Radeke et al., 1987) levels at birth were 120-fold higher than in the intact adult sciatic (Fig. 3).

There is a steady decrease in the levels of $mRNA^{rec}$ during the first 3 postnatal weeks. After transection of the adult nerve $mRNA^{rec}$ levels increase to levels exceeding those observed postnatally (fig. 3). The finding that specifically Schwann cells (and not other non-neuronal cells) re-express NGF-receptors (Taniuchi et al., 1986; Bandtlow et al.1987) and $mRNA^{rec}$ (R. Heumann et al., 1987b) after nerve transection opens the possibility of an autocrine function of NGF for Schwann cells located distally to the transection site. That these receptors are functional evolves from the recent observation from Seilheimer and Schachner, 1987, showing that in cultures of mouse Schwann cells NGF increases the levels of the cell attachment glycoprotein L1, whereas addition of anti-NGF antibodies decreases the levels of L1. Moreover, administration of NGF to cultured sciatic nerve segments resulted in an increase in c-fos-mRNA (D. Lindholm et al. unpublished observation). Thus, the function of low affinity NGF receptors on Schwann cells is not restricted to present NGF to the regenerating fibers as suggested by Taniuchi et al., 1986.

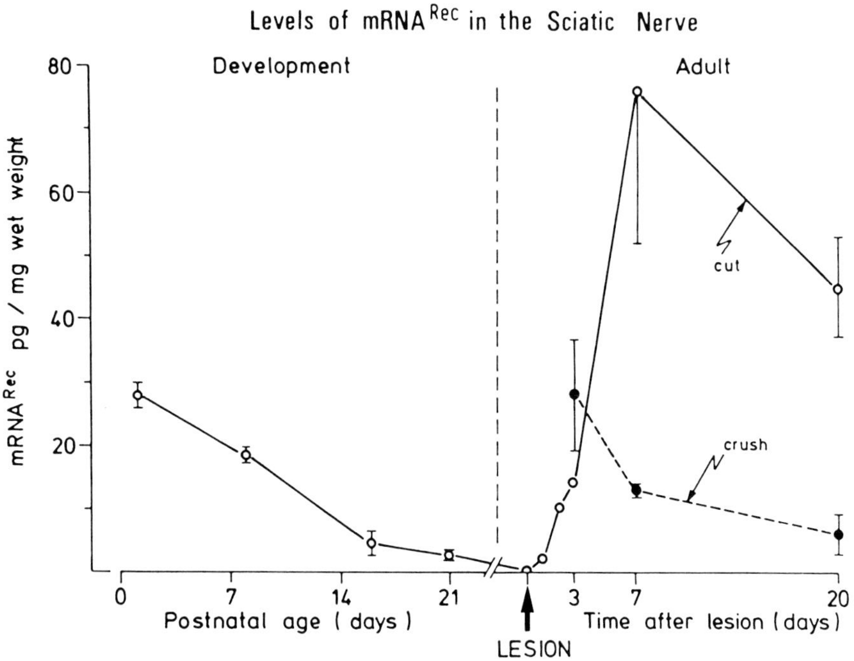


FIG. 3. Levels of mRNA$^{rec}$ during development (left panel) and in the adult animal (right panel). The sciatic nerve was lesioned (arrow) under conditions leading either to chronic denervation (cut) or regeneration of fibers into the distal stump.

In contrast to the regulation of mRNA$^{NGF}$ by a diffusible macrophage-derived substance, mRNA$^{rec}$ is not affected by the presence of macrophages (Heumann et al. 1987b) indicating a differential mechanism of regulation of NGF and its receptor. This is further supported by the comparison of the effects of regenerating fibers on mRNA$^{NGF}$ and mRNA$^{rec}$ levels after a crush lesion. As soon as the fibers contact the Schwann cells of the distal nerve stump mRNA$^{rec}$ decreases rapidly. Thus, 7 days after lesion the mRNA$^{rec}$ levels are 6-fold higher in the transected as compared to the crushed nerve. For the mRNA$^{NGF}$ levels, however, no difference is observed by day 7 (Heumann et al. 1987b). These results are consistent with the hypothesis that neuronal membranes are not only mitogenic for Schwann cells (see Salzer & Bunge, 1980) but that they also regulate the expression of NGF receptors as suggested by Taniuchi et al. 1986.

In conclusion, our results demonstrate that NGF synthesis is not directly regulated by contact between regenerating axons and non-neuronal cells. However, activated macrophages immigrating into the area of degenerating axons seem to play an essential role by releasing substance(s) which increase NGF synthesis in non-neuronal cells. NGF receptor synthesis, on the other hand, is not affected by macrophages. Axonal cell surface molecules appear to regulate NGF receptor expression by Schwann cells.

Acknowledgements: We are very grateful to Dr. G.D. Borasio for his help during the preparation of the manuscript.

REFERENCES

Abercrombie M Johnson ML (1946) Quantitative histology of Wallerian degeneration I. Nuclear population in rabbit sciatic nerve. J Anatomy 80:37-50

Bandtlow CE, Heumann R, Schwab ME, Thoenen H (1987) Cellular localization of nerve growth factor synthesis by in situ-hybridization. EMBO J 6:69-91

Beuche W, Friede RL (1986) Myelin phagocytosis in Wallerian degeneration of peripheral nerves depends on silica-sensitive, bg/bg-negative and Fc-positive monocytes. Brain Res 378:97-106

Cajal RY (1928) Degeneration of the peripheral stump. In: May RM (ed and transl) Degeneration and Regeneration of the Nervous System. University Press, Oxford, vol 1, pp 100-126

Davies AM, Bandtlow C, Heumann R, Korsching S, Rohrer H, Thoenen H (1987a) The site and timing of nerve growth factor (NGF) synthesis in developing skin in relation to its innervation by sensory neurones and their expression of NGF receptors. Nature 326:353-358

Greene LA, Shooter EM (1980) The nerve growth factor: biochemistry, synthesis, and mechanism of action. Ann Rev Neurosci 3:353-402

Hallpike JF, Adams CWM, Bayliss OB (1970) Histochemistry of myelin. IX. Neutral and acid proteinases in early Wallerian degeneration. Histochem J 2:209-218

Heumann R, Korsching S, Scott J, Thoenen H (1984a) Relationship between levels of nerve growth factor (NGF) and its messenger RNA in sympathetic ganglia and peripheral target tissues. EMBO J 3:3183-3189

Heumann R, Thoenen H (1986) Comparison between the time course of changes in nerve growth factor (NGF) protein levels and those of its messenger RNA in the cultured rat iris. J Biol Chem 261:9246-9249

Heumann R, Korsching S, Bandtlow C, Thoenen H (1987a) Changes of nerve growth factor synthesis in non-neuronal cells in response to sciatic nerve transection. J Cell Biol 104:1623-1631

Heumann R, Lindholm D, Bandtlow C, Meyer M, Radeke MJ, Misko TP, Shooter E, Thoenen H (1987b) Differential regulation of nerve growth factor (NGF) and NGF-receptor mRNA in the rat sciatic nerve during development, degeneration and regeneration; role played by macrophages. Proc Natl Acad Sci USA, in press

Johnson EM, Taniuchi M, Clark HB, Springer JE, Koh S, Tayrien MW, Loy R (1987a) Demonstration of the retrograde transport of nerve growth factor receptor in the peripheral and central nervous system. J Neurosci 7:923-929

Korsching S, Thoenen H (1983a) Nerve growth factor in sympathetic ganglia and corresponding target organs of the rat: correlation with density of sympathetic innervation Proc Natl Acad Sci USA 80:3513-3516

Korsching S, Thoenen H (1983b) Quantitative demonstration of the retrograde axonal transport of endogenous nerve growth factor. Neurosci Lett 39:1-4

Korsching S, Thoenen H (1985) Treatment with 6-hydroxydopamine and colchicine decreases nerve growth factor levels in sympathetic ganglia and increases them in the corresponding target tissues. J Neurosci 5:1058-1061

Levi-Montalcini R (1987) The nerve growth factor: thirty-five years later. EMBO J 6:1145-1154
Lumsden AGS, Davies AM (1983) Earliest sensory nerve fibres are guided to peripheral targets by attractants other than nerve growth factor. Nature 306:786-788
Müller HW, Gebicke-Härter PJ, Hangen DH, Shooter EM (1985) A specific 37,000-dalton protein that accumulates in regenerating but not in nonregenerating mammalian nerves. Science 228:499-501
Perry VH, Brown MC, Gordon S (1987) The macrophage response to central and peripheral nerve injury. J Exp Med 165:1218-1223
Purves D, Lichtman JW (1985) Principles of neural development. Sinauer Associates, Inc, Sunderland, MA, pp 131-178
Radeke MJ, Misko TP, Hsu C, Herzenberg LA, Shooter EM (1987) Gene transfer and molecular cloning of the rat nerve growth factor receptor: a new class of receptors. Nature 325:593-597
Rich KM, Luszczynski JR, Osborne PA, Johnson EM (1987) Nerve growth factor protects adult sensory neurons from cell death and atrophy caused by nerve injury. J Neurocytol 16:261-268
Rohrer H (1985) Nonneuronal cells from chick sympathetic and dorsal root sensory ganglia express catecholamine uptake and receptors for nerve growth factor during development. Dev Biol 111:95-107
Salzer JL, Bunge RP (1980) Studies on Schwann cell proliferation. I. An analysis in tissue culture of proliferation during development, Wallerian degeneration, and direct injury. J Cell Biol 84:739-752
Scheidt P, Waehneldt TV, Beuche W, Friede RL (1986) Changes of myelin proteins during Wallerian degeneration in situ and in millipore diffusion chambers preventing active phagocytosis. Brain Res 379:380-384
Seilheimer B, Schachner M (1987) Regulation of neural cell adhesion molecule expression on cultured mouse Schwann cells by nerve growth factor. EMBO J 6:1611-1616
Shelton DL, Reichardt LF (1984) Expression of the nerve growth factor gene correlates with the density of sympathetic innervation in effector organs. Proc Natl Acad Sci USA 81:7951-7955
Stoll G, Müller HW (1986) Macrophages in the peripheral nervous system and astroglia in the central nervous system of rat commonly express apolipoprotein E during development but differ in their response to injury. Neurosci Lett 72:233-238
Taniuchi M, Clark HB, Johnson Jr EM (1986) Induction of nerve growth factor receptor in Schwann cells after axotomy. Proc Natl Acad Sci USA 83:4094-4098
Thoenen H, Barde Y-A (1980) Physiology of nerve growth factor. Physiol Rev 60:1284-1335
Thoenen H, Bandtlow C, Heumann R (1987) The physiological function of nerve growth factor in the central nervous system: comparison with the periphery. Rev Physiol Biochem Pharmacol 109:145-178
Unanue ER, Allen PM (1987) The basis for the immunoregulatory role of macrophages and other accessory cells. Science 236:551-557
Webster HdeF, Martin JR, O'Connell MF (1973) The relationships between interphase Schwann cells and axons before myelination: A quantitative electron microscopic study. Dev Biol 32:401-416
Zimmermann A, Sutter A (1983) ß-nerve growth factor (ß-NGF) receptors on glial-cells - cell-cell interaction between neurons and Schwann-cells in cultures of chick sensory ganglia. EMBO J 2:879-885

# REGULATION OF GENE EXPRESSION IN NERVE CELLS: EFFECT OF GROWTH AND TROPHIC FACTORS.

A.M. Giuffrida Stella
Institute of Biochemistry
Faculty of Medicine
University of Catania
Viale Andrea Doria 6
95125 Catania, Italy

The regulation of gene expression in nerve cells has been widely studied and to some extent elucidated, although many aspects concerned with specialized functions of neuronal and glial cells in specific brain regions remain to be better investigated. The great progress made during the last few years by molecular neurobiology with the use of recombinant DNA and *in situ* hybridization techniques (Branks and Wilson, 1986) has been and, hopefully, will be very useful for the elucidation of many as yet unknown special features of gene expression regulation in nervous system.

As in all eukaryotic cells, this regulation could occur at transcriptional and/or at translational level. RNA synthesis and processing play a key role in the gene expression of nervous system in different conditions, such as development (Giuffrida et al., 1975; Lim, 1977; Serra et al., 1984; Giuffrida Stella, 1986), aging (for review see Giuffrida Stella and Lajtha, 1987) and regeneration (for review see

NATO ASI Series, Vol. H22
Neural Development and Regeneration
Edited by A. Gorio et al.

Giuffrida Stella and Lajtha, 1983; Alberghina and Giuffrida Stella, 1987).

A greater complexity of polyadenylated mRNAs expressed in mammalian brain than in other tissues (Bantle and Hahn, 1976; Chikaraishi, 1979) and remarkable changes of post-translational modifications of chromosomal proteins in various brain regions and in neuronal and glial cells, have been evidentiated (Serra and Giuffrida, 1986). The post-translational modifications of many chromatin-bound proteins may induce changes of DNA-protein interactions, modifying DNA conformation and affecting the binding of enzymes and proteins involved in the regulation of specific gene expression. Age-dependent changes of acetylation, phosphorylation and methylation of histones and non-histone proteins (NHPs) in various brain regions and cell types have been observed. During postnatal development an increasing phosphorylation of NHPs with molecular weight of about 90 kDa, in neuronal and glial nuclei has been found. It has been postulated that these proteins might be involved in the regulation of specific cell functions (Serra et al., 1986).

A number of polypeptide growth factors have a potential effect on nervous system, acting as mitogens, neuromodulators and neurotransmitters. Their role in the development, differentiation and function of neuronal and glial cells has been controversial.

Among the best known and characterized growth factors are: the nerve growth factor (NGF), the epidermal growth factor (EGF), the fibroblast growth factor (FGF) and the platelet derived growth factor (PDGF).

Recent advances to characterize NGF have given evidence for the critical role played by this factor in the development, maintenance and, in some cases, in the regeneration, collateral sprouting and establishment of new synaptic circuitry in the nervous system. This action for NGF, discovered by the pioneer work of R. Levi Montalcini, has been successively extended and investigated also at molecular levels by many Authors (Levi Montalcini and Angeletti, 1968; Greene and Shooter, 1980; Yankner and Shooter, 1982; Levi Montalcini, 1983; Gnahn et al., 1983; Perez-Polo and Haber, 1983; Levi Montalcini and Calissano, 1986; Stach and Perez-Polo, 1987).

The presence of NGF receptors in rodent brain and also in some specific areas of the central nervous system characterized by cholinergic innervation, (Taniuchi et al., 1986; Springer et al., 1987) has been recently demonstrated. NGF may serve as a trophic factor for magnocellular cholinergic neurons in the basal forebrain; it increases the activity of choline acetyltransferase in septum, hippocampus, striatum and cortex of neonatal rats and in cell cultures obtained from embryonic septal neurons (Gnahn et al., 1983; Hefti et al., 1985; Mobley et al., 1985). Endogenous levels of NGF and NGF receptors are present at higher concentrations in the basal forebrain. Messenger RNA level coding for NGF was found to be highest in the hippocampus and cortex (Korshing et al., 1985; Whittemore et al., 1986; Shelton and Reichardt, 1986).

FGFs are present in brain and pituitary which contain high

levels of these mitogenic proteins (Morrison, 1987). Brain preparations contain both acidic and basic activities. The two molecules are similar in mass (aFGF-1= 15.9 kDa, aFGF-2= 15.2 kDa, bFGF= 15.8 kDa). Acidic FGF is composed of 140 amino acids and does not express asparagine glycosylation sequences. The sequence of aFGF reflects homology with that of another growth factor, the interleukin-1 (IL -1). Analysis of the aFGF sequence showed a series of 10 amino acids with dibasic peptides (lys-lys) on both sides. These peptides are recognition sites for proteolytic enzymes, suggesting that the decapeptide might be released from a large molecule of precursor aFGF. This decapeptide sequence is similar to the sequence of many active neuropeptides (Gimenez-Gallego et al., 1985). Pituitary FGFs possess a mitogenic activity for astrocytes (Morrison and De Vellis, 1981; Pettmann et al., 1985) and oligodendrocytes (Saneto and De Vellis, 1985).

However, the cellular site of synthesis, the mechanism of release and the time of expression of these proteins _in vivo_ have not been determined.

It has been recently hypothesized that these mitogenic proteins might stimulate and coordinate cell proliferation, acting also as neurotrophic factors, maintaining neuronal survival and neurite extension (Gimenez-Gallego et al., 1985; Walicke et al., 1986; Morrison et al., 1986). The target neurons were obtained from hippocampus and cerebral cortex. Northern blot analysis of hypothalamic RNA suggests that bFGF is synthesized locally (Abraham et al., 1986). It is able to promote neuronal survival and neurite extension in picomolar concentration range. It is now necessary to extend the investigations on the effects at the molecular level to better understand its mode of action.

Despite the considerable advances made in the last decade, the exact mechanism of action of any polypeptide growth factor (PGF) has not been definitely clarified. The central problem is the importance of internalization of PGF-receptor complexes by endocytosis and the role played by intracellular receptors as messengers for further activity.

The relationship of polypeptide growth factors to human neoplastic diseases has been clearly established. The polypeptide growth factors elicit a specific hypertrophic and/or hyperplastic response in target cells resulting from the formation of a factor-receptor complex. Complexation with the receptor results in stimulation of cell metabolism and in modulation of specific gene expression either at the transcriptional or at the translational levels.

Although second messenger production, as a result of the formation of protein growth factor-receptor complex, is likely to occur, no evidence has been obtained till now. Cyclic nucleotides appear to be excluded.

Among the protein growth factors, insulin must be also considered, in spite of its classical hormonal activity, since it cannot be distinguished in most of its important features from other PGFs.

The serum iron-carrying protein, transferrin, is universally required in tissue culture systems, utilizing defined media. Transferrin might act as a trophic agent through its cell-surface receptors other than simply by supplying iron atoms. Among the rapid effects stimulated by polypeptide growth factors, phosphorylation of various intracellular proteins, including histones and non-histone proteins, has been observed (for review see James and Bradshaw, 1984).

The present study is mainly focused on the action of the epidermal growth factor (EGF) which has been studied extensively, but which needs further investigations to know how it elicits its action in nerve cells. It is a small polypeptide, originally isolated from salivary glands of the male mouse. It has become the best-characterized mitogenic polypeptide.

Taylor et al. (1972) reported the structure of EGF as a single peptide chain, constituted of 53 amino acid residues with three intramolecular disulfide bonds and isoelectric point at pH 4.6. The disulfide bonds in mouse EGF are required for its biological activity. EGF has been isolated as a component of high-molecular-weight complex of 74 kDa composed of 2 molecules of mEGF and 2 molecules of binding protein (Carpenter and Cohen, 1979). Evidence has been found that EGF forms a complex with plasma membrane receptors initiating a cascade of biochemical events ultimately eliciting cell growth response. EGF stimulates membrane protein phosphorylation. SDS polyacrylamide gel electrophoresis and autoradiography indicated that the enhanced phosphorylation of membrane associated proteins is mainly concerned with proteins of molecular weights of approximately 160, 80 and 22.5 kDa. These findings became clear successively when it was shown that the receptor molecule for EGF contains as an inherent part a tyrosin-specific protein kinase activity (for review see James and Bradshaw, 1984).

Prior to these observations protein kinase activity was found to be associated with the oncogenic products of actively transforming retroviruses. The cellular receptor for EGF is a 170 kDa membrane glycoprotein. The complete sequence of EGF receptor molecule, obtained by DNA sequencing technique, showed that it is constituted by a protein of 1186 amino acids, consisting of 621 amino acid extracellular component, a single short amino acid spanning region, and a 542 amino acid cytoplasmic region containing a sequence homologous to the v-erb-B oncogene protein kinase (Downward et al., 1984).

The effect of EGF in astrocytes and oligodendrocytes suggests that EGF may modulate glial interaction with CNS neurons.

In recent studies on the effect of EGF in primary rat astroglial cell cultures, maintained in serum-free basal medium supplemented with BSA, we confirmed and extended previous results (Avola et al., 1986, 1987) showing a stimulating action of EGF not only as mitogen (Simpson et al., 1982) but also on RNA metabolism. In particular, an increased synthesis of the major ribosomal RNA species and also of polyadenylated and non polyadenylated RNAs has been observed in cells treated with EGF (10 ng/ml culture medium).

The various RNA species were separated after phenol extraction by gel electrophoresis as previously described (Serra et al., 1983). Polyadenylated and non polyadenylated RNAs were obtained by oligo-dT cellulose separation.

As far as the population of polyadenylated and non polyadenylated RNAs in brain is concerned, it is worthwhile to recall that many non polyadenylated mRNAs have been found to be absent at birth in rodent brain and to increase during postnatal development (Chaudhari and Hahn, 1983). It has been postulated that they might serve for the synthesis of functional and structural brain polypeptides, such as receptor proteins, ion channel protein components, neuromodulators etc. However, the supporting evidence for this role is still lacking.

The use of in situ hybridization technique to identify cDNA clones of highly regulated mRNA species and to define their pattern of gene expression in brain at cellular levels, revealed that some mRNAs are differentially expressed by morphologically and functionally distinct neurons of specific brain regions (Branks and Wilson, 1986).

The increased synthesis of both polyadenylated and non polyadenylated RNAs by EGF treatment could be of great interest to understand the mode of action of EGF in nerve cells.

It is important to identify which proteins are codified by these mRNAs.

The content of cytoskeletal proteins such as actin, vimentin and GFAP has been measured in serum supplemented (SSM) or in chemically defined media (CDM) in glial cell cultures (Avola et al., 1987). It can be hypotesized that some of the increased mRNAs, found in the present study, might be involved in the synthesis of cytoskeletal proteins.

In the same experimental conditions, a marked increase of protein labeling from various subcellular fractions (nuclear, mitochondrial, microsomal and cytosolic), was found. Histones and NHPs were extracted from purified nuclei and analyzed by gel electrophoresis, as previously described (Serra et al., 1986). An increased labeling of histone proteins was found, while NHPs were not significantly affected by EGF treatment. The only non-histone proteins, which were highly labeled in cells treated with EGF, were proteins with Mws approximately 95-83 and 44 kDa.

The enhanced synthesis of histone proteins may be correlated to the increased DNA synthesis, since it is well known that these two biosynthetic processes are closely associated.

The role of the highly labeled NHPs, after EGF treatment, remains to be elucidated.

The regulation of gene expression in nerve cells through the modulation of molecular events by EGF needs also further investigations. EGF could act increasing the ability of ribosomes to bind mRNA in a functional manner, therefore enhancing protein synthesis. EGF may also increase RNA transport rate to the cytoplasm. These effects of EGF on the molecular events occurring during glial cell proliferation and differentiation, might be useful for modulating the growth, maintenance and probably repair of neuronal cells.

Recently the finding of a mRNA transcript, which is present in significantly high levels in rat cells transformed by polyoma virus or Rous sarcoma virus and which is rapidly induced by EGF, has provided new evidence of the existence of intracellular mechanisms common to the action of both growth factors and oncogenes (Matrisian et al., 1985).

In conclusion, although many progresses have been done, considerable work is required to elucidate how all the till now discovered growth and trophic factors exert their action on the target cells and to extend our knowledge on their effect on many phenomena, such as nerve cell proliferation, differentiation, regeneration and/or survival, occurring during development, aging, damage and repair.

Acknowledgements: This work has been accomplished by financial support of "Consiglio Nazionale delle Ricerche" (CNR), Italy. The skillful technical assistance of A. Costa and C. Reale, the accurate typing of the manuscript by P. Rapisarda, the preparation of line drawings by C. Desiderio and slides by G. Lo Re, is very much acknowledged. The great help of the Secretary, D. Blarasin is deeply appreciated.

REFERENCES

Abraham JA, Mergia A, Whang JL, Tumolo A, Friedman J, Hjerrild KA, Gospodarowicz D, Fiddes JC (1986) Nucleotide sequence of a bovine clone encoding the angiogenic protein, basic fibroblast growth factor. Science 233:545-548

Alberghina M, Giuffrida Stella AM (1987) The relationship between perikaryal synthesis and axonal transport during nerve regeneration. In: Tucek S (ed) Metabolism and Development of the Nervous System. Wiley and Sons, Chichester and Academia, Prague, pp. 219-228

Avola R, Serra I, Curti D, Lombardo B, Renis M, Condorelli DF, Giuffrida AM (1986) Nuclear and mitochondrial DNA synthesis and energy metabolism in primary rat glial cell cultures. Neurochem Res 11:789-800

Avola R, Condorelli DF, Surrentino S, Turpeenoja L, Costa A, Giuffrida Stella AM (1987) Effect of epidermal growth factor and insulin on DNA and RNA labeling in primary rat astroglial cell cultures. J Neurosci Res (submitted)

Bantle JA, Hahn WE, (1976) Complexity and characterization of polyadenylated RNA in the mouse brain. Cell 8:139-150

Branks PL, Wilson MC (1986) Patterns of gene expression in the murine brain revealed by in situ hybridization of brain-specific mRNAs. Mol Brain Res 1:1-16

Carpenter G, Cohen S (1979) Epidermal growth factor. Ann Rev Biochem 48:193-216

Chaudhari N, Hahn WE (1983) Genetic expression in the developing brain. Science 220:924-928

Chikaraishi DM, (1979) Complexity of cytoplasmic polyadenylated and nonpolyadenylated rat brain ribonucleic acids. Biochemistry 18:3249-3256

Downward J, Yarden Y, Mayes E, Scrace G, Totty N, Stockwell P, Ullrich A, Schlessinger J, Waterfield MD (1984) Close similarity of epidermal growth factor receptor and v-erb-B oncogene protein sequences. Nature 307:521-527

Gimenez-Gallego G, Rodkey J, Bennett C, Rios-Candelore M, Di Salvo J, Thomas K (1985) Brain-derived acidic fibroblast growth factor: Complete amino acid sequence and homologies. Science 230:1385-1388

Giuffrida AM, Cox D, Mathias AP (1975) RNA polymerase activity in various classes of nuclei from different regions of rat brain during postnatal development. J Neurochem 24:749-755

Giuffrida Stella AM, Lajtha A (1983) Perspectives for neural regeneration with changes in macromolecular metabolism. In: Haber B, Perez-Polo JR, Hashim G, Giuffrida Stella AM (eds) Nervous System Regeneration, vol XIX/4. Alan Liss, New York, pp. 23-32

Giuffrida Stella AM (1986) Regulation of gene expression in developing brain. Int J Dev Neurosci 4 suppl 1, S 18

Giuffrida Stella AM, Lajtha A (1987) Macromolecular turnover in brain during aging. Gerontology 33:121-131

Gnahn H, Hefti F, Heumann R, Schwab ME, Thoenen H (1983) NGF-Mediated increase of choline acetyl-transferase (ChAT) in the neonatal rat forebrain: Evidence for a physiological role of NGF in the brain. Dev Brain Res 9:45-52

Greene LA, Shooter EM (1980) The nerve growth factor: Biochemistry, synthesis, and mechanism of action. Ann Rev Neurosci 3:353-402

Hefti F, Hartikka J, Eckenstein F, Gnahn H, Heumann R, Schwab M (1985) Nerve growth factor increases choline acetyltransferase but not survival of fiber outgrowth of cultured fetal septal cholinergic neurons. Neuroscience 14:55-68

James R and Bradshaw R (1984) Polypeptide growth factors. Ann Rev Biochem 53:259-292

Korsching S, Auburger G, Heumann R, Scott J, Thoenen H (1985) Levels of nerve growth factor and its mRNA in the central nervous system of the rat correlate with cholinergic innervation. EMBO J 4:1389-1393

Levi Montalcini R, Angeletti PU (1968) Nerve growth factor. Physiol Rev 48:534-569

Levi Montalcini R (1983) The nerve growth factor-target cells interaction: A model system for the study of directed axonal growth and regeneration. In: Haber B, Perez-Polo JR, Hashim G, Giuffrida-Stella AM (eds) Nervous System Regeneration, vol XIX/4. Alan Liss, New York, pp 3-22

Levi Montalcini R, Calissano P, (1986) Nerve growth factor as a paradigm for other polypeptide growth factors. TINS 9:473-477.

Lim L, (1977) Regulation of RNA metabolism in the developing brain. In: Davison AN (ed) Biochemical correlates of brain structure and function. Academic Press, London, pp. 15-41

Matrisian LM, Glaichenhaus N, Gesnel MC, Breathnach R, (1985) Epidermal growth factor and oncogenes induce transcription of the same cellular mRNA in rat fibroblasts. EMBO J 4:1435-1440

Mobley WC, Rutkowski JL, Tennekoon GI, Buchannan K, Johnston MV, (1985) Choline acetyltransferase activity in striatum of neonatal rats increased by nerve growth factor. Science, 229:284-287

Morrison RS, de Vellis J (1981) Growth of purified astrocytes in a chemically defined medium. Proc Acad Sci USA 78:7205-7209

Morrison RS, Sharma A, de Vellis J, Bradshaw R.A.(1986) Basic fibroblast growth factor supports the survival of cerebral cortical neurons in primary culture. Proc Natl Acad Sci USA 83:7537-7541

Morrison RS (1987) Fibroblast growth factors: Potential neurotrophic agents in the central nervous system. J Neurosci Res 17:99-101

Perez-Polo JR, Haber B (1983) Neuronotrophic interactions. In: Rosenberg RN (ed) The Clinical Neurosciences, vol V, Churchill Livingstone Inc., New York, pp 37-51

Pettmann B, Weibel M, Sensenbrenner M, Labourdette G (1985) Purification of two astroglial growth factors from bovine brain. FEBS 189:102-108

Saneto RP, de Vellis J (1985) Characterization of cultured rat oligodendrocytes proliferating in a serum free, chemically defined medium. Proc Natl Acad Sci USA 82:3509-3513

Serra I, Cupello A, Gadaleta MN, Viola M, Ragonese P, Giuffrida AM (1983) Labeling of RNA in young and adult rat brain: evidence for different RNA processing. Neurochem Res 8:433-447

Serra I, Avola R, Vanella A, Lombardo B, Agodi A, Giuffrida AM (1984) RNA synthesis in neuronal and glial cell nuclei from rat cerebral hemispheres during early postnatal development. Neurochem Res 9: 1051-1063

Serra I, Giuffrida AM (1986) Post-translational modifications of chromosomal proteins in neuronal and glial nuclei from developing rat brain. In: Giuditta A, Kaplan BB, Zomzely-Neurath C (eds) Role of RNA and DNA in brain function; A molecular biological approach. Martinus Nijhoff Publishing Boston, USA, pp. 182-196

Serra I, Avola R, Condorelli DF, Surrentino S, Renis M, Kamiyama M, Hashim GM, Giuffrida AM (1986) Acetylation and phosphorylation of histones and nonhistone chromosomal proteins in neuronal and glial nuclei purified from cerebral hemispheres of developing rat brain. J Neurochem 46: 1881-1887

Shelton DL, Reichardt LF (1986) Studies on the expression of the β nerve growth factor (NGF) gene in the central nervous system: Level and regional distribution of NGF mRNA suggest that NGF functions as a trophic for several distinct populations of neurons. Proc Natl Acad Sci USA 83:2714-2718

Simpson DL, Morrison R, de Vellis J, Herschman HR, (1982) Epidermal growth factor binding and mitogenic activity on purified populations of cells from the central nervous system. J Neurosci Res 8:453-462

Springer JE, Koh S, Tayrien MW, Loy R (1987) Basal forebrain magnocellular neurons stain for nerve growth factor receptor: Correlation with cholinergic cell bodies and effects of axotomy. J Neurosci Res 17:111-118

Stach RW, Perez-Polo JR, (1987) Binding of nerve growth factor to its receptor. J Neurosci Res 17:1-10

Taniuchi M, Schweitzer JB, Johnson Jr EM (1986) Nerve growth factor receptor molecules in rat brain. Proc Natl Acad Sci USA 83:1659-1954

Taylor JM, Mitchell WM, Cohen S (1972) Epidermal growth factor: physical and chemical properties. J Biol Chem 247:5928-5934

Walicke P, Cowan WM, Ueno N, Baird A, Guillemin R (1986) Fibroblast growth factor promotes survival of dissociated hippocampal neurons and enhances extension. Proc Natl Acad Sci USA 83:3012-3016

Whittemore SR, Ebendal T, Larkfors L, Olson L, Seiger A, Stromber I, Persson H (1986) Developmental and regional expression of β nerve growth factor messenger RNA and protein in the rat central nervous system. Proc Natl Acad Sci USA 83:817-821

Yankner BA, Shooter EM (1982) The biology and mechanism of action of nerve growth factor. Ann Rev Biochem. 51:845-868.

# DEVELOPMENTAL ASPECTS OF MYELIN MEMBRANE PROTEIN SYNTHESIS: SPATIAL SEGREGATION OF POLYRIBOSOMES.

Colman, D., Bernier, L., Staugaitis, S., Salzer, J. and *Trapp, B.
Dept. of Cell Biology
N.Y.U. School of Medicine
550 First Avenue,
New York, 10016.

The rapid and precise construction of the myelin sheath is one of the most remarkable aspects of nervous system development and maturation. In the CNS, the myelinating cell is the oligodendrocyte, a cell with a small soma that supports via slender cytoplasmic "arms" thirty or more individual, flattened expanses of spirally-wrapped, tightly compacted myelin membrane. Thin section electron microscopy of the mature myelin sheath reveals an alternating pattern of thick (major dense, MDL) and thin (intraperiod, IDL) lines that represent the apposition of the cytoplasmic and extracellular aspects, respectively, of the oligodendrocyte plasma membrane bilayer (1). During rapid myelination, this cell generates vast quantities of plasma membrane, and inserts into this lipid matrix the myelin-specific polypeptides that presumably participate in the initial organization and subsequent maintenance of the mature sheath. How the oligodendrocyte precisely targets these proteins to the developing myelin domain of the plasma membrane is a challenging problem, especially since it is difficult to imagine that complete control of the local assembly process along individual myelin internodes resides solely in the cell soma, which comprises only a small fraction of the cell volume, and is for the most part located a considerable distance from the myelinating regions. In this short paper, we summarize the evidence that the oligodendrocyte controls the myelination process in part locally at each developing internode, by selectively segregating to the myelinating region those free polysomes engaged in synthesizing a specific set of major

*Dept. of Neurology, Johns Hopkins School of Medicine, 600 N. Wolfe St., Baltimore, MD 21205.

NATO ASI Series, Vol. H22
Neural Development and Regeneration.
Edited by A. Gorio et al.

myelin proteins, the myelin basic proteins. We believe that this phenomenon is an important aspect of the myelination program that may have evolved from a general cellular mechanism that places certain mRNAs near the sites of function of their encoded polypeptides (see refs. 2,3) and article by O. Steward, this volume).

Purified myelin can be shown to contain only a few abundant proteins (Fig. 1), two of which - the myelin basic proteins (MBPs) and the myelin proteolipid protein (PLP) are present in about a 1:1 proportion and together comprise about 70-80% of the total myelin protein:

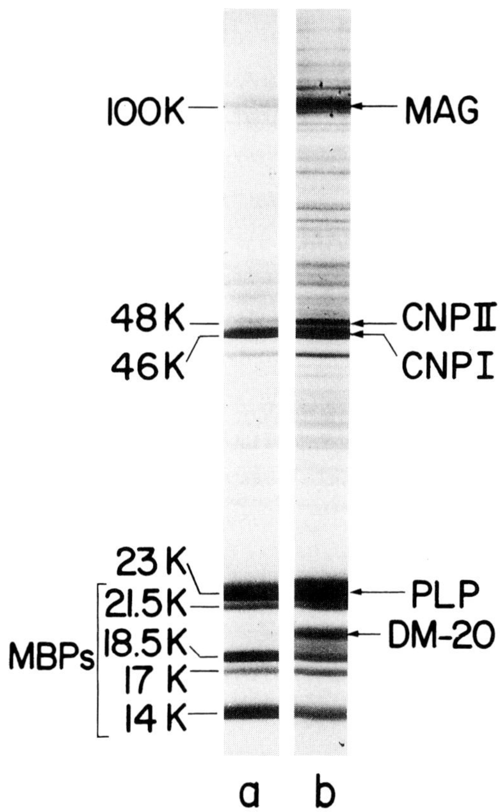


Fig. 1: The proteins of myelin: Highly purified rat myelin was prepared (12) and subjected to SDS PAGE (7-17% of acrylamide gradient). The major proteins of myelin are clearly demonstrated on Coomassie blue (lane a) and silver (lane b) staining. The myelin proteolipid protein (PLP, $M_r$ = 23 kd) and the family of myelin basic protein (MBPs, $M_r$ = 14 Kd, 17 Kd, 18.5 Kd and 21.5 Kd) constitute about 70% of the total protein. Other prominent bands include the 2'3' cyclic nucleotide 3' phosphodiesterases (CNPs, $M_r$ = 46 and 48 Kd, see ref. 14) and the myelin associated glycoproteins (MAGs, $M_r$ = 100 Kd, see ref. 15).

There is good evidence from studies on dysmyelinating mouse mutants that both the MBPs (4) and PLP (5) are essential for the normal formation of the myelin sheath.

The MBPs in the rat and mouse are a set of low molecular weight, highly charged peripheral membrane proteins that are rich in arginines and lysines. These proteins are first synthesized on free polysomes (6,7) and associate posttranslationally with the myelin membrane (7). The MBPs have been localized to the major dense line (8, 17) and they are cytoplasmically disposed in the bilayer. PLP on the other hand is a hydrophobic, transmembrane protein that is synthesized and inserted into the rough endoplasmic reticulum, and then incorporated into the forming myelin membrane (7). Ongoing studies with monospecific antibodies (8) and our own proteolysis studies (Colman, unpublished) reveal that portions of the PLP molecule are exposed on both sides of the bilayer and so can contribute to the formation of both the major dense and intraperiod lines.

We have shown that the initial association of PLP with the rough endoplasmic reticulum membrane is likely to be mediated by a portion of the PLP molecule that serves as a "signal" for insertion (7). It can be demonstrated by in vitro translation of total brain mRNA in the presence of dog pancreas microsomes (DPM) that this insertion process occurs strictly cotranslationally, and requires the presence of a specific cytoplasmic factor, (signal recognition particle, SRP; see ref. 10) as well as a specific membrane-bound receptor for the SRP-insertion signal complex in the RER (Fig. 2A). When SRP is omitted from the translation mixture, newly synthesized PLP behaves as if it were a soluble protein, and can therefore be completely recovered in the supernatant after sedimentation of the DPM:

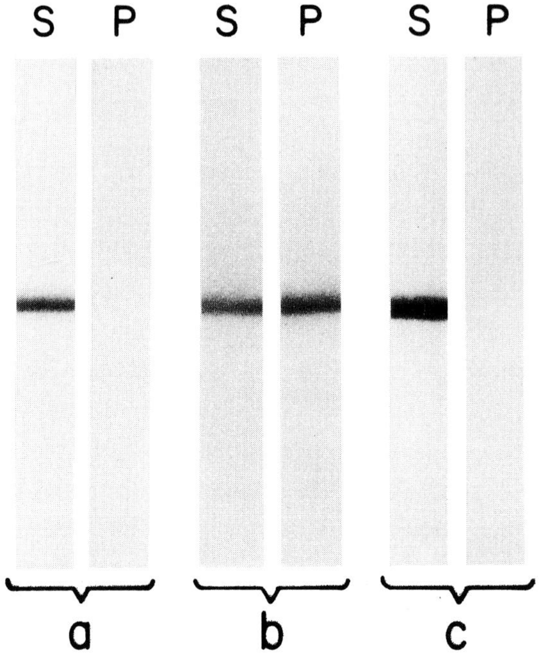


Fig. 2: Association of newly synthesized PLP and MBP with DPM: In vitro translations in the wheat germ system were programmed with brainstem mRNA. Samples (a, b, d, e) received DPMs at the start of the translation with (b, e) or without (a, d) added SRP. Another set (c and f) received the DPMs and SRP 2h after the translation had begun, and incubation was continued for an additional hour. Supernatants (S) and pellets (P) containing DPM were obtained from all samples after centrifugation (5 min., 13,000g) and were solubilized in detergents and immunoprecipitated sequentially first with PLP (Fig. 2A) and then MBP (Fig. 2B) antisera.

Fig. 2A: Insertion of PLP into DPM: In the absence of SRP, newly synthesized PLP remains in the translation mixture supernatant (a). With the addition of SRP, at least 50% of the PLP inserts into the DPM, and so can be recovered in the membrane pellet (b). By adding more SRP cotranslationally, more PLP can be inserted into the membranes (not shown). When SRP and DPM are added after translation is essentially complete, PLP cannot insert into the membranes (c), presumably because the first insertion signal in the molecule is inaccessible to SRP due to folding.

By contrast, in the same translation mixtures (which because they are programmed with total brain mRNA also synthesize the MBPs), MBP avidly associates with the surface of the DPM, even when SRP is absent or added posttranslationally:

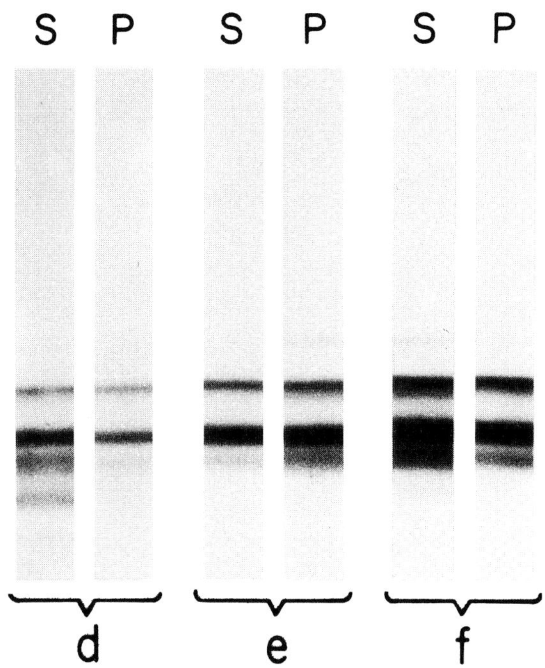


Fig. 2B: Association of MBPs with DPM: The same set of supernatants and pellets, when immunoprecipitated with MBP antisera reveal that MBP associates with the membranes irrespective of the cotranslational presence (e) or absence (d) of SRP. Posttranslational addition of SRP and DPM gave similar results (f).

In other experiments (data not shown), we have observed that newly synthesized MBP will bind with equal avidity to brain mitochondrial membranes and plasma membrane vesicles derived from Shiverer mouse brain.

Recently, we have succeeded in transfecting HeLa cells with a full length cDNA encoding the rat small MBP (14 Kd). In short term transient expression experiments, MBP could be mapped to perinuclear intracellular membrane systems despite the fact that the MBPs are synthesized on free polysomes (Fig. 3). Our interpretation of this is that as the MBP mRNA is released from the cell nucleus, it is immediately taken up into free polysomes and translated. The nascent MBP polypeptides, on emerging from the ribosomes, then rapidly bind to nearby membranes:

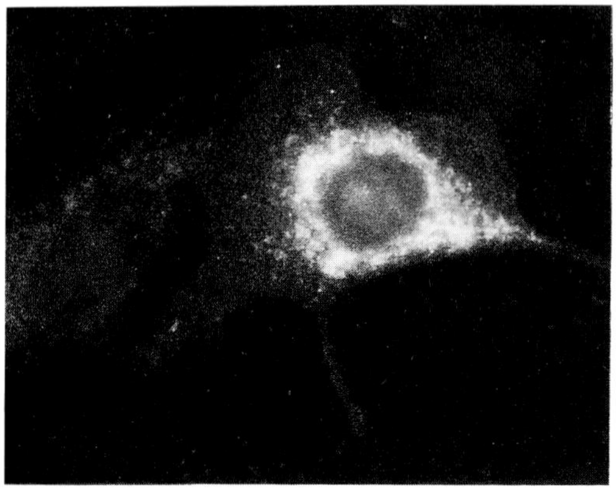

Fig. 3: Expression of MBP in HeLa cells: This HeLa cell was transfected with a MBP cDNA encoding the small (14 Kd) MBP. Twenty four hours after transfection the cell was fixed and treated first with MBP antibody, and then with rhodamine conjugated goat anti-rabbit IgG. Immunofluorescence is apparently confined to perinuclear membranes.

Both these data and the in vitro translation data (Fig. 2) would therefore indicate that unlike PLP, whose association with the RER is strictly regulated by SRP and membrane-bound factors, the MBPs can form non-specific, presumably ionic, associations with a variety of membranes from several sources.

The intensely reactive properties of the MBPs observed in vitro and in the HeLa cell experiments, would lead one to expect that the MBPs might be found distributed not only in compact myelin but throughout the oligodendrocyte cell body, and in other sites as well, such as the cell processes, where protein synthesis undoubtedly also occurs. Curiously, this does not seem to be the case. Immunocytochemical data reveal that oligodendrocytes with fully-formed processes stain for MBP only in the myelinating regions and not in the cell body (11). This suggests that the oligodendrocyte has developed a mechanism for ensuring that the MBPs become associated after synthesis only with the maturing myelin membranes. We have obtained the following evidence from cell fractionation studies that supports this hypothesis.

Myelin can easily be prepared by homogenization and flotation on a .85 M sucrose cushion (12). The homogenization procedure detaches cytoplasmic processes that apparently in many instances remain attached to contiguous compact myelin fragments or "pre-myelin membranes, which have a very high lipid:protein ratio and therefore are less dense than the homogenization medium. As the cytoplasmic processes break off and vesiculate, the content of the process becomes trapped within, and the vesicles so formed can ascend to the top of the .85M sucrose layer. We have found that these vesicles contain a large number of free polysomes (7). When these membranes are treated with guanidinium hydrochloride, a RNA population can be recovered that, when translated, yields about 20 times as much MBP as PLP (Fig. 4):

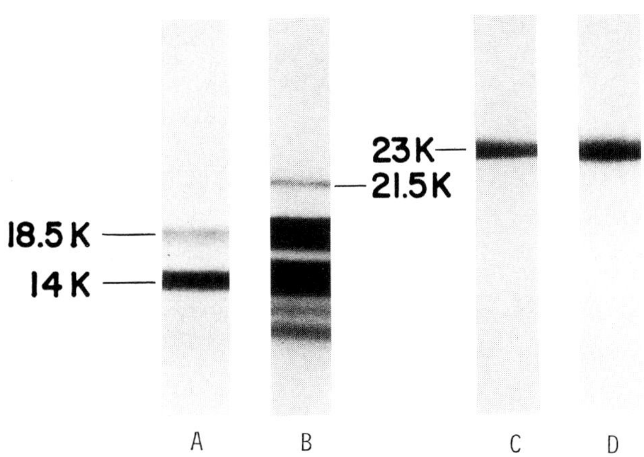


Fig. 4: MBP mRNAs are enriched in a crude myelin fraction: Total brainstem (a, c) and "myelin" mRNA was translated with $^{35}$S-methionine as the label and equal counts were immunoprecipitated with MBP (a, b) or PLP (c, d) antisera. As assessed in the in vitro translations, MBP mRNA sequences in the myelin fraction are much more abundant than MBP mRNA in total brainstem. PLP mRNA is not similarly enriched in the myelin fraction. A direct demonstration by Northern analysis of the relative amounts of MBP mRNAs in the myelin fraction versus brainstem mRNA has been presented elsewhere (16).

These biochemical data strongly suggest that the free polysomes synthesizing the MBPs are segregated in those peripheral regions of the oligodendrocyte cytoplasm that are most intimately and directly involved in myelin formation (7). Most recently, in situ hybridization of brain tissue sections with PLP and MBP cDNA probes (Fig. 5) have clearly demonstrated that the spatial segregation of MBP mRNAs to the cell periphery occurs in the intact oligodendrocyte (13).

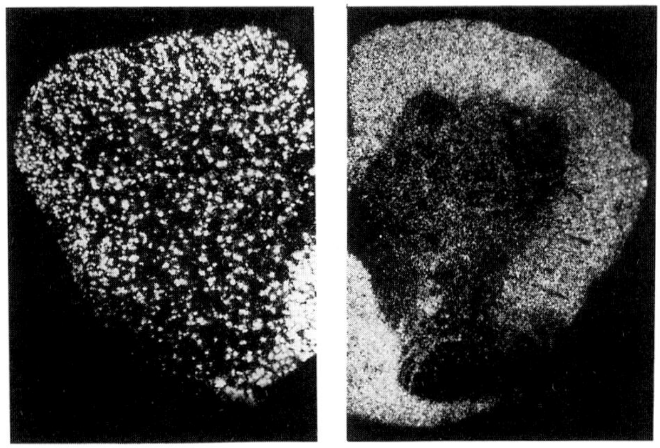

Fig. 5: In situ hybridization of adult rat spinal cord with cloned MBP and PLP cDNA probes: PLP mRNA is concentrated over oligodendrocyte cell bodies (left panel), while MBP mRNAs are distributed predominantly along myelinated fiber tracts (right panel).

We think that it is likely that this segregation of MBP-synthesizing polysomes within the myelinating "arms" prevents the non-specific association of the newly synthesized polypeptides with non-myelin intracellular membranes.

One can imagine several mechanisms that could establish and maintain this segregation. One possibility that we are currently considering is that sequences in the MBP mRNAs could specifically associate with cytoskeletal elements and migrate into the myelinating processes. Once the segregation is established, the nascent MBP polypeptides could directly interact with the sites of their deposition in the myelin sheath.

There are clearly a number of finely-tuned intracellular mechanisms that each oligodendrocyte must employ to rapidly and accurately construct so many myelin sheaths simultaneously. The availability of cloned probes for all the major myelin proteins now provides us with new tools that may help us to study these mechanisms at a molecular level.

Bibliography:


1. Peters A, Palay S, and DeF Webster H (1976) The fine structure of the nervous system. W. B. Saunders Co., Philadelphia, London, Toronto.
2. Cervera M, Dreyfuss G, and Penman S (1981) Messenger RNA is translated when associated with the cytoskeletal framework in normal and VSV infected HeLa cells. Cell 23: 113.
3. Fulton AB, Wan KM, and Penman S (1980) The spatial distribution of polyribosomes in 3T3 cells and the associated assembly of proteins into the skeletal framework. Cell 20: 849.
4. Kirschner DA, and Ganser AL, (1980) Compact myelin exists in the absence of basic protein in the shiverer mutant mouse. Nature (Lond.) 283: 207.
5. Gardinier MY, Macklin WB, Diniak AJ, Deininger PL (1986) Characterization of myelin proteolipid protein mRNAs in normal and Jimpy mice. Mol. Cell Biol. 6: 3755.
6. Campagnoni AG, Carey, and Yu Y (1980). In vitro synthesis of the myelin basic proteins: subcellular site of synthesis. J. Neurochem. 34: 677.
7. Colman DR, Kreibich G, Frey AB, and Sabatini DD. (1982). Synthesis and incorporation of myelin polypeptides in CNS myelin. J. Cell Biol. 95: 598.
8. Herndon RM, and Rauch H, and Einstein E (1973). Immunoelectron microscopic localization of the encephalitogenic basic protein in myelin. Immunol. Commun. 2: 163.
9. Hudson L, Dubois-Dalcq M, Behar T, Arnheiter H, and Lazzarini R (198) Orientation of the proteolipid protein in the oligodendrocyte membrane. J. Cell Biol. 105: 435a.
10. Walter P, and Blobel G (1980). Purification of a membrane-associated protein complex required for protein translocation across the endoplasmic reticulum. Proc. Natl. Acad. Sci. U.S.A. 77: 7112.
11. Sternberger NH, Itoyama Y, Kies MW, and Webster H deF. (1978) Myelin basic protein demonstrated immunocytochemically in oligodendroglia prior to myelin sheath formation. Proc. Natl. Acad. Sci. U.S.A. 75: 2521.
12. Norton WT, and Poduslo SE. (1973) Myelination in rat brain: Method of myelin isolation. J. Neurochem. 21: 749.
13. Trapp B D, Moench T, Pulley M, Barbosa E, Tennekoon G, and Griffin, J. (1987) Spatial segregation of mRNA encoding myelin-specific proteins. (In press, Proc. Natl. Acad. Sci., U.S.A.).
14. Bernier L, Alvarez F, Norgard EM, Raible DW, Mentaberry A, Sabatini DD, and Colman DR. (1987). Molecular cloning of a 2'3' cyclic nucleotide 3'-phosphodiesterase: mRNAs with different 5' ends encode the same set of proteins in nervous and lymphoid tissues. (In press, J. Neurosci.).
15 Salzer JL, Holmes WP, and Colman DR. (1987) The amino acid sequences of the myelin associated glycoprotein: Homology to the immunoglobulin gene superfamily. J. Cell Biol. 104: 957.
16. Mentaberry A, Adesnik M, Atchison M, Norgard EM, Alvarez F, Sabatini DD and Colman DR (1986) Small basic proteins of myelin from central and peripheral nervous systems are encoded by the same gene. Proc. Natl. Acad. Sci. 83: 1111.
17. Omlin FX, Webster H deF, Palkovits CG, and Cohen SR (1982) Immunocytochemical localization of basic protein in major dense line regions of central and peripheral myelin. J. Cell Biol. 95: 242.

# Cytotypic Specialization of the Neuronal Cytoskeleton and the Cytomatrix: Implications for Neuronal Growth and Regeneration.

**Scott T. Brady**
**Dept. of Cell Biology**
**University of Texas Southwestern Medical Center at Dallas**
**Dallas, Texas**
**U.S.A.**

The diversity of cell types in nervous tissue is one of its most remarkable attributes. Neurons are particularly striking in their many shapes, sizes, electrical properties, and biochemical compositions. Yet another aspect of neurons which varies with the type of neuron is the capacity for growth. In addition, the ability of a given neuron to grow and remodel its axonal and dendritic arbors changes during development and aging. Recently, work in many laboratories has begun to identify the some of the molecular mechanisms underlying neuronal growth. Such mechanisms include differential gene expression, regulation by growth factors and hormones, and changes in the extracellular environment, but in each of these cases neuronal growth must be mediated in part by the neuronal cytoskeleton. Therefore, an understanding of the composition and properties of the neuronal cytoskeleton is necessary before we can fully understand the mechanisms of neuronal development and regeneration.

Much has been learned about the neuronal cytoskeleton in recent years, particularly the axonal cytoskeleton. The importance of the axonal cytoskeleton is best appreciated by considering several special properties of neurons. Some of the features that distinguish neurons from other cell types are often overlooked when discussing the properties of the neuron. For example, neurons may be very large cells: the largest cells in the body. Much of the volume associated with a neuron is located in its axonal regions, which may be ten thousand times the length and contain as much as a thousand times the volume of the cell body. Neurons also have complex morphologies that are associated with particular functions and locations within the nervous system. A significant portion of these stereotyped morphologies come from the pattern of axonal branching and axonal connectivity characteristic of specific types of neurons. In fact, the size and shape of a neuron reflects the amount, composition, and distribution of the cytoskeletal elements in that neuron.

NATO ASI Series, Vol. H22
Neural Development and Regeneration
Edited by A. Gorio et al.

The large and complex morphologies of neurons are established during development and then the overall form is retained for the life of the organism. The general sequence of development in the nervous system is an initial period of growth and plasticity followed by stabilization of the overall patterns of axons, dendrites, and connections. One good example is found in the development of the visual system. Hubel and Wiesel were able to define a critical period during which the circuitry of the visual system is extremely sensitive to visual input (Hubel and Wiesel 1970). However, once this critical period has passed, the amount or type of visual input has little effect on the circuitry. While the timing of this critical period is well defined in various species (Hubel and Wiesel 1970, Lund and Lund 1972, 1976), relatively little is known about the cellular and molecular mechanisms that underlie this stabilization of neuronal connections. However, changes in the properties of the axonal cytoskeleton are known to occur at about this same time (Baittinger et al. 1984). Given the importance of the cytoskeleton in defining cellular morphology, changes in the properties of cytoskeletal elements in the neuron would be expected to play a role in any change in the dynamics of neuronal morphology. Consideration of the known features and functions for the neuronal cytoskeleton is a useful way to evaluate that role. However, even if we attempt to restrict our consideration to the neuronal cytoskeleton, the literature is too large for a detailed review, but with a judicious use of suitable examples, a real appreciation may be gained.

The Microtubule Cytoskeleton of Neurons.

Tubulin is the major protein of vertebrate brain, as much as a quarter of total brain protein in some cases (Anderson 1979, Hiller and Weber 1978, Bamberg et al. 1973). Tubulin in the form of MTs has many different functions, notably in the mitotic spindle, in cilia and flagella, and in cytoplasmic MTs (Dustin 1984). Although tubulin is a major constituent of almost all eukaryotic cells, few cell types devote as much of their protein synthesis to tubulin as neurons do. In nonneuronal cells, tubulin is generally 1-5% of total protein, but it may represent more than 25% of total protein in neurons (Anderson 1979, Hiller and Weber 1978). Since neurons are postmitotic cells and do not have motile cilia, neuronal tubulin synthesis must be directed towards the formation of cytoplasmic MTs. This is consistent with the large numbers of MTs in the axons and dendrites of neurons (Peters et al. 1976, Peters and Vaughan 1967, Zenker et al. 1975).

Cytoplasmic MTs generally have a number of different functions (Dustin, 1984). They represent a key element in the creation and maintenance of cellular morphology (Friede and Samorajski 1970, Hillman 1980, Solomon 1984). Similarly, they are involved in defining polarity and delineating compartments within the cytoplasm of a cell (Burton and Paige 1981, Chalfie and Thompson 1979, Heidemann et al. 1985). MTs appear to be necessary for the movement of cells or cellular extensions (such as neurites) across a surface (Lasek 1982, Yamada et al. 1971). Finally, cytoplasmic MTs are the substrate for transport of membranous organelles in intracellular transport (Brady 1987, Grafstein and Forman 1980, Schliwa 1984). Recent studies (for a brief review, see Brady 1987) have demonstrated the existence of a new molecular mechanism for microtuble-based movements that is the basis of fast axonal transport and begun characterization of the motor. All of these functions are important for neurons and are likely to be involved in the growth and development of the nervous system.

Consideration of neurite extension illustrates the involvement of MTs in neuronal growth. Neuronal MTs are essential for the extension of neurites and the movement of growth cones (Lasek 1982, Letourneau 1982, Shaw and Bray 1977, Yamada et al. 1971). During this stage, MTs serve to both supply additional plasma membrane to the growing tip by fast axonal transport and to stabilize the neurite extension. At later stages, branching of neurites and formation of presynaptic terminals requires reorganization of the underlying cytoskeleton (Lasek 1981, Hillman 1980). Axonal MTs provide polarity to axoplasm (Burton and Paige 1981, Heidemann et al. 1985) and, in association with microfilaments and neurofilaments, help define subcellular compartments associated with neuronal function, including the presynaptic terminal and domains for fast axonal transport. Axonal MTs are required for return of trophic substances and information via retrograde transport (Brady 1983). Finally, MTs participate in the stabilization of appropriate axonal morphologies and connections (Lasek 1981, Lasek and Morris 1982, Solomon 1984). Throughout this process, axonal MTs change in both composition and function. Moreover, at any one time, there is considerable heterogeneity in neuronal MTs.

Variation in composition, organization, and function of the cytoplasmic MT cytoskeleton have all been reported in different cell types. MTs vary in tubulin isotype (for examples, see Bond et al. 1984, Cumming et al. 1983, Field et al. 1984, Gozes 1982, Ginzberg et al. 1986, Hall et al.

1983, Lopata et al. 1983, ) and microtubule associated proteins (MAPs) (for examples, see Binder et al. 1984, Black and Kurdyla 1983, Bloom et al. 1984, Caceres et al. 1984a, 1984b, DeCamilli et al. 1984, Duerr et al. 1981, Huber and Matus 1984, Huber et al. 1985) relatively little was known about the functional consequences of these variations. Recently, studies have begun to associate particular changes in microtubule composition with specific structures and possible functions. For example, studies on ciliary and flagellar MTs led to the identification of polypeptides that make up dynein ATPase (Pfister et al. 1985, Pfister and Witman 1984) and indicate that ciliary alpha tubulins are acetylated (L'Hernault and Rosenbaum 1985, Piperno et al. 1987). As a result of these studies, our understanding of the molecular mechanisms underlying assembly and function of cilia was significantly advanced.

The microtubule cytoskeleton of the nervous system is particularly diverse. Tubulin is a multigene family (Cleveland 1983, Cowan and Dudley 1983, Ginzberg et al. 1986, Hall et al. 1983, Kemphues et al. 1980, Lopata et al. 1983) and some tubulin genes are preferentially expressed in nervous or other tissues (Bond and Farmer 1983, Bond et al. 1984, Cleveland 1983, Ginzberg et al. 1986, Kemphues et al 1980, 1982). There are also a number of posttranslational modifications of brain tubulin including acetylation (L'Hernault and Rosenbaum 1985, Piperno et al. 1987)(40,105,152), tyrosilation (Burgoyne and Norman 1986, Gunderson et al. 1984, Thomson 1982), phosphorylation (Goodman et al. 1970), and polyamination (Ambron and Kremzner 1982, Kremzner and Ambron 1982). In fact, more than 20 different isotypes of tubulin can be detected in vertebrate brain using biochemical methods (Field et al. 1984, George et al. 1981).

Cloning of the genes for beta tubulin have demonstrated that some beta tubulin genes are preferentially expressed in nervous tissue (Bond and Farmer 1983, Bond et al. 1984, Lopata et al. 1983, Hall et al. 1983). The study of alpha tubulin genes is not as far advanced, but it appears that expression of some alpha tubulin isotypes is also enriched in nervous tissue (Cumming et al. 1983, Ginzberg et al. 1986). Posttranslational modifications of tubulin such as tyrosilation (Gunderson et al. 1984) and acetylation (Piperno et al. 1987) have been demonstrated in the brain. Most of these specializations in tubulin appear to be widely distributed in nervous tissue, but the functional significance is in most cases unclear. The different isoforms of tubulin generally coassemble <u>in vitro</u> with essentially normal kinetics (see for example L'Hernault and Rosenbaum 1985,

Thompson 1982) and transport into the axon does not appear to be selective (Burgoyne and Norman 1986), so the functional significance of such modifications remains obscure.

One exception may be the cold insoluble form of tubulin which has been described in the axon. Traditionally, MTs are thought to be cold labile. However, a number of studies (Black et al. 1984, Brady 1981, Brady et al. 1984, Brady and Black 1986, Tashiro and Komiya 1983a, 1983b, Tashiro et al. 1983) have demonstrated that a large proportion of the tubulin in axons is cold insoluble. This cold insoluble tubulin is in the form of cold stable microtubule segments that appear to represent domains of longer MTs (Black et al. 1984, Brady and Black 1986, Joshi et al. 1986, Sahenk and Brady 1987). The tubulin in this insoluble form is different from the tubulin obtained by cycling from whole brain homogenates (Brady et al. 1982, 1984, Tashiro and Komiya 1983b). The alpha tubulin of these stable MTs appears to be posttranslationally modified and may also represent a distinct gene product (Brady et al. 1984). We have proposed that such stable microtubule segments represented a way of regulating and stabilizing axonal MTs (Brady et al. 1984, Brady and Black, 1986, Sahenk and Brady, 1987). Such a mechanism for regulating neuronal MTs is very different from the mechanisms that seem to function in fibroblasts, epithelial cells, and other nonneuronal cells (Mitchison and Kirschner 1984, Soltys and Borisy 1985). Indeed, the absence of microtubule organizing centers in the axon and the unusual resistance of axonal microtubules to depolymerization indicates that the axonal microtubule complex cannot be equivalent to that of a fibroblast.

Morphometric analyses of axonal microtubules in both longitudinal and cross-sections suggested that these stable microtubule segments were stable domains in longer microtubules (Sahenk et al. 1987, Sahenk and Brady 1987). Similar results have been obtained for neurons in culture (Black et al. 1984, Joshi et al. 1986), retinal ganglion cell axons (Sahenk and Brady 1987), and sciatic nerve axons (Sahenk et al. 1987). When retinal ganglion cell axons are incubated in the cold for an hour and examined in longitudinal sections (Sahenk and Brady 1987), the mean length for microtubule segments in a section was reduced from a control value of $0.84 \pm 0.67$ µm to only $0.45 \pm 0.36$ µm. The cold stable microtubule segments were also stable in the presence of the antimitotic agent podophyllotoxin, resulting in a reduction in mean segment length comparable to that for cold incubation. Combining cold and podophyllotoxin treatments reduced the mean segment length still further to 0.32±0.32 um, but did not eliminate axonal microtubules. By contrast, combination of the microtubule stabilizing drug taxol with cold treatment increased the mean segment length of microtubules to 0.61±0.

In order to be certain that the reduction in mean segment length was not the result of a change in microtubule orientation, both longitudinal and cross-sections were examined in the same populations of axons. Cold incubations reduced the density of microtubules by approximately 50% and podophyllotoxin reduced density to a slightly greater extent. Interestingly, these numbers were comparable to the amount of cold insoluble tubulin found in these axons. Although the axonal cytoskeleton was disorganized as a result of these treatments, it was clear that the remaining segments were surviving stable domains from longer axonal microtubules.

When similar experiments were conducted on sciatic nerve, using an in vivo incubation system with the antimitotic and cancer chemotherapeutic agent vincristine sulfate, similar results were obtained (Sahenk et al. 1987). Axonal diameters did not change significantly, but the mean length of microtubule segments in drug treated axons was 0.42±0.37 µm as compared to 0.67±0.55 µm in control axons. Just as in the retinal ganglion cell axons, the density of microtubules was significantly reduced. It is noteworthy that the mean length of microtubule segments in control axons was less than that found in optic nerve (0.84 µm in optic versus 0.67 µm in sciatic nerve). The results indicate that cold insoluble tubulin is found in stable domains within longer axonal microtubules. The presence of such stable microtubule segments has important implications for the regulation of the axonal cytoskeleton.

The differences between sciatic and optic nerve are intriguing because the insoluble fraction of axonal tubulin is smaller in sciatic nerve than in optic nerve (Brady and Black 1986 and see below). The disruption of fast axonal transport caused by vincristine would be greater in axons with more labile microtubules, so these observations are relevant to an understanding of the clinical side-effects of vincristine cancer chemotherapy. Sensory fibers of the sciatic nerve are the first to be affected by the peripheral neuropathy that is a common side effect of vincristine treatment (Sahenk et al. 1987). Our studies of axonally transported tubulin in ventral motor neurons (VM) and dorsal root ganglion sensory neurons (DRG) of the sciatic nerve indicate that DRG neurons have the greatest amount of tubulin associated with SCb (Oblinger et al. 1987, McQuarrie et al. 1986). Since the tubulin in SCb has a significantly smaller cold insoluble fraction, the microtubules in DRG axons are more labile. This observation provides a mechanism for differential sensitivity of two populations of axons in the same nerve (Sahenk et al. 1987 and unpublished observations).

In addition to these variations in tubulin, many MAPs have been shown to have distinctive distributions in the nervous system. For example, MAP2, one of the high molecular weight MAPs, is preferentially located in dendrites (Black and Kurdyla 1983, Caceres et al 1984, Huber and Matus 1984, Vallee 1982), while MAPs of the tau class are highly enriched in axons (Binder et al. 1984a, Black and Kurdyla 1983, Peng et al. 1986).

Progress has been slow in determining possible functions for specialized MTs. In many cases, the specialized form of microtubule protein can be detected in a variety of microtubules (Bloom et al. 1984, Kemphues et al. 1982, Piperno et al 1987). However, examples exist where different microtubule proteins are matched to distinct cellular locations. Tubulin isotypes may be associated with specific cellular or subcellular sites (Cumming et al. 1983, Gunderson et al. 1984). Such differences may be particularly apparent during development (Bond and Farmer 1984, Cumming et al. 1983, Kemphues et al. 1980).

The differential distribution of MAPs has been well documented (Binder et al. 1984a, Black and Kurdyla 1983, Bloom et al. 1984, Caceres et al 1984, DeCamilli et al. 1984, Huber et al. 1985, Huber and Matus 1984, Matus et al. 1981, Peng et al. 1986, Tytell et al. 1984, Vallee 1982). In vitro studies had shown that the addition of high molecular weight MAPs affected the packing density of MTs (Brown and Berlin 1985, Kim et al. 1979, Zingsheim et al. 1979). Serial section reconstruction of dendrites demonstrated that spacing of MTs in dendrites was consistent with the lengths of MAP2 (Sasaki-Sherrington et al. 1984). A recent study by Black (1987) takes this observation further by directly demonstrating that MAP2 alters the packing density of MTs, while the tau MAPs have no effect (see figure 1). Thus, differences in the MAP composition of neuronal MTs appears to be one mechanism for modulating the properties and functions of neuronal MTs. Moreover, the changes in MAPs of the brain during development of the nervous system (Binder et al 1984b, Drubin et al. 1984, Francon et al. 1982, Mareck et al. 1980) reinforce the importance of MAPs and microtubules in neuronal growth.

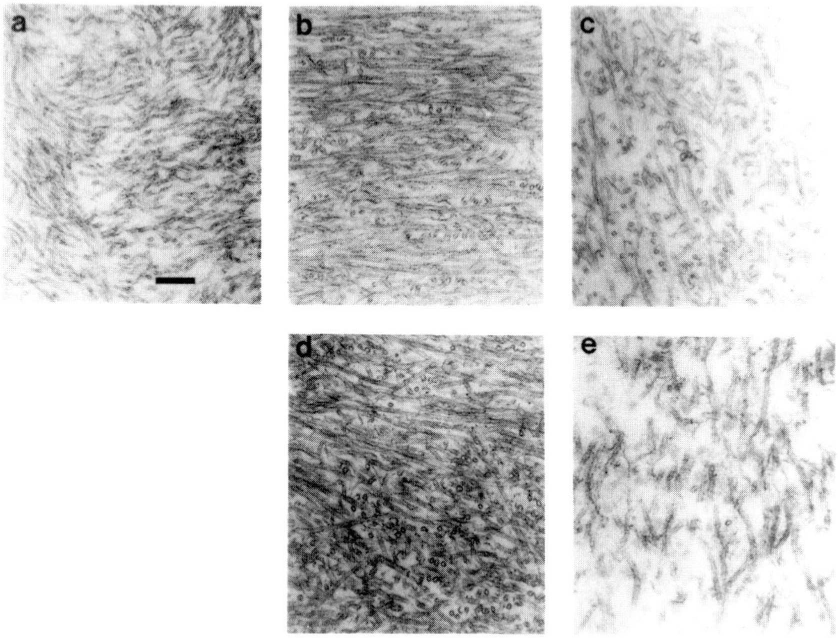


Figure 1. MAPs and the minimum packing density of microtubules. With taxol, microtubules can be assembled from solutions of tubulin alone (a) or in the presence of either tau (b and d) or MAP2 (c and e) microtubule associated proteins. In the absence of MAPs (a), microtubule pellets are very tightly packed. Addition of tau protein at a tubulin to tau ratio of 0.09 (b) or 0.15 (d) has no detectable effect on microtubule packing density, but addition of MAP2 at ratios of 0.09 (c) or 0.24(e) increases the spacing between microtubules in these pellets. Bar=0.2 $\mu$m (from Black (1987) Micrograph provided by Dr. M. M. Black.)

Variation in Neurofilaments. Neurofilaments (NF) are a member of the intermediate filament family of cytoskeletal proteins (Wang et al. 1985). Like other intermediate filaments, NF are long, unbranching 10 nm filaments. However, unlike other intermediate filaments, NF have several high molecular weight subunits. In mammals and many other vertebrates, there are three NF subunits, called the NF triplet (Hoffman and Lasek 1975). The two higher subunits appear to play a particular role in the formation of sidearms on the NF which are thought to crosslink the NF to each other or to other cytoskeletal structures. The cross bridges that can be seen between NF are a distinctive feature of NF bundles and are thought to affect the minimum packing density of NF (Hirokawa 1981, Hirokawa et al. 1984). The two higher molecular weight subunits are also subject to a considerable amount of phosphorylation (Sternberger and Sternberger 1983). *In vivo* the NF of the cell body and to some extent the dendrites are poorly phosphorylated, while the axonal NF are highly phosphorylated (Sternberger and Sternberger, 1983). The degree of phosphorylation is also thought to affect the minimum packing density of NF (Hirokawa et al. 1984) and may be altered in some neuropathologies that affect the cytoskeleton.

In an elegant series of studies, Hoffman and his associates (Hoffman et al. 1983, 1985a, 1985b) have demonstrated a dynamic relationship between the amount of NF in axonal transport and axonal caliber. Earlier studies had convincingly demonstrated that axonal diameter of large myelinated fibers was related to the number of NF in those axons (Friede and Samorajski, 1970). In smaller fibers with few NF, the contribution of MTs was more apparent (Friede and Samorajski, 1970, Parhad et al. 1987). During development, the amount of NF in a neuronal population changed as the caliber of their axons increased (Hoffman et al. 1983, 1985b, Willard and Simon 1983, Shaw and Weber 1982, Glicksman and Willard 1985). Hoffman et al. (1985a) found that during regeneration the diameter of the proximal axon decreased in a proximodistal direction and then gradually returned to normal as the regenerating fibers reestablished connections and began to mature. These changes were associated with changes in the amount of NF in the axon and reflected changes in the expression of the NF triplet by the corresponding neuronal cell bodies (Hoffman et al. 1985a).

Cytotypic variation in the composition and dynamics of the axonal cytoskeleton. In order to better understand the differences in the axonal cytoskeleton associated with different types of neurons, we have characterized the properties of the transported cytoskeleton in three classes of neurons: retinal ganglion cells (a CNS sensory neuron), ventral motor neurons (a PNS motor neuron), and dorsal root ganglion cells (a PNS sensory neuron). These three types of neurons have a number of interesting differences. In the sciatic nerve, the unmyelinated fibers contribute relatively little to the labeling in studies of slow axonal transport. As a result, the two peripheral neurons represent large myelinated fibers with associated Schwann cells. These fibers are among the largest in the mammalian nervous system and they regenerate well throughout the life of the animal. By contrast, the retinal ganglion cell axons are smaller fibers that are myelinated by oligodendroglia and have little capacity for regeneration in mammals.

The contrasts between sensory and motor neurons, central and peripheral environment, large and small myelinated fibers, and good and poor regenerating axons serve to define three distinct classes of neurons.

Common features may be noted and a number of differences can be described (McQuarrie et al. 1986, Oblinger et al. 1987). More slowly transported material was associated with SCa than SCb in both the DRG and the VM axons, while in the retinal ganglion cell (RGC) axons more material was associated with SCb than with SCa. Both SCa and SCb had higher rates of transport in DRG and VM than in RGC axons. The greatest difference was found with SCa where rates in DRG and VM axons (1-1.5 mm/day) were three to five fold greater than those in RGC axons (0.1-0.3 mm/day). The difference was not as great for SCb rates, but the SCb still moved twice as fast in the two peripheral nerves (4 mm/day) than in the optic nerve (2 mm/day).

During studies on transport rate, several differences between RGC and VM were noted in the composition of SCa and SCb (McQuarrie et al. 1986). The most obvious was that a substantial amount of tubulin moved with SCb in the VM axons, but not RGC axons. In addition, a fraction of some SCb proteins appeared to move with SCa. These differences were thought to be important for understanding the role of the axonal cytoskeleton in neurite growth, because all neurons examined that were able to readily regenerate axons had significant amounts of tubulin moving ahead of SCa and the neurofilaments. Therefore, we undertook a quantitative two dimensional electrophoretic analysis of the axonally transported cytoskeleton in RGC, VM, and DRG axons.

Each class of neurons was found to have a unique polypeptide composition for both SCa and SCb (Oblinger et al. 1987). As seen in figures 2 and 3, the differences between neurons were both quantitative (i.e. more labeled neurofilament protein in DRG and VM than in RGC) and qualitative (i.e. a major labeled polypeptide of 52 kilodaltons in RGC SCb, that was apparently absent from VM and DRG axons). Perhaps the most interesting differences, however, were in the microtubule proteins, where both qualitative and quantitative differences were apparent.

Our previous studies on axonal MAPs in RGC axons had identified two tau-like proteins in these axons (Tytell et al. 1984). The larger, more basic of these taus was preferentially found in the cold extractable fraction of axonal microtubules, while the other was present in all three fractions (Brady et al. 1984). The two RGC axonal taus were a subset of the MAPs identifiable in retina, which included two additional tau-like proteins and several high molecular weight MAPs (Tytell et al. 1984). No high molecular weight MAPs were detectable in axonal transport in RGC during these studies.

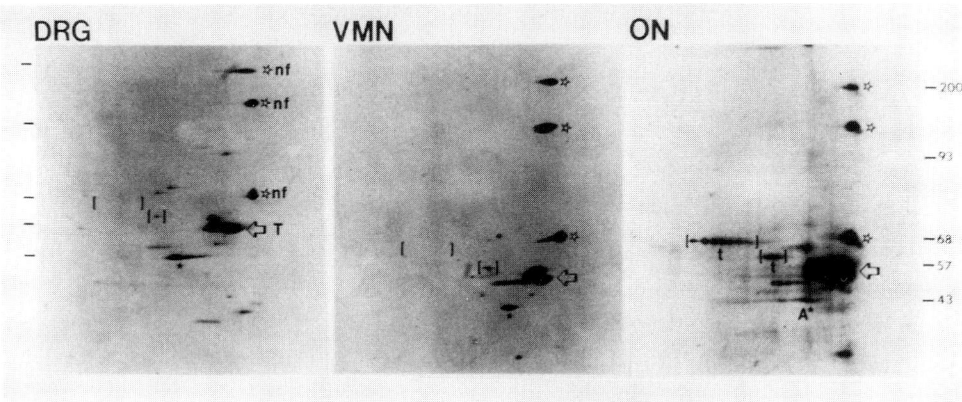


Figure 2. Comparison of polypeptide composition for Slow Component a in dorsal root ganglion sensory neurons (DRG), ventral motor neurons (VMN), and retinal ganglion cells (RGC). Fluorographs were exposed to give equivalent exposures for the neurofilament triplet (open stars, nf). Both quantitative and qualitative differences can be seen. For example, the ratio of tubulin (arrow, T) to neurofilament protein is significantly higher in the RGC axons. The composition of tau-like MAPs (t, brackets) and the relative amount of actin (A, filled star) is characteristic of each set of axons. (Figure from Oblinger et al. 1987)

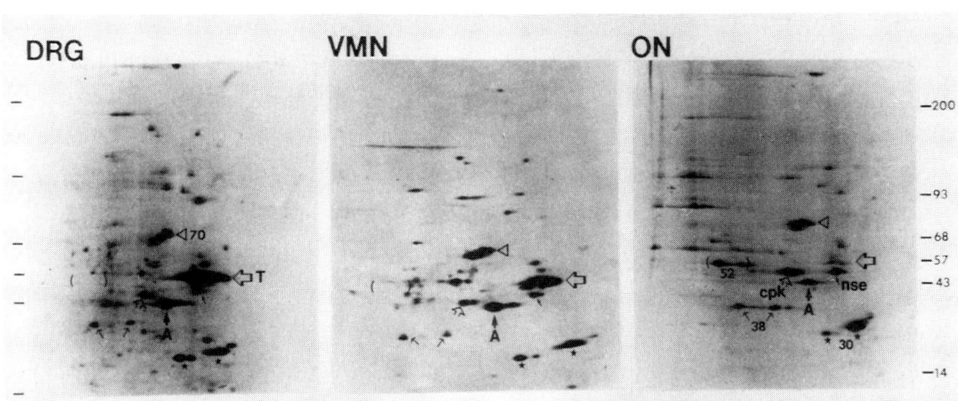


Figure 3. Comparison of polypeptide composition for Slow Component b in dorsal root ganglion sensory neurons (DRG), ventral motor neurons (VMN), and retinal ganglion cells (RGC). In this figure, fluorographs were exposed to give equivalent exposures for actin. The most striking difference is the presence of substantial amounts of tubulin (open arrow, T) in the DRG and VMN axons, but the absence of detectable tubulin in RGC axons. Numerous other differences can also be seen, making each axon population unique in the composition of its cytoskeletal elements (Figure from Oblinger et al. 1987)

Analysis of slow axonally transported proteins in DRG and VMN axons indicated that low levels of the smaller RGC axonal tau was present in SCa and possibly in SCb (Oblinger et al. 1987). The larger, more basic of the RGC axonal taus was not detected in either SCa or SCb of sciatic nerve axons. However,the two major tau-like proteins of retina appear to be present in both DRG and VMN axons (see figures 2 and 3). These two proteins of 67-70 kd seem to be in both SCa and SCb for the sciatic nerve axons, although there may be charge variants in different axons and rate components (unpublished observations). Although the functional significance of these differences in microtubule composition is not yet clear, the specificity of this cytotypic variation is striking. Additional studies on the properties of the axonal cytoskeleton in different neurons and during development using both axonal transport and specific probes of microtubule composition (such as monoclonal antibodies that distinguish between isotypes of tau) are needed.

Changes in the Neuronal Cytoskeleton during Development and Regeneration. The axonal cytoskeleton is particularly dynamic during growth. Changes in composition or organization of the microtubule cytoskeleton involve both tubulin (Bamberg et al. 1973, Bond and Farmer 1984, Cumming et al. 1983, Kemphues et al. 1980) and MAPs (Binder et al 1984b, Drubin et al. 1984, Francon et al. 1982, Mareck et al. 1980). Neurofilament structures change in amount and state of phosphorylation (Hoffman et al. 1983, 1985b, Willard and Simon 1983, Shaw and Weber 1982, Glicksman and Willard 1985). The amount of tubulin and neurofilament protein being transported as well as the rate of axonal transport for tubulin and neurofilaments differ when developing or regenerating axons are compared to mature neurons (Burrell et al. 1979, Hoffman et al. 1983, 1985b, Glicksman and Willard 1985, McQuarrie 1983, McQuarrie et al. 1986, Willard and Simon 1983).

The amount of particulate tubulin (i.e. insoluble tubulin) in chick brain changes from essentially zero to 25% of the total brain tubulin in adult chicken (Bamberg et al, 1973). The fraction of axonal tubulin that is cold insoluble continues to increase during aging in rat brain (Brady 1984, Brady and Black 1986). A substantial amount of the tubulin in developing neurons and in neurons capable of regenerating damaged axons moves with Slow Component b (SCb) (Brady and Black, 1986, Lasek et al. 1983, Wujek and Lasek, 1983). By contrast, in mammalian retinal ganglion cells which have little or no capacity to regenerate axons all of the tubulin moves at the slower rate of Slow Component a (SCa) (Black and Lasek 1980, Brady and Black 1986, Lasek and Brady 1982, McQuarrie et al. 1986, Oblinger et al. 1987). Interestingly, the cold insoluble fraction of the tubulin in SCb is significantly smaller than the cold insoluble fraction of SCa tubulin (Brady and Black 1986), which might reflect a more dynamic cytoskeleton in axons with SCb tubulin.

Implications for Neuronal Growth of Cytotypic Specialization in the Cytoskeleton.

The longterm goal of these studies is to gain an understanding of how changes in the neuronal cytoskeleton, particularly the microtubules, are related to the ability of neurons to grow and regenerate. In order to achieve this goal, we and others have been particularly interested in identifying factors that modify the axonal cytoskeleton in vivo by using or developing experimental models that have characteristic changes in the cytoskeleton. One such model is the axon during regeneration.

We are currently developing a paradigm for evaluating both changes during regeneration and the effects of the glial environment. Following an observation made by Aguayo et al. (1979), we are using the mutant mouse strain Trembler to examine the regulation of axonal caliber during myelination. The Trembler mutant has a defect in peripheral myelination that produces dysmelination and a reduction in axonal caliber. Initial studies on the axonal transport of the cytoskeleton in Trembler have already produced some surprising observations about the interaction between the axon and the Schwann cell (de Waegh and Brady 1988). Since the diameter of the axon is proportional to the amount of microtubules and neurofilaments in the axon (Friede and Samorajski 1970, Hillman 1980, Hoffman et al. 1985a, 1985b, Lasek 1981, Sasaki-Sherrington et al. 1984), as well as their rate of movement in slow transport (Hoffman et al. 1985b), a change in the dynamics of the axonal cytoskeleton was predicted. When Trembler and control profiles of slow axonal transport were examined in dorsal root ganglion sensory axons, there were both qualitative and quantitative differences in the transport of cytoskeletal proteins (DeWaegh and Brady 1987). The most striking effect was an increase of as much as 40% in the amount of tubulin moving with SCb. Changes in the transport of neurofilament protein and clathrin were also apparent.

Many questions remain about the specializations of the neuronal cytoskeleton during neuronal development and regeneration. Nevertheless, progress is being made in the determination of what features of the cytoskeleton are important for growth. Studies using Trembler mice and other model systems promise to illuminate many aspects of the roles played by the cytoskeleton and axonal transport in neuronal development and regeneration. As we define the functions and compositions of the cytoskeleton in various populations of neurons, it is likely that we will begin to comprehend the mechanisms by which the changes in neuronal environment, availability of growth factors, and developmental programs for gene expression are translated into the characteristic sizes and morphologies of neurons.

**Acknowledgements.** The author would like to thank Dr. Mark Black for the use of figure 1. Research described in this report were supported in part by grants from the National Institutes of Health (NS 23320 and NS 23868) and the Texas Neurofibromatosis Foundation.

## REFERENCES

Aguayo A, Bray G, Perkins S (1979) Axon Schwann cell relationships in neuropathies of mutant mice. Ann NY Acad Sci 317:512-531

Ambron R, Kremzner L (1982) Posttranslational modification of neuronal proteins: evidence for transglutaminase activity in R2, the giant cholinergic neuron of Aplysia. Proc Nat Acad Sci USA.

Anderson P (1979) The structure and amount of tubulin in cells and tissues. J Cell Biol

Baittinger C, Cheney R, Clements D, Glicksman M, Hirokawa N, Levine J, Meiri K, Simon C, Skene P, Willard M (1984) Axonally transported proteins in axon development, maintenance, and regeneration. Cold Spring Harbor Symp. Quant. Biol. 48:791-802

Bamburg J, Shooter E, Wilson L (1973) Developmental changes in microtubule protein of chick brain. Biochem 12:1476-1482

Binder L, Frankfurter A, Kim H, Caceres A, Payne M, Rebhun L (1984) MAP2 heterogeneity during brain development. Proc Nat Acad Sci USA 81:5613-5617

Binder L, Frankfurter A, Rebhun L (1984) A monoclonal antibody to tau factor localizes predominantly in axons. J Cell Biol 99:191a.

Black M (1987) Comparison of effects of MAP2 and tau on the packing density of assembled microtubules. Proc Nat Acad Sci USA (in press)

Black M, Lasek R (1980) Slow components of axonal transport: two cytoskeletal networks. J Cell Biol 86:616-623

Black M, Kurdyla J (1983) Microtubule associated proteins of neurons. J Cell Biol 97:1020-1028

Black M, Cochran M, Kurdyla J (1984) Solubility properties of neuronal tubulin: Evidence for extractable and stable microtubules. Brain Res 295:255-263

Bloom G, Schoenfeld T, and Vallee R (1984) Widespread distribution of MAP1 (microtubule associated protein 1) in the nervous system. J Cell Biol 98:320-330

Bond J, Farmer S (1983) Regulation of tubulin and actin mRNA production in rat brain: Expression of a new beta tubulin mRNA with development. Mol Cell Biol 3:1333-1342.

Bond J, Robinson G, Farmer S (1984) Differential expression of two neural cell-specific beta tubulin mRNA during brain development. Mol Cell Biol 4:1313-1319

Brady S (1987) Fast axonal transport in isolated axoplasm from the squid giant axon. Neurol Neurobiol 25:113-138

Brady S (1984) Increases in cold-insoluble axonal tubulin during aging. Soc Neurosci Abstr 10:273

Brady S. (1983) Basic properties of fast axonal transport and the role of fast transport in axonal growth. in Axonal Transport in Neuronal Growth and Regeneration (eds J Elam, P Cancalon) Plenum New York pp 13-29

Brady S (1981) Biochemical and solubility properties of axonal microtubules. J Cell Biol 91:333a

Brady S, Black M (1986) Axonal transport of microtubule proteins: Cytotypic variation of tubulin and MAPs in neurons. Ann NY Acad Sci 466:199-217

Brady S, Tytell M, Lasek R (1984) Axonal tubulin and axonal microtubules: Biochemical evidence for cold stability. J Cell Biol 99:1716-1724

Brown P, Berlin R (1985) Packing volume of sedimented microtubules: Regulation and potential relationship to an intracellular matrix. J Cell Biol 1492-15000

Burgoyne R, Norman K (1986) Alpha tubulin is not detyrosylated during axonal transport. Brain Res 381:113-120

Burrell H, Heacock A, Water R, and Agranoff B (1979) Increased tubulin messenger RNA in the goldfish retina during optic nerve regeneration. Brain Res 168:628

Burton P, Paige J (1981) Polarity of axoplasmic microtubules in the olfactory nerve of the frog. Proc Nat Acad Sci USA 78:3269-3273

Caceres A, Banker G, Steward O, Binder L, Payne M (1984) MAP2 is localized to the dendrites of hippocampal neurons which develop in culture. Dev Brain Res 13:314-318

Caceres A, Binder L, Payne M, Bender P, Rebuhn L, Steward O (1984) Differential subcellular localization of tubulin and the microtubule associated protein MAP2 in brain tissue as revealed by immunocytochemistry with monoclonal hybridoma antibodies. J Neurosci 4:394-410

Chalfie M, Thompson J (1979) Organization of neuronal microtubules in the nematode Caenorhabditis elegans. J Cell Biol 82:278-289

Cleveland D (1983) The tubulins: From DNA to RNA and back again. Cell 34:330-332

Cowan N, and Dudley L (1983) Tubulin isotypes and the multigene tubulin families. Intl Rev Cytol 85:147-173

Cumming R, Burgoyne R, Lytton N (1983) Axonal subpopulations in the central nervous system demonstrated using monoclonal antibodies against alpha tubulin. Eur J Cell Biol 31:241-248

DeCamilli P, Miller P, Navone F, Theurkauf W, Vallee R (1984) Distribution of microtubule associated protein 2 (MAP2) in the nervous system of the rat studied by immunofluorescence. Neurosci 11:819-846

de Waegh S K, Brady S (1988) Slow axonal transport in nerve from mice with a genetic myelin deficiency (Trembler). in Cellular and Molecular Aspects of Neuronal Development and Regeneration (eds B Haber, R Perez-Polo, J de Vellis, A Gorio) Springer Verlag Berlin this volume

Drubin D, Caput D, Kirschner M (1984) Studies on the expression of the microtubule associated protein, tau, during mouse brain development with newly isolated complementary probes. J Cell Biol 98:1090-1097

Duerr A, Pallas D, Solomon F (1981) Molecular analysis of cytoplasmic microtubules in situ: Identification of both widespread and specific proteins. Cell 24:203-211

Dustin P (1984) Microtubules Springer Verlag Berlin Heidelberg New York

Field D, Collins R, Lee J (1984) Heterogeneity of vertebrate brain tubulins. Proc Nat Acad Sci USA 81:4041-4045

Francon J, Lennon A, Fellous A, Mareck A, Pierre M, Nunez J (1982) Heterogeneity of microtubule associated proteins and brain development. Eur J Biochem 129:465-471

Friede R, Samorajski (1970) Axon caliber related to neurofilaments and microtubules in sciatic nerve fiber of rats and mice. Anat Rec 167:379-387

George H, Misra L, Field D, Lee J (1981) Polymorphism of brain tubulin. Biochem 20:2402-2409

Ginzberg I, Teichman A, Littauer U (1986) Isolation and characterization of two rat alpha tubulin isotypes. Ann NY Acad Sci 466:31-40

Glicksman M, Willard M (1985) Differential expression of the three neurofilament polypeptides. Ann NY Acad Sci 455:479-491

Goodman D, Rasmussen H, Dibella T, Guthrow C (1970) Cyclic adenosine 3'-5'-monophosphate stimulated phosphorylation of isolated neurotubule subunits. Proc Natl Acad Sci USA 67:652-659

Gozes I (1982) Tubulin in the nervous system. Neurochem Intl 4:101-120

Grafstein B, Forman D (1980) Intracellular transport in neurons. Physiol Rev 60:1167-1283

Gunderson G, Kalnoski M, Bulinski J (1984) Distinct populations of microtubules: Tyrosinated and nontyrosinated alpha tubulin are distributed differently in vivo. Cell 38:779-789

Hall J, Dudley L, Dobner P, Lewis S, Cowan N (1983) Identification of two human beta tubulin isotypes. Mol Cell Biol 3:854-862

Heidemann S, Hamborg M, Thomas S, Song B, Lindley S, Chiu D (1985) Spatial organization of axonal microtubules. J Cell Biol 99:1289-1295

Hiller G, Weber K (1978) Radioimmunoassay for tubulin: A quantitative comparison of the tubulin content of different established tissue culture cells and tissues. Cell 14:795-804

Hillman D (1980) Neuronal shape parameters and substructure as a basis of neuronal form. in The Neurosciences. 4th Study Program (eds F Schmitt, F Worden) MIT Press pp 477-498

Hirokawa N (1982) Cross-linker system between neurofilaments, microtubules, and membranous organelles in frog axons revealed by quick-freeze deep-etching method. J Cell Biol 94:129-142

Hirokawa N, Glicksman M, Willard M (1984) Organization of mammalian neurofilament polypeptides within the neuronal cytoskeleton. J Cell Biol 98:1523-1536

Hodge A, Adelman W (1983) in Structure and Function in Excitable Cells (eds D Chang, W Adelman, H Leuchtag) Plenum Press NY pp 75-111

Hoffman P, Lasek R (1975) The slow component of axonal transport. Identification of major structural polypeptides of the axon and their generality among mammalian neurons. J Cell Biol 66:351-366

Hoffman P, Lasek R, Griffin J, Price D (1983) Slowing of the axonal transport of neurofilament proteins during development. J Neurosci 3:1694-1700

Hoffman P, Thompson G, Griffin J, Price D (1985a) Changes in neurofilament transport coincide temporally with alterations in the caliber of axons in regenerating motor fibers. J Cell Biol 101:1332-1340.

Hoffman P, Griffin J, Gold B, Price D (1985b) Slowing of neurofilament transport and the radial growth of developing nerve fibers. J Neurosci 5:2920-2929

Hubel D, Wiesel T (1970) The period of susceptibility to the physiological effects of unilateral eye closure in kittens. J Physiol (Lond) 206:419-436

Huber G, Matus A (1984) Differences in the cellular distribution of two microtubule associated proteins, MAP-1 and MAP-2, in rat brain. J Neurosci 4:151-160

Huber G, Alaimo-Beuret D, Matus A (1985) MAP-3: Characterization of a novel microtubule associated protein. J Cell Biol 100:496-507

Joshi H, Baas P, Heidemann S (1986) The cytoskeleton of neurites after microtubule depolymerization. Exptl Cell Res 163:233-245

Kemphues K, Raff E, Raff R, Kaufmann T (1980) Mutation in a testis-specific beta tubulin in Drosophila: Analysis of its effects on meiosis and map location of the gene. Cell 21:445-451

Kemphues K, Kaufmann T, Raff R, Raff E (1982) The testis specific beta tubulin in Drosophila melanogaster has multiple functions in spermatogenesis. Cell 31:655-670

Kim H, Binder L, Rosenbaum J (1979) The periodic association of MAP2 with brain microtubules in vitro. J Cell Biol 80:266-276

Kremzner L, Ambron R (1982) Metabolism and axonal transport of polyamines in a single identified neuron of Aplysia californica J Neurochem 38:1719-1727

L'Hernault S, Rosenbaum J (1985) Chlamydomonas alpha tubulin is posttranslationally modified by acetylation on the epsilon amino group of a lysine. Biochem 24:473-478

Lasek R (1981) The dynamic ordering of neuronal cytoskeletons. Neurosci Res Prog Bull 19:7-32

Lasek R (1982) Translocation of the neuronal cytoskeleton and axonal locomotion. Phil Trans Roy Soc London B 299:313-327

Lasek R, McQuarrie I, Brady S (1983) Transport of cytoskeletal and soluble proteins in neurons. in Biological Structures and Coupled Flows (ed A Silberg) Academic/Balaban Press Rehovet pp329-347

Lasek R, Brady S (1982) The structural hypothesis of axonal transport: Two classes of moving elements in axoplasmic transport. in Axoplasmic Transport (ed D Weiss) Springer Verlag Berlin pp397-405

Lasek R, Morris J (1982) The microtubule-neurofilament network: The balance between plasticity and stability in the nervous system. in Biological Functions of Microtubules and Related Structures (eds H Sakai, H Mohri, G Borisy) Academic Press Tokyo pp 329-342

Letourneau P, (1982) Analysis of microtubule number and length in cytoskeletons of cultured chick sensory neurons. J Neurosci 2:806-814.

Lopata M, Havercroft J, Chow L, Cleveland D (1983)Four unique genes required for beta tubulin expression in vertebrates. Cell 32:713-724

Lund R, Lund J (1972) Development of synaptic patterns in the superior colliculus of the rat. Brain Res 42:1-20

Lund R, Lund J (1976) Plasticity in the developing visual system: Effects of retinal lesions made in young rats. J Comp Neurol 169:133-154

Mareck A, Fellous A, Francon J, Nunez J (1980) Changes in composition and activity of microtubule associated proteins during brain development. Nature 284:353-355

Matus A, Bernhardt R, Hugh-Jones T (1981) High molecular weight microtubule-associated proteins are preferentially associated with dendritic microtubules in brain. Proc Natl Acad Sci USA 78:3010-3014

McQuarrie I (1983) Role of the axonal cytoskeleton in the regenerating nervous system. in Nerve, Organ, and Tissue Regeneration: Research perspectives (ed F Seil) Academic Press NY

McQuarrie I, Brady S, Lasek R (1986) Diversity in the axonal transport of structural proteins: Major differences between optic and spinal axons in the rat. J Neurosci 6:1593-1605

Mitchison T, Kirschner M (1984) Dynamic instability of microtubule growth. Nature 312:237-242

Oblinger M, Brady S, McQuarrie I, Lasek R (1987)Cytotypic variation in the protein composition of the axonally transported cytoskeleton. J Neurosci 7:453-462

Parhad I, Clark A, Griffin J (1987) Effect of changes in neurofilament content on caliber of small axons: The 2,2'-iminodipropionitrile model. J Neurosci 7:2256-2263

Peng I, Binder L, Black M (1986) Biochemical and immunological analyses of cytoskeletal domains of neurons. J Cell Biol 102:252-262

Pfister K, Haley B, Witman G (1985) Labeling of Chlamydomonas 18s dynein polypeptides by 8-azidoadenosine 5'-triphosphate, a photoaffinity analog of ATP. J Biol Chem 260:12844-12850.

Pfister K, Witman G (1984) Subfractionation of Chlamydomonas 18s dynein into two unique subunits containing ATPase activity. J Biol Chem 259:12072-12080.

Piperno G, LeDizet M, Chang X (1987) Microtubules containing acetylated alpha tubulin in mammalian cells in culture. J Cell Biol 104:289-302

Sahenk Z, Mendell J, Brady S (1987) Studies on the pathogenesis of vincristine induced neuropathy. Muscle Nerve 10:80-84

Sahenk Z, Brady S (1987) Axonal tubulin and axonal microtubules: Morphological evidence for stable regions on axonal microtubules. Cell Motil Cytoskel (in press)

Sasaki-Sherrington S, Jacobs J, Stevens J (1984) Intracellular control of axial shape in nonuniform neurites: A serial electron microscopic analysis of organelles and microtubules in AI and AII retinal amacrine neurites. J Cell Biol 98:1279-1290

Schliwa M (1984) Mechanisms of intracellular organelle transport. Cell Muscle Motil 5:1-82

Shaw G, Bray D (1977) Movement and extension of isolated growth cones. Exptl Cell Res 104:55-62

Shaw G, Weber K (1982) Differential expression of neurofilament triplet proteins in brain development. Nature 298:27-279

Shaw G, Osborne M, Weber K (1981) An immunofluorescence microscopical study of the neurofilament triplet proteins, vimentin, and glial fibrillary acidic protein within the adult rat brain. Eur J Cell Biol 26:68-82

Solomon F (1984) Determinants of neuronal form. Trends Neurosci 7:17-20

Soltys B, Borisy G (1985) Polymerization of tubulin in vivo: Direct evidence for assembly onto microtubule ends and from centrosomes. J Cell Biol 100:1682-1689

Sternberger L, Sternberger N (1983) Monoclonal antibodies distinguish phosphorylated and nonphosphorylated forms of neurofilaments in situ. Proc Natl Acad Sci USA 80:6126-6130

Tashiro T, Komiya Y (1983) Two distinct components of tubulin transport in sensory axons of the rat recognized by dimethyl sulfoxide treatment. Biomed Res 4:443-450

Tashiro T, Komiya Y (1983) Subunit composition specific to axonally transported tubulin. Neurosci 4:943-950

Tashiro T, Kurokawa M, Komiya Y (1983) Two populations of axonally transported tubulin differentiated by their interactions with neurofilaments. J Neurochem 43:1220-1225

Thompson W (1982) The cyclic tyrosination/detyrosination of alpha tubulin. Meth Cell Biol 24:235-255

Tytell M, Brady S, Lasek R (1984) Axonal transport of a subclass of tau proteins: Evidence for the regional differentiation in neurons. Proc Natl Acad Sci USA 81:1570-1574

Vallee R (1982) A taxol dependent procedure for the isolation of microtubule and microtubule associated proteins (MAPs). J Cell Biol 92:435-442

Wang E, Fischman D, Liem R, Sun T (1985) Intermediate filaments. Ann. NY Acad Sci 455

Willard M, Simon C (1983) Modulations of neurofilament axonal transport during the development of rabbit retinal ganglion cells. Cell 35:551-559

Wujek J, Lasek R (1983) Correlation of axonal regeneration and slow component b in two branches of a single axon. J Neurosci 3:243-251

Yamada K, Spooner B, Wessels N (1971) Ultrastructure and function of growth cones and axons of cultured nerve cells. J Cell Biol 49:614-635

Zenker W, Mayr R, Gruber H (1975) Neurotubules: Different densities in peripheral motor and sensory nerve fibers. Experientia 31:318-320

Zingsheim H, Herzog W, Weber K (1979) Differences in surface morphology of microtubules reconstituted from pure brain tubulin using two different microtubule associated proteins: The high molecular weight MAP2 proteins and tau proteins. Eur J Cell Biol 19:175-183

# A cDNA CODING FOR RABBIT NEUROFILAMENT PROTEIN H: A WINDOW ON THE ROLE OF H IN NEURODEGENERATIVE DISEASES

by David Soifer[a,b], Kathryn Mack[a] and Henryk M Wisniewski[a]; Institute for Basic Research in Developmental Disabilities[a] and College of Staten Island CUNY[b]; Staten Island, NY[1]

Neurofilaments, the intermediate filaments of neurons, remain an enigma, in spite of the considerable effort that has been expended to understand their function. The proteins of neurofilaments are not uniformly expressed throughout the nervous system and are developmentally regulated. Certain neurodegenerative disorders, and the responses of neurons to some toxic substances, lead to the accumulation of tangles of neurofilaments. Neurofilament antigens have been reported to constitute part of the structure of the paired helical filaments of Alzheimer disease [1,2,5,16,18].

The proteins of intermediate filaments all share certain structural features. Each includes a central a-helical rod domain, flanked by N-terminal and C-terminal domains of varying sequence, size and structure [8,12,19a]. The sequence homologies of the rod domains of all intermediate filament proteins, and their common coiled-coil structures suggest that the rod regions are essential for the generation of the structure of the intermediate filament [12]. Neurofilaments are formed of three proteins, now generally called L, M and H. Each protein includes a rod domain with considerable sequence homology to other intermediate filament proteins. The C-terminal domains of the three neurofilament proteins are unique, although they do share certain features in common. The C-terminal tail regions of the M and H proteins include serine residues which are presumably phosphorylated in the course of the regulation of neurofilament function [11].

The presence of a common rod region with a variable C-terminal tail, has suggested the possibility that all three of the neurofilament proteins copolymerize to form the mature, cross-linked neurofilaments of the axonal cytoskeleton. The elongated C-terminal domains of M, and particularly of H, extend from the filament to form cross-bridges with adjacent filaments and with other constituents of the cytoskeleton. The developmental studies of Willard and Simon [25,26] demonstrated that the expression of H is necessary for the generation of a neurofilament lattice in the axoplasm. H includes a series of sites which may be phosphorylated. Antibodies which recognize the non-phosphorylated epitopes on H, generally react with perikarya, while antibodies against phosphorylated sequences generally demonstrate axonal localization [20,21]. When phosphorylation of H takes place in the perikaryon, accumulation of neurofilaments in the form of neurofibrillary

---------------

[1]Publication No. 1, CSI/IBR Center for Developmental Neuroscience

NATO ASI Series, Vol. H22
Neural Development and Regeneration
Edited by A. Gorio et al.

tangles may ensue, as is the case in aluminum intoxication [23]. Antibodies which recognize phosphorylated epitopes on H, have been reported to bind to the paired helical filaments characteristic of Alzheimer disease.

To study the regulation of synthesis of H, as well as the posttranslational events in the biology of this protein, it is useful to obtain molecular probes. Since multiple allelic forms of H were suggested from the several studies of rabbit neurofilament proteins, since the basic demonstration of developmental regulation of H was demonstrated in the rabbit retinal ganglion cell, and since rabbits are among the animals that respond to aluminum intoxication by the deposition of tangles of neurofilaments in neurons, we have been working with rabbits as an experimental system to study various aspects of neurofilament protein dynamics.

We prepared total RNA from rapidly frozen rabbit brain, [13,24]. Poly[A]$^+$ RNA, was obtained from the total brain RNA by three passes over oligo[dT]-cellulose [3]. cDNA was prepared by the procedure of Gubler & Hoffman [14], in which classical first-strand synthesis with reverse transcriptase is combined with the RNase H-DNA polymerase I-mediated second strand synthesis of Okayama & Berg [17]. The double stranded cDNAs were inserted into the unique EcoRI site in the DNA of the expression vector, bacteriophage lambda gt11 [29,30]. Following packaging of the insert-carrying phage DNA into infectious bacteriophage, the phage were plated on appropriate host strain bacteria (Y 1088 for amplification and to prevent restriction of foreign DNA prior to host modification; Y1090 for expression of the insert DNA). The total packaged library, before amplification, contained 2.33 x $10^6$ clear pfu, representing 71% of the total packaged phage.

The library was first screened with two polyclonal antisera. One of these, a gift of Gerry Shaw, was against rat sciatic nerve H. The second, generated at the Pocono Rabbit Farm against column purified bovine spinal cord H (prepared by Mazhar Malik) and screened by us, included antibodies which reacted with both M and H, but the anti-M activity could be removed by dilution. One plaque was selected, which contained a fusion protein that reacted with both antisera. This fusion protein could also be demonstrated to react with two monoclonal antibodies against non-phosphorylated epitopes on H (see below).

The selected phage (KMRH-1) was replated and reselected several times, to ensure clonality. The phage DNA was then extracted and purified and the insert was cut out of the phage DNA with EcoRI. Agarose gel electrophoresis showed the KMRH-1 insert to be about 900 base pairs long. The insert was subcloned into the EcoRI site of the polylinker region of phage M13mp18, a vector that is useful both for dideoxy-sequencing and for the generation of single-stranded probes. M13 clones were obtained which were tentatively identified to contain KMRH-1 inserts in both orientations, as was subsequently confirmed when they were sequenced.

To ensure that the KMRH-1 insert indeed is included in the rabbit genome, and that we were not working with an artifact, we prepared $^{32}P$ labelled insert cut out from the double stranded form of the M13 phage and labelled by multiple priming off small, random oligonucleotides with the Klenow fragment of DNA polymerase [6, 7]. The $^{32}P$-labelled probes were hybridized to Southern blots of EcoRI cut DNA (Fig 1). The presence of two bands on autoradiographs of these blots shows that there is indeed at least one homologous sequence to KMRH-1 in the rabbit geneome. The two bands reflect either the presence of more than one sequence or the presence within the homologous genomic DNA, of an intron, containing an EcoRI site.

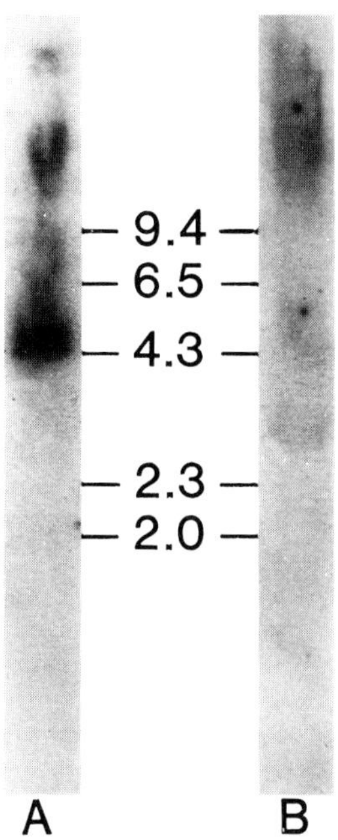


**Figure 1.** EcoRI cut Rabbit genomic DNA (30 ug/well) subjected to electophoresis on 0.8% agarose and transferred to nitrocellulose. A. $^{32}P$-KMRH-1 hybridized to DNA on filter. Filters washed in 0.1 x SSC/0.1% SDS at 55°C. Hybridized probes visualized by autoradiography. B. Rabbit tubulin probe hybridized to rabbit genomic DNA, washed at same stringency as A. Numbers indicate size, in kb of ds lambda phage DNA used as standard.

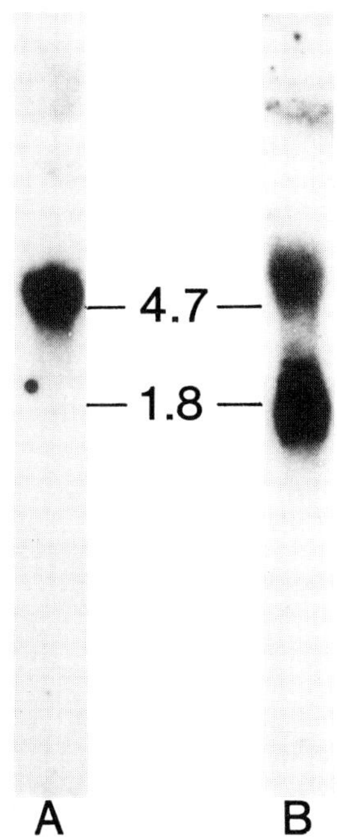


**Figure 2.** Northern blots of rabbit brain RNA (35 ug/well) probed with [A] KMRH-1, and [B] tubulin. RNA separated on 1% agarose gel in 6% formaldehyde and transferred to nitrocellulose. Following hybridization at 42° in 50% formamide, filters were washed at 55° in 0.1 x SSC/0.1% SDS. Hybridized probes visualized by autoradiography. Numbers indicate size of RNA in kb. Ribosomal RNA used as standard.

Northern analysis of rabbit brain RNA probed with KMRH-1 shows a single band indicating that H is coded for by a 4.7 kb mRNA (Fig 2). This large message is consistent with those recently reported for rat mRNAs [19].

Lambda gt11 phage from the cloned KMRH-1 were plated out on Y1090 on 100 mm plates to a plaque density of about 500 plaques per plate, and the fusion protein was expressed and blotted onto filters. The filters were cut into strips which could be screened with many different antibodies. Similar filters were generated with lambda gt11 containing no inserts, and with

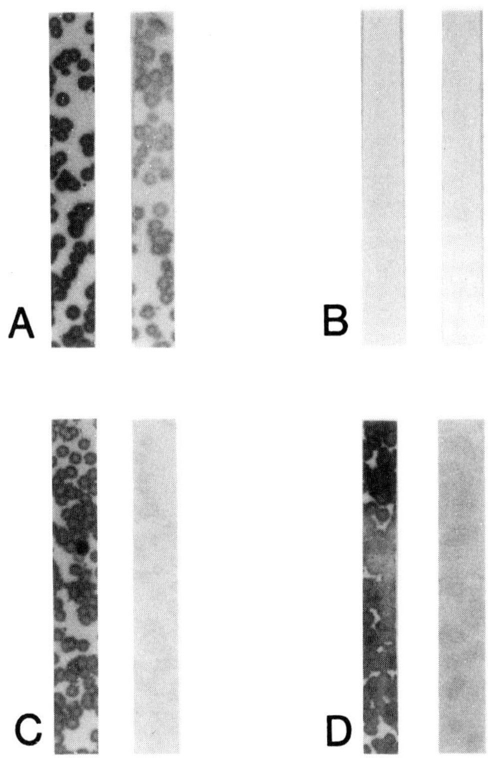


**Figure 3.** Immunoscreens of filter strips generated as described in the text. In each pair, the filter on the left includes fusion protein from KMRH-1 infected E. coli Y1090. The right filters are from control lambda gt11 infected Y1090. In each pair, both filters were incubated with the same antibodies, at the same dilutions. A. Rabbit anti-H serum (1:1000). High non-specific staining in the control is abolished following washing the filter in fetal calf serum. B. MAB 4502.135.12.1 (Sternberger) (1:300). C. MAB 4502.40.8.2 (Sternberger) (1:3000). D. MAB RMO 125.2 (Lee) (1:1000). Bound antibody was visualized with appropriate second antibody, labelled with alkaline phosphatase.

uninfected bacteria. The filter strips were incubated with two panels of monoclonal anibodies which react with various antigenic sites on neurofilament proteins [4, 21]. In each panel, only a single monoclonal antibody reacted with the filter-bound fusion protein. These positive antibodies have been found by the investigators who characterized them, to react with non-phosphorylated sites in the C-terminal domains of H (personal communications from N. and L. Sternberger and from V. Lee, who kindly provided the antibodies). Typical reactions are shown in Fig 3., which compares the reactions with three monoclonal antibodies, and the original antiserum used for the selection of KMRH-1. On the basis of these reactivities, we concluded that KMRH-1 codes for the C-terminal region of H. However, until the DNA sequence was obtained, the identification of KMRH-1 remained tentative.

```
  1  CCTGAGAAGG ACAAGTCCCC AGTGAAGGAG GAGGCCAAGT CCCCCGAGAA GGCCAAGTCC
 61  CCTGAGAAGG CCAAGTCCCC AGTGAAGGAG GAGGCCAAGT CCCCCGAGAA GGCCAAGTCC
121  CCAGTGAAGG AGGAGGCCAA GTCCCCCGAG AAGGCCAAGT CCCCAGTGAA GGAGGAGGCC
181  AAGTCCCCAG AGAAGGAGAC CCCCAAGAAG GAGGAGGTGA AAGTCAAAGA GCCCCCAAAG
241  AAGGTGGAGG AGACAGCCCC CGCCCCACCG AAAGTGGAGA AGGACAGCAA GAAAGACGAG
301  GCACCCAAGA AGGAGGCCCC AAAGCCTGCT GTAGAAAAGC CCAAAGAATC TACAGCTGAA
361  GCCAAGAAGG ACGAGGCTGA AGATAAGAAA AAAGCAGCTC CTGCCAAGAT GGAGGGGAAG
421  GAGGAGGCTA AACCCAAAGA GAAGACGGAG GTGGCCAAGA AGGAGCCGGA GATGCCAAGG
481  CCAAAGAACC CAGCAAACCC ACAGAGAAGG AGCCCGAGAA GCCAAAGAAG GAGGAGACCC
541  CCGCAGCCCC GGTGAAGAAG GAAGCCAAGG AGGAGGCCAG GAAGCCCGAG GAGAAACCCA
601  AGACGGAGCA AGGCCAAGGA GGATGACAAG GCCCTCTCAA AAGAGCCCAG CAAACCCAAG
661  ACGAGAAGGC AGAGAAATCC TCCAGCACGG ACCAGAAAGA TAGCAGGCTC CGGAGAAAGC
721  CACAGAAGAC AAGGCCGCCA AGGGGGAGAA ATAGAGCGGG AAGAGGGGAC AGTCCCAGAG
781  CAGCCAAAGA CATCGGGGGG AGGGTGGTCC TGGAACTCAA GGGCCGGTGT AAGGAATTTC
841  CCTTCCCTCC TCCCTTTTCT TTATGTAAGA AGAAACTCTG CTTAGACGG

   Sequence displayed from position    1 to end (position   889)
   Sequence numbered from position    1
```

**Figure 4.** The consensus DNA sequence of KMRH-1

The complete sequence of KMRH-1 (Fig. 4), obtained by dideoxy sequencing in both directions, using synthetic oligonucleotides as primers, showed considerable degrees of repetition, especially toward the 3' end. Indeed, the first 60 bases are repeated in positions 61 to 120, with the exception of position 11, where C is substituted for A. The sequence, starting at postion 34 {GCCAAGTCCCCCGAGAAG} is repeated four more times, at positions 52, 94, 136, and 178. Careful examination of the first 200 residues reveals several other repeating patterns which become even more apparent once the translated sequence is listed along with the base sequence (Fig. 5).

```
              10          20          30          40          50          60
               *           *           *           *           *           *
CCT GAG AAG GAC AAG TCC CCA GTG AAG GAG GAG GCC AAG TCC CCC GAG AAG GCC AAG TCC
Pro Glu Lys Asp Lys Ser Pro Val Lys Glu Glu Ala Lys Ser Pro Glu Lys Ala Lys Ser

              70          80          90         100         110         120
               *           *           *           *           *           *
CCT GAG AAG GCC AAG TCC CCA GTG AAG GAG GAG GCC AAG TCC CCC GAG AAG GCC AAG TCC
Pro Glu Lys Ala Lys Ser Pro Val Lys Glu Glu Ala Lys Ser Pro Glu Lys Ala Lys Ser

             130         140         150         160         170         180
               *           *           *           *           *           *
CCA GTG AAG GAG GAG GCC AAG TCC CCC GAG AAG GCC AAG TCC CCA GTG AAG GAG GAG GCC
Pro Val Lys Glu Glu Ala Lys Ser Pro Glu Lys Ala Lys Ser Pro Val Lys Glu Glu Ala

             190         200         210         220         230         240
               *           *           *           *           *           *
AAG TCC CCA GAG AAG GAG ACC CCC AAG AAG GAG GAG GTG AAA GTC AAA GAG CCC CCA AAG
Lys Ser Pro Glu Lys Glu Thr Pro Lys Lys Glu Glu Val Lys Val Lys Glu Pro Pro Lys

             250         260         270         280         290         300
               *           *           *           *           *           *
AAG GTG GAG GAG ACA GCC CCC GCC CCA CCG AAA GTG GAG AAG GAC AGC AAG AAA GAC GAG
Lys Val Glu Glu Thr Ala Pro Ala Pro Pro Lys Val Glu Lys Asp Ser Lys Lys Asp Glu

             310         320         330         340         350         360
               *           *           *           *           *           *
GCA CCC AAG AAG GAG GCC CCA AAG CCT GCT GTA GAA AAG CCC AAA GAA TCT ACA GCT GAA
Ala Pro Lys Lys Glu Ala Pro Lys Pro Ala Val Glu Lys Pro Lys Glu Ser Thr Ala Glu

             370         380         390         400         410         420
               *           *           *           *           *           *
GCC AAG AAG GAC GAG GCT GAA GAT AAG AAA AAA GCA GCT CCT GCC AAG ATG GAG GGG AAG
Ala Lys Lys Asp Glu Ala Glu Asp Lys Lys Lys Ala Ala Pro Ala Lys Met Glu Gly Lys

             430         440         450         460         470         480
               *           *           *           *           *           *
GAG GAG GCT AAA CCC AAA GAG AAG ACG GAG GTG GCC AAG AAG GAG CCG GAG ATG CCA AGG
Glu Glu Ala Lys Pro Lys Glu Lys Thr Glu Val Ala Lys Lys Glu Pro Glu Met Pro Arg

             490         500         510         520         530         540
               *           *           *           *           *           *
CCA AAG AAC CCA GCA AAC CCA CAG AGA AGG AGC CCG AGA AGC CAA AGA AGG AGG AGA CCC
Pro Lys Asn Pro Ala Asn Pro Gln Arg Arg Ser Pro Arg Ser Gln Arg Arg Arg Arg Pro

             550         560         570         580         590         600
               *           *           *           *           *           *
CCG CAG CCC CGG TGA AGA AGG AAG CCA AGG AGG AGG CCA GGA AGC CCG AGG AGA AAC CCA
Pro Gln Pro Arg ---

             610         620         630         640         650         660
               *           *           *           *           *           *
AGA CGG AGC AAG GCC AAG GAG GAT GAC AAG GCC CTC TCA AAA GAG CCC AGC AAA CCC AAG

             670         680         690         700         710         720
               *           *           *           *           *           *
ACG AGA AGG CAG AGA AAT CCT CCA GCA CGG ACC AGA AAG ATA GCA GGC TCC GGA GAA AGC

             730         740         750         760         770         780
               *           *           *           *           *           *
CAC AGA AGA CAA GGC CGC CAA GGG GGA GAA ATA GAG CGG GAA GAG GGG ACA GTC CCA GAG

             790         800         810         820         830         840
               *           *           *           *           *           *
CAG CCA AAG ACA TCG GGG GGA GGG TGG TCC TGG AAC TCA AGG GCC GGT GTA AGG AAT TTC

             850         860         870         880         890
               *           *           *           *           *
CCT TCC CTC CTC CCT TTT CTT TAT GTA AGA AGA AAC TCT GCT TAG ACG G


      Number of identified codons=  184
      Number of unidentified codons=    0
      Calculated Molecular Weight=  20573.58

      Translated in frame  1
      Translation stopped at termination codon (base no.  553)
      Sequence printed from base no.     1 to base no.  889
      Sequence numbered beginning with base no.    1
```

**Figure 5.** Translated sequence of KMRH-1.

Computer analysis of possible translated sequences was helped by the limited data available from Geisler et al.[11], indicating the presence of large numbers of glutamic acid, lysine, proline and alanine residues in the tail region of H. Translation in a single reading frame yielded a sequence of that sort. In the proper reading frame, the nucleotide sequence extends from the 5' end to the termination codon {TGA} at position 553. The remaining 334 bases in the 3' untranslated region, do not include a poly[A] tail, even though the original mRNA was selected by chromatography on oligo[dT]. This is not an unusual situation. There may be an EcoRI site in the sequence, so the poly[A] region would have been removed when the insert was originally cut out of the lambda gt11. Alternatively, the reverse transcription could have primed randomly, rather than from the oligo[dT] primer that was provided for the cDNA synthesis.

The complete translated sequence extends 184 amino acids from the C-terminal. The amino acid sequences coded for by the repeated sequences of the cDNA are indicated in Figure 5. It is immediately obvious that each of these repeated regions includes the sequence Lys.Ser.Pro. Indeed, preliminary analyses of conformational predictions, carried out in collaboration with David Bolton, suggest that these serine residues are positioned just before beta turns at each successive proline, creating a series of folds with the serines extending out from the polypeptide chain backbone, in convenient positions for phosphorylation.

The derived amino acid sequence may be aligned to highlight some of the repeated sequences (Fig. 6). The first 65 amino acids are involved in these nine repeats of KSP(V,E)K. The

```
     Translation of KMRH-1
     Translated from base     1 to base   556


  1 PEKDKSPVKEEAKSPEKA
              KSPEKA
      KSPVKEEAKSPEKA
      KSPVKEEAKSPEKA
      KSPVKEEAKSPEK

       ETPKK EEVKVKEPPK KVEETAPAPP KVEKDSKKDE APKKEAPKPA VEKPKESTAE
121 AKKDEAEDKK KAAPAKMEGK EEAKPKEKTE VAKKEPEMPR PKNPANPQRR SPRSQRRRRP
181 PQPR
```

**Figure 6.** The translated amino acid sequence of KMRH-1, aligned to emphasize the repeated KSP sequences. The first 65 amino acid residues from the amino terminal are involved in this repeating sequence.

limited amount of sequence information available for the rat C-terminal domain [19], also includes repeated Lys.Ser.Pro. sequences (Fig. 7). In one 16 residue stretch, there is a perfect match, except for position 4 in the rabbit sequence, where there is a D, as opposed to ET at the equivalent position in the rat sequence. Although the sequence KSP is indeed repeated in both proteins, at least in those portions already sequenced, the flanking amino acids are not the same. Since it is possible that we are not really comparing homologous regions of the rat and rabbit sequences at this point, we must be careful about claiming limited conservation of sequence in the C-terminal domains of neurofilaments. Nevertheless, the possibility of evolutionary divergence in the genes coding for H is of considerable interest.

| RABBIT | RAT |
|---|---|
| 1 PEKDKSPVKEEAKSPEKA | AS PEKETKSPVKEEAKSPA |
| KSPEKA | EAKSPA |
| KSPVKEEAKSPEKA | EAKSPA |
| KSPVKEEAKSPEKA | EAKSPA |
| KSPVKEEAKSPEK | EAKSPA |

**Figure 7.** Comparison of derived amino acid sequences from rabbit cDNA [KMRH-1] and rat cDNA [19] clones coding for the C-terminal tail region of H. Only the regions containing repeated KSP containing sequences are included.

When aluminum is administered intrathecally to mammals, they develop spiking activity, usually associated with seizures. In the case of rabbits, cats, and some other species, the treatment with aluminum is also followed by the accumulation of tangles of neurofilaments, in the perikaryon and proximal portions of dendrites and axons [15, 27, 28]. The filaments forming the tangles have recently been shown to contain H in a phosphorylated form which is generally restricted to the axon. In the case of rats, and other rodents, administration of aluminum brings about seizures without the neurofibrillary pathology. These preliminary sequence analyses, indicating that the C-terminal domains of rat and rabbit neurofilament protein H differ significantly in amino acid sequence, suggest the molecular basis for the differential responses of rats and rabbits to aluminum administration.

Acknowledgements: We thank Nancy and Ludwig Sternberger, Gerry Shaw, Mary Osborn and Virginia Lee, for making antibodies available to us; and Irith Ginzburg for the use of her tubulin clones. Julia Currie, Nina Casazza, Nick Robakis, Gloria Wolf, Mazhar Malik, Ash Shiekh, Ram Ramakrishnan, Yu-Wen Huang, David Miller and David Bolton have all contributed to the success of this work. The illustrations were prepared by Richard Weed and his capable staff. Supported, in part by the ALS Association and by the NY State Office of Mental Retardation and Developmental Disabilities.

REFERENCES

1. Anderton BH, Breinburg D, Downes MJ, Green PJ, Tomlinson BE, Ulrich J, Wood JN, Kahn J (1982) Nature 298:84-86
2. Autilio-Gambetti L, Gambetti P, Crane RC (1983) In:Katzman R (ed) Banbury Report 15:Biology of Alzheimer's Disease, Pp117-124
3. Aviv H, Leder P, (1972) PNAS 69:1408-1412
4. Carden MJ, Schlaepfer WW, Lee VM-Y (1985) J Biol Chem 260:9805-9817
5. Cork LC, Sternberger NH, Sternberger LA, Casanova MF, Struble RG, Price DL (1986) J Neuropath exptl Neurol 45:56-64
6. Feinberg AP, Vogelstein B (1983) Anal Biochem 132:6-13
7. Feinberg AP, Vogelstein B (1984) Anal Biochem 137:266-267
8. Fuchs E, Hanukoglu I (1983) Cell, 34:332-334
9. Geisler N, Kaufmann E,Fischer S, Plessmann U, Weber K (1983) EMBO J, 2:1295-1302
10.Geisler N, Fischer S, Vandekerckhove J, Plessmann U, Weber K (1984) EMBO J, 3:2701-2706
11.Geisler N, Fischer S, Vandekerckhove J, Van Damme J, Plessmann U, Weber K (1985) EMBO J,4:57-63
12.Geisler N, Weber K (1982) 1:1649-1656
13.Glisin VR, Crkvenjakov R, Byns C (1974) Biochemistry 13:2633-2637
14.Gubler U, Hoffman BJ (1983) Gene, 25:263-269
15.Klatzo I, Wisniewski H, Streicher E (1965) J Neuropath exp Neurol 26:427-436
16.Miller CJ, Brion J-P, Calvert R, Chin TK, Eagles PAM, Downes MJ, Flament-Durand J, Haugh M, Kahn J, Probst A, Ulrich J, Anderton BH (1986) EMBO J 5:269-276
17.Okayama H, Berg P (1983) Mol Cell Biol 2:161-170
18.Perry G, Rizzuto N, Autilio-Gambetti L, Gambetti, P (1985) PNAS, 82:3916-3920
19.Robinson PA, Wion D, Anderton BH (1986) FEBS Lett, 209:203-205
20.Sternberger LA, Harwell LW, Sternberger NH (1982) PNAS, 79:1326-1330
21.Sternberger LA, Sternberger NH (1983) PNAS, 80:6126-6130
22.Sternberger LA, Sternberger NH, Ulrich J (1985) PNAS, 2:4274-4276
23.Troncoso JC, Sternberger NH, Sternberger LA Hoffman PN, Price DL (1986) Brain Res, 364:295-300
24.Ullrich A, Shine J, Chirgwin J, Pictet R, Tischer E, Rutter WJ, Goodman HM (1977) Science 196:1313-1319
25.Willard MB, Meiri K, Glicksman M (1985) In:Edelman GM, Gall WE, Cowan WM (eds), Molecular Bases of Neural Development, Wiley, NY Pp 341-361
26.Willard M, Simon C (1983) Cell, 35:551-559
27.Wisniewski HM, Sturman JA, Shek JW (1982) Neurobiol Aging 3:11-22
28.Wisniewski HM, Shek JW, Gruca S, Sturman JA (1984) Acta Neuropath, 63:190-197
29.Young RA, Davis RW (1983) PNAS, 80:1194-1198
30.Young RA, Davis RW (1983) Science, 222:778-782

# STRUCTURE AND FUNCTION OF SOLUBLE NCAM

E. Bock, K. Edvardsen, D. Linnemann and O. Nybroe
The Protein Laboratory
University of Copenhagen
34, Sigurdsgade
DK-2200 Copenhagen N
Denmark

## INTRODUCTION

Specific nerve connections are generated by multiple steps in cell-cell interactions. These steps include cell proliferation, migration, aggregation, differentiation, synapse formation, cell death and elimination of synapses. Adhesive interactions between cell surfaces are of central importance during development of the nervous system. An understanding of the role of cell surfaces in cell recognition depends on the elucidation of the molecular mechanism involved. The neural cell adhesion molecule, NCAM, is presently the best characterized mammalian cell-cell adhesion molecule. NCAM has been shown to have a function in neuron-neuron, neuron-astrocyte and astrocyte-astrocyte adhesion (Rutishauser et al., 1976; Keilhauer et al., 1985), and in nerve-muscle cell recognition (Grumet et al., 1982).

NCAM mediated cell-cell adhesion occurs by a homophilic binding mechanism (Rutishauser et al., 1982), in which NCAM on the surface of one cell binds to NCAM on another cell. Cole et al. (1986) have shown that although NCAM mediated adhesion involves homophilic binding, the binding of cell surface heparan sulphate to NCAM is also required. The membrane associated forms of NCAM consist of three polypeptides which in SDS-polyacrylamide gels migrate with Mr's of ca.

NATO ASI Series, Vol. H22
Neural Development and Regeneration
Edited by A. Gorio et al.

190,000, 135,000 and 115,000 (hereafter referred to as polypeptides A, B, and C). The main difference between NCAM A and B is the size of their cytoplasmic domains (Gennarini et al., 1984; Nybroe et al., 1985; Murray et al., 1986). In contrast, NCAM C lacks a transmembrane domain (Nybroe et al., 1985) and is anchored in the membrane not by a stretch of hydrophobic amino acids, but by a phospholipid (He et al., 1986).

cDNA sequence data (Hemperly et al., 1986) indicate that NCAM is a member of the immunoglobulin gene superfamily. Members of this superfamily all share a common structure called the immunoglobulin homology unit. NCAM has probably at least four homology unit sequences, and it has been suggested (Hunkapiller and Hood, 1986) that the homophilic and polyvalent nature of NCAM may result from receptor-ligand binding analogous to the paired homology unit associations that generate the domain structure of other molecules of the superfamily.

Nearly all biochemical studies on NCAM have been performed on the membrane associated form. However, soluble forms of NCAM have been observed and quantified in human cerebrospinal fluid, amniotic fluid and serum (Jørgensen and Bock, 1975; Jørgensen and Nørgaard-Pedersen, 1981; Ibsen et al., 1983a). In cell culture supernatants the presence of NCAM was indicated by studies by Rutishauser et al. (1978) who produced antibodies against NCAM using chick retinal cell culture supernatants as source of antigen, and by Thiery et al. (1977) who were able to block the inhibitory effect of NCAM antibodies on cell-cell adhesion by means of soluble antigens from chick retinal cell culture supernatant. Schubert et al. (1983) showed that embryonic chick retinal cells release macromolecular aggregates, termed adherons, into their culture medium. Adherons promote cell-substratum attachment, and a polypeptide of apparent molecular weight (Mr) 170,000, immunochemically identical to NCAM, was demonstrated to be the cell-substratum adhesion molecule of the adherons (Cole and Glaser, 1986).

Even though the existence of soluble forms of NCAM in body-fluids and culture supernatants has long been recognized, little is known about the origin and structure of these components.

## NCAM IN CEREBROSPINAL FLUID AND AMNIOTIC FLUID

Due to the inaccessibility of the living human brain considerable efforts have been invested in attempts to demonstrate and quantify brain-derived proteins in cerebrospinal fluid, blood, urine and amniotic fluid. In the first study on NCAM in cerebrospinal fluid, patients suffering from a variety of neurological and psychiatric disorders (multiple sclerosis, inflammatory-degenerative neurological diseases, brain hemorrhage or thrombosis, manic-depressive psychosis and schizophrenia) were examined using an immunoprecipitation technique. However, no statistically significant changes were observed (Jørgensen and Bock, 1975). An enzyme linked immunosorbent assay (ELISA) was established using purified human brain NCAM and rabbit anti human brain NCAM antibodies (Ibsen et al., 1983b). The NCAM ELISA worked in the range 50-2000 ng/ml. Some results of the NCAM determinations obtained by this procedure are presented in Table 1.

Table 1. NCAM concentrations in cerebrospinal fluid (mean ± SEM). Data derived from Sørensen et al. (1983) and Massaro et al. (1987)

| Diagnosis | n | ng NCAM/ml |
|---|---|---|
| Controls | 24 | 641 ± 45 |
| Primary degenerative dementia | 14 | 658 ± 50 |
| Normal pressure hydrocephalus | 13 | 299 ± 48 |
| Multiple sclerosis acute phase | 20 | 589 ± 74 |
| Multiple sclerosis non-acute phase | 10 | 497 ± 95 |

The NCAM concentration in cerebrospinal fluid was found to be significantly lower in normal pressure hydrocephalus patients than in patients suffering from primary degenerative dementia ($p < 0.001$) and in controls ($p < 0.01$) (Sørensen et al., 1983). The subnormal NCAM concentration in cerebrospinal fluid in normal pressure hydrocephalus seems to be a unique finding. It is unknown whether the decreased NCAM concentration in normal pressure hydrocephalus reflects a defect in the brain of patients who might develop this disease, or is a result of the hydrocephalic state itself. However, the results indicate that measurement of NCAM in cerebrospinal fluid provides an additional diagnostic tool for discrimination between patients with normal pressure hydrocephalus and patients with hydrocephalus as part of a diffuse atrophy of the brain.

NCAM levels in cerebrospinal fluid have recently been studied in patients with multiple sclerosis (Massaro et al., 1987). All multiple sclerosis patients had two-three lumbar punctures performed at about one week intervals. No differences in NCAM concentrations in cerebrospinal fluids obtained by the first lumbar puncture could be demonstrated between acute and non-acute multiple sclerosis patients and controls. However, an increase of NCAM was shown, comparing the values of first (I) second (II), and third (III) lumbar puncture samples from the acute phase multiple sclerosis patients. Mean NCAM concentration of first (589 ng/ml), second (1.006 ng/ml) and third (1.065 ng/ml) lumbar puncture samples differed statistically significantly from each other ($p < 0.02$ comparing I and II; $p < 0.005$ comparing I and III; $p < 0.01$ comparing II and III). On the other hand no significant changes could be shown by the follow-up of the non-acute patients indicating a role for NCAM in the processes involved in acute demyelination and possibly in the following evolution of the sclerotic plaque (Massaro et al., 1987).

Jørgensen and Nørgaard-Pedersen (1981) demonstrated the correlation between raised NCAM concentration in amniotic fluid and neural tube defects. These authors found a 100% specificity of the screening procedure. Ibsen et al. (1983a) performed a more extensive study on amniotic fluids from pregnancies with neural tube defects and other malformations and found that using a cut-off level of 150 ng NCAM/ml amniotic fluid no false positive values were obtained. The sensitivity for detecting anencephaly was 100%, whereas the sensitivity for detecting spina bifida only was 75%. Ibsen et al. (1983a) also observed raised NCAM levels in amniotic fluids from fetuses with other defects, such as omphalocele, Meckel's syndrome, multiple malformations and intrauterine death. In normal pregnancies levels below 50 ng/ml were found.

## STRUCTURE AND ORIGIN OF SOLUBLE NCAM

### Immunochemical Comparisons Between Soluble and Membrane-Bound Forms of NCAM

In order to determine the immunochemical relationship between soluble and membrane-bound forms of NCAM Ibsen et al. (1983b) performed ELISA determinations of NCAM on serial dilutions of adult human brain, serum, cerebrospinal fluid and amniotic fluid. All dilutions resulted in plots that parallelled the curve obtained from the NCAM standard (derived from human fetal brain), implying immunochemical identity between the different NCAM antigens with regard to the employed antibody. Bock et al. (1987) collected conditioned medium from fetal rat brain neuronal cultures, detergent extract of rat brain membranes and supernatant from rat brain homogenates at postnatal days zero and 40. Serial dilutions of these five preparations all resulted in parallel dilution curves. Thus, the soluble forms of NCAM in brain, body fluids and medium from neuronal cultures carry the same epitopes as the membrane-bound forms. Using a specific polyclonal antibody, this means that approximately five to ten epitopes, each corresponding to ca. six to eight amino acids are identical in the various forms of NCAM.

## Amount of Soluble NCAM in Rat Brain

Soluble NCAM is a minor fraction of the proteins in brain. Bock et al. (1987) determined the amount in brains from rats at embryonic day 17, postnatal days 4, 15 and 40 (Table 2). The results are expressed relative to brain total protein or to total amount of NCAM. It appears from the table that the amount of soluble NCAM in rat brain varies from 85-194 µg/g total protein with the lowest value at embryonic day 17 and the peak value at postnatal day 15. For comparison the amount of total NCAM per g total protein was determined and soluble NCAM was expressed in percent of total NCAM. It can be seen that soluble NCAM constitutes a steadily increasing fraction during development from 0.7% at embryonic day 17 to 2.3% at postnatal day 40 (Table 2).

Table 2
Concentration of soluble NCAM in rat brain homogenate at various ages (mean ± SEM, n = 4) (Data derived from Bock et al., 1987)

| Age | µg/g total protein | % of total NCAM |
|---|---|---|
| Embryonic day 17 | 85 ± 8 | 0.7 ± 0.04 |
| Postnatal day 4 | 109 ± 3 | 0.8 ± 0.02 |
| Postnatal day 15 | 194 ± 6 | 1.5 ± 0.06 |
| Postnatal day 40 | 158 ± 4 | 2.3 ± 0.11 |

## Polypeptide Composition of Soluble NCAM in Brain

The polypeptide composition of soluble N-CAM in brain has been studied by radioiodination of supernatants obtained from homogenates of rat brains collected at postnatal days zero and 40. After labelling, NCAM was isolated by immunoprecipitation and submitted to SDS-polyacrylamide gel electrophoresis (Bock et al., 1987). The polypeptide composition of the soluble form differed from that of membrane associated NCAM. At postnatal day zero soluble NCAM is composed of a polypeptide of 170,000 Mr, whereas at postnatal day 40 soluble NCAM is composed of a polypeptide of 115,000 Mr. The 170,000 Mr soluble NCAM polypeptide had a migration distinctly different from the membrane-bound forms, whereas the 115,000 Mr soluble NCAM form in adult brain supernatant had a migration identical to the membrane associated form of the C polypeptide. Since it has been shown that the membrane associated form of NCAM of 190,000 Mr, polypeptide A, is an integral membrane protein with a cytoplasmic domain of ca. Mr 30,000 (Nybroe et al., 1985; Hemberly et al., 1986) it is unlikely that the soluble 170,000 Mr NCAM is derived from this molecule. On the other hand the soluble 115,000 Mr form presumably is identical to polypeptide C, which in vitro has been shown to be synthesized as a soluble protein (Nybroe et al., 1985).

## Polypeptide Composition of Soluble NCAM in Media from Neuronal Cultures

Since an 170,000 Mr NCAM form has been demonstrated in the so-called adheron fraction of media from chick retinal cells in culture (Cole and Glaser, 1986) Saermark et al., (1987) prepared adheron fractions from media from fetal rat brain neuronal cells in culture. They found that both the adheron fraction and the post-adheron supernatant contained a 170,000 Mr NCAM polypeptide.

## CONCLUSION

The soluble forms of NCAM demonstrated in brain and body fluids are probably actively secreted. Soluble NCAM is composed of at least two polypeptides at 170,000 and 115,000 Mr, the latter presumably representing a soluble subpopulation of the membrane-associated polypeptide C. We suggest that the functional role of extracellular NCAM in soluble form may be regulation of the adhesivity of neighbouring cells by binding to cell surface NCAM molecules, thereby changing their adhesive function. A consequence of such a binding may be a changed migratory capacity. The function of extracellular matrix-bound NCAM, so-called adheron-NCAM, on the other hand may be to act as an insolubilized chemotactic factor which guides migrating cells in specified directions. Thus, a possible target cell may secret soluble NCAM, which subsequently is bound to the extracellular matrix, and thereby create an insolubilized gradient of NCAM molecules around the secreting target cells. According to this theory NCAM's role in morphogenesis is expanded. NCAM may not only participate in cell-cell adhesion, but the secreted forms may modulate cell migration and create micratory pathways for NCAM expressing cells.

Acknowledgment

The financial support of The Danish Cancer Society (grants 84-104, 86-064, 86-078, 86-030) and The Danish Medical Research Council (grant 12-6517) is greatfully acknowledged.

REFERENCES

Bock E, Edvardsen K, Gibson A, Linnemann D, Lyles JM, Nybroe O (1987) Characterization of NCAM-related molecules secreted by neural cells. Submitted for publication

Cole GJ, Glaser L (1986) A heparin binding domain from NCAM is involved in neural cell-substratum adhesion. J Cell Biol 102:403-412

Cole GJ, Loewy A, Glaser L (1986) Neuronal cell-cell adhesion depends on interactions of NCAM with heparinlike molecules. Nature(Lond) 320:445-447

Gennarini G, Hirn M, Deagostini-Bazin H, Goridis C (1984) Studies on the transmembrane disposition of the neural cell adhesion molecule NCAM. Eur J Biochem 142:65-73

Grumet M, Rutishauser U, Edelman GM (1982) Neural cell adhesion molecule is on embryonic muscle cells and mediate adhesion to nerve cells in vitro. Nature 295:693-695

He H-T, Barbet J, Chaix J-C, Goridis C (1986) Phosphatidylinositol is involved in the membrane attachment of NCAM-120, the smallest component of the neural cell adhesion molecule.

EMBO J 5:2489-2494
Hemperly JJ, Edelman GM, Cunningham BA (1986) cDNA clones of the neural cell adhesion molecule (NCAM) lacking a membrane-spanning region consistent with evidence for membrane attachment via a phosphatidylinositol intermediate. Proc Natl Acad Sci USA 83:9822-9826
Hunkapiller T, Hood L (1986) The growing immunoglobulin gene superfamily. Nature 323:15-16
Ibsen S, Berezin V, Nørgaard-Pedersen B, Bock E (1983a) Quantification of D2 glycoprotein in amniotic fluid and serum from pregnancies with neural tube defects. J Neurochem 41:363-366
Ibsen S, Berezin V, Nørgaard-Pedersen B, Bock E (1983b) Enzyme-linked immunosorbent assay of the D2-glycoprotein. J Neurochem 41:356-362
Jørgensen OS, Bock E (1975) Synaptic membrane antigen D2 measured in human cerebrospinal fluid by rocket line immunoelectrophoresis. Determination in psychiatric and neurological patients. Scand J Immunol 1:3-16
Jørgensen OS, Nørgaard-Pedersen B (1981) The synaptic membrane D2-protein in amniotic fluid from pregnancies with fetal neural tube defects. Prenatal Diag 1:3-16
Keilhauer G, Faissner A, Schachner M (1985) Differential inhibition of neurone-neurone, neurone-astrocyte and astrocyte-astrocyte adhesion by L1, L2 and NCAM antibodies. Nature 316:728-730
Massaro A, Albrechtsen M, Bock E (1987) Determination of the neural cell adhesion molecule (NCAM) in cerebrospinal fluid from patients with multiple sclerosis. In: Rauf J, Lowenthal A (eds) Cellular and humoral components of CSF in multiple sclerosis. Plenum Press, New York, in press
Murray BA, Owens GC, Prediger EA, Crossin KL, Cunningham BA, Edelman GM (1986) Cell surface modulation of the neural cell adhesion molecule resulting from alternative mRNA splicing in a tissue-specific developmental sequence. J Cell Biol 103:1431-1439
Nybroe O, Albrechtsen M, Dahlin J, Linnemann D, Lyles JM, Møller CJ, Bock E (1985) Biosynthesis of the neural cell adhesion molecule: Characterization of polypeptide C. J Cell Biol 101: 2310-2315
Rutishauser U, Thiery JP, Brackenbury R, Sela BA, Edelman GM (1976) Mechanisms of adhesion among cells from neural tissues of the chick embryo. Proc Natl Acad Sci USA 73:577-581
Rutishauser U, Gall WE, Edelman GM (1978) Adhesion among neural cells of the chick embryo. IV. Role of the cell surface molecule CAM in the formation of neurite bundles in cultures of spinal ganglia. J Cell Biol 79:383-393
Rutishauser U, Hoffman S, Edelman GM (1982) Binding properties of a cell adhesion molecule from neural tissue. Proc Natl Acad Sci USA 79:685-689
Saermark T, Nybroe O, Gibson A, Bock E (1987) Endocytosis of the neural cell adhesion molecule (NCAM). Submitted for publication
Schubert D, LaCorbiere M, Klier FG, Birdwell C (1983) A role for adherons in neural retina cell adhesion. J Cell Biol 96:990-998

Sørensen PS, Gjerris F, Ibsen S, Bock E (1983) Low cerebrospinal fluid concentration of brain specific protein D2 in patients with normal pressure hydrocephalus. J Neurol Sci 62:59-65

Thiery J-P, Brackenbury R, Rutishauser U , Edelman GM (1977) Adhesion among neural cells of the chick embryo. II. Purification and characterization of a cell adhesion molecule from neural retina. J Biol Chem 252:6841-6845

# T H E M E III

## RESPONSES OF NERVOUS TISSUE TO TRAUMA

# Theme III - INTRODUCTION

The research field of nervous system trauma has developed greatly in recent years for several reasons ranging, from advances in basic neurosciences to increasing clinical relevance due to the increasing number of young patients every year who suffer traumatic injuries to the central nervous system (CNS).
Functional recovery after CNS damage may be accomplished by compensatory mechanisms developed by structures which survive or escape damage. The reorganization of both complex functional activity and anatomy is the basic mechanism which is utilized by CNS structures to achieve the restoration of functions. The processes of repair in the CNS of adult mammals take place in a highly defined anatomical and functional network with no possibility for repetition of developmental sequences to re-establish lost connections. However, there are a number of examples showing, that following degeneration of a given input, the vacated target area is reinnervated by sprouts originating from adjacent projections. These collateral sprouts can grow and form heterotypic synapses on the denervated neurons only for a distance of a few hundred microns. In spite of the nonspecificity of such a repair mechanism the anatomical rewiring is often accompanied by a behavioral recovery, which could be explained as resulting from the restored excitability of the formerly denervated neurons. On the other hand the true mechanisms of CNS repair are often unknown, since substitute processes, adaptative compensation and even restitution of functions due to redundant silent systems may take place at the same time. There is a strong need for a better understanding of the mechanisms underlying CNS repair. In this part of the symposium we have tackled the molecular and cellular aspects of CNS responses to trauma. The following questions were asked:

1) What is the role of extrinsic and intrinsic factors after neural injury?
2) How is nerve growth factor synthesis regulated?
3) What is the role of glial cell secreted proteins in neuronal regeneration?
4) Can neuronal regeneration occur in CNS?
5) What are the basic mechanisms and properties of CNS rewiring?
6) Can we improve neuronal survival and regeneration?
7) What are the ionic mechanisms triggered by neuronal damage?

The various authors have tried to respond to these basic questions during the symposium and the proceedings are a witness of their contribution.

# THE ROLE OF SCHWANN CELLS IN PERIPHERAL NERVOUS SYSTEM REGENERATION

H. David Shine
Department of Neuropathology
Harvard Medical School, and
Department of Neuroscience
Children's Hospital
300 Longwood Avenue
Boston, Massachusetts, 02115

## INTRODUCTION

The peripheral nervous system (PNS), unlike the central nervous system (CNS), has the ability for axonal regeneration after injury. As demonstrated by the grafting experiments of Aguayo and colleagues, PNS tissue supports regeneration of both PNS and CNS axons and provides evidence that the regenerative capacity of the PNS is a property of its environment and not its axons (Aguayo et al., 1983). Furthermore, their experiments demonstrate that failure of CNS regeneration is not intrinsic to CNS neurons but results from a non-permissive environment in CNS tissue. The difference in the cellular constituents of the two divisions of the nervous system (Schwann cells and fibroblasts in the PNS; oligodendrocytes and astrocytes in the CNS) is the basis for speculating that the regenerative capacity of the PNS, and its absence in the CNS, resides with a non-neuronal cell present in the PNS but absent in the CNS.

In order to identify the cellular constituent responsible for the regenerative capacity of the PNS and characterize the mechanism of action of this cell I have used a method to present a variety of cellular environments to injured PNS nerves under experimental conditions that would normally not result in effective regeneration and then observed the effects of these artificial environments on regeneration. The results of this experimental approach indicate that the living Schwann cell is the active agent that supports axonal regeneration in PNS tissue.

NATO ASI Series, Vol. H22
Neural Development and Regeneration
Edited by A. Gorio et al.

## MATERIALS AND METHODS

### Preparation of Cultured PNS Cells

Pure cultures of Schwann cells, fibroblasts, and sensory neurons and mixed cultures of the major cellular constituents of the PNS were derived from cultures of dorsal root ganglia (DRG) from C57BL/6J mouse embryos. The cultures were grown on a collagen substrate or in a collagen matrix in a medium consisting of human placental serum, glucose, antibiotics, and Nerve Growth Factor in minimal essential medium (Shine and Sidman, 1984; Shine et al., 1985). Cultures of DRG were prepared by enzymatic dissociation with trypsin and trituration. Schwann cells were prepared from dissociated DRGs of 18 day-old mouse embryos using a method, modified from Manthorpe et al. (1980), based on differential cell adhesion and preferential growth of Schwann cells in defined medium. The procedure yielded cultures of Schwann cells of greater than 95% purity. Sensory neurons were prepared from DRG cultures by a technique that relies on differential incorporation of 5-bromodeoxyuridine (5-BUdR) into DNA of dividing cells and amplification of photosensitivity of BUdR-substituted DNA by Hoechst dye 33258 (Stetten et al, 1976). The method removes all non-neuronal cells from DRG cultures but spares post-mitotic sensory neurons creating a pure population of sensory neurons (Shine and Sidman, 1984). Fibroblasts were cultured from DRG capsule tissue.

### Addition of cultured cells to Vitrogen 100 matrix and preparation of chambers

Cultured PNS cells were grown in a collagen matrix -- Vitrogen 100 -- before implantation. Vitrogen 100 is a commercially available solution of solubilized bovine dermal collagen prepared by pepsin digestion (Flow Labs, McLean, VA) that is liquid at $4^{o}$ C but gels at $36^{o}$ C. Cells were dispersed directly into a cold collagen/medium solution and then immobilized by warming the mixture until the solution gelled. The collagen/medium mixture was prepared by mixing 7 parts of Vitrogen 100 with 1 part of culture medium at 10 times concentration, plus 1 part 0.1 M NaOH and 22.0 mg/ml $NaHCO_3$. The collagen/cell mixture was placed in plastic cultureware and incubated at 36° C until the solution gelled. The Vitrogen 100 plus cell cultures were grown under standard conditions in the culture medium listed above. After approximately 20 days in vitro cultures were cut to size and drawn into polyethylene tubes (i.d. 0.76 mm ) with a fine wire. The tubes were cut to 7 mm lengths and one end was plugged with a glass bead to form a chamber (Figure 1).

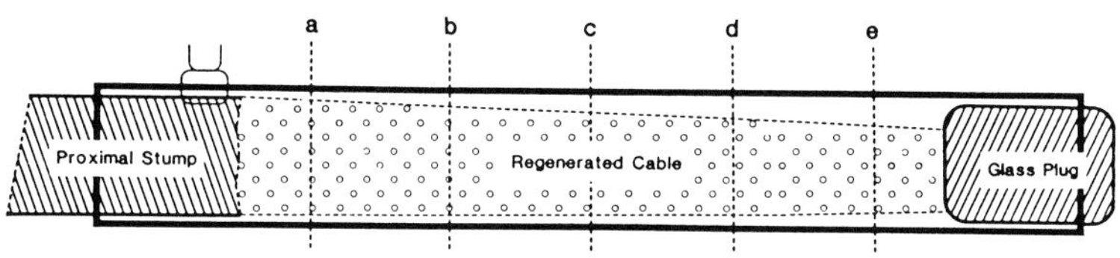


**Figure 1.** Diagram showing chamber configuration. Dashed lines, labeled a to e, mark points of sectioning and analysis.

In this manner chambers were filled with Vitrogen 100 containing microcultures of dissociated DRG cells (fibroblasts, sensory neurons, and Schwann cells; V+DRG), with pure microcultures of fibroblasts (V+F), with pure microcultures of sensory neurons (V+SN), or with pure microcultures of Schwann cells (V+SC). Additionally, chambers were filled with Vitrogen 100 that had been repeatedly saturated with fresh culture medium for 20 days (V+M) or Vitrogen 100 that had been repeatedly saturated at 36° C for 17 days with conditioned medium (V+CM) that had been removed from cultures of dissociated DRG.

**Chamber Implantation**

Adult C57BL/6J male mice were used as host animals for implantation experiments. The mice were anesthetized and sciatic nerves were exposed by a lateral incision. Under a dissecting microscope each nerve was transected at midthigh level and the proximal end of the cut nerve was inserted 1 mm into a chamber and held in place by a single epineurial stitch (Figure 1). The distal stumps were cut back at least 10 mm.

### Tissue Preparation and Analysis

In this series of experiments the implants remained in the animals for 4 weeks. After this time the host animals were systemically perfused under general anesthesia with paraformaldehyde and glutaraldehyde and the implants, with attached proximal stumps, were removed. The cable/stump units were then postfixed in $OsO_4$, dehydrated and embedded in epoxy. One micron transverse sections were cut at 1 mm points along the cable starting 0.5 mm from the cut surface of the proximal stump (Figure 1) and stained with alkaline toluidine blue for light microscopic examination. Myelinated axons were counted with the aid of an operator-interactive morphometric system interfaced with a Zeiss microscope with a computer-driven stage, video camera and digitizing tablet (Pearlstein et al., 1985). Thin sections were examined with a JEOL 100S transmission electron microscope.

## RESULTS AND DISCUSSION

The focus of this research was to answer the question, "What is the PNS cell type that establishes an environment permissive to axonal regeneration after injury?" To answer this question an experimental system -- microcultures in blind-ended chambers -- was created that permitted presentation of defined cellular and acellular environments to regenerating nerves. In effect, an experimental peripheral nerve that was undergoing regeneration was created; either in part, as when single cell types were included, or in whole, as when mixed cultures were implanted. The degree that axons grew into the chambers was taken as a measurement of the regenerative response to the defined environment since empty, blind-ended chambers will not support axon ingrowth (Williams et al., 1984). Those cellular additions that supported axonal growth into the chambers were considered influential for PNS regeneration.

Both neural and non-neural regenerative responses of severed peripheral nerves were influenced by the contents of the chambers. When chambers that contained only fluid (saline or culture medium) were implanted they remained empty except for a clear fluid after 4 weeks, but organized structures formed when the chambers contained Vitrogen 100 gel at the time of implantation. These organized structures, composed of Vitrogen 100 and tissue, had a characteristic morphology that did not differ appreciably with respect to the type of additives to the Vitrogen 100 gel. The presence of the collagen substrate appeared to be the critical factor in whether or not a cellular cable formed from proximal stump to the end of the chamber. The cable-like structures extended the length of the chamber and usually had a slight taper from the proximal end to the distal end resulting from a proximal to distal gradient of cell concentration. Each cable was well perfused by capillaries and consisted of a core of Vitrogen 100 with cells interspersed throughout surrounded by a cortex of fibroblast-like cells resembling a perineurial sheath (Figure 2).

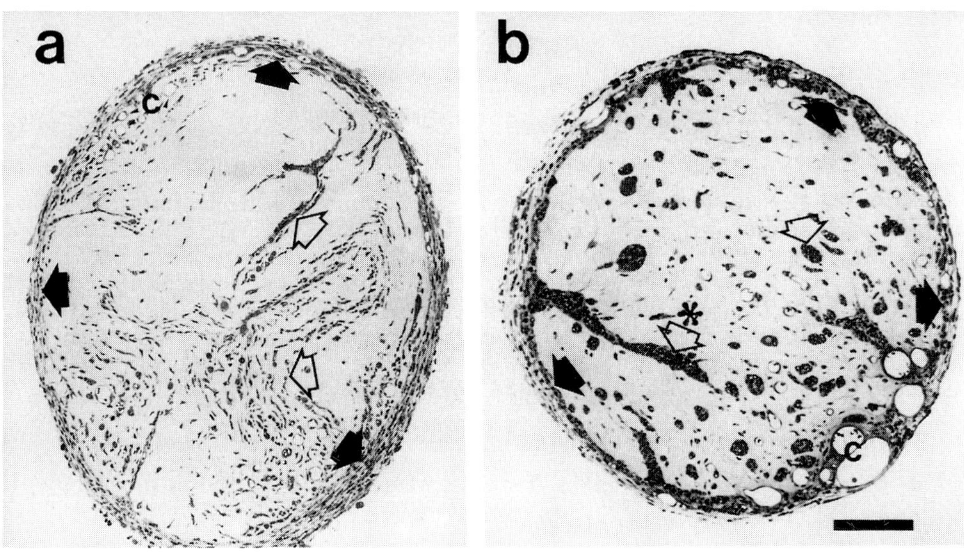


**Figure 2.** Light micrographs of cross sections of (a) a cable formed in a chamber that did not contain Schwann cells (V+M) and (b) one that contained Schwann cells at the time of implantation (V+DRG). A perineurial-like cortex (closed arrows), interspersed cells (open arrows) in the lightly staining collagen core, and capillaries (c) are visible in both sections. The sections were taken at midpoints of the chambers (section c) and stained with toluidine blue. The area indicated with an open arrow and asterisk is shown at higher power in Figure 3. (bar = 100 μm)

Cables that formed in chambers containing fibroblasts (V+F or V+DRG) had thicker perineurial-like sheaths and more cells within their collagen cores than cables not containing fibroblasts (V+M, V+CM, V+SN, V+SC). This presumably reflected a contribution of the implanted cells to the formation of the cellular structures. However, chambers that initially contained only Vitrogen 100 also formed cables indicating that cells from the proximal stumps readily migrated into chambers when an appropriate substrate was available.

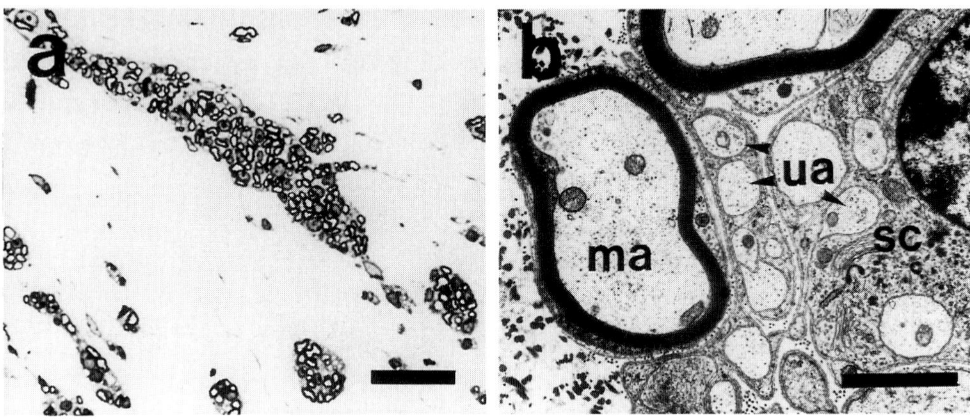


**Figure 3.** Light and electron micrographs showing greater detail of cable shown in Figure 2b (asterisk). (a) Light micrograph showing numerous large and small fascicles (arrows) that contain many myelinated axons (small darkly staining circular forms) in lighter staining Vitrogen 100. bar = 50 µm. (b) Electron micrograph showing components of a typical fascicular unit. Present are myelinated axons (ma), numerous unmyelinated axons (ua), and a Schwann cell (sc). bar = 2 µm.

While the regenerative behavior of non-neuronal cells from the proximal stumps was not appreciably influenced by the additives to the Vitrogen 100, the regenerative behavior of neuronal cells, as measured by the ingrowth of axons, was strictly governed by the chambers' cellular contents. Light and electron microscopic examination of cross sections of cables at 4 weeks revealed both myelinated and unmyelinated axons present at all 5 points when, and only when, Schwann cells were present at the time of implantation. Schwann cells had the same effect when implanted with other DRG cells (V+DRG) or as a pure population (V+SC). Axons were present in fascicular units comprised of several axons associated with Schwann cells that either formed myelin around a single axon or ensheathed several axons forming bundles of Remak (Figure 3). The fascicles were arranged in a longitudinal fashion aligned with the long length of the chamber. The ratio of myelinated to unmyelinated axons was approximately 1 to 6. Expect for fascicles of myelinated and unmyelinated axons, the cables appeared similar to cables formed in the absence of Schwann cells.

Quantification of the number of myelinated axons at 5 points along the length of the chambers (see Figure 1) verified the qualitative observation that the presence of Schwann cells was a prerequisite for growth of axons into and along the full length of the chambers (Figure 4). Every chamber, regardless of the additives, contained myelinated axons in the first two proximal-most cross sections (a & b in Figure 1). However, if Schwann cells were not included in the implant the number of myelinated axons dropped to almost zero after the 1.5 mm point (cross section b) and none were observed in the distal cross sections. When chambers contained Schwann cells, myelinated axons were present at all levels in decreasing numbers progressing proximal to distal.

Schwann cells may have influenced axonal growth into the chambers by releasing a diffusible factor or by providing an immobilized molecular cue. To determine whether Schwann cells released a long-lived soluble substance with a neurotropic or neurotrophic activity regenerating axons were presented with Vitrogen 100 saturated with conditioned medium from DRG cultures (V+CM). After 4 weeks, chambers that contained Vitrogen 100 and conditioned medium (V+CM) did not contain axons past the 1.5 mm analysis point indicating that the cultures did not release a diffusible substance into the culture medium that influenced axonal regeneration (Figure 4). Vitrogen 100 saturated with fresh culture medium (V+M), containing fibroblasts (V+F), sensory neurons (V+SN) and culture medium conditioned by these cells did not have an effect on the ingrowth of axons indicating that the effect was not a result of medium constituents such as serum or NGF. The absence of an effect of conditioned medium on axonal regeneration indicates that the Schwann cell's effect is not mediated by a long-lived soluble factor. However, these experiments do not rule out the possibility that Schwann cells effect axonal regeneration via a factor that does not remain active in the condition medium long enough to effect axonal regeneration.

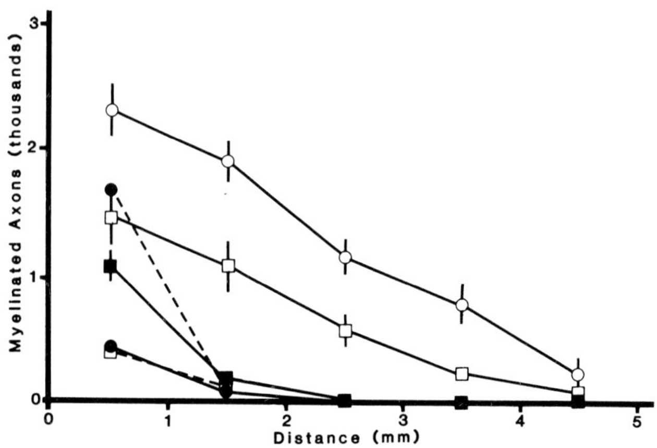


**Figure 4.** Number of myelinated axons along regenerated cables at points a through e as designated in Figure 1. Curves represent Vitrogen 100 with fresh culture medium ( □--□ ; V+M; n=2), Vitrogen 100 with conditioned medium ( ●--●; V+CM; n=3), Vitrogen 100 with Schwann cells (□—□; V+SC; n=5), Vitrogen 100 with fibroblasts ( ■—■; V+F; n=4), Vitrogen 100 with sensory neurons (●—● ; V+SN; n=4), and Vitrogen 100 with DRG cells (○—○ ; V+DRG; n=7). Error bars = SEM.

The lack of an effect of conditioned medium suggested that axonal regeneration was influenced through local interaction between a Schwann cell-associated structure and growth cones of the axons. Two candidates for such a structure are the Schwann cell basal lamina and the Schwann cell membrane. The growth of axons into and to the end of chambers containing pure populations of Schwann cells (V+SC; Figure 4) suggested that Schwann cell basal lamina is not required since basal lamina is not formed when Schwann cells are not cultured with neurons (Bunge et al., 1980). Therefore, axons initially growing into the chambers containing pure microcultures of Schwann cells would not encounter a basal lamina. To test whether Schwann cell basal lamina alone was sufficient to support axonal regeneration in blind-ended chambers, the effect of microcultures of DRG cells (V+DRG) that had been killed by repetitive freezing and thawing immediately preceding implantation were compared to the effect of living cultures. After 4 weeks, axons were not present in the distal levels of chambers that initially contained dead DRG microcultures although a typical cable formed, but axons were present at all levels of chambers that contained living cultures (Figure 5).

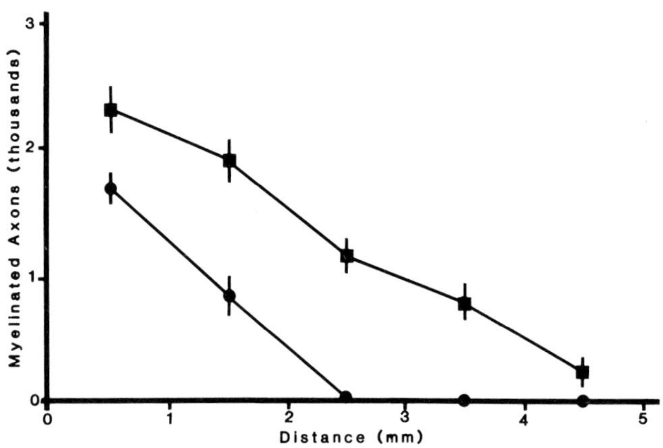


**Figure 5.** Number of myelinated axons present in chambers that contained living DRG cells ( ■—■ ; n=7) and chambers that contained dead DRG cultures ( ●—● ; n=5). Error bars = SEM.

Taken together, the positive influence of microcultures of living Schwann cells without basal lamina and the lack of an influence of microcultures of dead Schwann cells with basal lamina indicate that a structured basal lamina is not sufficient to support axonal regeneration, rather, only living Schwann cells have this influence. The unique ability of Schwann cells to influence axonal regeneration in this experimental system suggests that it is this cell that is solely responsible for the regenerative capacity of the PNS.

## ACKNOWLEDGEMENTS

The author would like to thank Paul G. Harcourt for technical assistance in tissue culture, surgery, and data acquisition, William M. Hamilton for technical assistance in electron microscopy, and William P. McIntosh for photographic assistance. The author thanks Richard L. Sidman for valuable discussions of this work. This work was supported by NIH Grants NS22223, NS20820, and HD18655 and by funds from Royal Insurance, St. Paul Insurance, and the Kemper Group.

## REFERENCES

Aguayo AJ, Benfey M, David S (1983) A potential for axon regeneration in neurons of the adult mammalian nervous system. In:Haber B, Perez-Polo JR, Hashim GA, Giuffrida Stella AM (eds) Nervous system regeneration. Alan R Liss,New York, p 327

Bunge MB, Williams AK, Wood PM, Uitto J, Jeffrey JJ (1980) Comparison of nerve cell and nerve cell plus Schwann cell cultures, with particular emphasis on basal lamina and collagen formation. J Cell Biol 84:184-202

Manthorpe M, Skaper S, Varon S (1980) Purification of mouse Schwann cells using neurite-induced proliferation in serum-free monolayer culture. Brain Res 196:467-482

Pearlstein RA, Kirschner L, Simons J, Machell S, White WF, Sidman RL (1986) A multimodal system for reconstruction and quantification of neurologic structures. Anal Quant Cytol 8:108-115.

Shine HD, Harcourt PG, Sidman RL (1985) Cultured peripheral nervous system cells support peripheral nerve regeneration through tubes in the absence of distal nerve stump. J Neurosci 14:393-401

Shine HD, Sidman RL (1984) Immunoreactive myelin basic proteins are not detected when Shiverer mutant Schwann cells and fibroblasts are co-cultured with normal neurons. J Cell Biol 98:1291-1295

Stetten G, Latt SA, Davidson RL (1976) 33258 Hoechst enhancement of the photosensitivity of bromodeoxyuridine-substituted cells. Som Cell Gen 2:285-290

Williams LR, Powell HC, Lundborg G, Varon S (1984) Competence of nerve tissue as distal insert promoting nerve regeneration in a silicone chamber. Brain Res 293:201-211

# REGENERATION OF SOMATIC NERVES IN PERMEABLE AND IMPERMEABLE TUBES

by

Richard E. Coggeshall, M.D. and Chung-Bii Jenq, Ph.D.

Marine Biomedical Institute
Departments of Anatomy & Neurosciences and
of Physiology & Biophysics
University of Texas Medical Branch
Galveston, Texas 77550-2772

Supported by the Muscular Dystrophy Association, NIH Grants 10161 and 11255 and a grant from the Florence and Marie Hall Endowment for Programs of Excellence in Education in the Medical Sciences.

NATO ASI Series, Vol. H22
Neural Development and Regeneration.
Edited by A. Gorio et al.

A goal of this symposium is to consider cellular aspects of neural regeneration. A major difficulty in such considerations is that the problem is so complex. The specific interactions of cells, extracellular matrices and soluble substances and the relative importance of each are not well understood, for example. This complexity is a major reason for using simplified regenerating systems such as dorsal root or sympathetic ganglion cells in culture where testing the effects of individual substances or cellular products on the rate of neurite extension can be done. Such studies are extremely important and have yielded many valuable insights, but if these insights are to be brought into the clinical realm, regeneration must also be studied _in vivo_. Simplification is even more necessary here, however. Our particular goal has been to study regeneration of transected rodent somatic nerves, and our method of simplification has been to place the stumps of the transected rat sciatic nerves in impermeable tubes (Jenq & Coggeshall, 1984; 1985a; 1985b; 1987). This method was first used as a method to guide and protect regenerating axons. The technique is not often used clinically, however, for reasons involving difficulties with vasculature, and permanence of the implant, but it provides an excellent experimental paradigm (Longo et al., 1983; Longo, Skaper et al., 1983; Longo et al., 1984; Lundborg et al., 1982; Lundborg, Dahlin et al., 1982; Politis et al., 1983; Scaravelli, 1985; Weiss & Taylor, 1944; Williams et al., 1983; 1985). From our particular point of view the usefulness of this paradigm is that it separates the area of regeneration from the rest of the organism and allows us to ask whether cells or soluble substances are more important in the regenerative phenomona we measure and also whether "factors" from the body in general have different effects than factors derived from the nerve stumps for these same phenomona.

## Materials and Methods

The experiments are done on adult (200-250 grams) rats of either sex. The basic procedure is to anesthetize the rats with nembutal, and when anesthesia is deep, to remove 8 mm or 16mm of sciatic nerve in the thigh.

The 2 resulting stumps are then placed in a silicone tube of appropriate diameter. The tubes are 1) unmodified (regular tube), 2) made completely permeable by cutting large holes in the side of the tube, (holey tubes), 3) made partially permeable by placing nucleopore filters with pore diameters of 5.0 μm over the large holes (5.0 μm tubes), and 4) made partially permeable by placing nucleopore filters with pore diameters of 1.2 μm over the large holes (1.2 μm filter tubes). The reason for the 2 pore sizes is that the 1.2 μm filters will allow only fluids to pass whereas the 5.0 μm filters will allow both fluids and cells to pass.

A sketch of these procedures is provided in Figure 1.

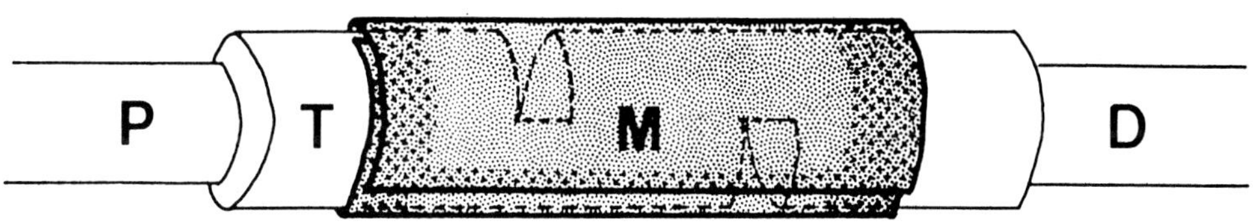


After 8 weeks of regeneration, the animals are perfused, the sciatic, sural and medial gastrocnemius nerves taken and embedded for light and electron microscopy. Further details of these methods are published in the reports cited from our laboratory (Jenq & Coggeshall, 1984; 1985a; 1985b; 1987). The data we will consider in this paper are the numbers of axons that have regenerated in the above nerves and the length of the gap the axons will span in the various tube paradigms.

## Results

### Length of the gap regenerating axons will span

Several investigators have reported that the maximum length between rodent sciatic nerve stumps that regenerating axons can cross when the stumps are placed in a tube is approximately 10 mm (Lundborg et al., 1982; Madison et al., 1985). Our work is confirmatory. By contrast, when the nerve stumps are placed in a permeable (holey) tube, they easily cross a gap of 16 mm. Thus making an impermeable tube completely permeable allows regenerating axons to cross a longer gap than if they regenerated in an impermeable tube.

### Numbers of regenerated axons

Criteria for recognizing myelinated and unmyelinated axons have been given (e.g. Jenq & Coggeshall, 1984). Numbers of regenerated axons in the gap between the stumps of the transected nerve, in the distal stump of the transected nerve, and in 2 tributary nerves, the sural nerve and the nerve to the medial gastrocnemious muscle in the various tube paradigms described above are shown in Table I. The numbers have been rounded off to the nearest 10 for the small nerve and to the nearest 50 for the larger nerves. The original data are given in the following papers (Jenq & Coggeshall, 1984; 1985a; 1985b; 1987). Note that the numbers of regenerated axons tend to be similar in the regular and 1.2 μm tubes, and also to be similar in the holey and 5.0 μm tubes. Also note in general that fewer axons have regenerated in the former group and that the numbers are closer to normal in the latter group.

A point important to the discussion is that the 1.2 μm tubes allow fluids but not cells to pass whereas the 5.0 μm tubes allow both cells and fluids to pass. The evidence for the 1.2 μm tubes is that fluids pass easily, as shown by injecting saline through the filter but cells do not pass as shown by histological examination (Fig. 2).

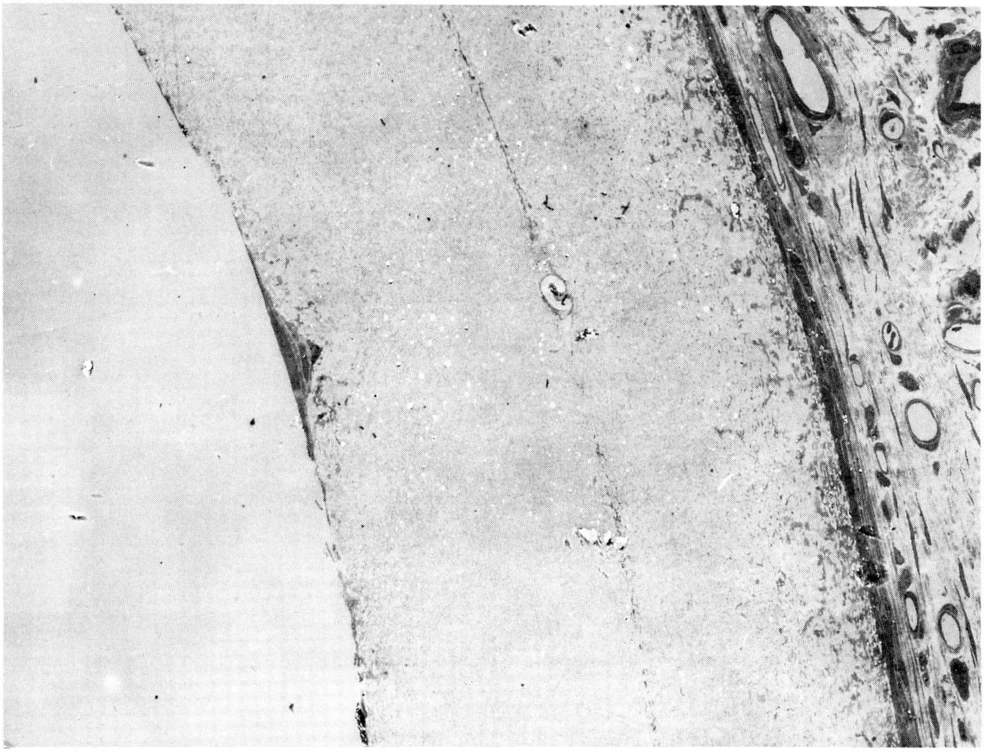

By contrast histological examination shows that cells as well as fluids pass through the 5.0 μm filter tubes.

Discussion

The first point is that regenerating axons span a longer gap and axonal numbers are closer to normal if regeneration occurs in a completely permeable (holey) as compared to a regular impermeable tube (Jenq & Coggeshall, 1987). Since 2 of the goals of therapy are to have axons cross maximal gaps and to have axon numbers return to normal (e.g. Sunderland, 1976), we feel justified in regarding these changes as improvements although functional correlates must be obtained to be certain. These findings are interesting because the focus of much work on nerve regeneration is on tropic substances or cells from the nerve stumps

(Denney-Brown, 1944; Ramon y Cajal, 1959; Sunderland, 1976; Thomas, 1966). Accordingly we would have predicted that regeneration would be better when substances and cells from the stumps are pooled around the regenerating axons, which is the situation with the impermeable tubes. The finding that permeable tubes led to better results for our parameters was essentially the starting point of this study. An obvious question is whether the changes we observed when a permeable tube was used are because cells from the body in general gain access to the regenerating axons or whether soluble substances (growth factors) are largely responsible. Because the improvements we observed, at least in terms of axonal numbers, were seen with the 5.0 μm tubes but not with the 1.2 μm tubes, we hypothesize that the improvements are correlated primarily with the access from cells of the general connective tissue to the regrowing axons. The reason for this conclusion is that soluble substances or nutrients could exchange with either the 1.2 or 5 μm tubes but cells could exchange only with only the 5.0 μm tubes. We have preliminary evidence that corroborates this conclusion in that proximal stumps placed in impermeable blind tubes or in blind tubes with a 1.2 μm filter over the distal end regenerate poorly or not at all whereas if the tube has a 5.0 μm filter over its distal end, the regeneration is robust.

The conclusion from the above is that cells from the general connective tissue improve those parameters of regeneration we measure when they are allowed access to regenerating axons. This conclusion needs to be corroborated by further research, and at present it is perhaps best simply to offer a few speculations as to directions for future research along this line. Perhaps the first question would concern the nature of the cells that improve regeneration in our paradigm. Since the cells concerned seem to come from the general connective tissue spaces of the body, it seems unlikely that they are Schwann cells. Thus the 2 obvious candidates are fibroblasts or reticuloendothelial cells. We favor the notion that they are fibroblasts because of the known role of these cells in fashioning extracellular matrices (e.g. Denny-Brown, 1944; Thomas, 1966). One way to get evidence would be to grow the appropriate cells in tissue culture and then place them in the tube at the time of transection to see which mimic the effects of using the permeable tube. This work is underway. Another obvious question is whether the improvements we see in morphology are accompanied by demonstrable improvements in function.

We would like to emphasize that our results do not imply that fibroblasts are the major factors in peripheral nerve regeneration, nor that cells or soluble substances from the nerve stumps are unimportant in regeneration nor that regeneration is optimal if permeable tubes are used. What we do suggest is that allowing cells from the general connective tissue access to the regenerating axons results in certain improvements that would not occur if they were denied such access. We would further like to suggest that, when these cells are identified, they be given consideration when devising procedures to maximize nerve regeneration.

As a summation, it has been shown previously that when the stumps of transected rodent sciatic nerves are placed in tubes to aid regeneration, the maximum length of the gap the axons can span is limited. Furthermore the numbers of axons that regenerate in the area of the gap, the distal stump and in certain tributary nerves at particular times is known. We have found that when the impermeable tubes are made completely permeable by cutting holes in their sides, the regenerating axons can span a much longer gap and axonal numbers are closer to normal at the times we measured them. The present article describes beginning experiments designed to get insights into the reasons for this improvement. The data indicate that the improvements occur when cells from the general connective tissue gain access to the regenerating axons. The next tasks are to identify the cells and to begin exploring the cellular and molecular mechanisms for these effects on axon regeneration *in vivo*.

## References


Denney-Brown DD (1944) Importance of neural fibroblasts in the regeneration of nerve. Arch Neurol Psych (Chicago) 55:171-215

Jenq CB, Coggeshall RE (1984) Regeneration of axons in tributary nerves. Brain Res 310:107-121

Jenq CB, Coggeshall RE (1985) Nerve regeneration through holey silicone tubes. Brain Res 361:233-241

Jenq CB, Coggeshall RE (1985) Numbers of regenerating axons in parent and tributary peripheral nerves in the rat. Brain Res 326:27-40

Jenq CB, Coggeshall RE (1987) Permeable tubes increase the length of the gap that regenerating axons can span. Brain Res 408:239-242

Longo FM, Manthorpe M, Skaper SD, Lundborg G, Varon S (1983) Neuronotrophic activities accumulate *in vivo* within silicone nerve regeneration chambers. Brain Res 261:109-117

Longo FM, Skaper SD, Manthorpe M, Williams LR, Lundborg G, Varon S (1983) Temporal changes in Neuronotropic activities accumulating *in vivo* within nerve regeneration chambers. Exp Neurol 81:756-769

Longo FM, Hayman EG, Davis GE, Ruoslahti E, Engvall E, Manthorpe M, Varon S

(1984) Neurite-promoting factors and extracellular matrix components accumulating *in vivo* within nerve regeneration chambers. Brain Res 309:105-117

Lundborg G, Dahlin LB, Danielsen N, Gelberman RH, Longo FM, Powell HC, Varon S (1982) Nerve regeneration in silicone chambers: influence of gap length and of distal stump components. Exp Neurol 76:361-375

Lundborg G, Gelberman RH, Longo FM, Powell HC, Varon S (1982) In vivo regeneration of cut nerve encased in silicone tubes, J Neuropathol Exp Neurol 41:412-422

Madison R, DaSilva CR, Dikkes P, Chiu TH, Sidman RL (1985) Increased rate of peripheral nerve regeneration using bioresorbable nerve guides and a laminin-containing gel. Exp Neurol 88:767-772

Politis MJ, Ederle K, Spencer PS (1983) Tropism in nerve regeneration in vivo. Attraction of regenerating axons by diffusible factors derived from cells in distal nerve stumps of transected peripheral nerves. Brain Res 253:1-12

Ramon y Cajal S (1959) Degeneration and Regeneration of the Nervous System, Hafner Publishing, New York, 769pp

Scaravelli F (1985) The influence of the distal environment on peripheral nerve regeneration across a gap. J Neurocyt 13:1027-1041

Sunderland SS (1978) Nerves and Nerve Injuries, 2nd edn. Churchill Livingston, Edinburgh, 1046pp

Thomas PK (1966) The cellular response to nerve injuries. The cellular outgrowth from the distal stump of the transected nerve. J Anat 100:287-303

Weiss P, Taylor AC (1944) Further experimental evidence against "neurotropism" in nerve regeneration. J Exp Zool 95:233-257

Williams LR, Longo FM, Powell HC, Lundborg G, Varon S (1983) Spatial temporal progress of peripheral nerve regeneration within a silicone chamber: parameters for a bioassay. J Comp Neurol 218:460-470

Williams LR, Varon S (1985) Modification of fibrin matrix formation *in situ* enhances nerve regeneration in silicone chambers. J Comp Neurol 231:209-220

## Table Legends

Table I. This table presents the numbers of myelinated (MY) and unmyelinated (UN) axons that regenerate in the gap between the nerve stumps, in the distal stump of the transected nerve, in the sural nerve and in the nerve to the medial gastrocnemius muscle (NMG) 8 weeks after the transection procedures described in the text.

## Figure Legends

Fig. 1. A sketch of surgical paradigm used in this study. The nucleopore filter (M) covers that part of the silicone tube (T) where large holes have been opened. The proximal (P) and distal (D) stumps of the transected nerve are also shown.

Fig. 2. A low power microscopic section of the 1.2 μm nucleopore filter covering a hole in a silicone tube. The lumen is to the left and the general connective tissue of the body to the right. Note that no cells penetrate the filter.

Summary

Previous work established certain parameters of regeneration when transected rodent sciatic nerves were placed in impermeable tubes. The work of the present report began with the observation that when the tube was made permeable these parameters improved. The present report is a review of experiments designed to get insight into the mechanisms of the improvement. The evidence obtained to date is consistent with the hypothesis that the improvement arises because cells from the general connective tissue of the body gain access to the regenerating axons. Further experiments to confirm this conclusion, to determine the nature of the cells and to begin to understand the mechanisms by which these changes come about are underway.

# ROLE OF FACTORS INTRINSIC AND EXTRINSIC TO CNS REGULATING INTRASPINAL DEGENERATIVE-ATROPHY FOLLOWING SCIATIC NERVE INJURY

ANNA MARIA DI GIULIO, ANTONELLA MANNAVOLA, BEATRICE TENCONI, PAOLO MANTEGAZZA and *ALFREDO GORIO

Department of Medical Pharmacology, University of Milano, Via Vanvitelli 32, Milano 20129, and *School of Pharmacology, Institute of Pharmacological Sciences, Via Balzaretti 9, Milano 20129, Italy.

## INTRODUCTION

Morphological, immunocytochemical, biochemical and electrophysiological correlates have indicated that the laminae I and II of the spinal cord dorsal horn constitute a complex system playing an important role in endogenous pain control mechanisms (1). The area contains a variety of neuroactive peptides which, as shown by immunocytochemical studies are distintly located in the axon terminals of the peripheral sensory imputs, in a wide population of local interneurons and in the central descending pathways (1,2,3,4,5). Such a complex anatomical organization displays a remarkable capacity of rearrangements. Peripheral nerve lesions cause profound changes in the sensory maps of the dorsal horn (6), suggesting alterations of both sensory imputs and local interneurons. It was, indeed, shown that section of the sciatic nerve induces a significant drop of substance P sensory imput and of met-enkephalin contained in

NATO ASI Series, Vol. H22
Neural Development and Regeneration
Edited by A. Gorio et al.

dorsal horn interneurons (5,7).

The early findings on the central substance P depletion caused by the lesion of the peripheral portion of the sensory axons have stimulated a very broad interest in the biochemical and morphological plasticity of the dorsal horn. Our interest on investigating enkephalin and subtance P stems from two obvious reasons: a) enkephalin is present in interneurons of the Substantia Gelatinosa (8) and , when injected in the dorsal horn laminae I and II, displays a powerful antinociceptive activity (9); b) peripheral nerve lesions are often associated with pain sensations . A most dramatic example is the phantom limb pain. The causes of such sensations are commonly related to the presence of unmyelinated sprouting axons in damaged or pathologically and functionally altered nerves or to an abnormal firing rate (10,11). We have tested, therefore, the above hypotheses and the mechanisms intrinsic and extrinsic to CNS in experimental conditions of chronic nerve lesions associated with neuroma formation (5, 12).

## SUBSTANCE P AND MET-ENKEPHALIN ALTERATIONS IN THE DORSAL HORN OF THE LUMBAR SPINAL CORD

The specimens were analysed with immunocytochemistry and radioimmunoassay (RIA) techniques and with a specific histological stain for the fluoride resistant acid phosphatase (FRAP). Figure 1 shows a series of sections from various experimental animals stained with the FRAP technique, which darkly outlines some sensory imput to lamina II of the dorsal horn (13). As already reported (13) it is clear that also this sensory

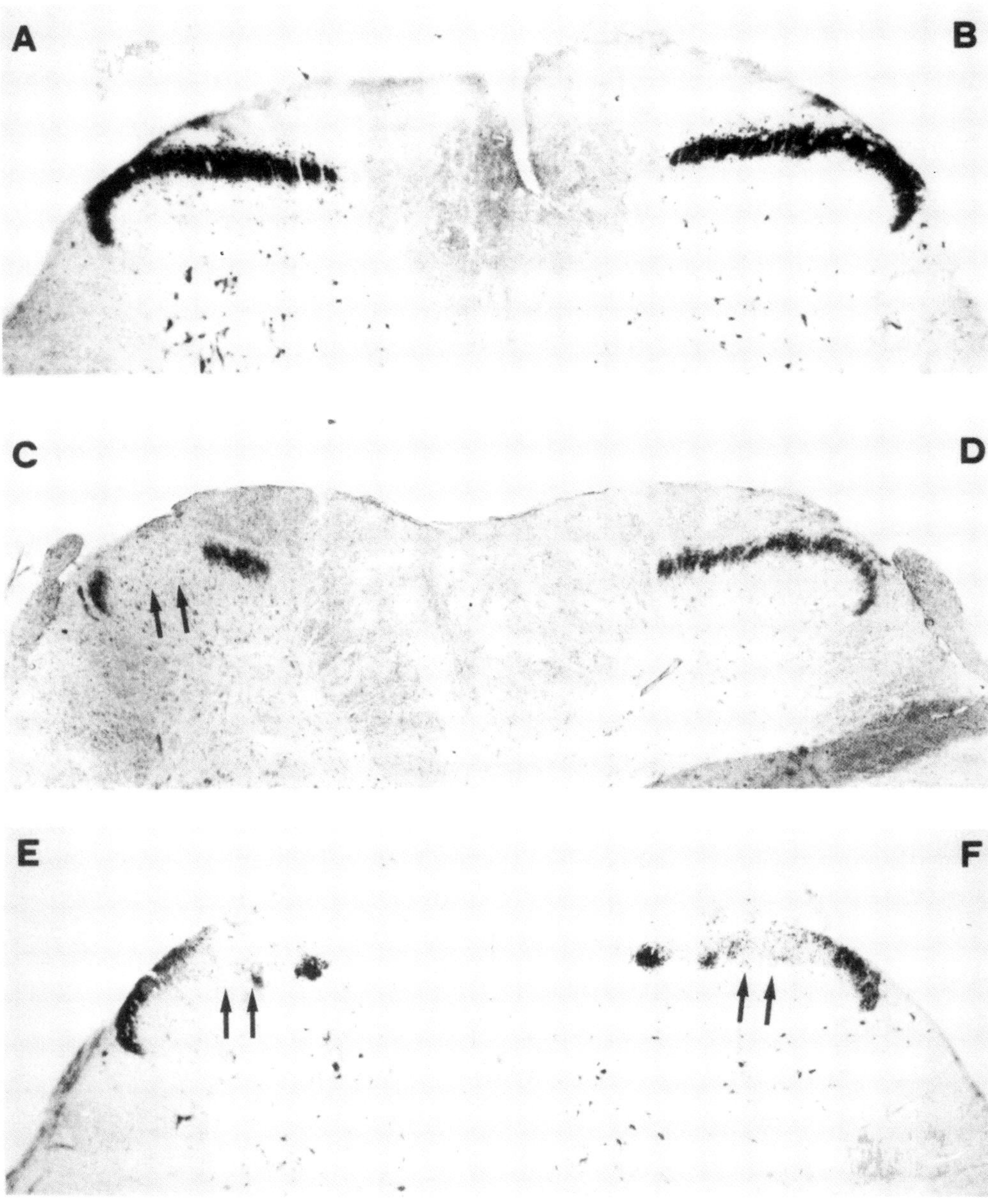


Fig.1 Fluoride resistant acid phosphatase (FRAP) stain is present in lamina II of the dorsal horn (A), and disappears (arrows) ipsilaterally to the lesioned nerve (B, left panel). The contralateral side is unaffected (B, right panel). Section of both sciatic nerves causes a bilateral loss (arrows) of FRAP stain (C) which is, in each horn, as intense as after monolateral lesion. Reprinted from ref. 12 with permission of authors and editors.

imput undergoes degenerative atrophy following peripheral nerve section. Ipsilaterally to the lesion site there is a marked loss of staining. Immunocytochemical staining with specific antibodies has revealed that a similar localized loss of staining also occurs for substance P and met-enkephalin ipsilaterally to the lesioned nerve (5,12). RIA for both peptides shows a significant decrease in peptide levels. Thirty days after sciatic nerve resection, the lumbar spinal cord shows a drop of substance P (from 10.3 to 4.9 ng/mg of protein) and met-enkephalin (from 3.8 to 2.0 ng/mg of protein). If the lumbar spinal cord is subdivided in dorsal and ventral portions, it is evident that the decrease occurrs only dorsally and ipsilaterally to the lesion (7,14), while the ventral horn concentration of both peptides is unaffected (7,14).Such a localized loss is confirmed by quantitative immunocytochemistry for met-enkephalin containig boutons. By applying a computer-assisted integrative image analysis, described in reference 14, it is evident that the density per unit area of met-enkephalin containing boutons present in laminae I and II decreases significantly ipsilaterally to the lesion (14). The extent of loss of stained boutons is equivalent to the peptide decrease as detected by RIA.

Figure 1 also shows that if the sciatic nerve resection is performed bilaterally, the loss of FRAP staining is also bilateral. Both dorsal horn bear the normal extent of decreased staining. On the other hand RIA for substance P and met-enkephalin indicated that following bilateral lesioning the peptidergic decrease in the lumbar spinal cord was similar to that detected after monolateral nerve lesions, with loss (12).

These results all toghether show that peripheral deafferentation of dorsal root ganglion sensory neurones causes degenerative atrophy of the central branches beginning 7-10 days after sciatic nerve resection. Such a loss of imput is correlated with a simultaneous degenerative atrophy of met-enkephalin containing interneurones, displayed as a decreased nerve terminal density per unit area, in laminae I and II of the dorsal horn. Such anatomical alterations of the local interneuronal opiate system may be responsible of the pain sensations which are often associated to peripheral nerve injuries. In addition, the results obtained after bilateral sciatic nerve resection have shown that the nerve injury is the trigger mechanism for the observed intraspinal changes, but the extent of peptide loss may be intraspinally regulated.

## SEROTONINERGIC ROLE IN INTRASPINAL ALTERATIONS CAUSED BY PERIPHERAL NERVE LESIONS

One of the intraspinal candidates for regulating the peptide loss, triggered by sciatic nerve lesions, was the complex descending serotoninergic pathway, which is presumably involved in the endogenous pain control system (1). We monitored the lumbar cord levels of 5-HT and its main metabolite 5-HIAA at various times after sciatic nerve resection. It was found that although 5-HT levels do not change at 1, 2, 4, and 10 days following nerve injury, 5-HIAA levels are significantly increased within 24 hours and decline to control levels only at day 10 (14). It is remarkable that the restoration of normal 5-HIAA levels is timely correlated with the intraspinal peptidergic loss. In order to investigate 5-HT role we depleted the amine store by treating the animals with para-chlorophenilalanine (p-CPA) prior to sciatic nerve lesion (14). As shown in figure 2, p-CPA-induced serotonin depletion does not interfere with substance P loss but, successfully, prevents the trans-synaptic met-enkephalinergic interneuron atrophy. It is conceivable that the descending serotoninergic pathways are involved in regulating both the profound

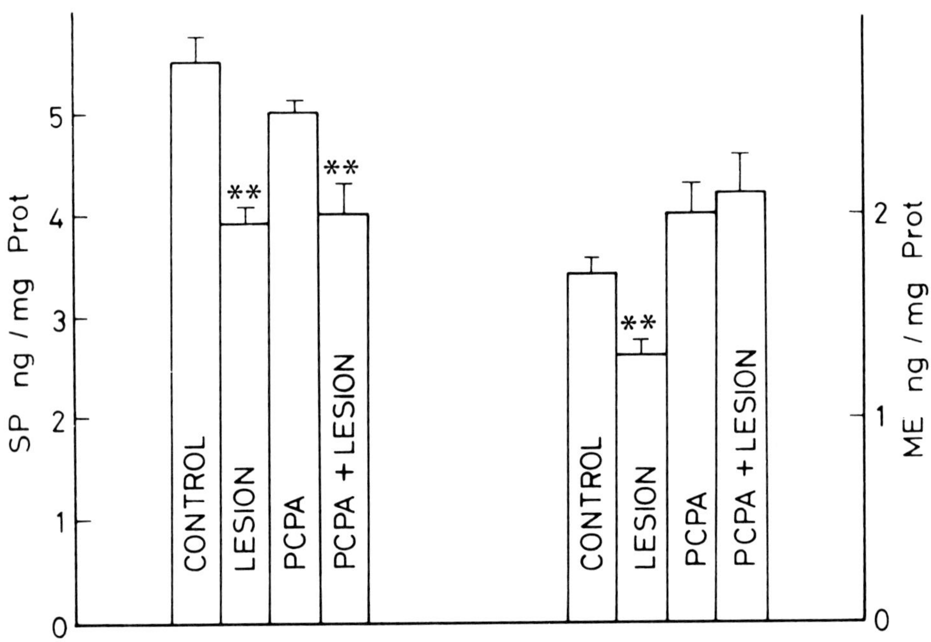


Fig.2 Effect of p-chlorophenylalanine (PCPA) treatment on rat lumbar spinal cord substance P (SP) and met-enkephalin (ME) loss induced by sciatic nerve lesion. Each bar represents the mean+SEM of 8-10 independent determinations. **$p<0.01$ vs control ( Student t-test). Reprinted from reference 14 with permission of authors and editors.

rearrangements occurring in the dorsal horn following peripheral sensory deafferentation and the often associated pain sensations, such as the case of phantom limb pain. The cellular mechanisms involved in these processes could be related to serotonin modulated neuronal plasticity.

REFERENCES


1. Basbaum A.I., and Fields H.l. (1984). Endogenous pain control Systems: Brainstem spinal pathways and endorphins circuitry. Annual Rev. Neurosc. 7:309-338
2. Gibson S.J., Polak J.M., Bloom S.R., and Wall P.D. (1981). The distribution of nine peptides in the rat spinal cord with special emphasis on the substantia gelatinosa and on the area around the central canal (lamina X). J. Comp. Neurol. 201:65-79
3. Seybold V., and Elde R. (1980). Immunohistochemical studies of peptidergic neurons in the dorsal horn of the spinal cord. J. Histochem. Cytochem. 28:367-370
4. Sasek C.A., Seybold V.S., and Elde R. (1984). The immunohistochemical localization of nine peptides in the sacral parasympathetic nucleus and the dorsal gray commissure in rat spinal cord. Neuroscience 12:855-873
5. Di Giulio A.M., Mantegazza P., Dona' M., and Gorio A. (1985). Peripheral nerve lesions cause simultaneous alterations of substance P and enkephalin in the spinal cord. Brain Res. 342:405-408
6. Devor M., and Wall P.D. (1978). Reorganization of of spinal cord sensory maps after peripheral nerve injury . Nature (London) 276:75-76
7. Jessel T., Tsunoo A., Kanazawa I., Otsuka M (1979). Substance P: depletion in the dorsal horn of the spinal cord after section of peripheral processes of primary sensory neurons. Brain Res. 168:247-259
8. Hunt S.P., Kelly J.S., and Emson P.C. (1980). The electron microscopic localization of methionine-enkephalin within the superficial layers (I and II) of the spinal cord. Neuroscience 5:1871-1890
9. Duggan A.W., Hall J. G., Headley P.M. (1977). Enkephalins and dorsal horn neurons of the cat: effect on responses to noxious and innocuous skin stimuli. Brit. J. Pharmacol. 61:399-408
10. Brown M.J., Martin J.R., and Asbury A.K. (1976). Painful diabetic neuropathy. A morphometric study. Arch. Neurol. 33:164-171
11. Culp W.J. (1984). Abnormal impulse generation. In Serratrice G. et al. (eds), Neuromuscular Diseases, Raven Press, New York, 303-308
12. A.M. Di Giulio, Borella F., Mantegazza P., Hong J.-S., Panozzo C., Zanoni R., and Gorio A. (1985). Structural and biochemical alterations in the dorsal horn of the spinal cord caused by peripheral nerve lesions. Peptides 6: 249-256

13.Devor M., and Claman D. (1980). Mapping and plasticity of acid phosphatase afferents in the rat dorsal horn. Brain Res. 190:17-28

14.Di Giulio A.M., Tenconi B., Mannavola A., Mantegazza P., Schiavinato A., and Gorio A. (1987). Spinal cord interneuron degenerative atrophy caused by peripheral nerve lesions is prevented by serotonin depletion. J. Neurosc. Res. 18:3, in press

# INTRASPINAL SPROUTING OF PRIMARY AFFERENTS AFTER SPINAL DENERVATION AND TREATMENT WITH ANTIBODIES TO NERVE GROWTH FACTOR

C. E. Hulsebosch
Marine Biomedical Institute and Department of Anatomy & Neurosciences
University of Texas Medical Branch
Galveston, Texas 77550-2772

Spinal cord injury is accompanied by a loss of sensation and motor control below the level of the lesion. If such distressing injuries are to be controlled and an effective therapy instituted it is essential to understand the result of injury on sensory and motor systems. One possible response of the nervous system to injury which may be enhanced is sprouting.

Several types of sprouting have been described in both central and peripheral nervous systems. One example of sprouting is the neurite outgrowth from injured neurons following transection of their dendrites or axons. The response to this pruning stimulis may be growth and is termed pruning, wherein the injured neuron gives rise to numerous sprouts (Stelzner et al., 1972). A fiber population lesion, on the other hand, may create another kind of sprouting. This results in adjacent unlesioned fibers sprouting presumably to fill vacated postsynaptic sites. This sprouting phenomenon is termed collateral sprouting. Both of these sprouting phenomenon may also be termed branching, since in the pruning paradigm, the injured neuron emits more branches and in the collateral sprouting paradigm, the adjacent uninjured neural populations emit more branches. Both pruning and collateral sprouting may take place over several microns, that is at considerable distance from the denervated site and may or may not result in the formation of synapses. Another category of sprouting which occurs close to the denervated site, is called terminal sprouting. In this paradigm, either injured or adjacent uninjured neural processes emit a very fine neurite which forms a new synapse within a few microns.

The hypothesis that I propose to account for the sprouting phenomenon is that the delicate balance of neurotrophic factors, which by definition is necessary to maintain appropriate neural connections, is disrupted. Neurotrophic factors are substances produced by target tissues or supporting cells which are taken up by a nerve process and retrogradely

NATO ASI Series, Vol. H22
Neural Development and Regeneration
Edited by A. Gorio et al.

transported back to the nerve soma (Hendry et al., 1982; Perez-Polo, 1985). Subsequent interaction of this substance, either through a second messenger system or by direct regulation of the genome, informs the nerve cell that the neural connections are appropriate and are to be maintained. If the transport of the neurotrophic factor is blocked, the nerve cell perceives that it is denervated and either dies or sprouts, depending on the requirements of that cell for the deprived factor. For example, nerve cells whose processes are severed are deprived of information produced by their target and may respond to this denervation by sprouting (Hulsebosch and Coggeshall, 1981; Liu and Chambers, 1958). However, the neurotrophic interactions are not just all or none but in some systems may be graded. If a neural population is lesioned, adjacent neural terminals from uninjured neural populations suddenly find excess neurotrophic substances (Korsching and Thoenen, 1985) which may elicit sprouting into the denervated territory. One of the best characterized neurotrophic factors is Nerve Growth Factor (NGF). More will be discussed on the involvement of NGF and sprouting later in this chapter.

In this chapter, I will describe the results of experiments on central projections of primary sensory neurons into the spinal cord. I present evidence that supports the interpretation of intraspinal sprouting of primary afferent fibers after spinal cord denervation in the first section. In the second section, I show evidence which supports the interpretation of intraspinal sprouting of primary afferent fibers in a Nerve Growth Factor deprived environment. In both sections the notion of the involvement of neurotrophic factors, and NGF in particular, will be discussed.

## Intraspinal Sprouting After Surgical Denervation

The sprouting of uninjured neurons or collateral sprouting in the mammalian spinal cord after surgical denervation was first described in 1958 by Liu and Chambers using modified Golgi techniques. They reported significant sprouting of sensory axons in the spinal cord of adult cats after neighboring dorsal roots were sectioned (Liu and Chambers, 1958). Subsequent studies either confirmed (Beattie et al., 1981; Cotman, 1978; Goldberger and Murray, 1974; Hulsebosch and Coggeshall, 1981; Murray and Goldberger, 1986; Stelzner et al., 1972; Tessler et al., 1980; Tessler et al., 1984) or denied (Kerr, 1972; Kerr, 1975; Rodin and Kruger, 1984; Rodin et al., 1982; Stelzner and Weber, 1979) these early interpretations by using various techniques including horseradish peroxidase (HRP) and peptide markers. The use of HRP is problematical since small diameter fibers are difficult to fill completely and this technique fills a great number of medium and large diameter fibers (Sarter, 1986; Zenker et al., 1980). The peptide markers for primary afferents are also problematical since many of these peptides, for example substance P and somatostatin, are also localized in intrinsic neurons of the spinal cord and in descending pathways (Hunt, 1983; Stine et al., 1982; Tessler et al., 1980; Tessler et al., 1984). For these reasons, a significant increase in the number of myelinated or unmyelinated fibers or a significant amount of terminal sprouting might be masked.

In this laboratory we repeated the spared root paradigm of Liu and Chambers and used ultrastructural techniques to count the number of primary afferent axons in dorsal roots on the denervated side of the spinal cord and compared these counts to counts of roots on the contralateral side of the cord. We demonstrated 17 to 20% more unmyelinated axons (or C-fibers) in the roots on the denervated side compared to the contralateral side. We interpreted this increase in axon numbers to be collateral sprouting or branching of primary afferent neurons elicited by spinal deafferentation (Hulsebosch and Coggeshall, 1981; 1983). While this technique allows quantitation of sprouting in the dorsal root, several millimeters from the denervated site in the spinal cord, our data do not address the extent of primary afferent terminal sprouting or synaptogenesis within the spinal cord. Therefore, we chose to test intraspinal sprouting of primary afferents using the fluoride resistant acid phosphatase reaction (FRAP) which is specific to small diameter primary afferents and their terminals (Coimbra et al., 1974; Dodd et al., 1984; Hunt, 1983; Knyihar, 1971; Knyihar et al., 1974; Knyihar-Csillik and Csillik, 1981; Palerman et al., 1981).

Unilateral chronic, followed 28 days later by contralateral acute dorsal rhizotomies were done three segments above and below a spared segment (T9) in seven, one month old, Sprague-Dawley rats. Following perfusion 4 days later with 4% paraformaldehyde, frozen T9 spinal cords were serially sectioned (20 μm thick) and reacted by a modified Gomori procedure for FRAP reactivity (Hunt, 1966; Knyihar-Csillik and Csillik, 1981; McNeill and Hulsebosch, 1987). Sections were taken every 100 μm and viewed for density and distribution of reaction product by light microscopy. No shrinkage of grey matter occurred as determined by area measurements made with an acoustic stylus coupled to a PDP 11/44 computer.

To test for normally occurring asymmetrical FRAP projections, acute bilateral spared root surgery was done on sixty day old rats. No asymmetrical FRAP projections were found.

The dorsal horn on both the chronic and the acutely denervated sides had FRAP deposition from only the spared primary afferents of T9 and thus appears lightly stained (Fig. 1). The FRAP reaction product, which stains primary afferent terminals, is located principally in lamina II and on the acute side, and is primarily in the midsection of the dorsal horn. The FRAP reaction on the chronic side is also found principally in lamina II but is more dense and extends more medially and laterally in the dorsal horn on the chronic side in all seven animals (McNeill and Hulsebosch, 1987).

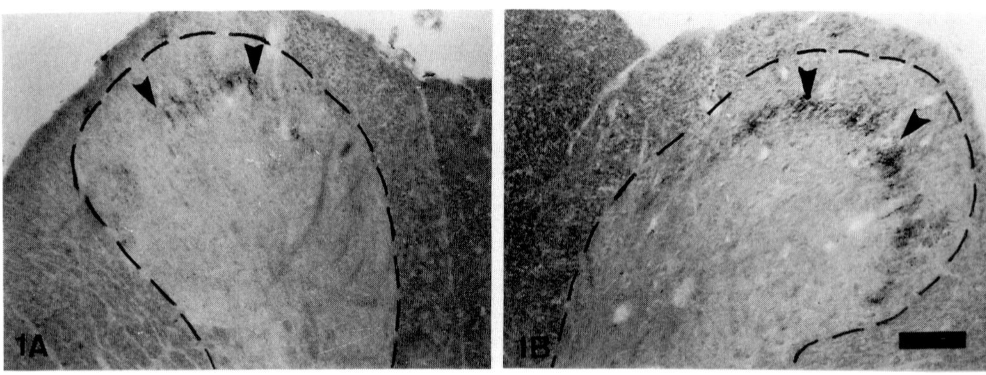


Figure 1. FRAP enzyme activity from primary afferents in the dorsal horn (dashed-outlined) of the T9 spinal segment 4 days following acute surgery to remove fibers from adjacent segments "sparing" the T9 primary afferents (1A). Identical section, contralateral side, 34 days following chronic surgery (1B). Note that the FRAP reaction product on the chronically denervated side is more dense and extends more medially and laterally (arrows), principally in laminae II.

Bar = 0.1mm

We interpret the increased and extended reaction product in the chronic dorsal horn to be sprouting of T9 primary afferent terminals as a result of the denervation provided by eliminating the primary afferent input for three segments above and below the sprouted segment. Since the acute dorsal rhizotomies were done four days prior to sacrifice, this allowed for degeneration of FRAP containing primary afferents (Knyihar-Csillik and Csillik, 1981) above and below T9 on the acute side but was not enough time for sprouting to have occurred. Therefore, the FRAP deposition on the acute side of the dorsal horn represents the normal projection pattern for the T9 primary afferents, while the FRAP deposition on the chronic side represents an extended terminal projection pattern as a result of sprouting of primary afferent terminals. The process of synaptogenesis after spinal deafferentation has been reported (Murray and Goldberger, 1986); however, the contribution of the current study is the identification of the sprouting population as primary afferent fibers. The mediolateral distribution of synaptogenesis after spinal deafferentation has not been previously reported.

What is the stimulus that induces sprouting of adjacent uninjured primary afferents? To review the anatomy of the primary afferent fibers, axons enter the spinal cord and separate into fine (C and Aδ) and coarse (Aβ) fiber tracts. The fine fibers travel longitudinally in the tract of Lissauer and the coarse fibers travel longitudinally in the dorsal columns. Each fiber of both tracts sends periodic elaborate networks into the neuropile of the dorsal horn over several segments (Brown, 1981) and ultimately ascends to synapse in the cunneate or gracilis nucleus in the medulla (Carpenter, 1972). The important point for this discussion is that adjacent spinal segments of primary afferent fibers have considerable synaptic overlap in the dorsal horn. It is reasonable to predict that deafferentation will alter a delicate balance of interactions of neurotrophic factors produced by postsynaptic structures, surrounding glial elements, as well as factors produced by the neuron which interact with surrounding cells and surfaces.

In the spared root paradigm, a "spared group" of primary afferent soma responds to the imbalance of neurotrophic factors by emitting supernumerary branches (Hulsebosch and Coggeshall, 1981; 1983; Hulsebosch et al., 1986) and greatly elaborating and expanding terminal fields within the dorsal horn (present study). The collateral sprouting in the dorsal root (Hulsebosch and Coggeshall, 1981; 1983) and the terminal sprouting within the cord may be the same population of C-fibers or may be two different mechanisms of response by two different C-fiber populations. Nonetheless, the reported sprouting is a restorative phenomenon which restablishes a novel neurotrophic set of interactions in the dorsal horn with new presynaptic elements (from the sprouted primary afferents) onto existing previously vacated postsynaptic elements. To test the importance of neurotrophic substances and involvement in primary afferent sprouting it would be desireable to manipulate the endogenous levels of neurotrophic factors by either addition of exogenous factors or by biologically blocking factors.

Intraspinal Sprouting after ANTI-NGF Treatment

Since earlier studies in my laboratory (Hulsebosch and Coggeshall, 1981; Hulsebosch and Coggeshall, 1983a; 1983b; Hulsebosch, 1985) and others (Beattie et al., 1981; Cotman, 1978; Goldberger and Murray, 1974; Murray and Goldberger, 1986; Stelzner et al., 1972; Tessler et al., 1980; Tessler et al., 1984) demonstrate that primary afferent fibers exhibit collateral and terminal sprouting, it seemed desireable to determine if this sprouting response could be manipulated by altering levels of a neurotrophic factor. The factor of choice is Nerve Growth Factor (NGF) since this protein is known to stimulate sprouting of sympathetic and sensory neurons *in vitro* (Levi-Montalcini, 1982), is well characterized (Greene et al., 1980) and can be purified in a stable form (Varon, 1972). This means that the pure protein can be used to generate reliable antibodies (Johnson et al., 1980; Perez-Polo, 1985; Zaimis, 1972).

In addition, there is data to support the concept of Nerve Growth Factor as a neurotrophic factor for mammalian sensory nerve cells as well as to suggest that the central projections of primary afferents may be trophically dependent on Nerve Growth Factor produced in central nervous system cells. Recent work has shown substantial levels of mRNA for NGF in the midbrain and spinal cord (Shelton and Reichardt, 1986), both sites of synaptic contacts of the primary afferent fibers. The ability of dorsal root ganglia cells to retrogradely transport NGF both from central and peripheral sources (Johnson and Yip, 1985; Yip and Johnson, 1984) has been documented. Furthermore, if primary afferents are severed from their central connections, subsequent neuronal death can be prevented with the addition of exogenous Nerve Growth Factor (Yip et al., 1984).

To test the involvement of NGF in the sprouting of primary afferent fibers, newborn rats were divided into four groups. All groups were given hemisections at birth, a paradigm which elicits sprouting of the central projections of primary afferents in dorsal roots on the denervated side (Hulsebosch and Coggeshall, 1983). (It might be noted that a hemisection paradigm cuts the primary afferent fibers in the cord so sprouting in the root may be a result of pruning and/or collateral sprouting). Three groups were given daily subcutaneous injections, near the dorsal fat pad, for a period of one month of the following substances. The first group was given NGF, 1.5 μl/gm body weight of purified 7S NGF at a concentration of 10 ng/ml phosphate buffer solution, the second was given antibodies to NGF (ANTI-NGF) in whole sera, 3 μl/gm body weight, [generated in rabbit against 7S NGF purified from mouse submaxillary glands (Varon et al., 1972) and assayed as was the NGF before during and after the 1 month injection period using bioassays of chick sensory ganglia and human neuroblastoma cells (Perez-Polo, 1982)], the third group was given preimmune whole sera from the same rabbits used to generate the antibodies, and the fourth group was hemisected with no further treatment. Since a consequence of sprouting is more fibers, then a test for sprouting is to quantitate fiber number. Accordingly, the number of axons were counted in dorsal roots of the hemisected side and compared to the number in roots of the contralateral side.

In the first, third and fourth groups, a 13 to 20% increase in the number of unmyelinated fibers in the dorsal roots on the denervated side of the cord was reported. We interpret this increase to be sprouting of primary afferents in roots on the denervated side. In the ANTI-NGF rats, by contrast, the unmyelinated axons were numerically greater by 7% than the roots of the sprouted side in hemisected untreated rats. In addition, the unmyelinated counts of roots from the unsectioned side were greater by approximately 50%. The myelinated population was little affected (Hulsebosch et al., 1984).

Since the above paradigm was complicated with surgical treatment, we repeated the treatment schedule with ANTI-NGF in neonatal rats which had no surgical manipulation. The numbers of neurons in T4-T6 dorsal root ganglia and the numbers of axons in the dorsal roots from the same animals were counted and compared to normal littermates. The ANTI-NGF rats had 38% fewer neurons in thoracic ganglia but 17% more myelinated and 40% more unmyelinated fibers than the untreated littermates. Furthermore, it is the small diameter DRG soma population which is decreased in number which we interpret as a disproportionate loss of small cells (Hulsebosch et al., 1987b). We interpret this data to indicate that dorsal root ganglion cells, principally small ones, die when endogenous NGF is unavailable and remaining cells emit more processes than normal. Furthermore, the ANTI-NGF induced increase in myelinated and unmyelinated fibers persist for the life of the rat suggesting permanent synaptic contacts (Hulsebosch et al., 1987a).

The results are surprising since the addition of exogenous NGF did not increase the sprouting response observed after hemisection alone with no additional treatment. Presumably, this is a result of sufficient levels of endogenous NGF produced as a consequence of hemisection in amounts appropriate to induce primary afferent sprouting. The addition of exogenous NGF appears to be ignored by the system since the response is not different than the untreated group of rats. Conversely, the addition of ANTI-NGF leads to a decline in dorsal root ganglion cells but an increase in dorsal root axon numbers for thoracic segments in the rat. The mechanism by which this occurs is of considerable interest. In this regard, it is thought that NGF is produced by target tissues, retrogradely transported to the sensory cell body (Hendry et al., 1982; Korsching and Thoenen, 1985; Yip and Johnson, 1984), where one of its functions might be to "signal" that the cell is still attached to its appropriate target. Thus, if NGF is removed we postulate that the cells could interpret this as a sign of axon detachment and begin sprouting. If we add the further complication that some rat sensory neurons require this compound postnatally to survive, than the result of its withdrawal would be a decrease in cell numbers but an overall increase in axon numbers, which is what is observed.

In the specific case of primary afferent sensory neurons, the two "peripheral" structures with which these neurons interact are: 1) sensory transducers at the periphery and 2) neurons in the midbrain and spinal cord. I hypothesize that the sprouting observed after NGF deprivation is a response mediated by central nervous system factors and is not a response to either a NGF deprivation occuring at the periphery or a generalized response to the 38% DRG soma loss. To test the possible involvement of peripheral denervation and/or DRG cell loss on sprouting of primary afferent axons, forelimbs of neonatal rats were amputated at birth and examined one month later. Amputation removes the peripheral structures and results in a subsequent, 30% loss of DRG soma. In contrast to the ANTI-NGF primary afferents, there was a 16% decrease in fiber number in the dorsal root (Heath et al., 1986) and not unexpectedly a 30% decrease in fiber number in Lissuaer's tract (unpublished observation), a tract in the white matter which contains principally unmyelinated and small diameter myelinated primary afferents and some propriospinal fibers.

To determine if the supernumerary fibers in the dorsal roots after ANTI-NGF treatment enter the spinal cord, the number of unmyelinated and myelinated fibers in Lissauer's tract were counted in the T3-T4 segments of the same ANTI-NGF treated rats used in the study described previously. The results are shown in Table 1. The number of fibers in Lissauer's tract is

49% greater in the ANTI-NGF treated rats compared to untreated littermates. Since the same ANTI-NGF rats demonstrated a 38% decrease in small diameter soma, one would predict a decrease in the numbers of fibers in Lissauer's tract (as in the amputation paradigm) unless sprouting occurred in either the primary afferents or the propriospinal neurons. We hypothesize that axonal branching occurred in the white matter as a result of NGF deprivation and that the primary afferent population is the sprouting population. Current studies are in progress to determine the origin and extent of synaptogenesis of the sprouted fibers in Lissauer's tract in the NGF deprived rats.

TABLE I

Number of Fibers in Lissauer's Tract

| | ANTI-NGF | | | CONTROL | | |
|---|---|---|---|---|---|---|
| | MY | UN | TOTAL | MY | UN | TOTAL |
| | 1833 | 11946 | 13779 | 1711 | 7929 | 9640 |
| | 1584 | 10210 | 11794 | 2226 | 7354 | 9580 |
| | 2037 | 10963 | 13000 | 1418 | 5225 | 6643 |
| | 1908 | 10171 | 12079 | 1522 | 6589 | 8111 |
| Mean | 1841 | 10822 | 12663 | 1719 | 6774 | 8493 |
| ±S.E. | ± 95 | ± 416 | ± 402 | ±179 | ±584 | ±711 |

Table I. The number of myelinated (MY) and unmyelinated (UN) fibers in Lissauer's tract in the T3-T4 segment of ANTI-NGF rats compared to untreated littermates (CONTROL) is shown as are the total fiber counts (TOTAL) from each entry. The means ± standard errors (S.E.) are given as the last row. There is not a statistical difference in the myelinated fiber populations; however, there are 60% more unmyelinated fibers and a 49% increase in total fibers in the ANTI-NGF rats compared to control values. These differences are statistically significant. (Student's T-Test: $p < .002$, $p < .003$, respectively).

An important note is the observation that axon-myelin sheath relationships in ANTI-NGF treated animals are different when compared to controls (Fig. 2). Thus, in both normal and ANTI-NGF animals we find a linear relationship between axon size and myelin sheath thickness in the dorsal root, but the slope of this linear correlation is steeper in ANTI-NGF animals. This means that the myelin sheath is thinner for small diameter fibers in the ANTI-NGF animals. This finding presumably indicates that the removal of NGF affects supporting cells in addition to primary sensory neurons and axons. These effects might be mediated by receptors to NGF that exist on primary sensory axons (Richardson and Riopelle, 1984) and Schwann cells (Taniuchi et al., 1986).

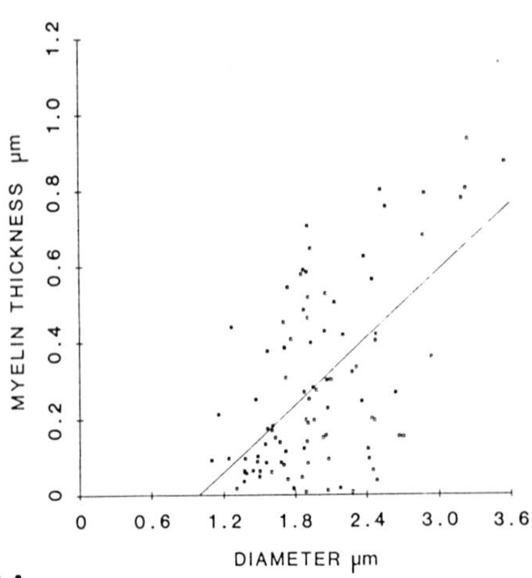


2A

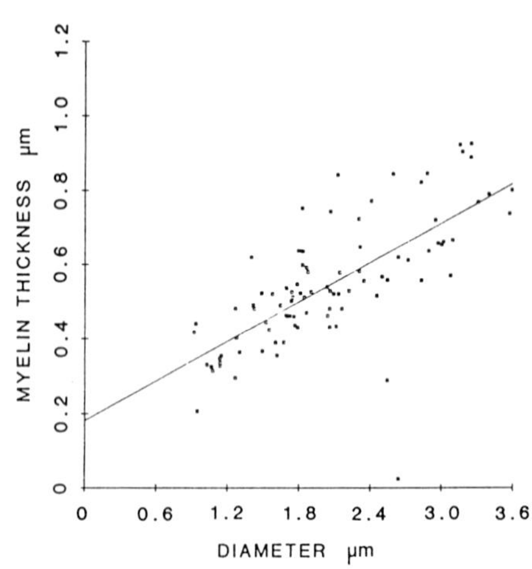


2B

Figure 2. Scattergram of myelin thickness as a function of fiber diameter from dorsal roots of rats treated with ANTI-NGF (2A) and untreated littermates (2B). The equation for the regression line in A is Y = (0.29)X - 0.030 and for B is Y = (0.18)X + 0.19. Thus, small diameter fibers have thinner myelin in the ANTI-NGF group.

## Conclusion

To summarize, these experiments support the hypothesis of intraspinal sprouting of primary afferents in the spinal cord after denervation, and as a result of NGF deprivation. The interaction of primary afferent neurons and other neurons, is dependent on a precise balance of neurotrophic factors provided by the appropriate supporting cells, target tissues and extracellular milieu. If the balance of neurotrophic factors is disrupted, as is the case in denervation or biological inactivation of a known neurotrophic factor, then the affected neuronal population may be altered similar to an earlier period in development. Wherein neurons trophically dependent on a specific factor die if this need is not met (Perez-Polo, 1985). Concurrently, populations of neurons not requiring the factor, interpret the interruption of a specific neurotrophic factor as a signal for sprouting and axonal elongation in response to other factors. Presumably, the resulting axonal sprouting and elongation would re-establish appropriate target connections, stimulated by factors in supporting cells, target cells and/or the extracellular matrix. Specifically, the types of primary afferent sprouting described in this chapter; pruning, collateral sprouting and terminal sprouting, are regenerative mechanisms which are elicited by denervation or inactivation of NGF. Finally, on a broader scale, as neurotrophic factors are defined for different subclasses of neurons, the use of the antibodies against those factors may be important therapeutically, toward inducing sprouting in select populations of neurons.

## LITERATURE REFERENCES


Beattie MS, Bresnaham JC, Liussi FJ (1981) Aberrant axons from the dorsal roots after chronic spinal hemisection in the cat. Soc Neurosci Abstr 7:626

Brown AG (1981) Organization in the spinal cord: The anatomy and physiology of identified neurones. Springer-Verlag, New York

Carpenter MB (1972) Core Text of Neuroanatomy. The Williams & Wilkins Co, Baltimore

Coimbra A, Sodre-Borges BP, Magalhaes MM (1974) The substantia gelatinosa Rolandi of the rat. Fine structure, cytochemistry (acid phosphatase) and changes after dorsal root section. J Neurocytol 3:199-217

Cotman CW (1978) Neuronal Plasticity. Raven Press, New York

Dodd J, Jahr CE, Jessell TM (1984) Neurotransmitters and neuronal markers at sensory synapses in the dorsal horn. In: Kruger L, Liebskind JC (eds) Advances in Pain Research and Therapy, Vol. 6. Raven Press, New York, pp. 105-121

Goldberger ME, Murray MM (1974) Restitution of function and collateral sprouting in the cat spinal cord: the deafferented animal. J Comp Neurol 158:37-53

Greene LA, Shooter EM (1980) The nerve growth factor: biochemistry, synthesis and mechanisms. Ann Rev Neurosci 3:353

Heath III DD, Coggeshall RE, Hulsebosch CE (1986) Axon and neuron numbers after forelimb amputation in neonatal rats. Exp Neurol 92:220-233

Hendry IA, Bonyhady RE, Hill CE (1982) The role of target tissue in development and regeneration - retrophins. In: Haber B, Perez-Polo JR,

Hashim GA, Stella AMB (eds) Nervous System Regeneration. Alan R Liss, New York, pp 263

Hulsebosch CE (1985) The influence of denervation and nerve growth factor on dorsal root axonal sprouting. In: Correia MJ, Perachio AA (eds) Contemporary Sensory Neurobiology. Alan R Liss, New York pp. 163-169

Hulsebosch CE, Coggeshall RE (1981) Sprouting of dorsal root axons. Brain Res 224:170-174

Hulsebosch CE, Coggeshall RE (1983a) A comparison of axonal numbers in dorsal roots following spinal cord hemisection in neonate and adult rats. Brain Res 265:187-197

Hulsebosch CE, Coggeshall RE (1983b) Age related sprouting of dorsal root axons after sensory denervation. Brain Res 288:77-83

Hulsebosch CE, Coggeshall RE, Chung K (1986) Numbers of rat dorsal root axons and ganglion cells during postnatal development. Dev Brain Res 26:105-113

Hulsebosch CE, Coggeshall RE, Perez-Polo JR (1984) Effects of nerve growth factor and its antibodies on sprouting of sensory axons following spinal cord hemisection. Brain Res 323:1-10

Hulsebosch CE, Coggeshall RE, Perez-Polo JR (1987a) Persistence of anti-NGF induced dorsal root axons: possible penetration into the mammalian spinal cord. Brain Res 411:267-274

Hulsebosch CE, Perez-Polo JR, Coggeshall RE (1987b) In vivo ANTI-NGF induces sprouting of sensory axons in dorsal roots. J Comp Neurol 259:445-451

Hunt SP (1966) Microscopic histochemical methods for the demonstration of enzymes. In: Thompson S (ed) Selected Histochemical and Histopathological Methods. C.C. Thomas, Springfield

Hunt SP (1983) Cytochemistry of the spinal cord. In: Emson PC (ed) Chemical Neuroanatomy. Raven Press, New York

Johnson E, Gorin P, Brandies L, Pearson J (1980) Dorsal root ganglion neurons are destroyed by exposure in utero to maternal antibody to nerve growth factor. Sci 210:916-918

Johnson Jr EM, Yip HK (1985) Central nervous system and peripheral nerve growth factor provide trophic support critical to mature sensory neuronal survival. Nature 314:751-752

Kerr FWL, (1972) The potential of cervical primary afferents to sprout in the spinal nucleus of V following long term trigeminal denervation. Brain Res 43:547-560

Kerr FWL (1975) Neuroplasticity of primary afferents in the neonatal cat and some results of early deafferentation of the trigeminal spinal nucleus. J Comp Neurol 163:305-329

Knyihar E (1971) Fluoride-resistant acid phosphatase system of nociceptive dorsal root afferents. Experientia 27:1205-1207

Knyihar E, Laszlo I, Tornyos S (1974) Fine structure and fluoride resistant acid phosphatase activity of electron dense sinusoid terminals in the substantia gelatinosa Rolandi of the rat after dorsal root transection. Exp Brain Res 19:520-544

Knyihar-Csillik E, Csillik B (1981) Frap: Histochemistry of the primary nociceptive neuron. Prog Histochem Cytochem 14:1-137

Korsching S, Thoenen H (1985) Nerve growth factor supply for sensory neurons: site of origin and competition with the sympathetic nervous system. Neurosci Lett 54:201-205

Levi-Montalcini R (1982) Developmental neurobiology and the natural history of nerve growth factor. Ann Rev Neurosci 5:341

Liu CN, Chambers WW (1958) Intraspinal sprouting of dorsal root axons. Arch Neurol Psychiat 79:46-61

McNeill DL, Hulsebosch CE (1987) Intraspinal sprouting of rat primary afferents after deafferentation. Neurosci Lett-In Press

Murray M, Goldberger ME (1986) Replacement of synaptic terminals in lamina II and Clarke's nucleus after unilateral lumbosacral dorsal rhizotomy in adult cats. J Neurosci 6:3205-3217

Palerman NN, Brown KH, Smith DL (1981) Selective neurotoxic action of capsaicin on glomerular C-type terminals in rat substantia gelatinosa. Brain Res 208:506-510

Perez-Polo JR (1985) Neuronotrophic factors. In: Bottenstein JE, Sato G (eds) Cell Culture in the Neurosciences. Plenum Publishing Corporation, pp. 95-123

Richardson PM, Riopelle RJ (1984) Uptake of nerve growth factor along peripheral and spinal axons of primary sensory neurons. J Neurosci 4:1683-1689

Rodin BE, Kruger L (1984) Absence of intraspinal sprouting in dorsal root axons caudal to a partial spinal hemisection: A horseradish peroxidase transport study. Somatosensory Res 2:171-192

Rodin BE, Sampogna SL, Kruger L (1982) An examination of intraspinal sprouting in dorsal root axons with the tracer horseradish peroxidase. J Comp Neurol 215:187-198

Sarter M (1986) Denervation-induced collateral sprouting: no case for tracing methods. Intern J Neurosci 29:65-72

Shelton DL, Reichardt LF (1986) Studies on the expression of the B nerve growth factor (NGF) gene into the central nervous system: Level and regional distribution of NGF mRNA suggest that NGF functions as a trophic factor for several distinct populations of neurons. Proc Natl Acad Sci USA 83:2714-2718

Stelzner DJ, Weber ED (1974) A lack of dorsal root sprouting found after spinal hemisection in neonatal or weanling rat. Soc Neurosci 4:437

Stelzner DJ, Weber ED, Prendergast J (1979) A comparison of the effect of mid-thoracic spinal hemisection in the neonatal or weanling rat on the distribution and density of dorsal root axons in the lumbosacral spinal cord of the adult. Brain Res 172:407-426

Stine SM, Yang H, Costa E (1982) Evidence for ascending and descending intraspinal as well as primary sensory somatostatin projections in the rat spinal cord. J Neurochem 38:1144-1150

Taniuchi M, Clark HB, Johnson Jr EM (1986) Induction of nerve growth factor receptor in Schwann cells after axotomy. Proc Nat'l Acad Sci 83:4094-4098

Tessler A, Glazer E, Artymyshyn R, Murray M, Goldberger ME (1980) Recovery of substance P in the cat spinal cord after unilateral lumbosacral deafferentation. Brain Res 191:459-470

Tessler A, Himes BT, Soper K, Murray ME, Goldberger ME, Reichlin S (1984) Recovery of substance P but not somatostatin in the cat spinal cord after unilateral lumbosacral dorsal rhizotomy: A quantitative study. Brain Res 305:95-102

Varon SJ, Nomura JR, Perez-Polo JR, Shooter EM (1972) The isolation and assay of nerve growth factor proteins. In: Fried R (ed) Methods in Neurochemistry. Dekker, New York, p 203

Yip HK, Johnson Jr EM (1984) Developing dorsal root ganglion neurons require trophic support from their central processes. Evidence for a role of retrogradely transported nerve growth factor from the central nervous system to the periphery. Natl Acad Sci USA 81:6245-6249

Yip HK, Rich KM, Lampe PA, Johnson CM (1984) The effects of nerve growth factor and its antiserum on the postnatal development and survival after injury of sensory neurons in rat dorsal root of ganglia. J

Neurosci 4:2986-2992
Zaimis E (1972) Nerve Growth Factor and its Antiserum. Athlone Press, London pp 59-70
Zenker W, Mysicka A, Neuhuber W (1980) Dynamics of the transganglionic movement of horseradish peroxidase in primary sensory neurons. Cell Tissue Res 207:479-489

ACKNOWLEDGEMENTS

This work was supported by NIH grants NS20091 and NS11255, the Spinal Cord Research Foundation of the Paralyzed Veterans of America and the Florence and Marie Hall Endowment for Programs of Excellence in Education in the Medical Sciences.

# ROLE OF NERVE GROWTH FACTOR IN NEURONAL INJURY AND SURVIVAL

J. Regino Perez-Polo and K. Werrbach-Perez.
Department of Human Biological Chemistry and Genetics
University of Texas Medical Branch
Galveston, Texas, 77550

The response of the central and the peripheral nervous system to injury has several common elements. In particular, the population of molecules that serve as intercellular signals among neurons and glial elements is altered. The intracellular environment changes in response to the injurious event itself, directly, or to secondary events associated with the disruptive events and permeability changes at the interface of the endothelial barrier to the circulatory and lymphoid systems. It has been demonstrated for the hippocampal region of the CNS and the sciatic nerve in the PNS that injury results in synthesis, secretion and accumulation of neuronotrophic substances, and that glial cells proliferate and, with microglia in CNS or satellite cells in PNS, actively carry out phagocytosis and eventually participate in glial scar formation (Hendry, 1975; Nieto-Sampedro & Cotman, 1985; Rich et al, 1987). Also, CNS glial cells have been shown to actively respond to and synthesize lymphokines like interleukin 1 and 2 (Saneto et al; Giulian et al, this volume). This lesion induced development of immunological properties by CNS glia may be the result of interactions with invading lymphoid cells and/or circulating factors, interruption of molecular exchanges with surrounding neurons or, as is more likely, varying degrees of all these phenomena. That glia respond to interleukins and, conversely, that splenic mononuclear cells have receptors and respond to neurotransmitters, such as opiates and growth factors like NGF, would only suggest that active intercellular communication between the nervous and immune system is not limited to post-lesion events; but rather, is also likely to play a significant role in neuronal development and homeostasis (Thorpe et al, this volume).

The evidence that such a broad spectrum of lesion induced events takes place is substantiative although in most instances the individual molecular events are not fully understood (Nieto-Sampedro & Cotman, 1985). However, it would appear that the early events that trigger

NATO ASI Series, Vol. H22
Neural Development and Regeneration
Edited by A. Gorio et al.

secondary responses might be predictive of outcome of recuperative and regenerative events (Perez-Polo & Werrbach-Perez, 1985). The need for explanations at the molecular level would suggest that there is a need for lesion paradigms that minimize the heterogenous nature of morphological disruption, using mechanical crush or impact techniques on neuronal tissues in vivo (Khan et al, In Press), and focus on molecular events associated with chemical disruption of energy metabolism and/or the generation of toxic substances.

An early event associated with cellular injury, as experienced in stroke, spinal or head trauma, is the generation of oxyl and hydroxyl radicals that can generate lipid peroxides in cellular membranes due to ferrous ion mediated generation of free radicals upon interaction with hydrogen peroxide. Both for the ischemic and membrane disruptive events associated with injury there is a dramatic increase in the generation of free radicals that in the case of hydroxyl radicals can be augmented in the lipid environment of neural membranes. Hydroxyl radicals can initiate lipid peroxidation by abstracting a methylene hydrogen from polyunsaturated fatty acids in a chain reaction of lipid peroxidation that can yield intracellularly, increasing amounts of aldehydes. The aldehydes thus generated can inactivate proteins and nucleic acids.

An advantage of using free radical generators as sources of injury is that lesions can be induced in a controlled manner in vitro with well defined neural primary cultures or established cell lines. There is the caveat that dissociated primary cultures are in themselves a regenerating system whereas established cell lines may have altered metabolisms selected for their compatibility with cell culture (Martin et al, 1987). However, such model systems do provide specific hypotheses that can be further tested in vivo.

For certain peripheral nervous system neurons it has been demonstrated that the nerve growth factor protein (NGF) is necessary for successful regeneration to take place or for protection from either chemically induced axotomy or surgical section of the sciatic nerve (Hendry, 1975; Rich, 1987). Although in the central nervous system NGF has not been found to have trophic or neurite inducing effects, it has been found to have a trophic or sparing effect following lesions to some cholinergic tissues (Whittemore & Seiger, 1987). These findings would suggest that the protective trophic effects of NGF are relevant to neuronal injury. The human neuroblastoma line SK-N-SH-SY5Y and the rat pheochromacytoma line PC12 have been found to be two useful model systems to study the role of NGF in recuperative and regenerative events in vitro (Greene & Shooter, 1980; Perez-Polo et al, 1982). In particular, both SY5Y and PC12 respond to NGF and meet most requirements of an NGF-responsive neuron (Table 1). As an example, NGF treatment causes dramatic increases in cellular volume and protein content of SY5Y cells (Fig. 1), accelerates rates of attachment of these cells, induces neurite outgrowth, increases fasciculation of neurites and confers electrical excitability to these cells (Perez-Polo, 1982). Here we will focus our discussion on the SY5Y line and those NGF effects that are pertinent to regeneration and cell viability.

Table 1

Minimal Requirements of NGF-response neuronal line.

1. That cells be genetically stable.
2. That cells display saturable and specific NGF receptors.
3. That NGF induce cellular hypertrophy.
4. That NGF induce neurite outgrowth.
5. That NGF stimulate protein synthesis.
6. That NGF accelerate rate of cell attachment.
7. That NGF stimulate metabolite uptake process.
8. That NGF treated cells become electrically excitable.
9. That NGF potentiate induction of neurotransmitter synthesis.

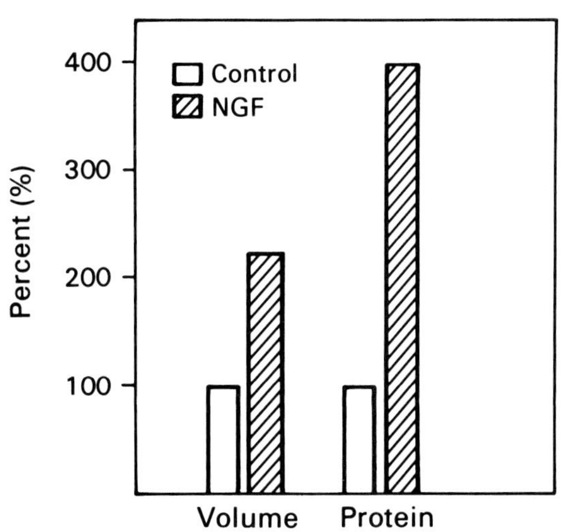


Figure 1. Effect of NGF treatment on SY5Y cells. Adapted from Perez-Polo et al, 1979.

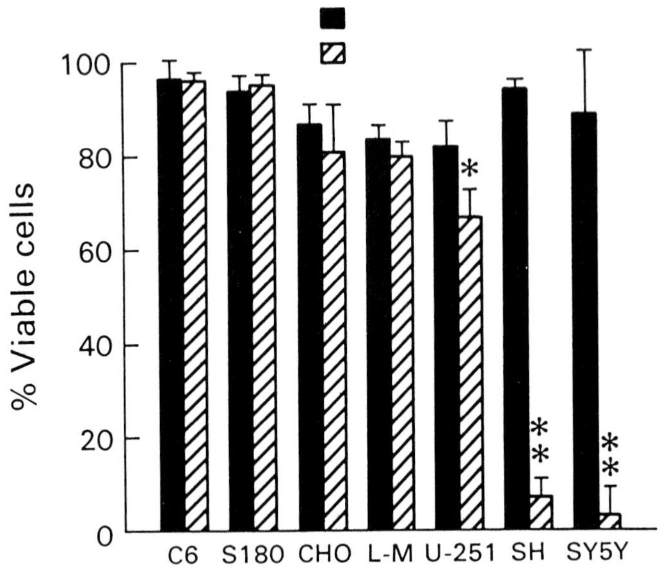


Figure 2. Effect of 6-OHDA (crosshatched) on rat glioma (C6), mouse sarcoma (S180), hamster fibroblast (CHO), mouse fibroblast (6-M), mouse glioma (U-251) and human neuroblastoma lines (SH and SY5Y). Adapted from Perez-Polo et al, 1983.

A reliable and physiologically relevant agent for the induction of neuronal injury in vitro is 6-hydroxydopamine (6-OHDA). The SY5Y clone of SK-N-SH is very sensitive to 6-OHDA treatment compared to other non-neuronal cell lines (Fig. 2, 3). This sensitivity is shared by most human neuroblastoma lines irrespective of whether the neurotransmitters being expressed are common to their sympathetic progenitors. At physiological pH, 6-OHDA spontaneously reacts with oxygen in solution and yields 1,4-para-quinone, hydrogen peroxide, as well as superoxide and hydroxyl radicals. The formation of hydroxyl radicals can be catalyzed from the breakdown of $H_2O_2$ by iron ions (Haber & Weiss 1934; Heikkila & Cohen, 1973).

The toxic effects of 6-OHDA can be detected as early as 3 hours after the addition of 6-OHDA to the culture media by a number of different criteria (Fig. 4,5). However, there is no appreciable quinone formation or effects of NGF on quinone formation under those in vitro conditions that demonstrated NGF protection from 6-OHDA (Tiffany-Castiglioni et al, 1982). Thus, the mechanism of toxicity by 6-OHDA and NGF protection from 6-OHDA could be due to effects of $H_2O_2$ directly or to secondary effects as a result of the interruption of the specific uptake machinery of catecholamines by SY5Y, since 6-OHDA is a dopamine analogue (Saner & Thoenen, 1970; Thoenen et al, 1987). These latter effects could be disruptive of NGF binding, uptake and retrograde transport to cell soma.

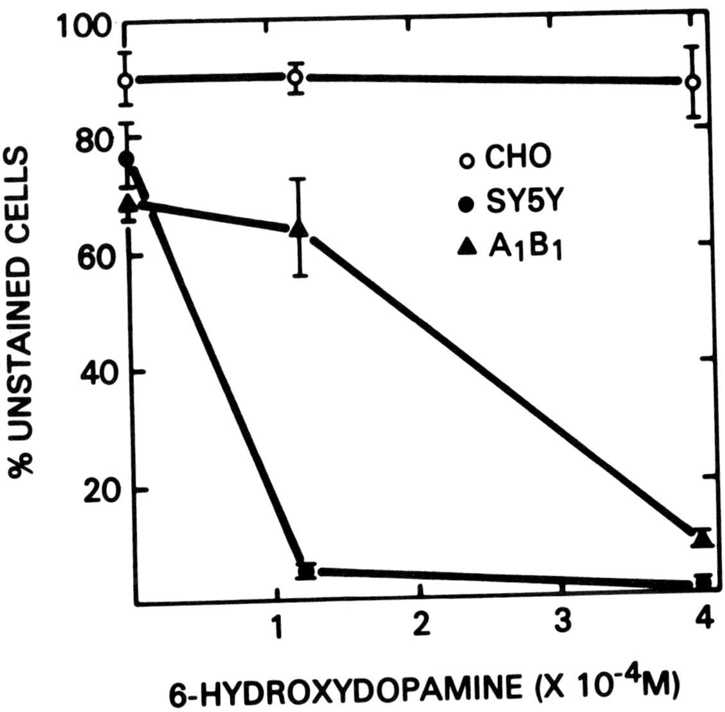


Figure 3. Dose response of 6-OHDA treatment on CHO, SY5Y and a huma glioma line (A1B1). Adapted from Perez-Polo et al, 1983.

These data are in agreement with the hypothesis that neuronal cell death induced by 6-OHDA has two components. One due to the specific and saturable uptake of dopamine that can be abolished using cocaine as a dopamine uptake inhibitor (Fig. 6) and another effect due to the generation of hydrogen peroxide and hence hydroxyl in vitro. When SY5Y are exposed to dibutyryl cyclic AMP, they extend neurites that are not stable. These neurites do not fasciculate and there is no effect on the rates of cell attachment to culture dishes (Perez-Polo et al, 1979; Schulze and Perez-Polo, 1982). As shown in Figure 7, the protection from

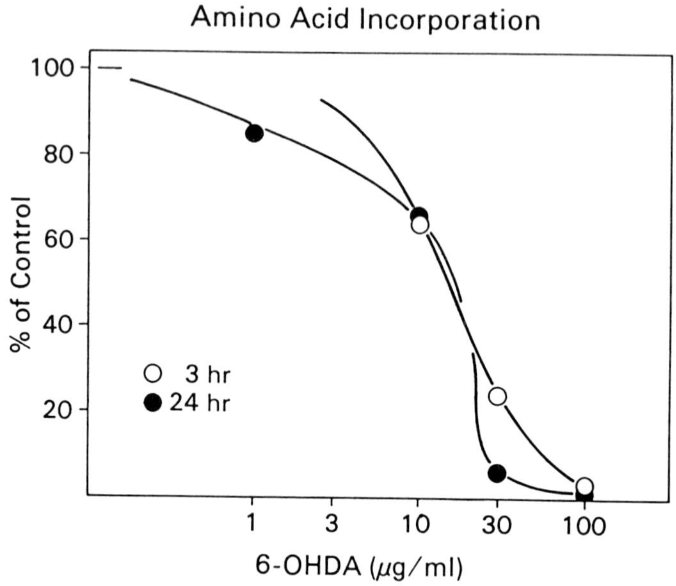


Figure 4 Dose response of 6-OHDA on SY5Y amino acid incorporation 3 and 24 hours after treatment. Adapted from Tiffany-Castiglioni & Perez-Polo, 1980.

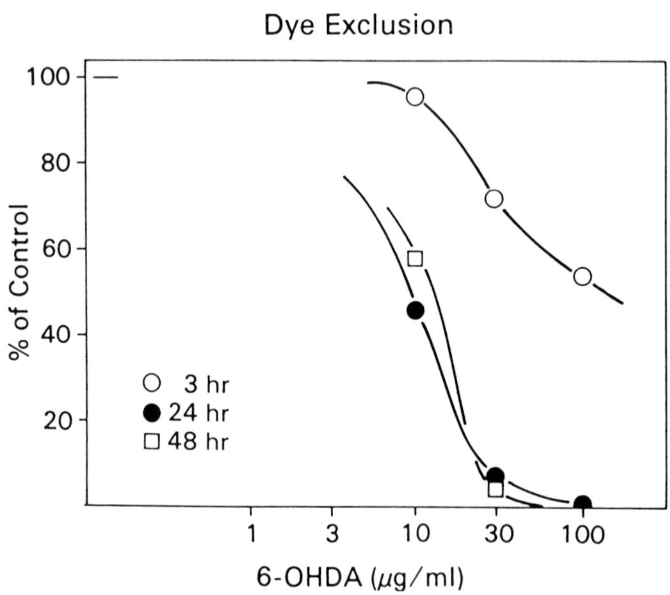


Figure 5 Dose response of 6-OHDA effect on SY5Y viability as determined by Trypan blue dye exclusion. Adapted from Tiffany-Castiglioni & Perez-Polo, 1980.

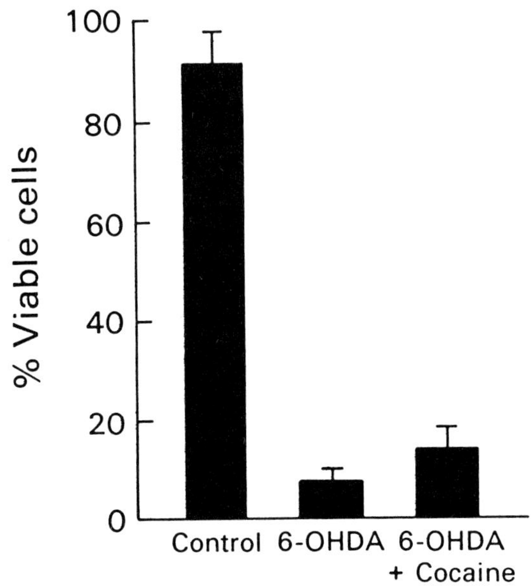


Figure 6 Effect of 6-OHDA on SY5Y cell viability in the presence and absence of equimolar concentrations of cocaine under conditions similar to those described in Tiffany-Castiglioni et al, 1982.

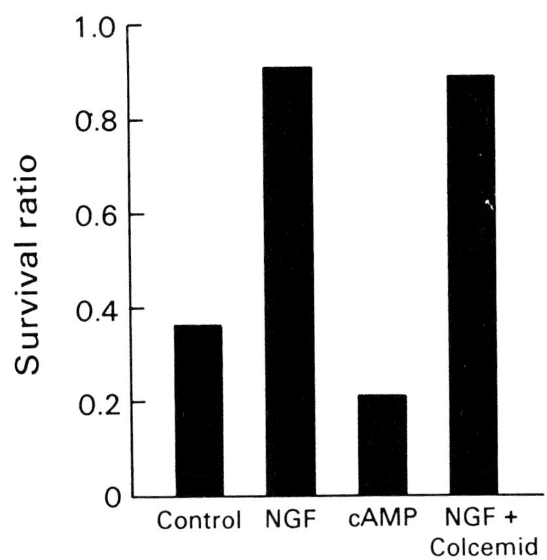


Figure 7 Role of transport processes and neurite in NGF protection of SY5Y from 6-OHDA. Adapted from Perez-Polo et al, in press.

6-OHDA by NGF is independent of neurite extension since dibutyryl cyclic AMP offered no protection and NGF application in the presence of colcemid, at non-toxic concentrations, that nevertheless disrupt microtubules to the extent that retrograde transport and neurite outgrowth are blocked, did not prevent NGF protection from the 6-OHDA insult suggesting that NGF protection was independent of transport processes and morphological consequences of axotomy.

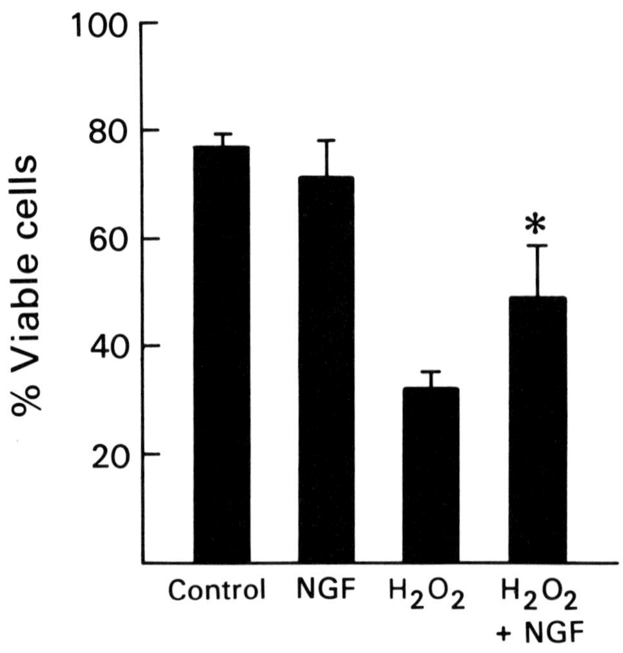


Figure 8 NGF protection of SY5Y from $H_2O_2$. Adapted from Tiffany-Castiglioni et al, 1982.

Table 2

| Treatment | Catalase (%) | SOD (%) |
|---|---|---|
| Control | 100 $\pm$ 7 | 100 $\pm$ 14 |
| NGF | 400 $\pm$ 23 | 107 $\pm$ 11 |

NGF was also found to protect againt $H_2O_2$ at concentrations equivalent to those generated by the concentrations of 6-OHDA used earlier (Fig. 8). Since catalase is the enzyme that converts $H_2O_2$ to $H_2O$, it is not surprising that it offered the most protection (Fig. 9). The protection by catalase is at the extracellular level and involves prevention of the accumulation of hydroxyl radicals and their interaction with the cell membrane. Evidence that the mechanism of action of NGF protection involves regulation of catalase activity comes from the finding that NGF induced catalase in a specific fashion in SY5Y (Table 2) and that NGF protection was abolished by aminotriazole, AZ, a catalase inhibitor (Table 3).

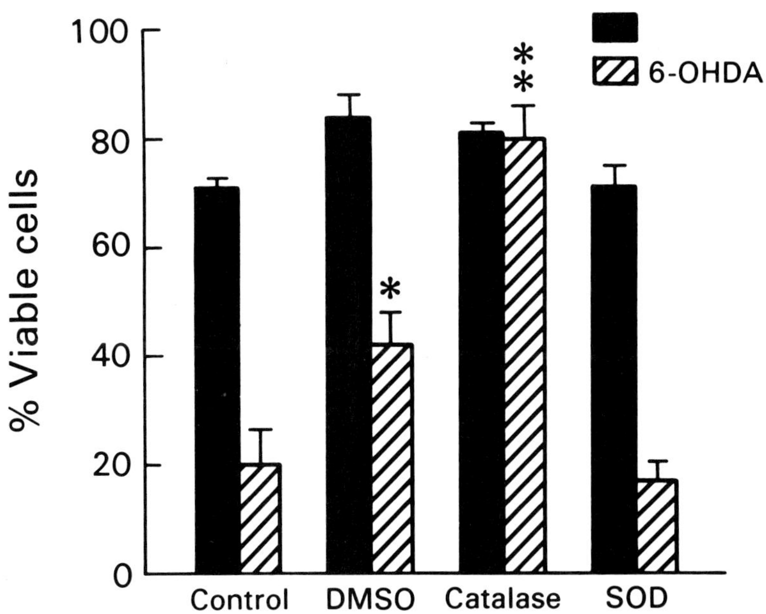


Figure 9 Protection of SY5Y from 6-OHDA by DMSO, catalase and superoxide dismutase. Adapted from Tiffany-Castiglioni et al, 1982.

Table 3

| Treatment | % Viable Cells |
|---|---|
| Control | 100 ± 2 |
| $H_2O_2$ +NGF | 43.2 ±7.8 |
| $H_2O_2$ +NGF+AZ | 17.6 ±1.8 |

In a limited sense these results would support the hypothesis that neuronal cell lines in vitro are rescued from free radical damage by NGF through the specific induction of catalase by NGF. In a somewhat broader sense, it is of interest that similar results can be obtained with the PC12 cell line (Perez-Polo et al, 1986) and that in the absence of NGF protection, aminotriazole treatment results in decreases of cell survival by neurons when challenged by $H_2O_2$ in a dose dependent fashion (Jackson, et al, in preparation). This may be because neuronal lines have low endogenous levels of catalase and glutathione peroxidase in comparison to non-neuronal lines (Table 4).This is in agreement with the hypothesis that, in vitro, catalase plays a central role in predicting cell survival in response to $H_2O_2$ lesions. If it is taken into account that there is ample evidence that neuronal cell death is a prime determinant of specificity in neuronal embryogenesis and that NGF is, at least for many peripheral structures, the prime regulator of cell death, one could speculate that the regulation of catalase by NGF may play a critical role in providing the mechanistic explanation of cell death (Perez-Polo, 1985; Oppenheim, 1987).

TABLE 4

| CELL LINE | CATALASE | GSH-Px |
|---|---|---|
| SY5Y | 100% | 100% |
| A1B1 | 518% | 325% |
| CHO | 524% | 275% |

NGF levels in target tissues, in vivo, are such that there is not enough NGF available to saturate NGF receptors on target neurons (Whittemore & Seiger, 1987; Thoenen et al, 1987) making these neurons exquisitely sensitive to fluctuations in NGF levels. Since endogenous catalase levels are low in these cells, it is plausible that competition for target derived NGF would provide sufficient extra NGF to induce catalase and assure survival of those properly connected neurons which receive NGF from target tissues by retrograde transport. Also, following injury of adult neurons, exogenous NGF could induce catalase and allow cellular recuperative metabolism, highly oxidative in nature, to insure recuperation through the regenerative process. If these hypothesis can be substantiated in vivo, they may provide a molecular interpretation of the regulation of neuronal death by neuronotrophic factors in development and regeneration.

Acknowledgements: This research was supported by grants from the NIH and Moody Foundation. Thanks to C. Beck for expert technical assistance and to D. Masters for manuscript preparation.

## References

Giulian D and JF Krebs (this volume) Glia-promoting factors and control of oligodendroglial growth during brain development and regeneration. In: Haber B, deVellis J, Gorio A, Perez-Polo JR (eds.) Cellular and Molecular Aspects of Neural Development and Regeneration. Springer Verlag, Heidelberg.

Greene LA and Shooter E (1980) The nerve growth factor: Biochemistry, synthesis, and mechanism of action. Ann. Rev. Neurosci. 3:353-402.

Haber F, Weiss J (1934) The catalytic decomposition of hydrogen peroxide by ion salts. Proc R. Soc Lond(A), 147:332-340.

Heikkila RE, Cohen G (1973) 6-hydroxy dopamine: Evidence for superoxide radical as an oxidative intermediate. Science, 181:456-457.

Hendry IA (1975) The response of adrenergic neruons to axotomy and nerve growth factor. Brain Res. 94:87-97.

Jackson G, Apffel L, Werrbach-Perez K and Perez-Polo JR, manuscript in preparation.

Khan T, Green B and Perez-Polo JR (to be published) Effect of injury on nerve growth factor uptake by sensory ganglia. J. of Neurosci Res.

Martin EME, Skaper SD and Varon S (1987) Catalase protection of neuronal survival in vitro is not directed to the accumulation of peroxides in the culture medium. Int. J. Devl. Neurosci. 5:1-10.

Nieto-Sampedro M and Cotman CW (1985) Growth factor induction and termporal order in central nervous system repair. In: Cotman CW (ed) Ch. 14 Synaptic Plasticity, The Guilford Press, New York, pp. 407-455.

Oppenheim RW (1987) Muscle activity and motor neuron death in the spinal cord of the chick embryo. In: Selective neuronal death. Ciba Foundation Symposium 126, Wiley and Sons, New York, pp. 96-112.

Perez-Polo JR, Werrbach-Perez K and Tiffany-Castiglioni E (1979) A human clonal cell line model of differentiating neurons. Dev. Biol. 71:341-355.

Perez-Polo JR, Tiffany-Castiglioni E, Ziegler M, Reynolds CP, Schulze I and Werrbach-Perez K (1982) NGF effects on human neuroblastoma lines: A model system. In: Coulter J, Haber B, and Perez-Polo JR (eds.), Proteins in the Nervous System: Structure and Function, Alan R. Liss, New York, pp.285-299.

Perez-Polo JR, Tiffany-Castiglioni E and Werrbach-Perez (1983) Model clonal system for study of neuronal cell injury. In: Haber B,

Perez-Polo JR, Hashim GA and Giuffrida-Stella AM (eds.) Birth Defects: Original Article Series, vol. 19(4), March of Dimes Foundation Alan R. Liss, New York, pp. 201-220.

Perez-Polo JR (1985) Neuronotrophic Factors. In: Bottenstein J and Sato G (eds.), Cell Culture in the Neurosciences, vol 3. Plenum Publishing Comp. pp:95-123.

Perez-Polo JR, Werrbach-Perez K (1985) Effects of nerve growth factor on the in vitro response of neurons to injury. In: Eccels J, Dimitrijevic MR (eds.) Recent Achievements in restorative neurology upper motor neuron functions and dysfunctions, vol 30, Karger pp. 321-337.

Perez-Polo JR, Apffel L and Werrbach-Perez (1986) Role of CNS and PNS trophic factors on free radical mediated aging events. Clinical Neuropharmacology 9(4):98-100.

Perez-Polo JR, Beck C, Marchetti D, Morgan B, Thorpe LW and Werrbach-Perez (In Press) Role of NGF receptors in intercellular communication In: International Society For Myochemistry, John Libbey Eurotext Ltd, France.

Rich KM, Luszczynski JR, Osborne PA and Johnson EM (1987) Nerve growth factor protects adult sensory neurons from cell death and atrophy caused by nerve injury. J. of Neurocytol. 16:261-268.

Saner A, Thoenen H (1970) Model experiments on the molecular mechanism of action of 6-hydroxydopamine. Mol. Pharmacol. 7:147-154.

Saneto RP, Altman A, Knobler RL, deVellis J (this volume) Immune System Growth Factor Modulation of Neonatal Oligodendrocyte Growth In Vitro In: Haber B, de Vellis J, Gorio A, and Perez-Polo JR (eds.) Cellular and Molecular Aspects of Neural Development and Regeneration. Springer Verlagn Heidelberg.

Schulze I and Perez-Polo JR (1982) Nerve growth factor and cyclic AMP: Opposite effects on neuroblastoma-substrate adhesion. Jour. of Neurosci. Res. 8:393-411.

Thoenen H, Barde YA, Davies AM and Johnson JE (1987) Neuronotrophic factors and neuronal death In: Ciba Foundation Symposium 126, Wiley and Sons, New York pp. 82-95.

Thorpe LW, Morgan B, Werrbach-Perez K, Beck C and Perez-Polo JR (this volume) Nerve Growth Factor and the Immune System In: Haber B, deVellis J, Gorio A, and Perez-Polo JR (eds.) Cellular and Molecular Aspects of Neural Development and Regeneration, Springer Verlag Heidelberg.

Tiffany-Castiglioni E, Saneto RP, Proctor PH, Perez-Polo JR, (1982) Participation of active oxygen species in 6-hydroxydopamine toxicity to a human neuroblastoma cell line. Biochem. Pharmacol. 31:181-188.

Whittemore S and Seiger A (1987) The expression, localization and functional significance of Beta-Nerve growth factor in the central nervous system. Brain Res Rev. In press.

# GLIAL-DERIVED SUBSTANCES ASSOCIATED WITH CNS REGENERATION

by M. Schwartz[1], A. Harel[1], A. Cohen[1], C. Stein-Izsak[1], M. Fainaru[2], M. Rubinstein[3], M. Belkin[4], A. Solomon[4]
[1]Department of Neurobiology
The Weizmann Institute of Science
Rehovot 76100, Israel

Axonal injury stimulates two complimentary systems, the axon and its surrounding non-neuronal cells which operate in synchrony. Our results suggest that the non-neuronal cells response to injury have an impact on the subsequent ability of the axon to grow and elongate. In this chapter we review some of our observations related to the components which interplay in this process. One example for biochemical manifestations of an early response to injury in CNS of a regeneration system (i.e. fish visual system) is the accumulation of a 28 kDa polypeptide which we identified as apolipoprotein-A-I (apo-A-I). The accumulation of primarily one isoform of apo-A-I, may be due to a need created by the injury for a particular stable and functional isoform. These observations are similar to those reported in adult rat sciatic nerves where a 37 kDa polypeptide showed an elevation after injury and was identified as apo-E. We attribute to apo-A-I a role in removal of dead tissue to pave the way for regeneration. Subsequent regeneration depends on the accessibility to growth supportive substances and organized and proper extracellular matrix. We found that soluble substances originating from regenerating fish optic nerves and newborn rabbit optic nerves contain factors which acti-

---

[2]Kaplan Hospital, Rehovot; [3]Department of Virology, The Weizmann Institute of Science, and [4]Maurice and Gabriela Goldschleger, Eye Research Institute, Tel- Aviv Sackler School of Medicine, Sheba Medical Center, Tel-Hashomer, Israel.

NATO ASI Series, Vol. H22
Neural Development and Regeneration
Edited by A. Gorio et al.

vate neurons and may modulate the glial response to injury. These factors when applied to injured adult rabbit optic nerves cause in the later biochemical alterations in the retinas and acquisition of a growth supportive surface including accumulation of laminin by the surrounding non-neuronal cells. A non-regenerative system either does not provide these factors, or keeps them inaccessible at the critical time but has the machinery to respond to these factors. Our results suggest that the response to injury of non-neuronal cell is not different from the response to injury of any other damaged tissue and may therefore obey to the same set of rules governing proliferation and differentiation of other cells. The possible involvement of protooncogenes in their response to injury was therefore examined. The protooncogenes fos and myc were found to be constitutively expressed in these cells and an elevation was found after injury. These protoncogenes may have a role in the plasticity of this system, an issue which is currently being further investigated.

## 1. Introduction

The loss of function which results from damage to the central nervous system (CNS) of higher vertebrates, including man, is often irreversible (Attardi and Sperry, 1943; Guth and Windle, 1970; Kiernan, 1979), due to their low regenerative potential. By contrast, the adult peripheral nervous system has a substantial ability to regrow and to reach peripheral targets after injury. Similarly, the central nervous system of lower vertebrates is also able to re-establish functional connections following injury (Attardi and Sperry, 1943).

Recent observations, from our laboratory and others, have offered new clues as to why the adult CNS fails to regenerate (Aguayo *et al.*, 1978a; Hadani *et al.*, 1984; Kao *et al.*, 1977; Neuman *et al.*, 1983; Nieto-Sampedro *et al.*, 1983; Schwartz *et al.*, 1985; Williams and Varon, 1985). These studies have demonstrated that the environment of injured neurons determines the ability of the axon to regenerate following injury.

The first observation that the environment can either facilitate or inhibit axonal regeneration was made by Ramon Y. Cajal (1928). More recently nerve transplantation experiments demonstrated that the neuronal environment should be conducive for regeneration to occur. For example, spinal and brain axons regenerate readily through columns of Schwann cells in peripheral nerves but, usually, fail to enter grafted CNS nerve segments (Aguayo et al., 1978a,b; David and Aguayo, 1981; Richardson et al., 1982; Richardson and Issa, 1984). These in vivo studies were confirmed lately by in vitro experiments in which the growth of neurites showed preference towards co-cultured sciatic nerves (Schwab & Thoenen, 1985) and regenerating fish optic-nerves (Carbonetto et al., 1987), rather than optic nerves of adult mammals (Schwab and Thoenen, 1985).

Among the elements that the environment may provide are diffusible substances and extracellular matrix components (David and Aguayo, 1981; Longo et al., 1982; 1983; Lundborg et al., 1982; Manthorpe et al., 1982; Manthorpe et al., 1983; Nieto-Sampedro et al., 1982; Richardson et al., 1982; Richardson and Issa, 1984; Williams & Varon, 1985).

## 2. The system

Studies in our laboratory have focused on the influence of soluble substances from the environment on regeneration of the CNS using the visual system as a model (Goldberg, 1976). The advantage of the visual system is multifold: the optic nerve is part of the CNS yet both axons and cell bodies are accessible to experimentation; cell body and axon in the visual system are well separated and thus can be individually studied; studies in the regenerative visual system of lower vertebrates have established certain characteristic features of successful regeneration, including increased RNA

(Burrell *et al.*, 1978; Murray, 1973) and protein synthesis in the cell body (Agranoff *et al.*, 1980; Benowitz *et al.*, 1983; Grafstein and McQuarrie, 1978; Kohshaka *et al.*, 1981); increased synthesis and transport of specific polypeptides (Skene and Willard, 1981a-c; Willard and Skene, 1982); and sprouting of new fibers from the retina in culture (Landerth and Agranoff 1976, 1979).

Our studies were initiated by suggestions drawn from the available data that environmental elements, both soluble and non-soluble, determine the fate of the neuron after injury.

To get an insight as to the nature of these environmental elements, we began by studying soluble substances originating from the fish visual system (a model for a regenerative CNS) in the form of conditioned media (CM) derived from either injured or non-injured fish optic nerves (Rachailovich and Schwartz, 1984). We reasoned that these soluble substances, in the CM, would largely derive from the surrounding non-neuronal cells with the contribution of axoplasmic proteins leaking from the axon being, at most, minute. Such CM are likely comprised of multiple constituents, some of which may participate in the regenerative response to injury, by acting in concert or in a synchronized fashion, as occurs in other growth processes. Such components may include neuronal factors (Mizrachi *et al.*, 1986), glial factors (Giulian *et al.*, 1986), proteases and their inhibitors (Monard *et al.*, 1983), and other substances which may neutralize inhibitors. Our results provide evidence that indeed, injury causes changes both in the type and amount of substances originating from the non-neuronal cells (Harel et al., 1987; Rachailovich and Schwartz, 1984; Schwartz *et al.*, 1985).

In this chapter, a few of the soluble components of the CM which have been isolated in our laboratory will be discussed, with emphasis on their possible physiological relevance to the process of regeneration and the mechanism which regulates their production, activation, and accessibility.

## 3. Results and Discussion

### 3.1. Apolipoproteins in response to injury - putative scavengers of degradation products

Among the prominent changes in soluble substances (i.e. CM) derived from non-neuronal cells, which occur following optic nerve injury in the fish, is the increased labeling of a 28 kDa polypeptide in CM of regenerating nerves (Rachailovich and Schwartz, 1984). In the rat sciatic nerves, a 37 kDa polypeptide, showing increased labeling under similar conditions (Muller _et al._, 1985; Skene and Shooter, 1983) has been identified as apolipoprotein-E (apo-E) (Ignatius _et al._, 1986; Snipes _et al._, 1986). This polypeptide was found to be accumulated in the regenerating PNS in contrast to its increased synthesis without accumulation in the non-regenerating CNS (Muller _et al._, 1985).

We hypothesized that the fish 28 kDa polypeptide may also be an apolipoprotein. We found that fish plasma contains a 28 kDa polypeptide which, based on its molecular weight, amino acid composition and microheterogeneity is apo-A-I (apo-E is absent from fish plasma, Harel _et al._, 1987a). Antibodies were raised against the isolated and purified fish plasma apo-A-I, as no immunological cross-reactivity could be detected between fish and rodent apo-A-I. Using these antibodies we were able to show, by Western blot of two-dimensional gels, that in non-injured fish optic nerves there are two isoforms of fish apo-A-I whereas in the injured nerves there is an additional isoform (Fig. 1). This expression of a particular isoform in injured fish optic nerves was also accompanied by an overall increase in the amount of accumulated apo-A-I in the injured fish optic nerves. The plasma apo-A-I isoforms (pI 5.7 - 6.5) and nerve apo-A-I isoforms (6.5-6.7) were found to be different except for a possible similarity in one isoform. In other systems differences between plasma and glial derived apolipoproteins were observed as well. For example, apo-E derived from rat brain and astrocytes in culture were found to be different in the degree of their sialic acid residues when compared with plasma-drived apo-E (Pitas et al., 1987). These differences may be related to the changes in stability and functional activity of these apolipoproteins.

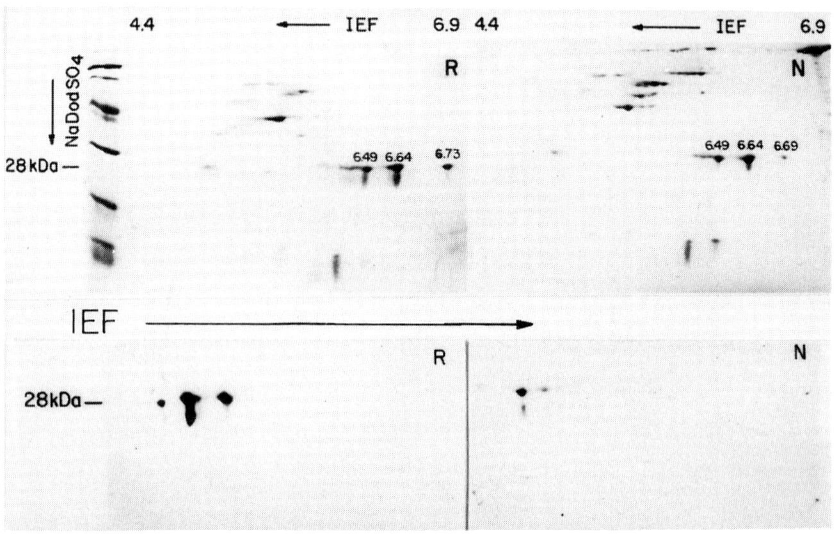


Fig. 1. Injury in the fish optic nerve is accompanied by increased expression of one isoform of apo-A-I Media conditioned by non-injured (normal, N) and injured (regenerating, R) fish optic nerves (50 g protein) were analyzed by two dimensional gel electrophoresis. For the first dimension, tube gels were prepared in denaturing solution containing 9.5 M Urea, 2% NP-40, 2% ampholines (1.6% pH 5-7, 4% pH 3.5-10) and 5% 2-mercaptoethanol (O'Farrell, 1975). The gels from the first dimension were applied to slab gels and were further analyzed by SDS-PAGE (15% acrylamide). One set of gels (shown at the top of the figure) of injured and non-injured nerves were then fixed, stained, and photographed. The second set was then blotted onto nitrocellulose (0.45 m; Schleicher & Schuell, Germany) for 2 h, 200 mA in transfer buffer (15.6 mM Tris-HCl, 120 mM glycine, pH 8.3). The blotted nitrocellulose was then incubated overnight at room temperature in PBS containing 0.3% Tween-20. The immunological reaction was carried out sequentially; incubation for 1 h with the primary antibodies, wash, incubation with horseradish peroxidase conjugated to protein A (Radiochemical Center, Amersham International), wash, and incubation with 4-chloro-1-naphthol. The gels were then photographed and are shown at the bottom of the figure. The polypeptides of interest corresponding to a molecular weight of 28 kDa are marked by their pI values in the Coomassie blue stained photographs and were the only polypeptides which were stained by the specific anti-plasma apo-A-I antibodies. Note the appearance of three spots of 28 kDa molecular weight (pI 6.49, 6.64, 7.75) which are apo-A-I positive in the preparation obtained from the regenerating nerve and two apo-A-I positive spots in the preparation of the intact nerve (pI 6.49, 6.64) (From Harel et al., 1987a).

The functional activity of apo-A-I in the nervous system is not known. An increase in apo-E and apo-A-I synthesis after injury was observed in rat and avian optic nerves, respectively, a two non-regenerating systems (Dawson et al., 1986). It is possible that after injury apo-A-I is involved in the elimination of myelin degradation products (especially cholesterol) which otherwise may impede regeneration (McConnell and Berry, 1982). It is reasonable to assume that the apo-A-I in the fish CNS (the present study) and apo-E in regenerating PNS of mammals (Ignatius et al., 1986; Snipes et al., 1986) are performing similar roles. Binding studies using $^{125}$I-labeled apo-A-I liposomes revealed no specific binding of apo-A-I to apo-B/E receptors, in contrast to specific apo-E binding (Fainaru et al. in preparation). We therefore assume that the apolipoproteins which accumulate in injured nerves may be involved in eliminating myelin degradation products. Although the apolipoproteins are involved in degeneration, a seemingly destructive process, their role might be to form an essential bridge for the subsequent constructive process of regeneration, leading to the formation of new tissue. The cellular origin of apo-A-I in this system might be glial cells and as such might be part of the glial response to the injury, an issue which is discussed below.

## 3.2 Glial maturation factors in the response to injury

In the absence of an appropriate control mechanism, the non-neuronal cells in mammalian CNS will form a glial scar which may impede or at least will not support regrowth. An appropriate glial response should involve a well-controled process to activate the glial cells to acquire regeneration-supportive properties at the right time. This response may include production of soluble factors and extracellular components, needed for neuronal survival, neurite growth and elongation.

Both the available data and our own results indicated a correlation between the ability of a nerve to grow and the composition of its environment. Therefore, we reasoned that both regenerating and growing nerves possess the machinery to stimulate the appropriate response in the neuron, as well as in the environment, needed for regeneration. Accordingly, we developed an experimental model using the adult rabbit (mammalian) visual system, which allowed application of exogenous soluble substances to crush-injured rabbit optic nerves (Solomon et al., 1985, see Figure 2). As an exogenous source for soluble substances we used CM of regenerating fish optic nerves assuming that the molecules involved in growth stimulation may not be species specific.

Our previous studies have shown that the application of these active substances to injured optic nerve of adult rabbit results in biochemical changes, reminiscent of regeneration, in the corresponding rabbit retinas (Hadani et al., 1984; Schwartz et al., 1985; Solomon et al., 1985; Stein-Izsak et al., 1985). These include a general increase in protein synthesis and elevation in labeling of a few polypeptides. Similar activity was observed when media conditioned by developing mammalian optic nerves (i.e. newborn rabbit optic nerves) were examined. These factors were therefore named collectively as growth associated triggering factors, GATFs (Hadani et al., 1984). A 300 dalton molecule isolated from fish CM was found to be responsible for the biochemical effect (Harel et al., unpublished data; Stein-Izsak et al., 1986b).

These biochemical changes in the retinas were accompanied also by morphological changes in the nerves as manifested by the survival of injured fibers and the appearance of growth cones in the treated injured nerves. The growth cones were observed adjacent to glial surfaces in regions in which large extracellular spaces were seen (Lavie et al., 1987). Similar morphological relationship between glial organiza-

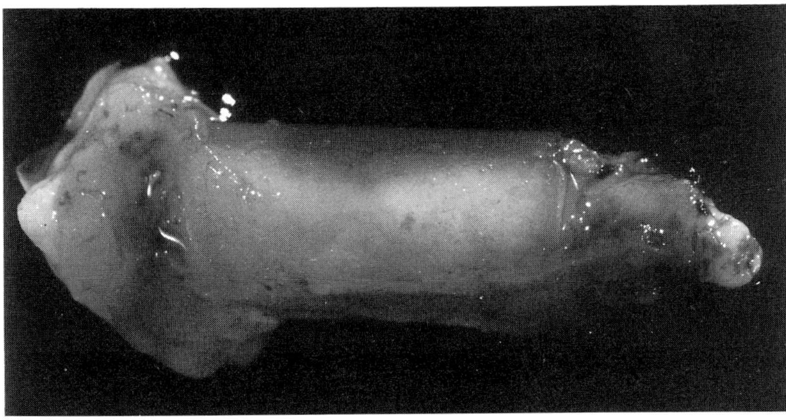

Fig. 2. Silicone tubes wrapped around an injured optic nerve of adult rabbit. The pictures show an excised nerve three weeks after the operation (For detailed experimental procedure see Solomon *et al.*, 1985)

tion, growth cones and extracellular spaces were seen in developing nerves (Schwartz *et al.*, 1987). The apparent changes in the glial cell surface caused by the active CM stimulated us to look for the presence of supportive elements at the surface of the glial cells.

Cell surface elements supportive of growth may include extracellular matrix components like collagen (Bunge *et al.*, 1980); laminin (Rogers *et al.*, 1983; Sanes, 1983); fibronectin (Schachner *et al.*, 1978); and glycosaminoglycans (Margolis and Margolis, 1979) which are pivotal for regeneration. *In vivo* and *in vitro* studies carried out in both the CNS and the PNS have provided evidence that laminin is one of the extracellular matrix components which has a key role in growth and regeneration (Carbonetto *et al.*, 1983; Carbonetto *et al.*, 1987; Evercooren *et al.*, 1982; Schwab and Thoenen, 1985). Moreover, a correlation was found between the ability of nerves to grow and the presence of an organized extracellular matrix which includes laminin. For example, in the fish visual system, similarly to PNS of mammals, laminin is continuously expressed and injury causes elevation in its level (Hopkins *et al.*, 1986; Leisi *et al.*, 1984a; Leisi, 1985).* The absence of laminin in the CNS of adult mammals was proposed as a reason for their poor ability to regenerate (Leisi *et al.*, 1983, 1984b). We therefore examined whether our observed morphological alterations, in the injured implanted rabbit optic nerves, expressed by apparent changes in glial cell surface, are associated with laminin.

Our results revealed that in intact adult rabbit optic nerves, laminin immunoreactive sites appeared in the epinerium and around the sparsley distributed blood vessels. Following injury, laminin immunoreactivity could be detected in the epinerium, in connective tissue surrounding blood vessels and in the scar tissue. However, after injury and implantation of media conditioned by regenerating fish optic nerves, the pattern of laminin immunoreactivity was changed and additional laminin-immunoreactive sites were detected. These appeared as a fine network coursing throughout the matrix of the nerves (Zak *et al.*, 1987). These results agree with the assumption that the absence of laminin, may be a cause for a poor inherent capacity to regenerate. These results also suggest that factor(s) in the CM may, at least partially, counteract this deficit.

The aforementioned studies suggest that the glial cells of mammals may be amenable to activation and that the non-neuronal cells of a regenerative system, like the fish optic nerve may contain the appropriate activators. In contrast, the injured mammalian CNS may not contain these activators or contain them but in an inaccessible form or at an inappropriate time. To test this hypothesis we have established an *in vitro* assay system where the ability to activate glial cells directly by active substances from fish can be tested and the isolation of the active components should thus be feasible (A. Cohen and M. Schwartz, in preparation).

--------------------

Analysis by light and electron microscopy of the fish optic nerves further supported the notion that the fish optic nerves are behaving like a peripheral nerve (Murray, 1976).

## 3.3 Regulation of the non-neuronal cell response to injury and proto-oncogenes

It has by now been well established that the response of the non-neuronal cells to nerve injury has an impact on the subsequent regeneration of the axon. Little is yet known, however, about the mechanisms regulating non-neuronal cell regenerative response. When the axon is injured, normal growth processes continue and additional regrowth processes are recruited. We hypothesized that the non-neuronal cells may require a compensatory mechanism for operating efficiently during transient changes in growth factor requirements created by the injury.

Cellular proto-oncogenes have been postulated to function in normal cellular proliferation and differentiation (see review by Bishop, 1985). We explored the possibility that they may also contribute to the regulation of regrowth of axons after axonal injury.

Our studies showed that non-neuronal cells surrounding intact fish optic nerves express sequences homologous to two nuclear proto-oncogenes, namely, fos and myc (Fig. 3). In response to injury the expression of these oncogenes is increased (Stein-Izsak *et al.* 1986) as was measured by dot blot of hybridization of fos probe to poly$(A)^+$ RNA from non-neuronal cells surrounding intact and regenerating fish optic nerves.

The constitutive expression of fos and myc might be attributable to the continuous growth of the retinas and optic nerves throughout the lifespan of the fish causing the visual system to behave, in part, as continuously developing tissue. The expression of fos and myc in the non-neuronal cells surrounding the fish optic nerves may be cell-specific or may be restricted to a certain nerve region, adjacent to the injury. This issue is currently being studied by the method of *in situ* hybridization.

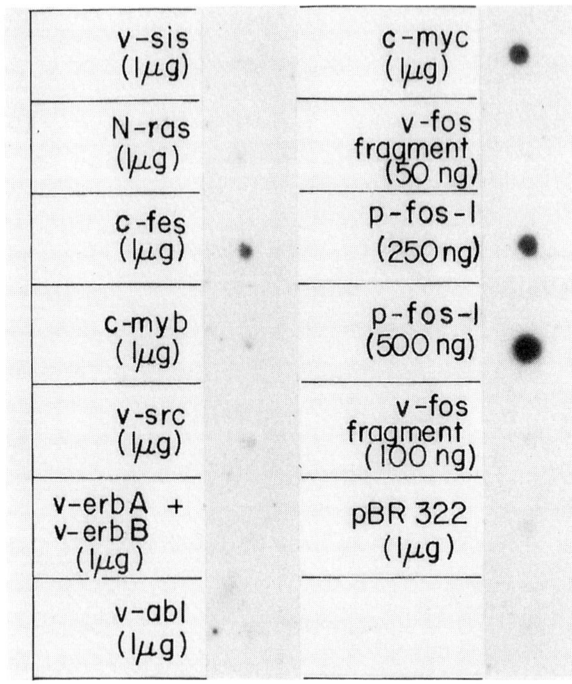


Fig. 3. Expression of the cellular proto-oncogenes *fos* and *myc* in non-neuronal cells from regenerating carp optic nerves. Dot blots of v-oncogene and c-oncogene plasmids or purified fragments were bound to nitrocellulose paper and hybridized with $^{32}$P-labelled cDNA probe from mRNA of regenerating carp optic nerves. A strong hybridization signal was obtained with *fos* and *myc* relative to the non-specific signal obtained for pBR322. At this exposure, hybridization with *fos* fragment (50ng; spot 9) could not be detected and was weakly visible with 100 ng (spot 12). No significant hybridization occurred to non-specific DNA such as pBR322 (spots 13 and 14). The irregular spot in the area of c-fes is due to non-specific hybridization. The oncogene plasmids used were: *c-fes*, human 3.9 Kb BamH1 fragment in P26 plasmid (Franchini *et al.* 1982); *c-myb*, human 2 Kb EcoR1 fragment in F8 plasmid; *v-src* 0.8 Kb PvuII fragment; PAE11, *v-erbA + v-erbB*, 5.5 Kb EcoR1 fragment; *v-abl*, HindIII-HincII 1.7 + 1.1Kb fragments; *c-myc*, *myc* 5PP, 2.2 Kb Pst 1 fragment (Dalla Favera et *al. 1982*); *p-fos*-1 is the clone of pFBJ2 (Curran *et al.* 1982).

The oncogene fragments used were: *v-sis*, 6 Kb BamH1 fragment (Gelman *et al.* 1981), *v-fos*, 1.0 Kb Pst 1 fragment (Curran *et al.* 1982).

Differential expression of fos has been found during embryonal and postnatal development of the mouse (Muller *et al.*, 1982, 1983, 1984). Similarly, transient increases in myc mRNA levels have been reported in neurons of the developing mouse cerebellum (Ruppert *et al.*, 1986). Experiments *in vitro* have demonstrated that expression of both fos and myc may be modulated by proliferative signals, including epidermal growth factor (EGF), platelet derived growth factor (PDGF) and nerve growth factor (NGF) stimulation (Bravo et al., 1985; Kruijer et al., 1984, 1985; Millbrandt, 1986). It is conceivable that factors whose presence or activity are injury-dependent and are involved in reciprocal interactions of axon-glial are part of the observed injury-induced modulation of these protooncogenes.

## 4. Conclusions

We have shown that after injury both the neurons and their surrounding non-neuronal cells are activated. The early response might be similar to a reparative response in any other proliferative tissue. This includes among many other early destructive events release of peroxides, activation of proteases and an active degradation (see Fig. 4). Efficient neutralization of peroxides by anti peroxidases, inhibition of proteases by protease inhibitors; and elimination of degradation products by the aid for example of apolipoproteins (presented in this work), are essential for paving the way for regeneration by bringing the system to a permissive stage (see Fig. 4).

The inability of the non-neuronal cells of mammals to achieve a reactive state and thereby to provide the needed substances to support growth at the right time may be a cause for the poor subsequent ability to regenerate. Perhaps, as our results indicate, the triggering factors provided by non-neuronal cells of growing nerves (regenerating or developing) can modulate and activate the "scar forming glial cells" in mammalian injured optic nerves. One manifestation for such activation is our observation of the appearance of laminin in the extracellular matrix of the injured rabbit optic nerves which had been treated with triggering factors from fish non-neuronal cells (Lavie et al., 1987; Zak et al., 1987). As laminin is absent from the CNS of adult mammals but is continuously expressed in the fish CNS, it is suggested that the absence of laminin might be a cause for the poor regenerative ability of CNS, and that it may be overcome by the active factors. Our recent preliminary results using glial cells in culture, indicate that the CM contains components which can directly activate glial cells to produce laminin (Cohen and Schwartz, in preparation).

The mechanism which regulate glial cell response to injury is as yet unknown. One such may require the involvement of protooncogenes which may participate in the response to injury and their protein products may be relevant to plasticity.

Further characterization of active components from the non-neuronal cells will give us means to increase their accessibility to the injured nerve in the right temporal sequence. We intend to further analyze the mode of action of these substances to determine the extent of anatomical regeneration and establish more efficient means for their application.

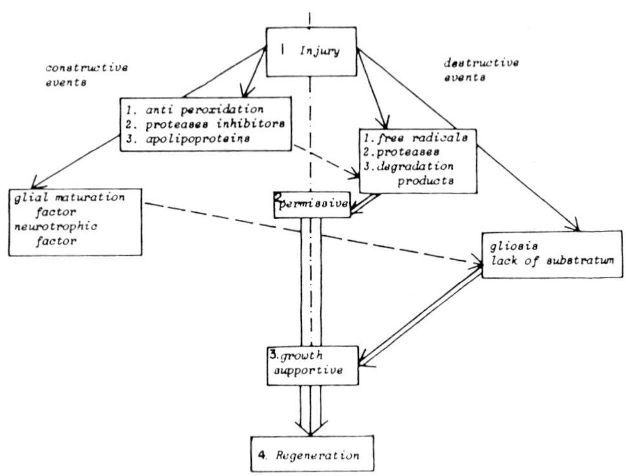


Fig. 4. Mile stones in the process of response to injury leading to regeneration.

Acknowledgment. This study was supported by U.S. Army Medical Research and Development command and by the Spinal Cord Injury Association-California Chapter given to M.S.

Literature


Agranoff BW, Feldman AM, Heacock AM, Schwartz M (1980) The retina as a biochemical model of the central nervous system regeneration. Neurochem 1:487.

Aguayo A, Samuel D, Dickson R, Trecarten Y (1978a) Axonal elongation in peripheral and central nervous system transplantations. Neurosci Lett 9:97.

Aguayo A, Samuel D, Richardson P, Bray G(1978b) Axonal elongation in peripheral and central nervous system transplantations. Adv Cell Neurobiol 3:215-221.

Attardi DG, Sperry RW (1963) Preferential selection of central pathways by regenerating optic nerve. Exp Neurol 7:46-64.

Benowitz LI, Yoon MG, Lewis ER, (1983) Transported proteins in regenerating optic nerve: Regulation by interactions with the optic tectum. Science 222:185.

Bishop MJ (1985) Viral oncogenes (review) Cell 42:23-28.

Bravo R, Burckhardt J, Curran T, Muller R (1985) Stimulation and inhibition of growth by EGF in different A-431 cell clones is accompanied by the rapid induction of c-fos and c-myc protooncogenes. EMBO J 4:1193-1197.

Bunge MB, Williams AK, Wood PM, Uitto J, Jeffrey JJ (1980) Comparison of nerve cell cultures with particular emphasis on basal lamina and collagen formation. J Cell Biol 84:184-202.

Burrell HR, Dokas LA, Agranoff BW (1978) RNA metabolism in the goldfish retina during optic nerve regeneration. J Neurochem 31:289.

Carbonetto S, Evans D, Cochard P (1987) New fiber growth in culture on tissue substrata from central and peripheral nervous system. J Neurosci 7:610-620.

Carbonetto S, Gruver MM, Turner DC (1983) Nerve fiber growth in culture on fibronectin, collagen, glycosaminoglycan substrates. J Neurosci 3:2324-2335.

Curran T, Peters, G., Van Beveren C, Teich NM and Verma IM (1982) FBJ murine osteosarcoma virus: Identification and molecular cloning of biologically active proviral DNA. J Virol 44:674-682.

Dalla Favera R, Gelmann EP, Martinotti S, Franchini G, Papas TS, Gallo RC and Wong-Staal F (1982) Cloning and characterization of different human sequences related to the onc gene (v-myc) of avian myelocytomatosis virus (MC29). Proc Natl Acad Sci USA 79:6497-6501.

David S, Aguayo AJ (1981) Axonal elongation into peripheral nervous system "bridges" after central nervous system injury in adult rats. Science 214:931-933.

Dawson PA, Schechter N, Williams DL (1986) Induction of rat E and chicken A-I apolipoproteins and mRNAs during optic nerve degeneration. J Biol Chem 261:5681-5684.

Franchini G, Gelmann EP, Dalla Favera R, Gallo RC and Wong-Staal F (198) Human gene (c-fes) related to the onc sequences of Snyder-Theilen feline sarcoma virus. Mol and Cell Biol 2:1014-1019.

Gelmann EP, Wong-Staal F, Kramer RA and Gallo RC (1981) Molecular cloning and comparative analyses of the genomes of Simian sarcoma virus and its associated helper virus. Proc. natl. Acad. Sci. USA 78:3373-3377.

Giulian D, Allen RL, Baker TJ, Tomozawa Y (1986) Brain peptides and glial growth. I. Glia-promoting factors as regulator of gliogenesis in the developing and injured central nervous system. J Cell Biol 102:803.

Goldberg S (1976) Central nervous system regeneration and ophtalmology. Ophtalmol 20:261.

Grafstein B, McQuarrie IG (1978) Role of nerve cell body in axonal regeneration. In, Neuronal plasticity (C.M. Cofman, ed.) New York, Raven Press, New York, 155.

Guth L, Windle W (1970) The enigma of central nervous system regeneration. Exp Neurol Suppl 5:1-43.

Hadani M, Harel A, Solomon A, Belkin M, Lavie V, Schwartz M (1984) Substances originating from the optic nerve of neonatal rabbit induce regeneration-associated response in the injured optic nerve of adult rabbit. Proc Natl Acad Sci USA 81:7965-7969.

Harel A, Fainaru M, Shafer Z, Schwartz M (1987) Optic nerve regeneration in adult fish is associated with accumulation of apolipoprotein-A-I manifested preferentially in one isoform. Submitted.

Harel A, Rubinstein M, Solomon A, Belkin M, Schwartz M (1987) Isolation of a growth associated triggering factor from regenerating optic nerve. J Neurochem (Abst) in press.

Hopkins JM, Ford-Holevnski TS, McCoy JP, Agranoff BW (1985) Laminin and optic nerve regeneration in the goldfish. J. of Neurosci 5:3030-3038.

Ignatius MJ, Gebicke-Harter PJ, Skene JHP, Schilling JW, Weisgraber KH, Mahley RW, Shooter EM (1986) Proc Natl Acad Sci USA 83:1125-1129.

Kao CC, Chang LW, Bloodworth JMB Jr (1977) Axonal regeneration across transected mammalian spinal cords: An electron microscopic study of delayed microsurgical grafting. Exp Neurol 54:591-615.

Kiernan JA (1979) Hypotheses concerned with axonal regeneration in the mammalian nervous system. Biol Rev 54:155-197.

Kohsaka S, Schwartz M, Agranoff BW (1981) Increased activity of ornithine decarboxylase in goldfish following optic nerve crush. Dev Brain Res 1:391.

Kruijer W, Schubert D, Verma IM (1985) Induction of the protooncogenes fos by nerve growth factor. Proc Natl Acad Sci USA 82:7330-7334.

Landerth GE, Agranoff BW (1976) Explant culture of adult goldfish retina, effect of prior optic nerve crush. Brain Res 118:299.

Landerth GE, Agranoff, BW (1979) Explant cultures from adult goldfish retina, a model for the study of CNS regeneration. Brain Res 161:39.

Lavie V, Harel A, Doron A, Solomon A, Lobel D, Belkin M, Benbasat S, Sharma S, Schwartz M (1987) Morphological response of injured adult rabbit optic nerve to implant containing neonatal derived substances. Brain Res in press.

Liesi P (1985) Laminin-immunoreactive glia distinguish regenerative adult central nervous systems form non-regenerative ones. EMBO J 4:2505-2511.

Liesi P, Dahl D, Vaheri A (1983) Laminin is produced by early rat astrocytes in primary culture. J Cell Biol 96:920-924.

Liesi P, Dahl D, Vaheri A (1984a) Neurons cultured from developing rat brain attach and spread preferentially to laminin. J Neurosci Res 11:241-251.

Liesi P, Kaakola S, Dahl D, Vaheri A (1984b) Laminin is induced in astrocytes of adult brain by injury. EMBO J 3:683-686.

Longo FM, Skaper SD, Manthorpe M, Lundborg G, Varon S (1983) Temporal changes in neuronotrophic activaties accumulate in vivo within nerve regeneration chambers. Brain Res 261:109.

Longo FM, Manthorpe M, Varon S (1982) Spinal cord neurotrophic factors (SCNTFs), 1. Bioassay of schwannoma and other conditioned media. Dev Brain Res 3:277.

Lundborg G, Longo FM, Varon S (1982) Nerve regeneration model and trophic factors in vivo. Brain Res 232:157-161.

Manthorpe M, Engrall E, Ruoslahti E, Longo FM, Davis GE, Varon S (1983) Laminin promotes neuritic regeneration from cultured peripheral and central neurons. J Cell Biol 97:1882-1890.

Manthorpe M, Longo FM, Varon S (1982) Comparative features of spinal neurotrophic factors in fluids collected in vitro and in vivo. J Neurosci Res 8:241-250.

Margolis RV, Margolis RK (1979) Complex carbohydrates of nervous tissue. Plenum Press New York.

McConnell P, Berry M (1982) Regeneration of ganglion cell axons in the adult mouse retina. Brain Res 241:362-366.

Milbrandt J (1986) Nerve growth factor rapidly induces c-fos mRNA in PC 12 rat pheochromocytoma cells. Proc Natl Acad Sci USA 83:4789-4793.

Mizrachi, Y., Rubinstein, M., Kimhi, Y. and Schwartz, M. (1985) Neurotrophic factor derived from goldfish brain: characterization and purification. J. Neurochem. 46, 1675-1682.

Monard D, Niday E, Limat A, Solomon F. (1983) Inhibition of protease activity can lead to neurite extension in neuroblastoma cells. Prog Brain Res 58:359-365.

Muller HW, Gebicke-Harter PJ, Hangen DH, Shooter EM (1985) A specific 37,000-dalton protein that accumulates in regenerating but not in non-regenerating mammalian nerves. Science 228:499-501.

Muller R, Bravo R, Burckhardt J, Curran T (1984) Induction of c-fos gene and protein by growth factors precedes activation of c-myc. Nature 716-720.

Muller R, Slamon DJ, Thrembray JM, CLine MJ, Verma IM (1982) Differential expression of cellular oncogenes during pre- and post-natal development of the mouse. Nature 299:640-644.

Muller R, Verma IM, Adamson ED (1983) Expression of c-onc genes: c-fos transcripts accumulate to high levels during development of mouse placenta, yolk sac and amnion. EMBO J 2:679-684.

Murray M (1973) $^{3}$H-Uridine incorporation by regenerating retinal ganglion cells of goldfish. Exp Neurol 39:489.

Murray M (1976) Regeneration of retinal axons into the goldfish optic tectum. J Comp Neurol 168:175.

Neumann D, Yerushalmi A, Schwartz M (1983) Inhibition of non-neuronal cell prolfieration in the goldfish visual pathway affects the regenerative capacity of the retinas. Brain Res 272:237-245.

Nieto-Sampedro M, Lewis ER, Cotman CW, Manthorpe M, Skaper SD, Brabi G, Longo FM, Varon S (1982) Brain injury causes a time-dependent increase in neurotrophic activity at the lesion site. Science 217:860-861.

Nieto-Sampedro M, Manthorpe M, Barbin G, Varon S, Cotman CW (1983) Injury-induced neuronotrophic activity in adult rat brain: Correlation with survival of delayed impalnsts in the wound cavity. J Neurosci 3:2219-2289.

Pitas RE, Boyles JK, Lee SH, Foss D, Mahley RW (1987) Astrocytes synthesize apolipoprotein E and metabolize apolipoprotein-containing lipoproteins. Biochem Biophys Acta 917:148-161.

Rachailovich I, Schwartz M (1984) Molecular events associated with increased regenerative capacity of the goldfish retinal ganglion cells following X-irradiation: decreased level of axonal growth inhibitors. Brain Res 306:149-155.

Ramon y Cajal S (1928) Degeneration and regeneration of the nervous system. English translation and reprint (1959) Hafner Press, New York.

Richardson PM, Issa VMK (1984) Peripheral injury enhances central regeneration of primary sensory neurons. Nature 309:791-793.

Richardson PM, McGuinness UM, Aguayo AJ (1982) Peripheral nerve autografts to the rat spinal cord: Studies with axonal tracing methods. Brain Res 237:147-162.

Rogers SL, Letourneau PC, Palm SL, McCarthy J, Furcht LT (1983) Neurite extension by peripheral and central nervous system neurons in response to substratum-bound fibronectin and laminin. Dev Biol 98:212-220.

Ruppert C, Goldowitz D, Willie W (1986) Proto-oncogene c-myc is expressed in cerebellar neurons of different developmental stages. EMBO J 5:1897-1901.

Sanes JR (1983) Roles of extracellular matrix in neural development. Ann Rev Physiol 45:581-600.

Evercooren Baron-van A, Klienman HK, Ohno S, Marangos D, Schwatz JP, Dubois-Dalcq ME (1982) Nerve growth factor, laminin, and fibronectin promote neurite growth in human fetal sensory ganglia cultures. J Neurosci Res 8:179-193.
Schachner M, Schoonmaker G, Hynes RO (1978) Cellular and subcellular localization of LETS protein in the nervous system. Brain Res 158:149-158.
Schwab, ME, Thoenen H (1985) Dissociated neurons regenerate into sciatic but not optic nerve explants in culture irrespective of neurotrophic factors. J of Neurosci 5:2415-2423.
Schwartz M, Belkin M, Harel A, Solomon A, Lavie V, Hadani M, Rachailovich I, Stein-Izsak C (1985) Regenerating fish optic nerves and regeneration-like response in injured optic nerve of adult rabbits. Science 228:600-603.
Schwartz M, Harel A, Stein-Izsak C, Solomon A, Bawnik Y and Belkin M (1987) Growth associated triggering factors and central nervous system response to injury. in "Pharmacological Approaches to the Treatment of Brain and Spinal Cord Injuries" (edited by Drs. DG Stein and B Sabel. Plenum Publishing Corporation NY) in press.
Skene JHP, Shooter EM (1983) Denervated sheath cells secrete a new protein after nerve injury. Proc Natl Acad Sci USA 80:4169-4173.
Skene JHP, Willard M (1981a) Changes in axonally transported proteins during axon regeneration in toad retinal ganglion cells. J Cell Biol 89:86-95.
Skene JHP, Willard M (1981b) Axonally transported proteins associated with axon growth in rabbit central and peripheral nervous systems. J Cell Biol 89:96-103.
Skene JHP, Willard M (1981c) Characteristics of growth associated proteins (GAPs) in regenerating toad retinal ganglion axons. J Neurosci 1:419-425.
Snipes GJ, McGuire CB, Norden JJ, Freeman JA (1986) Proc Natl Acad Sci USA 83:1130-1134.
Solomon A, Belkin M, Hadani M, Harel A, Rachailovich I, Lavie V, Schwartz M (1985) A new transorbital approach to the rabbits optic nerve. J Neurosci Metho 12:259-262.
Stein-Izsak C, Harel A, Solomon A, Belkin M, Schwartz M (1985) Alterations in mRNA translation products are associated with regenerative response in the retina. J Neurochem 45:1754-1760.
Stein-Izsak C, Brener O and Schwartz M (1986) Expression of the proto-oncogenes fos and myc in optic nerve regeneration. Abst. Neurosci., 12, 12.
Willard M, Skene JH (1982) Molecular events in axonal regeneration In: Repair and regeneration of the nervous system (Nicholls JG ed) Dahlem Konferenzen, Springer-Verlag Berlin Heidelberg New York 71.
Williams LR, Varon S (1985) Modification of fibrin matrix formation in situ enhances nerve regeneration in silicone chambers. J Comp Neurol 231:209-220.
Zak NB, Harel A, Bawnik Y, Benbasat S, Vogel Z, Schwartz M (1987) Laminin immunoreactive sites are induced by growth-associated triggering factors in injured rabbit optic nerve. Brain Res, in press.

Abbreviations: CNS, central nervous system; PNS, peripheral nervous system; CM, conditioned media; GATF, growth-associated triggering factor; apo-A-I, apolipoprotein-A-I; kDa, kilodaltons, IEF, isoelectrofocusing.

# NEURONAL RESCUE IN CEREBELLAR CULTURES

Fredrick J. Seil
Neurology Research (151N)
Veterans Administration Medical Center and
Department of Neurology
Oregon Health Sciences University
Portland, Oregon 97201
USA

## INTRODUCTION

Cerebellar explants derived from neonatal mice and maintained in Maximow chambers for 2-3 weeks develop many of the features of cerebellum *in vivo* (Seil, 1979). The 5 major classes of cortical neurons are proportionally represented, including Purkinje, Golgi, basket, stellate and granule cells, the last being the only excitatory neurons in the cerebellar cortex (Eccles *et al.*, 1967). Normal synaptic relationships develop between these cortical neurons *in vitro* (Seil, 1979; Herndon *et al.*, 1981; Blank and Seil, 1982). The expected neuron-glia interactions also occur in this culture system, and Purkinje cell somata and dendrites are ensheathed by astrocytes, and oligodendrocytes myelinate myelin-receptive axons. The normal extracerebellar afferents, are not, however, present in significant numbers in these isolated explants.

We have developed a tissue culture model of neural plasticity by taking advantage of the fact that granule cell precursors are dividing neuroblasts at the time of explantation (Seil *et al.*, 1980). The granule cell precursors are therefore destroyed by exposure to cytosine arabinoside (Ara C), a DNA synthesis inhibitor. The Ara C is incorporated into the nutrient medium in a 5-10 ug/ml

NATO ASI Series, Vol. H22
Neural Development and Regeneration.
Edited by A. Gorio et al.

concentration for the first 5 days *in vitro* (DIV). After this period, the cultures are maintained in normal nutrient medium. Such granuloprival cultures can be observed for organizational changes that take place among the remaining neuronal groups to compensate for the missing elements.

A secondary effect of Ara C exposure is the destruction of some of the glial population and an arrest of maturation of the surviving glia (Seil *et al.*, 1980; Blank *et al.*, 1982). The lack of functional glia also plays a prominent role in the organizational changes that occur in granuloprival cerebellar cultures.

## GRANULOPRIVAL CEREBELLAR CULTURES

A striking feature at the light microscopic level of examination of granuloprival cultures from about 9 DIV on is the presence of a great number of closely packed large cortical neurons, which are predominantly Purkinje cells (Seil *et al.*, 1980). There is an associated paucity of smaller nuclei and a lack of cortical lamination. In quantitative terms, the number of large cortical neurons in Ara C treated cultures is 3-4 times the number in normal cerebellar explants (Seil, 1987).

Equally remarkable is the tremendous increase in the number of neurites observed in silver stained preparations of granuloprival cultures (Seil *et al.*, 1980). By fiber tracing, these increased neurites prove to be primarily sprouted Purkinje cell recurrent axon collaterals, which are present in an excess number per Purkinje cell. That these sprouted recurrent axon collaterals are functional is indicated by extracellular electrophysiological recording. Retrograde stimulation of Purkinje cells produces a dramatic inhibition of spontaneous cortical activity in Ara C treated explants, as compared with no remarkable change or a transient increase in cortical spontaneous activity (disinhibition) in normal cultures.

At the ultrastructural level (Blank *et al.*, 1982) most of

the numerous Purkinje cell dendritic spines, which are normally occupied by granule cell axon (parallel fiber) terminals, now make synapses with Purkinje cell recurrent axon collateral terminals. A few spines remain unattached. Purkinje cell somata and proximal dendrites have no or incomplete astrocytic sheaths, and the somata are hyperinnervated by excess recurrent axon collateral terminals. Another manifestation of the Ara C effect on glia is the absence of myelin in Ara C treated cultures.

The changes related to Purkinje cells, granule cells and astrocytes that take place in Ara C treated as compared with normal cerebellar cultures are presented diagrammatically in Fig. 1 (upper two panels). The normal Purkinje cell has an astrocytic sheath (stippled) and projects recurrent axon collaterals to nearby Purkinje cells. Not shown is the projection of the Purkinje cell axon, which for most Purkinje cells is to the intracerebellar (deep) nuclei, as this is not germane to the studies presented here. Granule cells are present, and their axons (dashed lines) contact the Purkinje cell dendritic spines. The granule cells are absent in the Ara C treated culture, and 3-4 times as many Purkinje cells survive _in vitro_. The Purkinje cells are not or are only minimally ensheathed by astrocytes. There is a sprouting of Purkinje recurrent axon collaterals, which make heterologous synapses with most Purkinje cell dendritic spines in the absence of parallel fibers and extracerebellar afferents, and which hyperinnervate unensheathed Purkinje cell somata.

## TRANSPLANTED GRANULOPRIVAL CULTURES

After Ara C treated cerebellar cultures have become reorganized in response to a lack of granule cells and functional glia, the missing elements can be fully or partially restored by transplantation with granule cells and glia, or with glia alone. Such cultures can be observed for further organizational changes as a consequence of transplantation.

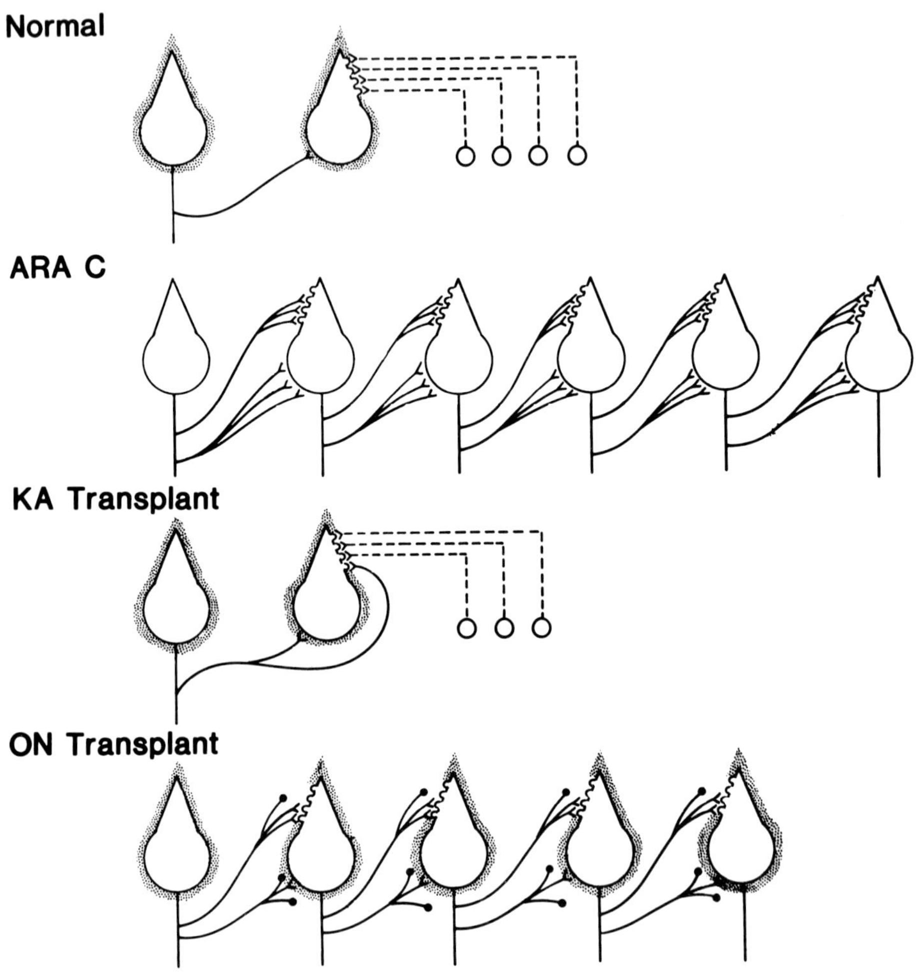


Fig. 1 Schematic representation of relations between granule cells (small circles), Purkinje cells (large circles with cones) and astrocytes (stippled regions around Purkinje cells) in normal cerebellar cultures, cerebellar cultures treated with cytosine arabinoside (Ara C) and Ara C treated cultures transplanted with cerebellar explants exposed to kainic acid (KA transplant) or with fragments of optic nerve (ON transplant). Granule cell axons (parallel fibers) are indicated by dashed lines and Purkinje cell axons and axon collaterals are indicated as solid lines. Only proximal portions of Purkinje cell axons are shown, to just beyond the

Transplantation with Granule Cells and Glia

Exposure of cerebellar cultures to $10^{-4}$ M kainic acid, a glutamate analog, for the first 5 DIV results in destruction of all cortical neurons except granule cells (Seil et al., 1979). Glia remain intact in such preparations. Kainate exposed cerebellar cultures are thus complementary to granuloprival explants, in that the former contain the granule cells and functional glia not present in the latter. Kainic acid treated cultures can be detached from their collagen substrates at 9 DIV and superimposed upon 9 or 16 DIV host granuloprival explants (Seil et al., 1983).

Axonal myelin is visible 3-5 days after transplantation in 80% of cultures observed in the living state (Seil and Blank, 1981). The number of large cortical neurons is reduced to normal (Seil, 1987). The excess sprouted Purkinje cell axon collaterals are also remarkably reduced (Seil et al., 1983). Functionally, inhibition of spontaneous cortical discharges is no longer obtainable with retrograde stimulation of Purkinje cell axons. At the ultrastructural level (Blank and Seil, 1983), most Purkinje cell dendritic spines make synaptic contact with parallel fiber terminals, although occasional recurrent axon collateral-dendritic spine synapses remain. Purkinje cells are ensheathed by astrocytes, and the Purkinje cell somata and proximal dendrites are no longer hyperinnervated by recurrent axon collateral terminals.

origins of the recurrent axon collaterals. Purkinje cell somata are diagrammed as circular and Purkinje cell dendrites as conical elements, with dendritic spines represented by projections from the cones. Synapse forming terminals are indicated as "Y" shaped, and non-synapsing terminals in bottom panel as dots. Please see text for details.

Some of the changes induced by transplantation with granule cells and glia are schematized in the third panel of Fig. 1 (KA transplant). Granule cells are restored in the host explants, although in probably less than normal numbers. Their axons synapse with most of the Purkinje cell dendritic spines, while occasional recurrent axon collateral-dendritic spine synapses persist. The Purkinje cell number is reduced to normal and Purkinje cells are ensheathed by astrocytes. The number of sprouted recurrent axon collaterals is reduced to normal or near normal, and the collaterals no longer hyperinnervate Purkinje cell somata.

## Transplantation with Glia Alone

Mouse optic nerve constitutes a source of glia without granule cells. Fragments of 7-8 day optic nerve are superimposed upon 13 or 14 DIV granuloprival cultures. Axonal myelination is also observed in such transplanted granuloprival cultures, but less frequently than when transplanted with kainate treated explants. The large cortical neuron population is reduced by approximately 25% (Seil, 1987), and the excess sprouted recurrent axon collaterals in the host explants are not appreciably reduced (Meshul and Seil, 1987). Purkinje cells are ensheathed by astrocytes, and the number of axosomatic synapses on Purkinje cells is markedly reduced (Meshul *et al.*, 1987), in spite of the persistence of excess recurrent axon collaterals. Moreover, the number of synapses (predominantly axospinous) in the neuropil is also reduced, though to a lesser degree (Meshul and Seil, 1987).

These changes are summarized in the lowest panel in Fig. 1 (ON transplant). The Purkinje cell population is modestly reduced and the Purkinje cells are ensheathed by astrocytes. Excess Purkinje cell recurrent axon collaterals persist, but both axosomatic and axospinous synapses formed by the terminals of these axons are reduced.

## DISCUSSION AND CONCLUSIONS

There is an interesting interplay between Purkinje cells, granule cells and astrocytes in these tissue culture models. Astrocytes can effect a reduction of both axosomatic and axospinous synapses when added to granuloprival cultures, and thus play a role in synapse regulation. The presence of granule cells, however, appears to be necessary to reduce to normal the large cortical neuron population and the number of sprouted Purkinje cell recurrent axon collaterals, both of which are present to great excess in granuloprival cultures.

The question can then be posed as to why increased numbers of Purkinje cells survive in granuloprival cultures, and why they sprout excess recurrent axon collaterals. We have postulated (Seil et al., 1980; Seil, 1987) that both of these phenomena are related to available synaptic sites (Purkinje cell dendritic spines) resulting from destruction of the granule cells. The availability of Purkinje cell somatic sites for hyperinnervation by recurrent axon collateral terminals in the absence of functional astrocytes in Ara C treated cultures seems to be a less important stimulus for sprouting. When cerebellar cultures are exposed to Ara C preparations that do not inhibit astrocyte maturation, with resulting astrocytic ensheathment of Purkinje cells and the presence of a normal number of axosomatic synapses, excess neurites are nevertheless present (Seil, F.J. and Meshul, C.K., unpublished observations).

Purkinje cells develop dendritic spines autonomously in the absence of afferent innervation (Herndon, et al., 1971; Hirano and Zimmerman, 1973; Jones and Gardner, 1976). Although not indicated in correct proportion in Fig. 1, many more synaptic sites are available on dendritic spines than on somata or proximal dendrites. In the absence in granuloprival cultures of parallel fibers that normally contact these spines, and of climbing and mossy fiber afferents that, if present, might have priority for synapsing with Purkinje cell dendritic spines (Llinas et al., 1973), the spines are occupied by Purkinje cell recurrent axon collateral terminals (Blank _et al._, 1982). Thus Purkinje cell dendritic spine sites made available by the destruction of granule cells constitute a tremendously expanded target field for the axon collaterals of other Purkinje cells, resulting in increased Purkinje cell survival. This is analogous to the rescue of neurons from naturally occurring cell death during development by increasing the size of the target with which synaptic connections are made (Hollyday and Hamburger, 1976; Cowan _et al._, 1984; Oppenheim, 1985). The analogy is not strict, however, for in the _in vitro_ situation the Purkinje cells are being rescued from an "artificially occurring cell death," as it is estimated that only about 25% of the starting population of neurons survives in the culture environment (Sobkowicz et al., 1968; Seil, 1979, 1987).

The argument that increased numbers of Purkinje cells survive _in vitro_ because available Purkinje cell dendritic spines form an expanded target field for heterologous synapse formation with Purkinje cell recurrent axon collateral terminals seems circular. However, it is supported by the fact that the Purkinje cell numbers in granuloprival cultures return to normal after transplantation with granule cells and the subsequent appearance of parallel fiber-Purkinje cell dendritic spine synapses.

In that the projecting neurons that are "rescued" and the target neurons are one and the same, other factors that might contribute to neuronal rescue, such as retrogradely transported, target supplied trophic factors (Cowan _et al._, 1984; Oppenheim, 1985), would seem not to be important in this model. It is possible, however, that the astrocyte induced synapse reduction described with optic nerve transplantation (Meshul _et al._, 1987; Meshul and Seil, 1987) may contribute to the modest reduction (25%) of Purkinje cells observed in such cultures (Seil, 1987).

Because the projecting and target neurons are the same cells in this _in vitro_ model, the conditions that promote neuronal survival may be more limited than those that prevail in most _in vivo_ systems. The tissue culture model presented here does, however, emphasize the importance of the size of the target field (as indicated by the number of available synaptic sites) in determining the proportion of the projecting neuronal population that survives.

## ACKNOWLEDGMENTS

Supported by the Veterans Administration and by NIH grant NS 17493.

## REFERENCES

Blank NK, Seil FJ (1982) Mature Purkinje cells in cerebellar tissue cultures: An ultrastructural study. J Comp Neurol 208:169-176

Blank NK, Seil FJ (1983) Reorganization in granuloprival cerebellar cultures after transplantation of granule cells and glia. II. Ultrastructural studies. J Comp Neurol 214:267-278

Blank NK, Seil FJ, Herndon RM (1982) An ultrastructural study of cortical remodeling in cytosine arabinoside induced granuloprival cerebellum in tissue culture. Neuroscience 7:1509-1531

Cowan WM, Fawcett JW, O'Leary DDM, Stanfield BB (1984) Regressive events in neurogenesis. Science 225:1258-1265

Eccles JC, Ito M, Szentagothai J (1967) The cerebellum as a neuronal machine. Springer, Berlin Heidelberg New York

Herndon RM, Margolis G, Kilham L (1971) The synaptic organization of the malformed cerebellum induced by perinatal infection with the feline panleukopenia virus (PLV). II. The Purkinje cell and its afferents. J Neuropathol Exp Neurol 30:557-570

Herndon RM, Seil FJ, Seidman C (1981) Synaptogenesis in mouse cerebellum: A comparative <u>in vivo</u> and tissue culture study. Neuroscience 6:2587-2598

Hirano A, Zimmerman HM (1973) Aberrant synaptic development. Arch Neurol (Chicago) 28:359-366

Hollyday M, Hamburger V (1976) Reduction of the naturally occurring motor neuron loss by enlargement of the periphery. J Comp Neurol 170:311-320

Jones MZ, Gardner E (1976) The pathogenesis of methylazoxymethanol-induced lesions in the postnatal mouse cerebellum. J Neuropathol Exp Neurol 35:413-444

Llinas R, Hillman DE, Precht W (1973) Neuronal circuit reorganization in mammalian agranular cerebellar cortex. J Neurobiol 4:69-94

Meshul CK, Seil FJ (1987) Transplanted astrocytes reduce synaptic density in the neuropil of cerebellar cultures. Submitted for publication

Meshul CK, Seil FJ, Herndon RM (1987) Astrocytes play a role in regulation of synaptic density. Brain Res 402:139-145

Oppenheim RW (1985) Naturally occurring cell death during neural development. Trends Neurosci 8:487-493

Seil FJ (1979) The cerebellum in tissue culture. In: Schneider DM (ed) Reviews of neuroscience, vol 4. Raven, New York, p 105

Seil FJ (1987) Enhanced Purkinje cell survival in granuloprival cerebellar cultures. Submitted for publication

Seil FJ, Blank NK (1981) Myelination of central nervous system axons in tissue culture by transplanted oligodendrocytes. Science 212:1407-1408

Seil FJ, Blank NK, Leiman AL (1979) Toxic effects of kainic acid on mouse cerebellum in tissue culture. Brain Res 161:253-265

Seil FJ, Leiman AL, Woodward WR (1980) Cytosine arabinoside effects on developing cerebellum in tissue culture. Brain Res 186:393-408

Seil FJ, Blank NK, Leiman AL (1983) Reorganization in granuloprival cerebellar cultures after transplantation of granule cells and glia. I. Light microscopic and electrophysiological studies. J Comp Neurol 214:258-266

Sobkowicz HM, Guillery RW, Bornstein MB (1968) Neuronal organization in long term cultures of the spinal cord of the fetal mouse. J Comp Neurol 132:365-395

# AXONAL REGENERATION IN THE CONTEXT OF SPINAL CORD TRAUMA

A. R. Blight
Departments of Neurosurgery
and Physiology & Biophysics
New York University Medical Center
550 First Avenue
New York, NY 10016

The possibility of repairing spinal cord injuries remains an important practical stimulus for studies in the basic cell biology of axonal regeneration. Much phenomenology of degeneration and regeneration in the central nervous system (CNS) has derived from attempts to produce in higher vertebrates the kind of spontaneous recovery of function seen following complete spinal cord transection in lower vertebrate species. The history of those attempts is sometimes not the stuff of scientific textbooks, though it includes illuminating examples of the response of the mind when faced with a complex intellectual barrier to an apparently achievable goal held up by Nature. There is perhaps a rough analogy with the history of aviation before the twentieth century. It may not be wise at this stage, therefore, to deprecate too fiercely the potential contribution of inventive approaches, nor to follow blindly the scientific tradition of overestimating the necessity of basic understanding for practical implementation (Kuhn, 1971). As scientists, we are faced with dismantling the intellectual barrier, but it would be obviously of great advantage if some more empirical approach were first to find a way around it.

Studies of regeneration in the CNS have been reviewed extensively by others (e.g. Berry, 1979; Kiernan, 1979; Veraa and Grafstein 1981; Reier et al. 1983). The purpose of this short account is primarily to draw attention to some contextual features of spinal cord trauma that affect the questions to be asked of axonal regeneration and the ways that they may be addressed. Those who study cellular mechanisms of neurite growth are used to considering the transected spinal cord as a single example from the wider field of development and regeneration. Similarly, from the viewpoint of those interested primarily in the spinal cord and its reaction to injury, axonal regeneration is only one of several possible avenues of approach to minimizing deficits and promoting recovery of function. Though it seems potentially the most important approach, it may not be the most attainable, nor by itself necessarily sufficient for the desired clinical end.

NATO ASI Series, Vol. H22
Neural Development and Regeneration
Edited by A. Gorio et al.

*Ugly pathology and the clean experiment*

Our knowledge of the cell biological context of human spinal cord injuries is unfortunately limited and what we know is unpleasant from the scientific point of view. Injuries vary widely in type, position and extent and there is no satisfying classification (e.g. Kakulas and Bedbrook 1976; Jellinger 1976). They invite neither painstaking pathological reconstruction nor accurate experimental modelling. Two main experimental approaches have been taken to examining the elements of this pathology. Contusive or compressive (crushing) lesions of a short length of the cord have been the preferred means of testing experimental methods of reducing putative acute secondary damage. Attempts to promote regenerative responses, on the other hand, have relied mostly on cutting spinal tracts, particularly on cutting the entire spinal cord. The reasons for this dichotomy are methodologically sound. A crushing lesion is essential for studying secondary effects associated with crushing but it is quite unsatisfactory if we wish to know precisely the extent of the primary lesion. To identify regenerating axons it is usually necessary to know that they must have been severed originally. Total cord transection, on the other hand, limits the questions that can be asked and results in lesions that are different in kind from the 'typical' clinical case.

These differences are not trivial. The cut usually transects the major longitudinal blood vessels, which the contusion does not, yet it produces more restricted primary neuronal damage than the crush. A transection also completely separates the tissue environments of the proximal and distal segments of the cord. This immediately sets up a requirement for some kind of bridge between the proximal and distal CNS compartments if regrowth of axons is to proceed. First, there may be a mechanical requirement to bind the two ends of the cord together against the tendency of body movements and spinal cord elasticity to separate them. Secondly, there is the need for a substrate for growth. Therefore the transection model has already introduced an inessential first step in the problem of studying and promoting regeneration - the goal of achieving a mechanical and parenchymal bridge. A number of studies have successfully demonstrated an ability to provide such a bridge, at least for limited growth into the distal stump, of which peripheral nerve grafts have provided the most striking example (Kiernan 1979; David and Aguayo 1981; Richardson et al 1984)), though embryonic tissue grafting also shows considerable promise (Nornes et al. 1983; Reier et al. 1983, 1985; Bregman and Reier 1986). Recently, human amnion membrane has also been reported to act as an effective substrate for axonal bridging in the CNS (Davis et al. 1987). These in themselves have been highly significant steps, with potential practical implications, but they remain somewhat supplementary to the issue of axonal regeneration *within* the adult CNS.

*Observations from complete transection*

The effect of complete transection of the mammalian spinal cord has been studied in detail in a number of species (see Ramón y Cajal 1928; Matthews et al 1979b; Reier et al. 1983). Some consistent effects of spinal cord transection may be enumerated as follows:
1) The two ends of the severed spinal cord may separate a short distance immediately, as a result of residual tension in the tissue and its normal tendency for movement along the vertebral canal.
2) Over the course of several days, the two ends undergo additional necrosis and axons die back a few millimeters, though there is often fusing of pia-arachnoid elements across the gap.
3) The CNS tissue surrounding the lesion becomes vacuolated and invaded by peripheral and meningeal elements - Schwann cells, fibroblasts, and a few peripheral nerve collaterals.
4) The plane of transection is eventually occupied by a dense transverse collagenous scar.
5) The limited regenerative responses that occur in a small proportion of axons do not generally lead to bridging of the scar, and they are often later displaced entirely by cystic expansion at the lesion site.
6) There may be considerable loss of neurons remote from the lesion as a secondary effect of axotomy or massive deafferentation (Feringa 1984; Eidelberg 1986).

*Observations from Contusion Injuries*

Despite their general unsuitability as tools for studying regeneration, contusion models can provide useful insight into the cell biology of spinal cord trauma. The chronic pathology of contusion injuries is similar to many naturally occurring lesions described in the clinical literature, albeit at the relatively gross structural level available there (see Kakulas and Bedbrook 1976; Jellinger 1976; Bresnahan et al. 1976; Blight 1983, 1985; Blight and DeCrescito 1986). Some characteristics of the chronic contusion lesion may be enumerated as follows:
1) Central necrosis often results in cystic cavitation that can be longitudinally extensive and both radially and longitudinally highly variable in extent.
2) In all but the most extreme cases, there is some survival of CNS tissue - axons and glial cells - around the outer rim of the cord throughout the lesion. The degree of chronic functional recovery associated with these surviving pathways can be quite variable, and clearly does not involve a simple linear relationship between surviving axon number and functional outcome.

3) The large volume of tissue necrosis involved in the initial lesion results in intense phagocytic activity in the first weeks after injury and a large contingent of phagocytic macrophages remains in the area, effectively permanently.

4) There is widespread demyelination and only partial remyelination of surviving axons crossing through the lesion.

5) In areas where the glia limitans has broken down in the early stages of the injury, the tissue is invaded by peripheral elements and axons are locally remyelinated by Schwann cells.

6) Most of the severed axons die back at least several millimeters; a few show limited and aberrant growth responses, though there is no evidence of effective regrowth across or around the lesion under normal circumstances, even along the track of those axons which survive, together with their central glial environment, in the sub-pial rim.

The full physiological significance of cystic cavitation in the injured cord is not clear, but it does mean that the gray matter territory, with its specific cell types and high rate of blood flow are generally completely lost at the lesion site, and replaced by a fluid filled space or by a dense astroglial and collagenous scar. One significance of the surviving rim of CNS tissue is that there is in such injuries no obvious requirement for a structural bridge across a gap. Instead, we are faced directly with the issue of restrictions on axonal growth in the adult mammalian CNS, perhaps particularly in the white matter territory. Inflammatory responses in the nervous system are poorly understood, yet they almost certainly impinge on the acute regenerative response of both axons and glia (though see Berry 1979 for a review of evidence against a direct immunological blockade of regeneration). Both regenerative and inflammatory responses would be expected to peak at about the same time, in the first week after injury (Blight 1985). The associated problem of demyelination and inappropriate or incomplete remyelination is important in limiting the ultimate recovery of electrophysiological and behavioural function, but it also indicates underlying restrictions on accurate cell-cell interaction in the adult CNS. Invading Schwann cells, on the other hand, appear to be more competent for remyelination but their migration through the tissue is strictly limited by competing glial cells, particularly by the astrocytic basal lamina (Blakemore 1977; Duncan et al. 1981).

Comparison of the morphology of the chronic lesion with functional outcome is useful in that it gives an impression of the potential effectiveness of limited axonal connection. This is relevant to the planning of experiments on axonal regeneration. Complex functions like coordinated standing and walking, do not recover independetly except in the presence of several tens of thousands of surviving axons in the cat (Blight and DeCrescito 1986 and unpublished observations), and they are unlikely to be noticeably restored by artificial reconnection of a few thousand regenerated fibers, unless they are specifically targetted and matched to the function. There seems to be much greater hope of demonstrating functional effects of limited regenerative responses if it is possible to select limited behavioural functions, the underlying circuitry of which is relatively well localized. Comparative morphometric studies also highlight the fact that the mere presence of axons is not sufficient to mediate functional recovery but that those axons must also be physiologically competent (Blight 1983b). Severe behavioural deficits often remain in the presence of large numbers of surviving axons in the cord. The factors that determine the ability of axons to conduct through the lesion are not fully characterized, though it is expected that the pattern and extent of myelination play significant parts. Even profuse regeneration of axons is therefore not likely to be sufficient for function without concomitant effective myelination.

*The use of partial transection*

Partial transection of the spinal cord offers a valuable compromise between the contusion and compression models on the one hand and complete transection on the other. It is easier to define the extent of primary damage with a cutting lesion, though not as precisely as with a complete transection, while it maintains the advantage of the crushing lesion in that it leaves potential pathways for axonal growth within the intact part of the cord. In fact, partial sections have an additional advantage over the crushing injury in that they allow us to examine the accessibility of gray matter as well as white matter territories to axonal growth.

Hemisection of the spinal cord has been used to examine effects on synaptic or axonal rearrangement in surviving systems (Bernstein and Bernstein 1971; Murray and Goldberger 1974; Blight and Precht 1981; Hulsebosch et al. 1984) but partial sections have also been used effectively to examine axonal responses (Lampert and Cressman 1964; Gilson and Stensaas 1974; Bernstein et al. 1978; Guth et al. 1978; Bregman and Reier 1986). There is no evidence that regeneration occurs more readily in the partially transected cord than in complete sections or contusion injuries. The morphological responses of severed axons in the spinal cord, so far as they are available, appear similar in partial, complete and crushing injuries, though some recent studies with very small lesions in the mammalian brain have indicated that there may be more regrowth of axons with very restricted lesions and in young animals (Foerster, 1982; Kawaguchi et al. 1986). These approaches lead us to a recent attempt to examine regeneration in the spinal cord with restricted dorsal column lesions, using an implanted wire marker to define the lesion boundary (Borgens et al. 1986a). This did not produce qualitatively different axonal responses from those seen with transection or contusion. There was no growth of severed axons either through or around the lesion in the absence of further intervention.

*Results of interventive techniques*

The literature on regeneration in the spinal cord suggests a remarkable degree of success in overcoming the limitations on growth by various interventive techniques. Many of the currently *promising* approaches, however, were familiar to Ramón y Cajal when writing his monograph on Degeneration and Regeneration more than 60 years ago, and "success" at this time connotes no more than the ability to demonstrate important principles

Of the empirical approaches that have been tried to the problem of enhancing the feeble regenerative activity of mammalian spinal cord axons, many have concentrated on the glial scar as a possible physical barrier to growth and have attempted to modify its character accordingly (reviewed by Reier et al. 1983). Others have relied on the fact that growth of axons outside the CNS environment is much more pronounced, whether the axons themselves are central or peripheral in origin. It is widely felt that there is some feature of the CNS environment which inhibits growth, though it is also possible that this reflects a lack of stimulus to growth. The ability of axons to extend long distances in the peripheral nervous system has provided the means of bridging the gap in the spinal cord created by complete transection. The technique of peripheral nerve grafts to the CNS has been pursued by a succession of investigators (reviewed by Kiernan 1979; Aguayo et al. 1982). The mechanism of surface selectivity by growing neurites seems best addressed, however, by studies in tissue culture, which are beginning to dissect out some of the relevant molecular information (Schwab and Thoenen 1985; Carbonetto et al. 1987).

*Effects of electric fields*

Like the effect of peripheral nerve elements, the possible role of electrical fields in axonal development was raised early in the century (Ingvar 1920, and reviewed by Ramón y Cajal 1928), though clear and careful demonstration of the phenomenology has only been obtained recently (Hinckle et al. 1981; Patel and Poo 1982; McCaig 1986) and we are still lacking a definite mechanistic understanding. Demonstration of effects of applied electric fields *in vivo* required axonal tracing techniques that have also only recently become available. It has now been shown that applied fields enhance the regenerative responses of severed axons in the nerve cord of the lamprey (Borgens et al. 1981) and in spinal cord of adult guinea pigs (Borgens et al. 1986). These studies have previously shown only morphological effects of applied fields on regenerative responses and much interest logically attends the possibility of functional benefit from such manipulation. In recent experiments we have been concerned to address this problem by selecting a functional spinal cord system that should be ideally suited for sensitive detection of regenerative responses at the functional level (Borgens et al. 1987).

The skin of the back in many quadrupeds can be twitched, or contracted more tonically, by the underlying cutaneous trunci muscle (CTM) which originates from the bicipital arch in the axillary region on either side, and spreads backwards in a thin, broad sheet closely applied to the dermis. Reflex activation of this muscle has been studied in some detail in the rat (Nixon et al. 1984). Cutaneous stimulation on the back of the animal produces a local contraction of the skin. The sensory arm of the reflex is produced by axons in the local dorsal cutaneous nerves of thoracic and lumbar cord. The motoneurons innervating the muscle, however, are located primarily in the cervical cord, projecting in the lateral thoracic nerve of the brachial plexus. The sensory pathway within the cord projects ipsilaterally in the lateral tracts. The reflex in the guinea pig is qualitatively similar to that of the rat, though it differs quantitatively in some respects. The guinea pig reflex occurs at a lower threshold, responding to light tactile stimulation with a phasic twitch, whereas the rat requires a relatively strong pinch with activation of A-$\partial$ and C fibers (Nixon et al. 1984) and produces a more tonic contraction. The guinea pig skin is also less mobile than that of the rat but movements are similarly related to the site of stimulation, with preservation of 'local sign'. The reflex is conveniently quite resistant to pentobarbital anesthesia in both species.

This reflex has a number of advantages as a means of testing functional regeneration of spinal axons:

1) Lateral hemisection of the mid thoracic cord results in permanent loss of the reflex response to cutaneous stimulation ipsilateral and caudal to the hemisection.

2) The dependency of the reflex on the lateral tracts of the cord appears to be based on the sensory projection alone and is therefore unidirectional.

3) This function appears to be organized at the propriospinal level and should not require regenerative responses beyond the spinal cord itself. It is clear from the results of peripheral nerve grafting that regenerative responses of cells near to the lesion are much stronger than those of fibers from distant parts of the nervous system (Richardson et al. 1984).

4) Because the sensory stimulus is very slight, the reflex is probably a very sensitive indicator of the integrity of sensory tracts in the spinal cord, with amplification at the level of the motor center.

5) The response is both visible and easily electrically recorded with subcutaneous emg electrodes. It can also be electrically elicited with stimulation of the dorsal cutaneous nerves.

Over the last year, Richard Borgens, Eugene McGinnis and I have studied the effect of applied electric fields on guinea pigs with thoracic spinal cord hemisections and have found a striking recovery of function in the CTM reflex in 25% of experimental animals at more than 50 days post section (Borgens et al. 1987). The methods used for field application were essentially similar to those in our recent anatomical study of dorsal column section (Borgens et al. 1986b), though the applied current was increased from 10 to 35 μA. At the present time, 28 experimental and 29 control animals implanted with sham batteries have been followed for up to 120 days post section. Distinct recovery of the CTM reflex below the lesion has been recorded in 7 of the animals exposed to 35 μA current for approximately 4 weeks, beginning immediately at the time of hemisection. No recovery of the reflex was detected in any of the animals implanted with sham batteries. More prolonged study of other animals with lateral hemisection but no battery implantation indicates that the loss of CTM responsiveness below the lesion is normally permanent. The recovery of function seen following field application appears to be based on the kind of regenerative response we have seen in the dorsal column in adult guinea pigs, though here it probably involves the lateral funiculus. The possibility that fields might affect the peripheral innervation of the skin rather than central projections has been eliminated by confirming that the reflex responses are appropriately abolished by selective section of dorsal cutaneous nerves below the level of the hemisection.

### *The Example from Lower Vertebrates*

The most encouraging observations on the capacity of complex nervous systems to recover from spinal transection derive from a variety of lower vertebrate species - cyclostomes, selachians, teleosts and urodeles - (reviewed by Anderson and Waxman 1983). Large numbers of axons grow through a complete transection of the cord, and some degree of locomotor function is effectively restored by axonal reconnection in these animals. On the other hand, it is clear that only a proportion of the original axon population regenerates through a thoracic lesion, and that most of these do not regrow to their orginal targets, but have more restricted projections in the distal segment of the cord, and probably make a number of inappropriate connections (Bernstein and Gelderd 1973; Wood and Cohen 1981). The behavioural recovery produced by this naturally occurring regeneration may be equally limited in extent, but is difficult to quantify.

*Is the initial goal of spinal cord regeneration achieved but unrecognized?*

The initial goal of mammalian spinal cord regeneration research might logically be expressed as the intention to produce in a mammalian system the kind of axonal regeneration seen in lower vertebrate preparations. This is the goal initially "held up by Nature" as being apparently attainable. The question that may now be asked is whether we would recognize the achievement of that goal once attained. Would the kind of regeneration enjoyed by the teleost or the cyclostome be sufficient to produce wholesale recovery of function in rat, cat or man? It is important to recognize that the locomotory activity of lower vertebrates is likely to depend much less on specific interconnections at long distances than it is on local segmental interactions. The locomotion of fishes depends not only on relevant activity in the nervous system but also on the interaction of fluid dynamics and subtle adaptation of body mechanics (Blight 1977). Relatively weak and unspecific interactions between proximal and distal parts of the spinal circuitry can be responsible for surprisingly adaptive behaviour - as was discovered by a number of 19th century physiologists who found it difficult to determine the effect of acute spinal section on the swimming behaviour of selachians. Recently, the locomotory behaviour of regenerated lampreys has been analyzed in more detail and shows distinct quantitative deficits, especially in adult animals (Ayers et al. 1980, 1981, and in preparation), despite the fact that the motor coordination problem is made relatively simple by the aquatic environment, the nature of the movements and the body form. Even the basic quadrupedal locomotion of urodeles is heavily dependent on a mechanical linkage of side-to-side body movements with appropriate placement of limbs rather than a complex integration of posture and locomotion. How different this is from the kind of motor control problems faced by cursorial quadrupeds.

A number of groups have applied techniques that appear to promote significant axonal regeneration in the adult mammalian spinal cord, some of them documented several times, like Piromen® (Clemente and Windle 1954; Thulin 1960; Puchala and Windle 1977, Matthews et al. 1979b). Peripheral nerve grafts have shown extensive morphological signs of enhanced regeneration (Kao et al. 1977; Richardson et al. 1984). Electric field application now seems both theoretically and practically exciting. Yet clearly we do not yet have any means of effecting truly significant functional recovery following spinal cord injury. To what extent is this because the regeneration that has been achieved is still not as extensive as that found in lower vertebrates? To what extent is it because we have rarely looked at recovery of function with sufficient refinement to detect changes in propriospinal systems rather than more dramatic descending and ascending pathways to the brain? And to what extent may other factors than axonal regeneration be involved in maintained dysfunction? The presence of regenerated axons is not sufficient by itself, they must also function effectively, which requires sufficient remyelination and synaptic integration at the target systems. The lesson from contusion injuries of the cat spinal cord is clear in this respect. It is possible to have tens of thousands of axons surviving across the injury site without any obvious recovery of gross behavioural function (Blight and DeCrescito 1986). We would not expect more from equal numbers of axons regenerating relatively short distances into inappropriate areas of the nervous system.

Nonetheless, there is reason to be optimistic of the eventual practical success of interventive approaches. We have hardly begun, for example, to explore the possibilities offered by the burgeoning field of growth factors, which is examined in detail by many of the other contributors to this symposium. There is a particular need to try combining the most effective elements of techniques that have already shown value in principle. It will remain necessary to pursue such studies with comparative experimental strategies and analytical subtlety, while actively seeking underlying mechanisms and maintaining a respectful awareness of the peculiarities of the mammalian system. To fly like a bird may have been the original goal of aviation research but it was not achieved, nor could it have been. Seeing history in context, it is clearly easier in some respects to fly like a man.

## REFERENCES:


Aguayo A J, Richardson P M, David S, Benfy M (1982) Transplantation of neurons and sheath cells - a tool for the study of regeneration. In: Nicholls J G (ed) Repair and Regeneration of the nervous system Springer Verlag, Berlin, pp. 91-105.

Anderson M J, Waxman S G (1983) Regeneration of spinal neurons in inframammalian vertebrates: morphological and developmental aspects. J Hirnforsh 24: 371-398.

Ayers J, Carpenter G, Currie S, Kinch J (1980) Quantitative analysis of normal and regenerating behaviours in the sea lamprey. Soc Neurosci Abst 6: 466.

Ayers J, Carpenter G, Currie S, Kinch J (1981) Behavioural analysis of spinal cord regeneration in the sea lamprey. Soc Neurosci Abst 7: 681.

Bernstein J J, Bernstein M E (1971) Axonal regeneration and formation of synapses proximal to the site of lesion following hemisection of the rat spinal cord. Exp Neurol 30: 336-351.

Bernstein J J, Gelderd J B (1973) Synaptic reorganization following regeneration of goldfish spinal cord. Exp Neurol 41: 401-410.

Bernstein J J, Wells M R, Bernstein M E (1978) Effect of puromycin treatment on the regeneration of hemisected and transected rat spinal cord. J Neurocytol 7: 215-228.

Berry M (1979) Regeneration in the central nervous system. In: Smith W T, Cavanaugh J B (eds) Recent advance in neuropathology. Churchill Livingstone, New York, pp 67-111.

Blakemore W F (1977) Remyelination of CNS axons by Schwann cells transplanted from the sciatic nerve. Nature (Lond) 266: 68-69.

Blight A R (1977) The muscular control of vertebrate swimming movements. Biol Rev 52: 181-218.

Blight A R, Precht W (1981) Primary afferent synaptic modulation as a mechanism of behavioural compensation following spinal cord lesions in the frog. In: Flohr H, Precht W (eds) Lesion-Induced Neuronal Plasticity in Sensorimotor Systems. Springer Verlag, Berlin, pp. 117-129.

Blight A R (1983) Cellular morphology of chronic spinal cord injury in the cat: analysis of myelinated axons by line sampling. Neuroscience 10: 521-543.

Blight A R (1983) Axonal physiology of chronic spinal cord injury in the cat: intracellular recording in vitro. Neuroscience 10: 1471-1486.

Blight A R (1985) Delayed demyelination and macrophage invasion: a candidate for "secondary" cell damage in spinal cord injury. Cen Nerv Syst Trauma 2: 299-315.

Blight A R, DeCrescito V (1986) Morphometric analysis of experimental spinal cord injury in the cat: the relation of injury intensity to survival of myelinated axons. Neuroscience 19: 321-341.

Borgens R B, Blight A R, McGinnis M E (1987) Behavioural recovery in an intersegmental spinal reflex induced by an applied electric field following spinal cord hemisection in adult guinea pig. (submitted for publication).

Borgens R B, Blight A R, Murphy D J (1986) Axonal regeneration in spinal cord injury: a perspective and new technique. J comp Neurol 250: 157-167.

Borgens R B, Blight A R, Murphy D J, Stewart L. (1986) Transected dorsal column axons within the guinea pig spinal cord regenerate in the presence of an applied electric field. J comp Neurol 250: 168-180.

Borgens R B, Roederer E, Cohen M J (1981) Enhanced spinal cord regeneration in lamprey by applied electric fields. Science 213: 611-617.

Bregman B S, Reier P J (1986) Neural tissue transplants rescue axotomized rubrospinal cells from retrograde death. J comp Neurol 244: 86-95.

Bresnahan J C King J S, Martin G F, Yashon D (1976) A neuroanatomical analysis of spinal cord injury in the rhesus monkey (Macaca mulatta). J Neurol Sci 28: 521-542.

Carbonetto S, Evans D, Cochard P (1987) Nerve fiber growth in culture on tissue substrata from central and peripheral nervous systems. J Neurosci. 7: 610-620

Clemente C D, Windle W F (1954) Regeneration of severed nerve fibers in the spinal cord of the adult cat. J comp Neurol 101: 691-731.

David S, Aguayo A J (1981) Axonal elongation into peripheral nervous system "bridges" after central nervous system injury in adult rats. Science 214: 931-933.

Davis G E, Blaker, S N, Engvall E, Varon S, Manthorpe M, Gage F (1987) Human amnion membrane serves as a substratum for growing axons in vitro and in vivo. Science 236: 1106-1109.

Duncan I D, Aguayo A J, Bunge R P, Wood P M (1981) Transplantation of rat Schwann cells grown in tissue culture into mouse spinal cord. J Neurol Sci 49: 241-252.

Eidelberg E (1986) Spinal cord injury causes loss of distant motoneurones. Soc Neurosci Abst 12: 1422.

Feringa E R (1984) Histological evidence for death of cortical neurons after spinal cord transection. Neurology 34: 1002-1006.

Foerster A (1982) Spontaneous regeneration of cut axons in adult rat brain. J comp Neurol 210: 335-356.

Gilson B C, Stensaas L J (1974) Early axonal changes following lesions of the dorsal columns in rats. Cell Tissue Res 149: 1-20.

Guth L, Bright D, Donati E J (1978) Functional deficits and anatomical alterations after high cervical spinal hemisection in the rat. Exp Neurol 58: 511-520.

Hinckle L, McCaig C D, Robinson K R (1981) The direction of growth of differentiating neurons and myoblasts from frog embryos in an applied electric field. J Physiol (Lond) 314: 121-135.

Hulsebosch C E, Coggeshall R E, Perez-Polo J R Effects of nerve growth factor and its antibodies on sprouting of sensory axons following spinal cord hemisection. Brain Res 323: 1-10.

Ingvar S (1920) Reaction of cells to the galvanic current in tissue cultures. Proc Soc exp Biol Med 17: 198-199.

Jellinger K (1976) Neuropathology of cord injuries. In Vincken P J, Bruyn GW, Braakman R (eds) Handbook of clinical neurology, injuries of the spine and spinal cord. North Holland, Amsterdam, Vol 25, part 1, pp 43-121.

Kakulas B A, Bedbrook G M (1976) Pathology of injuries of the vertebral column. In Vincken P J, Bruyn GW, Braakman R (eds) Handbook of clinical neurology, injuries of the spine and spinal cord. North Holland, Amsterdam, Vol 25, part 1, pp 27-42.

Kao C C, Chang L W, Bloodworth J M B (1977) Axonal regeneration across transected mammalian spinal cords: an electron microscopic study of delayed microsurgical nerve grafting. Exp Neurol 54: 591-615.

Kawaguchi S, Miyata H, Kato N (1986) Regeneration of the cerebellofugal projection after transection of the superior cerebellar peduncle in kittens: morphological and electrophysiological studies. J comp Neurol 245: 258-273.

Kiernan J A (1979) Hypotheses concerned with axonal regeneration in the mammalian nervous system. Biol Rev 54:153-197.

Kuhn T S (1971) The relations between history and the history of science. Daedalus 100: 271-304.

Lampert P W, Cressman M (1964) Axonal regeneration in the dorsal columns of the spinal cord of adult rats. Lab Invest 13: 825-839.

Matthews M A, StOnge M F, Faciane C L, Gelderd J B (1979a) Spinal cord transection: A quantitative analysis of elements of the connective tissue matrix formed within the site of lesion following administration of piromen, cytoxan or trypsin. Neuropath appl Neurobiol 5: 161-180.

Matthews M A, St.Onge M F, Faciane C L, Gelderd J B (1979b) Axon sprouting into segments of rat spinal cord adjacent to the site of a previous transection. Neuropath appl Neurobiol 5: 181-196.

McCaig C D (1986) Dynamic aspects of amphibian neurite growth and the effects of an applied electric field. J Physiol (Lond) 375: 55-69.

Murray M, Goldberger M E (1974) Restitution of function and collateral sprouting in the cat spinal cord: the partially hemisected animal. J comp Neurol 158: 19-36.

Nixon B J, Doucette R, Jackson PC, Diamond J (1984) Impulse activity evokes precocious sprouting of nociceptive nerves into denervated skin. Somatosensory Res 2: 97-126.

Nornes H A, Bjorklund A, Stenevi U (1983) Reinnervation of the denervated adult spinal cord of rats by intraspinal transplants of embryonic brain stem neurons. Cell Tissue Res 230: 15-35.

Patel N, Poo M M (1982) Orientation of neurite growth by extracellular electric fields. J Neurosci 2: 483-496.

Puchala E, Windle W F (1977) The possibility of structural and functional restitution after spinal cord injury. A review. Exp Neurol 55: 1-42.

Ramón y Cajal S (1928) Degeneration and Regeneration in the Nervous System. Hoffner, New York.

Reier P J, Bregman B S, Wujek J R (1986) Intraspinal transplantation of embryonic spinal cord tissue in neonatal and adult rats. J comp Neurol 247: 275-296.

Reier P J, Perlow M J, Guth L (1983) Development of embryonic spinal cord transplants in the rat. Dev Brain Res 10: 201-219.

Reier P J, Stensaas L J, Guth L (1983) The astrocytic scar as an impediment to regeneration in the central nervous system. In: Kao C C, Bunge RP, Reier P J (eds) Spinal cord reconstruction. Raven Press, New York, pp 163-195.

Richardson P M, Issa V M K, Aguayo A J (1984) Regeneration of long spinal axons in the rat. J Neurocytol 13: 165-182.

Schwab M, Thoenen H (1985) Dissociated neurons regenerate into sciatic but not optic nerve explants in culture irrespective of neurotrophic factors. J Neurosci 5: 2415-2423.

Thulin C-A (1960) Bioelectrical characteristics of regenerated fibers in the feline spinal cord. Exp Neurol 2: 533-546.

Veraa R P, Grafstein B (1981) Cellular mechanisms for recovery from nervous system injury: A conference report. Exp Neurol 71: 6-75.

Wood M R, Cohen M J (1981) Synaptic regeneration and glial reactions in the transected spinal cord of the lamprey. J Neurocytol 10: 57-79.

# NEUROFILAMENT PROCESSING IN TRAUMA AND DISEASE

Ludwig A. Sternberger, Jurg Ulrich, Lloyd Guth,
Charles P. Barrett, and Nancy H. Sternberger

Departments of Neurology, Pathology and Anatomy
University of Maryland School of Medicine
Baltimore, Maryland 21201

and

Neuropathology Division, Department of Pathology
Universitat Basel, CH 4003 Basel, Switzerland

Address for Correspondence:

Ludwig Sternberger, M.D.
Department of Neurology
University of Maryland Hospital
22 South Greene Street
Baltimore, Maryland 21201

NATO ASI Series, Vol. H22
Neural Development and Regeneration
Edited by A. Gorio et al.

Monoclonal antibodies provide opportunity to purify known antigens, discover and purify new antigens, characterize their submolecular structure, collect, in favorable cases, relevant cDNA from multiple clones obtained from an expression vector, and finally study normal and pathologic interactions of antigens in situ. Our work had been initiated as a "peche a la ligne" expedition, using whole brain homogenate as bait to the immune system of mice and fishing out from the pool of fused immune B cells those that produced antibodies of special interest, while discarding antibodies that were irrelevant. Special interest imposed a limitation to include antibodies that reacted at high specificity and selectivity. The requirement was fulfilled when the antibodies detected only one antigen, previously known or unknown, to the exclusion of any other antigen in the same host. This type of analysis could be carried out when the antibodies produced by clones derived from fusions of immune spleen cells with myeloma cells were analyzed by immunocytochemistry, which does not require prior knowledge of the antigens searched for, in contrast to the more commonly performed kinds of analysis, such as enzyme-linked or radioimmunoassay, which utilize the specific antigen looked for.

In our approach we selected antibodies that detected given structures on paraffin sections of brain without reacting with other structures. Such selection included, for example, antibodies that visualized blood-brain barrier endothelium, but not endothelia in other tissues or in brain regions deficient in blood-brain barrier, and did not react with any other cells in the organism (Sternberger and Sternberger, 1987). Absence of reaction in these other sites was defined by absence of background staining, so that the unstained tissue section is invisible in light microscopy unless special optics, such as Nomarski optics, are used. Absence of background staining by any monoclonal antibody not only assures high specificity to given cells and structures, but also high affinity of the antibody, as low cross reactivity is equivalent to high affinity (Sternberger, 1986). An important prerequisite for this type of selection procedure is the entire absence of background from the immunocytochemical staining method alone, and not only from the degree of specificity of the monoclonal antibody used as first antibody. This can be accomplished by adherence to the principle of unlabeled, rather than labeled antibody as second antibody (Sternberger and Sternberger, 1986) and detection by peroxidase-antiperoxidase complex made from monoclonal antiperoxidase (ClonoPAP).

A large number of monoclonal antibodies produced by fusions from mice immunized with whole brain fulfilled the criteria of specificity for given cells or structures. On the basis of their immunocytochemical staining patterns these antibodies could be divided into major groups. Within each of the neuron-specific groups minor differences in staining patterns denoted epitope heterogeneity. Two of the neuron-specific groups were of relevance to the subject of the present paper.

One group of these antibodies reacted only with axons, leaving cell bodies and dendrites unstained (Fig. 1). On immunoblots these antibodies reacted with the 200 Mr neurofilament protein (NfH). In contrast, a second group of antibodies reacted with neuronal cell bodies and dendrites, and only some axons, particularly proximal and thick axons (Fig.2). Despite the paucity of overlap of staining with antibodies of the first group, these antibodies, on immunoblots, also reacted with NfH. To explain this apparent paradox we assumed that our antibodies detected a post-translational change in neurofilaments. Among a number of posttranslational changes examined, we explored the possibility that the antibodies detected modifications dependent upon phosphorylation, since Mushinski's group has discovered earlier that neurofilaments are extensively phosphorylated (Julien and Mushinsky 1981, 1982).

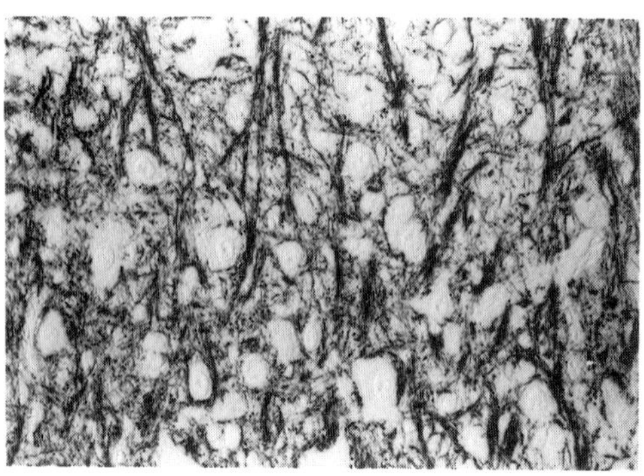

Fig. 1 Rat nucleus ruber, paraffin section, stained with anti-PNf 07-5. x200.

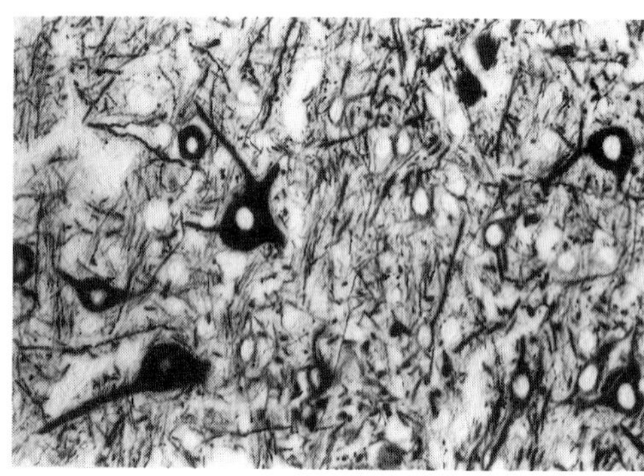

Fig. 2 Rat nucleus ruber, paraffin section stained with anti-nPNf 10-1. X200

We found that:

A. Immunocytochemical staining of antibodies reactive with axons is suppressed in the presence of phosphate, acting as a hapten, while staining with antibodies reactive with cell bodies and dendrites is unaffected (Sternberger and Sternberger, 1983).

B. On two-dimensional electrophoresis transblots of cytoskeletal preparations, most but not all antibodies, reacting with axons detected only an acidic protein (nI 5.1) at 200 Mr (Goldstein et al, 1987a). Antibodies reacting with cell bodies and dendrites stained a streak extending from a 200 Mr, pI 5.1 position to a 170 Mr, pI 6.0 position. Julien and Mushinsky (1982) have shown that hypophosphorylated NfH has a higher apparent electrophoretic mobility in sodium dodecyl sulfate than the extensively phosphorylated form. Consequently, antibodies that stained cell bodies revealed neurofilaments in various stages of low degrees of phosphorylation.

C. Treatment of immunoblots with phosphatase abolished reaction of the antibodies that stained axons, but enhanced reaction of antibodies that stained cell bodies and dendrites (Sternberger and Sternberger, 1983) The effect of phosphatase was abolished by inorganic phosphate and aminophylline, both inhibitors of phosphatase.

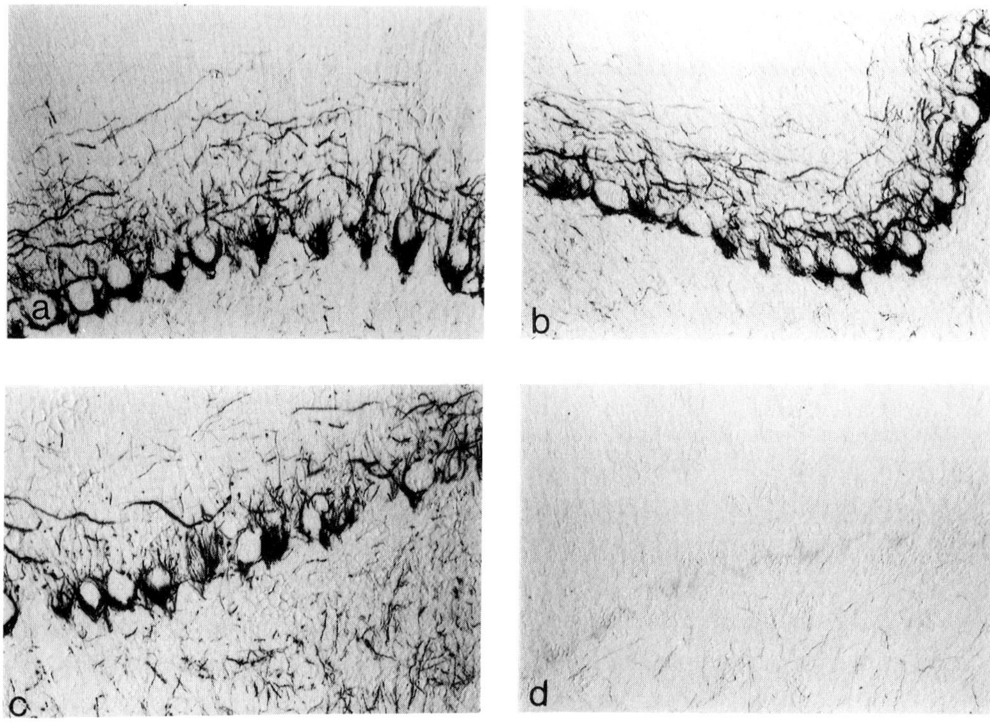


Fig. 3 Rat cerebellum, paraffin section, stained with anti-PNf 06-17 after treatment with a) buffer b) phosphatase c) trypsin d) trypsin followed by phosphatase. X400.

These three lines of evidence suggested that antibodies that stained axons reacted with phosphoepitopes in neurofilaments (anti-PNf) while antibodies that stained cell bodies and dendrites revealed nonphosphorylated or hypophosphorylated neurofilaments (anti-nPNf). However, attempts to dephosphorylate neurofilaments in paraffin sections were, at first, unsuccessful. Thus, staining with any of the anti-PNf was unaffected by pretreatment of sections with phosphatase (Fig. 3a,b) nor was it affected by trypsin (Fig. 3c). However, when sections were first treated with trypsin and then with phosphatase staining became diminished (Fig. 3d). The effects of trypsin in preparing sections for dephosphorylation by phosphatase were nonspecific. Other proteolytic enzymes or even hydrochloric acid could be substituted for trypsin.

On vibratome sections phosphatase abolished the staining (Fig. 4a,b,d) even in the absence of proteolytic enzyme pretreatment. Trypsin left staining unaffected (Fig. 4c).

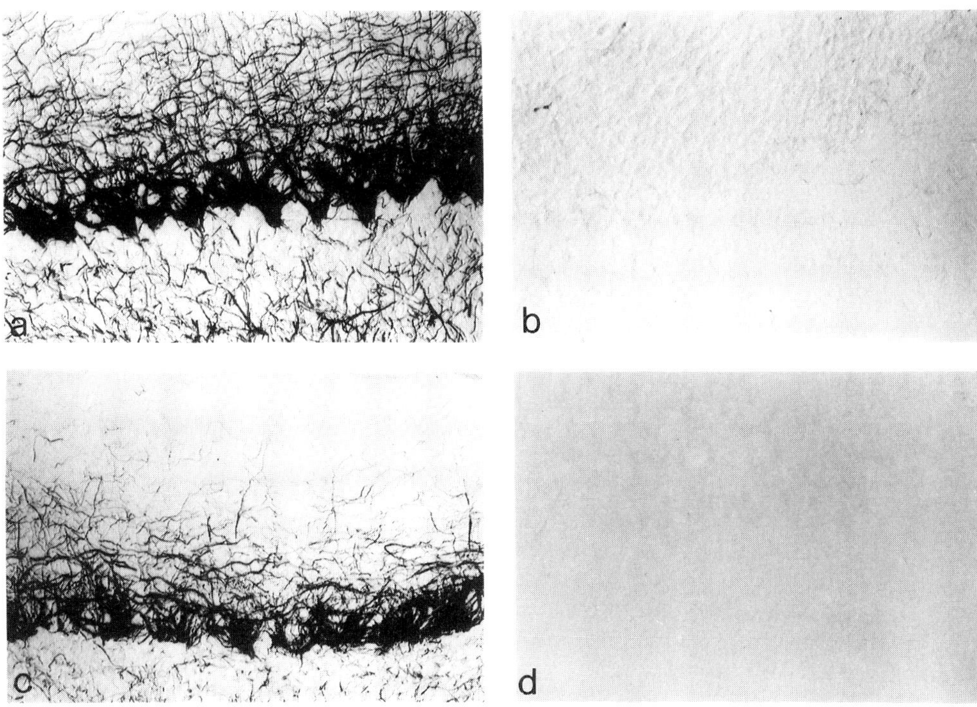


Fig 4. Rat cerebellum, vibratome section, stained with anti-PNf 06-17 after treatment with a) buffer b) phosphatase c) trypsin d) trypsin followed by phosphatase. x100

With regard to antibodies to nonphosphorylated neurofilaments (anti-nPNf), staining on paraffin (Fig. 5a,b) or vibratome sections (Figs. 6a,b) was unaffected by pretreatment with phosphatase, as expected. In contrast to anti-PNf, staining with anti-nPNf was abolished by trypsin. Staining could be restored if trypsin treatment was followed by phosphatase. However, in the process the staining had been converted from a cell body-dendrite pattern characteristic of nPNf, to an axonal pattern, characteristic of PNf. The effects were trypsin-specific and could not be substituted for by other proteolytic enzymes.

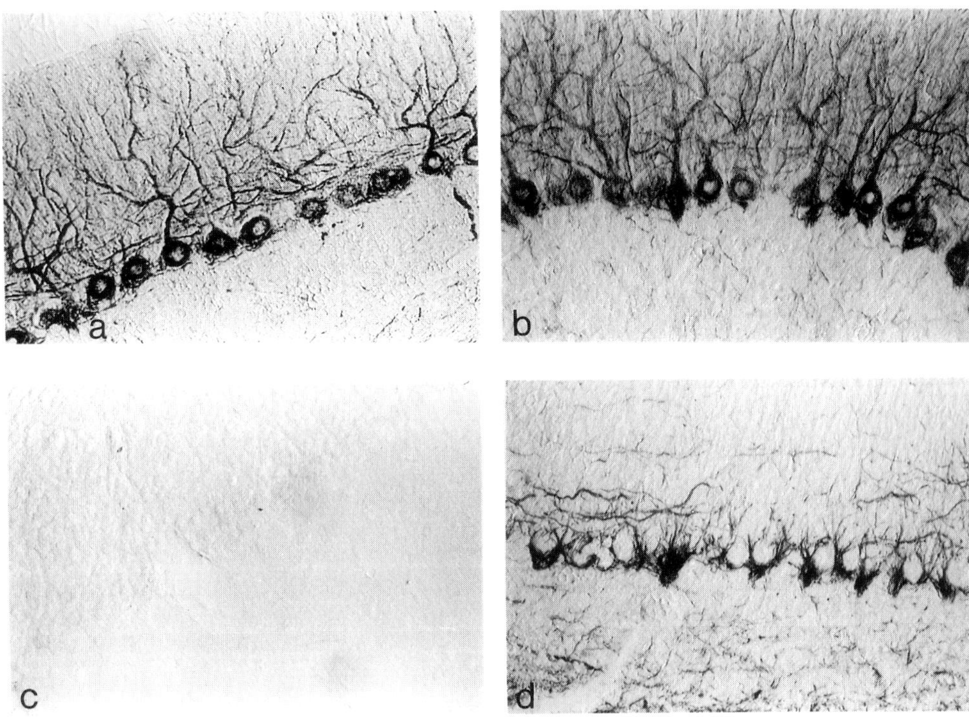


Fig. 5 Rat cerebellum, paraffin section, stained with anti-nPNf 02-135 after treatment with a) buffer b) phosphatase c) trypsin d) trypsin followed by phosphatase. x400

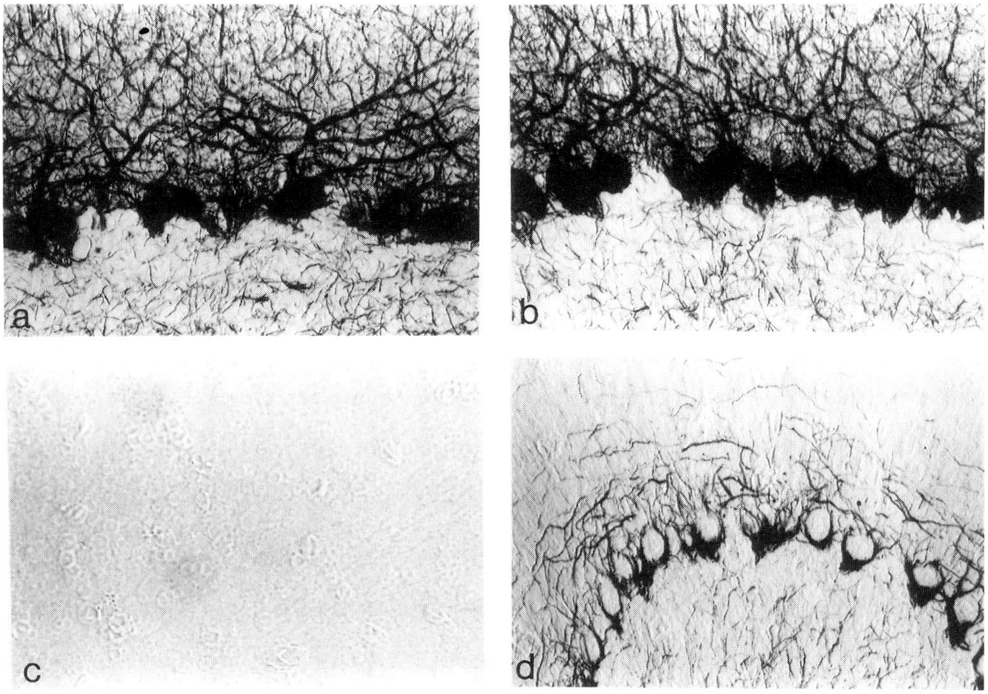

Fig. 6 Rat cerebellum, vibratome section stained with anti-nPNf 02-135 after treatment with a) buffer b) phosphatase c) trypsin d) trypsin followed by phosphatase. x100

These data, as well as other examinations on immunodots and immunoblots led to the conclusion that nPNf epitopes contained a trypsin-sensitive lysine and/or arginine group which is in proximity to a serine group, that phosphorylation protects the nPNf epitope against accessibility of both trypsin or antibodies, and that one function of neurofilament phosphorylation is impairment of flexibility of the molecule. This impairment can occur either by interaction with other proteins or by interaction with self, since it can be demonstrated even in electrophoretically separated NfH. It may be responsible for the lower electrophoretic mobility of PNf as compared to nPNf in sodium dodecyl sulfate gels as first reported by Julien and Mushinsky (1982).

In other experiments (Goldstein et al, 1987b) we have shown that phosphorylation protects neurofilaments against proteolysis and that dephosphorylated neurofilaments are rapidly degraded by proteases. These proteases appear to be cytoskeleton-associated nonspecific proteases, in contrast to the calcium-activated protease of Schlaepfer (1971, 1987) that may well exhibit selectivity for neurofilaments. Protection against phosphorylation is probably one of the least important functions of normal neurofilament phosphorylation, but it seems to assume some significance in pathologic conditions as discussed below.

It now appears from emerging data of several investigators that neurofilaments react in nearly every neurologic disorder amined by accumulated or dammed-up phosphorylation: while normally cell bodies contain only nPNf, in pathologic conditions selected perikarya are replete with PNf. All phosphoepitopes for which antibodies are available, are involved. Thus, Forno et al (1986) as well as Galloway et al (1987) have shown that Lewy bodies, a perikaryonal structure associated with Parkinsonism, are phosphorylated, and so are Pick bodies (Forno, 1987). A number of current studies reveal that selected neuronal cell bodies in amyotrophic lateral sclerosis possess PNf. Several cerebellar disorders, including ceroid lipofuscinosis, crossed cerebellar atrophy, cerebellar hemiagenesis, Menko's disease and hypertrophy of the inferior olive, reveal PNf in cell bodies (Shiurba et al 1987). As shown by Cork et al (1987) motorneuron disorders in a variety of vertebrate species reveal PNf containing cell bodies, while Wiley et al (1987) have described perikaryonal phosphorylation in a case of an infantile neurodegenerative disorder resembling juvenile amyotrophic lateral sclerosis. Gold et al (1987) observed PNf in dorsal root ganglia in a number of experimental neuropathies, and Rosenfeld et al (1987) have shown that early after peripheral nerve transection PNf accumulate in ganglion cells. In these instances each of the phosphoepitopes for which there exist monoclonal antibodies is involved in the premature or ectopic phosphorylation. The generality of perikaryonal neurofilament phosphorylation in a large variety of disorders and specifically the phosphorylation of Purkinge cells in Lhermitte-Duclos disease (Shiurba et al 1987b) a disorder that seems to involve granule cells primarily and Purkinje cells secondarily, have led Urich to suggest that aberrant neurofilament phosphorylation in cell bodies may be a reactive rather than a degenerative process.

An exception to the indiscriminate perikaryonal neurofilament phosphorylation widely observed in pathologic conditions and even in normal aging is provided by the selective neurofilament phosphorylation in Alzheimer tangles and in aluminum intoxication tangles, both of which are perikaryonal structures. In Alzheimer disease (Sternberger and Sternberger, 1985) only one phosphoepitope is involved in perikaryonal phosphorylation, while in aluminum poisoning (Troncoso et al, 1986) two epitopes, distinct from that participating in Alzheimer disease, are phosphorylated prematurely. This finding suggests that Alzheimer disease may be a disturbance of phosphorylation and that incorporation of neurofilaments in tangles may only be one of the consequences of aberrant phosphorylation, while other proteins may also be involved in a similarly based pathologic process.

To explore the question of premature perikaryonal phosphorylation in the majority of neurologic disorders as a reactive rather than degenerative process, we examined the consequences of spinal crush injury in the rat with particular attention to the relation of any premature perikaryonal neurofilament phosphorylation in injured neurons as compared to that in any uninjured interneurons that might be involved in a reactive or secondary manner. These studies provide a continuation of earlier work by Guth et al (1985a, b) on spinal cord injury.

With anti-PNf, normal spinal cord reveals the usual axonal staining pattern with cell bodies and dendrites unstained (Fig. 7). With anti-nPNf, the majority of cell bodies are stained (Fig. 8). Following and persisting after crush injury most anti-PNf and anti-nPNf-detectable structures in the lesion itself have disappeared (Fig. 9 and 10) except for the presence of degenerative products in the form of amorphous droplets. These droplets are more prominent with anti-nPNf than with anti-PNf.

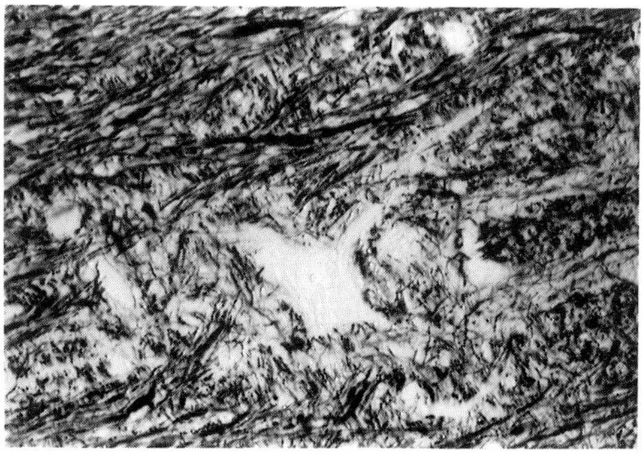

Fig. 7

Normal rat spinal cord, paraffin section stained with anti-nPNf 06-17.

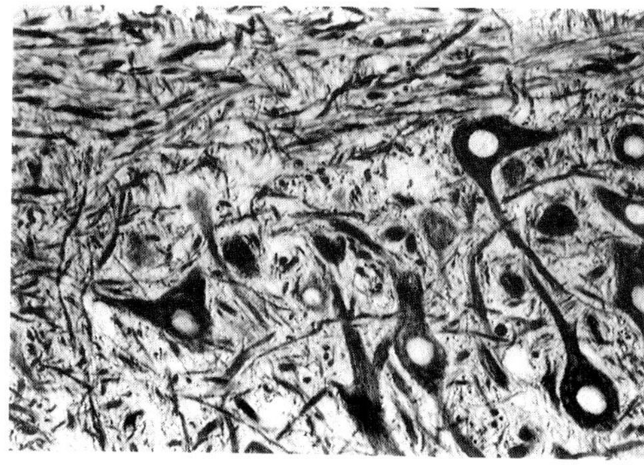

Fig. 8

Section adjacent to that of Fig. 7, stained with anti-nPNf 02-135. x200.

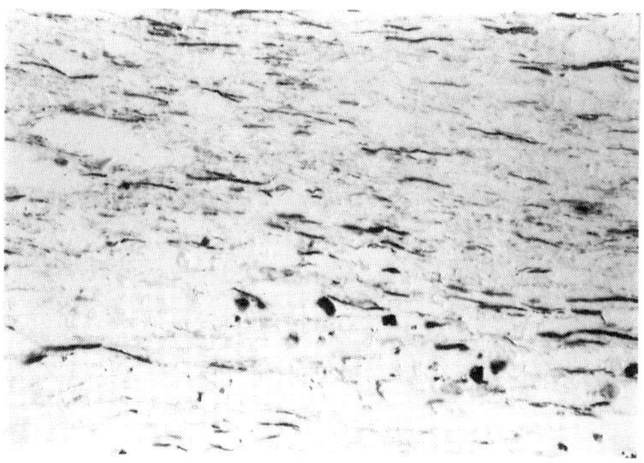

Fig. 9

Crush lesion of rat spinal cord, paraffin section stained with anti-nPNf 06-17.

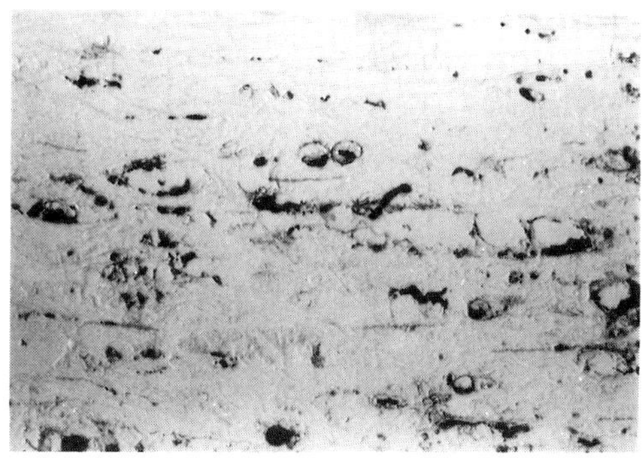

Fig. 10

Section adjacent to that of Fig. 9, stained with anti-nPNf 02-135. x200.

Proximal to the lesion, a few cell bodies belonging to interneurons of largely local circuitry react with all of the anti-NPNf (Fig. 11). Only a minority of neurons are involved, as revealed by the larger number of cell bodies stained with anti-nPNf (Fig. 12).

Motorneuron cell bodies are not phosphorylated in the proximal segment. Also, there is no evidence of PNf degradation (Fig. 11), and only a moderate degree of nPNf degradation (Fig. 12) is revealed.

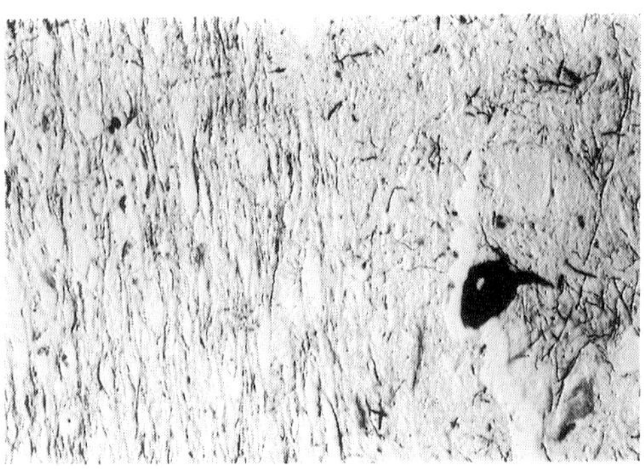

Fig. 11

Rat spinal cord, two segments proximal to the site of crush injury, paraffin section stained with anti-PNf 06-17. x200.

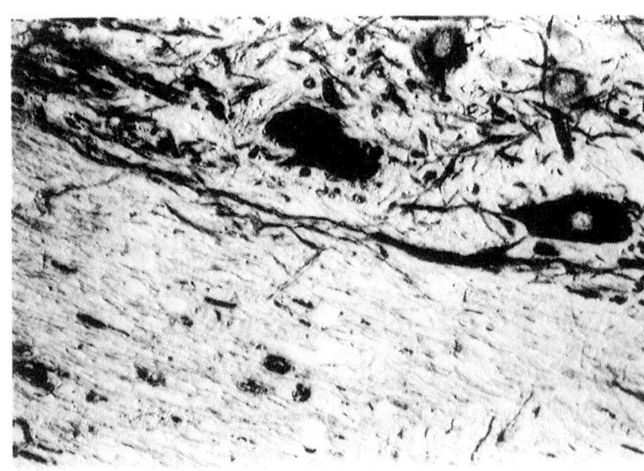

Fig. 12

Section adjacent to that of Fig. 11, stained with anti-nPNf 02-135. x200.

In the distal segment we find not only phosphorylation of cell bodies of interneurons, but also that of an occasional motorneuron (Fig. 13). There is some degree of PNf degradation as revealed by the presence of amorphous droplets. However, upon staining with anti-nPNf (Fig. 14) extensive degradation of NPNf is revealed.

Cell bodies of the dorsal root ganglion that project into the lesion appear normal and do not contain PNf (Fig. 13) while most of them are revealed with anti-nPNf as expected (Fig. 14).

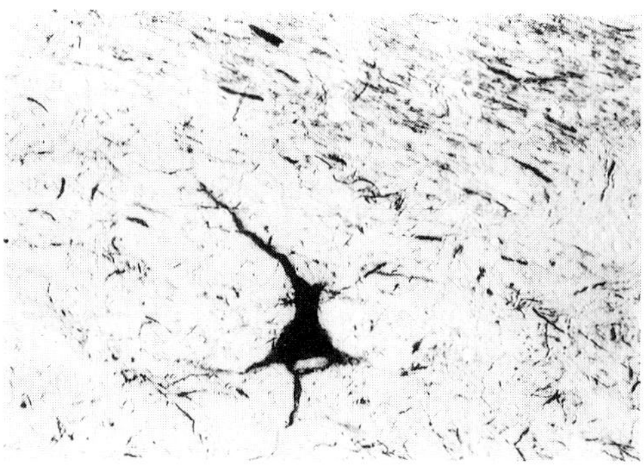

Fig. 13

Rat spinal cord, two segments distal to site of crush injury, paraffin sections stained with anit-PNf 06-17. x200.

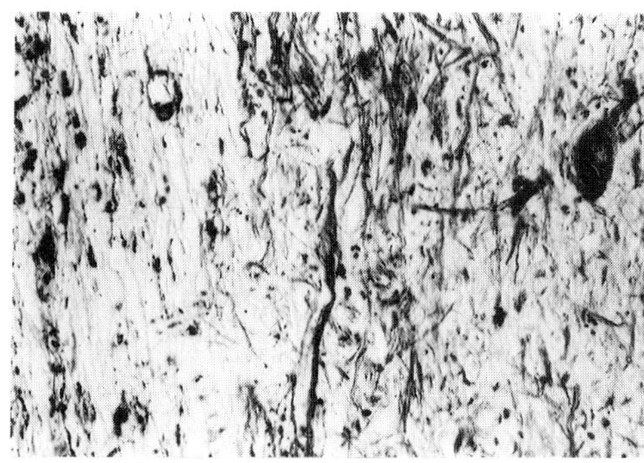

Fig. 14

Section adjacent to that of Fig. 13, stained with anti-nPNf 02-135. x200.

These data suggest that perikaryonal neurofilament phosphorylation is not necessarily restricted to injured neurons, but may be a response of cells that receive input from injured neurons, such as interneurons that are proximal or distal to a crush lesion and motorneurons that are distal, but not proximal to the site of injury. Dorsal root ganglion cells whose projections into the lesion are injured, are free of PNf.

The proteolysis that accompanies spinal cord crush (Guth et al, 1985a) seems to affect mainly nonphosphorylated or dephosphorylated neurofilaments, while PNf are largely protected.

Conceivably, cell death may be associated with the presence of nPNf in normal neurons, while cells that have responded by perikaryonal neurofilament phosphorylation may be protected.

## REFERENCES

Cork LC, Troncoso JC, Klarano GG, Johnson ES, Sternberger NH, Sternberger LA, Price DL (1987): Neurofilamentous pathology in motor neurons in spontaneously occurring animal diseases. J Neuropath Exp Neural, submitted.

Forno LS, Sternberger LA, Sternberger NH, Strefling MA, Swanson K, Eng LF (1980): Reaction of Lewy bodies with antibodies to phosphorylated and non-phosphorylated neurofilaments. Neurosci Let 64:253.

Forno LS (1987): The locus cerulus in Pick's disease. Am Assn Neuropath 63:127

Galloway P, Grundke-Lqal I, Autilio-Gambetti L, Gambetti P, Perry G (1987): Neuronal cytoskeleton involvement in Lewy body formation. Am Assn Neuropath 63:120.

Gold BG, Price DL, Griffin JW, Rosenfeld J, Hoffman PH, Sternberger NH, Sternberger LA (1987): Neurofilament antigens in acrylamide neuropathy. Am Assn Neuropath 63:65.

Goldstein ME, Sternberger LA, Sternberger NH (1987a): Varying degree of phosphorylation determine microheterogeneity of the heavy neurofilament peptide (Nf.H). J Neuroimmunol 14:138, 1987.

Goldstein MF, Sternberger NH, Sternberger LA (1987b): Phosphorylation protects neurofilaments against proteolysis. J Neuroimmunol 14:149.

Guth L, Barrett CP, Donati EJ, Anderson FD, Smith MV, Lifson M (1985a): Essentiality of a specific cellular terrain for growth of axons into a spinal cord lesion. Exp Neurol 88:1.

Guth L, Barrett CP, Donati EJ, Smith MV, Lifson M, Roberts E (1985b): Enhancement of axonal growth into a spinal cord lesion by topical application of triethanolamine and cytosine arabinoside. Exp Neurol 88:44.

Julien J-P, Mushynski WE (1982): Multiple phosphorylation within mammalian neurofilament polypeptides. J Biol Chem 257:10467.

Julien J-P, Mushyniski WE (1981): The distribution of phosphorylation sites among identified proteolytic fragments of mammalian neurofilaments. J Biol Chem 258:4019.

Rosenfeld J, Dorman ME, Griffin JW, Sternberger LA, Sternberger NH, Price DL (1987): Distribution of neurofilament antigens after axonal injury. J Neuropath Exp Neurol, in press.

Schlaepfer WW (1971): Experimental alterations of neurofilaments and neurotubules by calcium and other ions. Exp Cell REs 67:73.

Schlaepfer WW (1987): Neurofilaments: Structure, metabolism and implications in disease. J Neuropath Exp Neurol 46:117.

Shiurba RA, Eng LF, Sternberger NH, Sternberger LA, Urich H (1987): The cytoskeleton of the human cerebellar cortex. Brain Res 107:205.

Shiurba RA, Gessaga EC, Eng LF, Sternberger LA, Sternberger NH, Urich H (1987): Lhermitte-Duclos disease: An immunohistochemical study of the cerebellar cortex. Acta Neuropath, in press.

Sternberger NH, Sternberger LA (1987): Blood-brain barrier protein recognized by monoclonal antibody. Proc Natl Acad Sci USA, in press.

Sternberger LA (1986): Immunocytochemistry, 3rd Ed. John Wiley and Sons, New York, (524 pp).

Sternberger LA, Sternberger NH (1986): The unlabeled antibody method. Comparison of peroxidase-antiperoxidase with avidin-biotin complex by a new method of quantification. J Histochem Cytochem 34:399.

Sternberger LA, Sternberger NH (1983): Monoclonal antibodies distinguish phosphorylated and non-phosphporylated forms of neurofilaments *in situ*. Proc Natl Acad Sci USA 80:6126.

Sternberger NH, Sternberger LA, Ulrich J (1983): Aberrant neurofilament phosphorylation in Alzheimer disease. Proc Natl Acad Sci (USA) 82:4147.

Tronscoso JC, Sternberger NH, Sternberger LA, Hoffman PH, Price DL (1986): Immunohistochemical studies of neurofilament antigens in neurofibrillary pathology indjuced by aluminum. Brain Res 364:295.

Wiley CA, Love S, Skoglund RR, Lampert PW (1987): Infantile neurodegenerative disease with accumulation of phosphorylated neurofilaments. Acta Neuropath 72:369.

# THE PROCESS OF REINNERVATION OF CNS NEURONS; EVIDENCE FOR LOCAL SYNTHESIS OF SYNAPTIC CONSTITUENTS AT POSTSYNAPTIC SITES

O. Steward[1], G. A. Banker[2], L. Davis[1], and L. L. Phillips[1]
[1]Departments of Neuroscience and Neurosurgery
University of Virginia School of Medicine
Charlottesville, VA 22908
U.S.A.

and

[2]Department of Anatomy
Albany Medical College
Albany, NY 12208
U.S.A.

## INTRODUCTION

When neuronal connections are interrupted as a result of injury, complete reconstruction requires not only the regrowth of axons, but also successful reconnection of the growing axons with their targets. A great deal has been learned recently about the regulation of axon growth; relatively little is known however, about how reinnervation is regulated. In large measure, our ignorance about the process of reinnervation is because successful regeneration of CNS axons is so rare. For this reason, situations where reinnervation does occur are of special interest.

Perhaps the best studied example of reinnervation of CNS neurons following injury involves the granule cells of the dentate gyrus of rats after damage to the ipsilateral entorhinal cortex. Complete destruction of the entorhinal cortex leads to the degeneration of about 90% of the synapses upon distal dendrites of the dentate granule cells. Over time, these synapses are replaced as a result of the proliferation of several afferent systems that survive the lesion (for a review, see Cotman and Nadler, 1978, and Steward, 1986a).

As a result of a number of studies, a data base is available regarding the cellular and molecular correlates of

NATO ASI Series, Vol. H22
Neural Development and Regeneration
Edited by A. Gorio et al.

the reinnervation process in the dentate gyrus. 1) Quantitative electron microscopic studies have revealed that the reinnervation process involves a substantial proliferation of presynaptic processes; this begins between 4 and 6 days postlesion, and the period of maximal growth is between 6 and 12 days (Steward and Vinsant, 1983); 2) Golgi and electron microscopic studies have indicated that there is a loss and re-growth of spines and distal dendritic segments with denervation and reinnervation (Caceres and Steward, 1983, Steward, 1986a). The rapid phase of reinnervation between about 6 and 12 days postlesion seems to involve the formation of new contacts on dendritic segments that are preserved following deafferentation; the later slower phase of synapse replacement may involve in part the growth of new dendrites (Steward et al., in press). In both cases, it seems that many of the reinnervating fibers innervate newly constructed postsynaptic membrane specializations rather than old sites. 3) Electron microscopic studies have demonstrated that there is a substantial increase in the protein synthetic machinery (polyribosomes) beneath synaptic sites during reinnervation (Steward, 1983a); 4) Autoradiographic studies following intraveneous injections of labeled protein precursors have revealed increases in protein synthesis in the portion of the neuropil containing the denervated dendrites; the increases in protein synthesis occur during the same period as the increases in polyribosomes (Fass and Steward, 1983, Phillips et al., in press).

These observations have led us to propose that reinnervation occurs as the result of the sequence of events illustrated in Fig. 1. As synaptic terminals degenerate, they are removed by glia. The membrane specializations may be internalized in the dendrite. Either simultaneously with (Fig. 1C) or shortly after the removal of the degenerating terminal (Fig. 1D) a new synaptic site is constructed. Some of the new sites are at the base of existing spines (Steward, et al., in press). Polyribosomes accumulate at these sites during the time that the new contacts are being made; their numbers decline as the synapses mature.

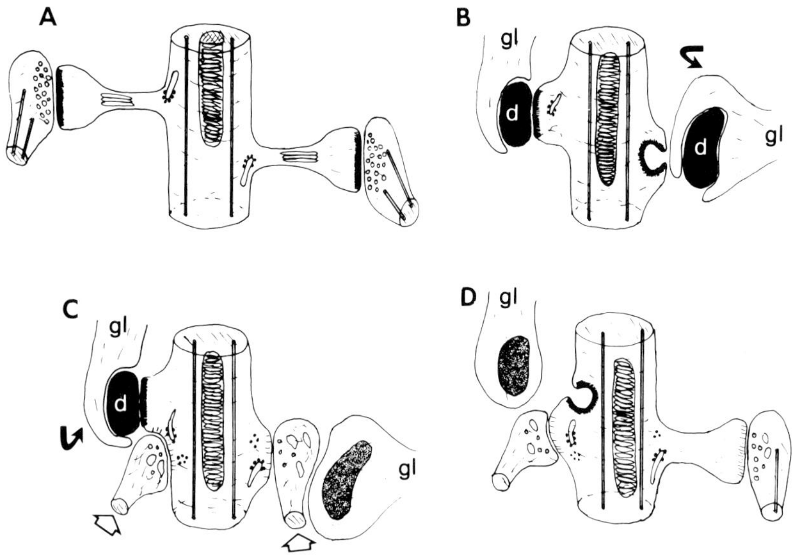


Figure 1. The process of reinnervation on dendritic segments that are preserved after denervation. A) Entorhinal fibers terminate principally on dendritic spines in the intact dentate gyrus. B) As terminals degenerate (d), they are removed by glia (gl). C) Simultaneously with the removal of degenerating terminals, or shortly thereafter, new synaptic sites are constructed. Some of the new sites are at the base of existing spines. D) With time new spines develop.

These observations suggest that proteins synthesized on dendritic polyribosomes may play an important role in the reinnervation process (Steward, 1983b, 1986a,b).

Quantitative electron microscopic studies in developing animals have revealed that polyribosomes are even more prominent beneath developing synaptic contacts (Steward and Falk, 1986). These studies have also provided some indication about when in the course of synapse development the polyribosomes are most prominent. The polyribosomes could be important at three stages of the synaptogenic process: 1) for the initial stages of contact formation (producing growth factors or recognition molecules); 2) for maturation of the synaptic site (producing protein constituents of the synaptic junction itself); or 3) for the construction of spines

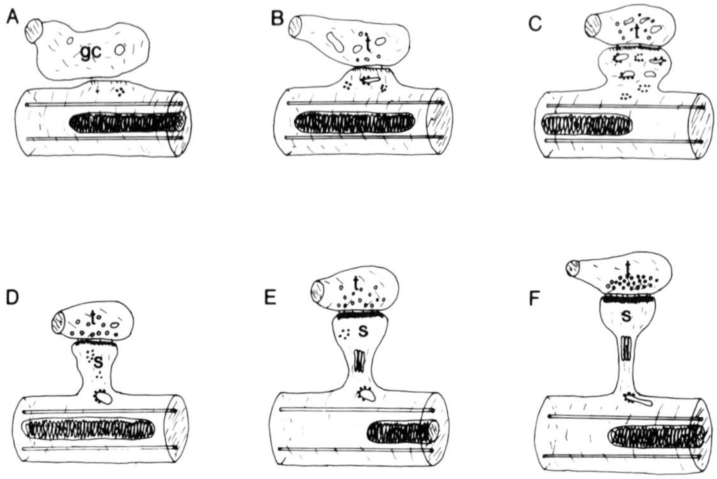


Figure 2. A summary of the relationship between polyribosomes and developing synapses. A-F illustrate the proposed sequence of synaptic maturation. Note that polyribosomes are most prominent during the time that primitive contacts differentiate into mature-appearing synapses.

(producing structural proteins). Each of these hypotheses leads to different predictions regarding when the polyribosomes would be most prevalent. Thus, if polyribosomes played a role in initial contact formation, they should be most prominent before the onset of synaptogenesis, when growing axons first contact their targets. If the polyribosomes synthesized proteins that played a role in the construction of the synapse, then they should be most prominent when primitive contacts differentiate into mature synapses. If the polyribosomes synthesized molecules for the spine, they should be most prominent when spines were being elaborated. In fact, polyribosomes appeared to be most prominent sometime after initial contact formation, during the time when primitive contacts develop into mature synapses (Fig. 2). Taken together, these studies thus suggest that the local synthesis of proteins within dendrites plays a particularly important role during the construction of synaptic junctions.

## Evidence for Local Synthesis of Protein Within Dendrites

Direct evidence for protein synthesis within dendrites has been obtained through studies of protein synthesis by neurons grown in culture. Hippocampal neurons can be grown in low density cultures permitting the complete visualization of the dendritic trees of individual neurons (Bartlett and Banker, 1984a and see Fig. 3A). The dendrites of these neurons can be unambiguously identified by immunostaining for the dendrite-specific microtubule-associated protein MAP2 (Caceres et al., 1986, and see Fig. 3B). These neurons form numerous synaptic contacts with one another (Bartlett and Banker, 1984b), and many of the synapses are on dendritic spines (Fig. 3B and C). Polyribosomes are often accumulated beneath the spines, as is also true *in situ* (Fig. 3C). These neurons continue to elaborate axons and dendrites for 2-3 weeks in culture, providing an opportunity to study neurons during the time that they are constructing synapses.

When hippocampal neurons in such low density cultures are exposed for 15 minutes to a medium containing 3H-leucine, and then are fixed and prepared for autoradiography, silver grains are found not only over the cell bodies, but also over dendrites (see Fig. 4). There is, however, no labeling over the thin axonal processes.

Fifteen minutes is much too short a time for material to be synthesized in the cell body and transported into the dendrites. Even if dendrites possessed the machinery for rapid transport, in all systems that have been studied to date, there is a 45-60 minute delay between synthesis and the first appearance of recently synthesized protein in neuronal processes (Droz and Leblond, 1963). Indeed, with the 15 minute pulse, there was no evidence whatsoever for labeling of the axons, which presumably do possess the machinery for rapid transport. Thus, the labeling that is observed over the dendrites almost certainly reflects local protein synthesis within the dendrites.

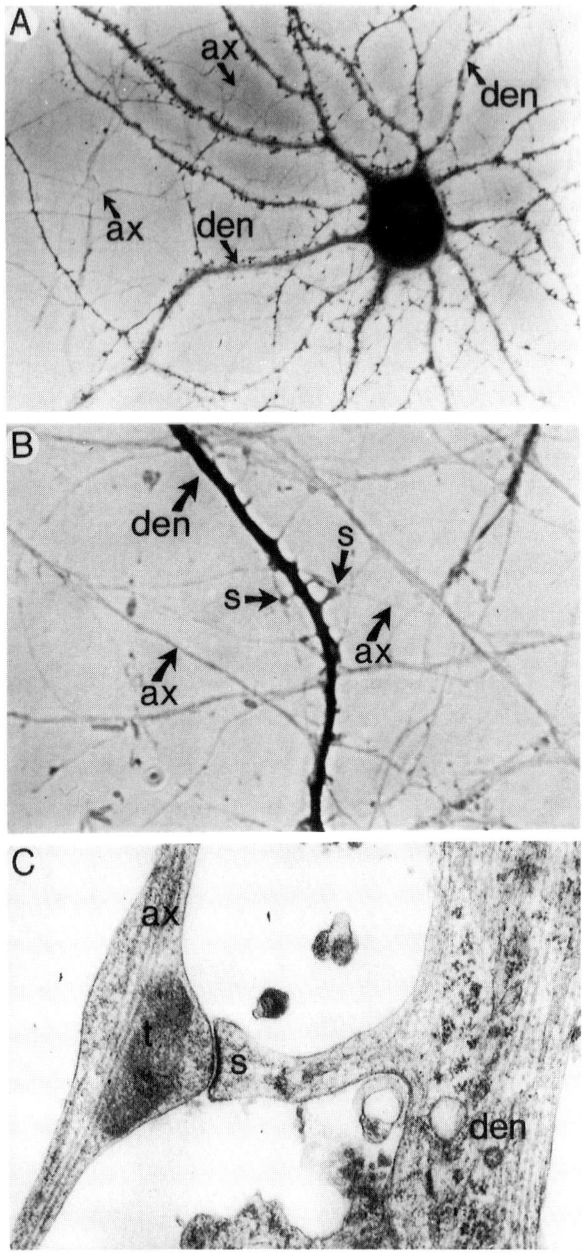


Figure 3. A) A hippocampal neuron in low density culture immunostained for MAP2. Note that the thick, tapering dendrites (den) are stained, while the thin axons (ax) are not. B) A higher magnification of a MAP2 stained dendrite with spines (s) and surrounding axons. C) Electron micrograph of a spine contacted by a synaptic terminal (t) in a hippocampal neuronal culture. Note presence of polyribosomes.

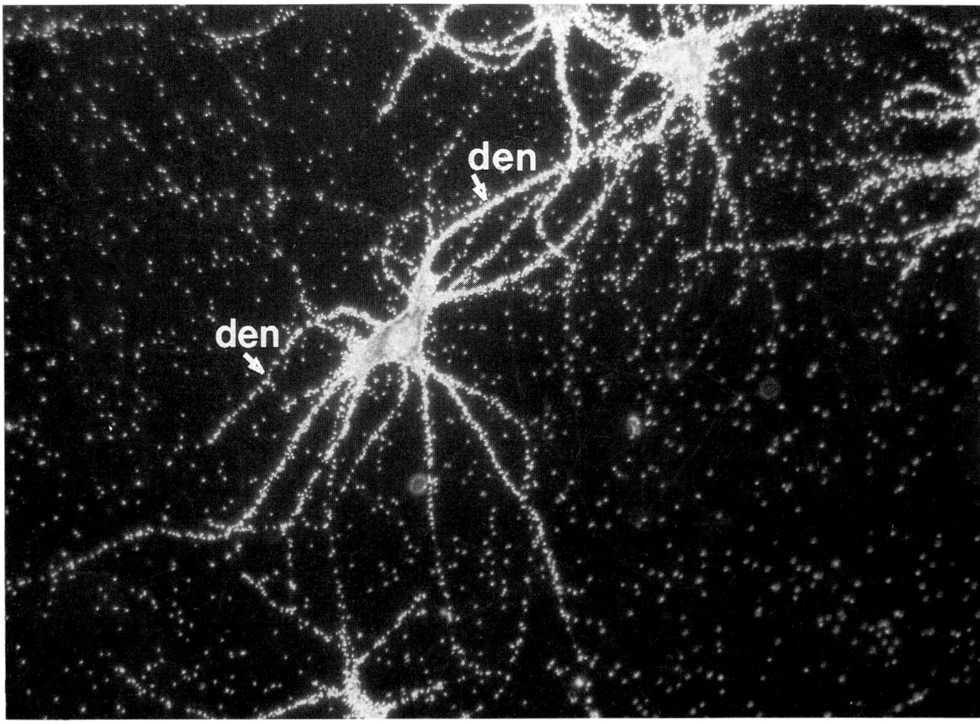


Figure 4. Pattern of labeling of hippocampal neurons in culture after a 15 minute pulse with 3-H leucine. Note dense accumulations of silver grains over cell bodies and dendrites (den). Numerous axons (not visible in darkfield) crisscross the field and are unlabeled.

## Evidence that Proteins of the Synaptic Junction are Synthesized Locally at the Synaptic Site

If there is local synthesis of protein within dendrites, and if this synthesis is particularly important during periods of synapse construction, then an obvious question is whether the polyribosomes actually synthesize protein constituents of the synaptic junction. To address this question, we have used pulse-labeling techniques in combination with subcellular fractionation. If recently synthesized proteins appeared in synaptic junctions more rapidly than could be explained by transport from the cell body, this would be consistent with their local synthesis. As noted above, recently synthesized proteins that move via transport systems do not usually begin to be transported until 45-60 minutes after their synthesis

(Droz and Leblond, 1963). Thus, if recently synthesized proteins are incorporated into synaptic junctions within 45 minutes, this would suggest local synthesis.

In order to obtain a sufficiently high level of labeling of recently synthesized proteins, pulse-labeling with protein precursors was carried out in vitro. Hippocampal slices were prepared from adult male Sprague-Dawley rats, and incubated for 15-60 minutes in a medium containing 3H-leucine (1mCi/ml). The slices were then homogenized in 0.32M sucrose, and synaptic junctional complexes (SJC) were isolated according to the method of Cotman and Taylor (1972). About 80 slices were pooled for each isolation, and 4 isolations were typically carried out simultaneously (three labeled preparations and one for electron microscopic analysis).

For these initial studies, we used slices from mature animals; this deserves some comment. On the basis of the results reviewed above, one would clearly expect higher levels of local synthesis during periods of synapse growth. However, polyribosomes are present beneath synaptic sites in the mature nervous system, and clearly there should be some turnover of synaptic constituents at steady state. Thus, if the polyribosomes do synthesize proteins for the synaptic junction, it should be possible to demonstrate this using tissue from the mature CNS. The advantage of using tissue from the mature CNS is that the subcellular fractionation techniques are better characterized.

The SJC fractions obtained after Triton X-100 treatment of synaptic plasma membranes have been characterized extensively. At the electron microscopic level, much of the material is amorphous in appearance and stains darkly with osmium. However, many of the profiles have the size and shape of postsynaptic densities (psd's) often having a small slip of membrane attached (Fig. 5). Cytochemical studies of such fractions using ethanolic phosphotungstic acid have provided evidence for the identity of the electron dense material as psd's (Cotman and Taylor, 1972).

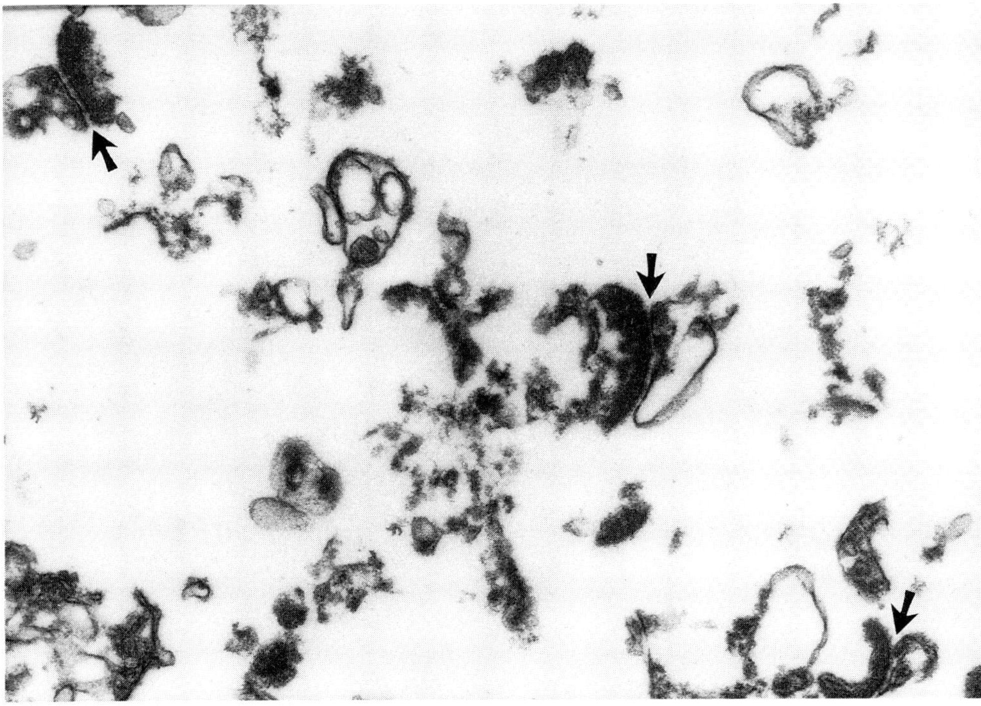

Figure 5. Electron microscopic appearance of the synaptic junctional complex (SJC) fraction isolated according to the method of Cotman and Taylor (1972).

The rate of appearance of recently synthesized proteins in the SJC fraction is illustrated in Figure 6. In order to combine data from several different experiments, the values for each time point are expressed as a percentage of the 30 minute value. As is evident, there is a linear increase in the cpm/mg protein in the SJC fraction over the first 45 minutes. Interestingly, the extent of incorporation at 60 minutes is more than would be predicted by a linear extrapolation of the line of the 15, 30, and 45 minute values. It is still too early to be certain of the significance of this nonlinearity, but one interpretation is that the increased rate of appearance of recently synthesized proteins after 45 minutes reflects the appearance of material that had been synthesized in the cell body and transported to the synaptic site.

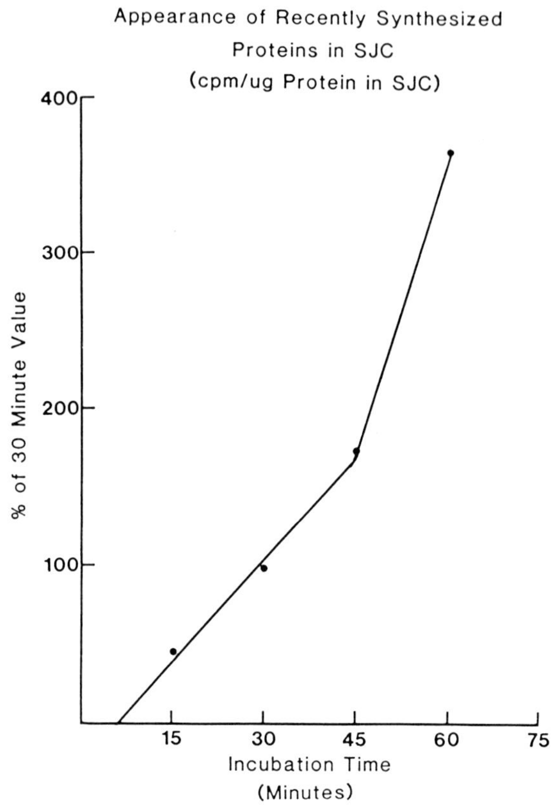


Figure 6. Rate of accumulation of recently synthesized proteins in SJC fractions prepared from hippocampal slices after various pulse intervals.

**CONCLUSION**

It is certainly not surprising that reinnervation would require a coordinated interaction between pre- and postsynaptic partners. On the postsynaptic side, the junctional specializations associated with degenerating contacts must be removed; the dendrite must be maintained temporarily in the denervated state; finally, new membrane specializations must be constructed for the reinnervating fibers. Even if some membrane specializations are re-used, it seems likely that some renovation would be required to accomodate the new synapses. Our studies suggest that an important part of the latter process involves the positioning of protein synthetic machinery beneath the new synaptic sites.

If this model is correct in general, then a number of very interesting questions arise. For example, it is clear that polyribosomes are selectively positioned beneath synaptic sites, but we do not know how this comes about. One issue is how the ribosomes and their associated mRNA are transported into dendrites. A separate issue is how the machinery is selectively positioned beneath synaptic sites. Information on these processes will be important for our understanding of how neurons accomplish the task of constructing, maintaining, and modifying their complex receptive surfaces. Such information may also suggest the means to facilitate the re-establishment of CNS connections following injury.

ACKNOWLEDGEMENTS: Thanks to P. M. Falk for technical help, and A. Pollack and A. Rao for their contributions to the subcellular fractionation studies. Supported by NIH grant NS12333 to O.S. and grant NS23094 to G.B. and O.S.

## REFERENCES

Bartlett WP, Banker GA (1984a) An electron microscopic study of the development of axons and dendrites by hippocampal neurons in culture: I. Cells which develop without intercellular contacts. J Neurosci 4:1944-1953

Bartlett WP, Banker GA (1984b) An electron microscopic study of the development of axons and dendrites by hippocampal neurons in culture: II. Synaptic relationships. J Neurosci 4:1954-1965

Caceres AO, Banker GA, Binder L (1986) Immunocytochemical localization of tubulin and microtubule-associated protein 2 during the development of hippocampal neurons in culture. J Neurosci 6:714-722

Caceres AO, Steward O (1983) Dendritic reorganization in the denervated dentate gyrus of the rat following entorhinal cortical lesions: a golgi and electron microscopic analysis. J Comp Neurol 214:387-403

Cotman CW, Nadler JV (1978) Reactive synaptogenesis in the hippocampus. In: Cotman CW (ed) Neuronal plasticity. Raven, New York, p 227

Cotman CW, Taylor D (1972) Isolation and ultrastructural studies on synaptic complexes from rat brain. J Cell Biol 55:696-711

Droz B, Leblond CP (1963) Axonal migration of proteins in the central nervous system and peripheral nerves as shown by radioautography. J Comp Neurol 121:325-346

Fass B, Steward O (1983) Increases in protein-precursor incorporation in the denervated dentate gyrus during reinnervation. Neurosci 9:653-664

Phillips LL, Nostrandt SJ, Chikaraishi DM, Steward O (to be published) Increases in ribosomal RNA within the denervated neuropil of the dentate gyrus during reinnervation: evaluation by in situ hybridization using DNA probes complementary to ribosomal RNA. Mol Brain Res

Steward O (1983a) Alterations in polyribosomes associated with dendritic spines during the reinnervation of the dentate gyrus of the adult rat. J Neurosci 3:177-188

Steward O (1983b) Polyribosomes at the base of dendritic spines of central nervous system neurons: their possible role in synapse construction and modification. Cold Spring Harbor Symp Quant Biol 48:745-759.

Steward O (1986a) Lesion-induced synapse growth in the hippocampus: in search of cellular and molecular mechanisms, In: Isaacson RL, Pribram KH (eds) The Hippocampus, vol 3. Plenum, New York London, p 65

Steward O (1986b) Making and modifying synapses in the mammalian CNS: towards a molecular biology of synapse growth and plasticity. In: Ruben RW (ed) The biology of change in otolaryngology. Elsevier, Amsterdam, p 235

Steward O, Caceres AO, Reeves TM (to be published) Rebuilding synapses after injury: remodeling the postsynaptic cell's receptive surface during reinnervation. In: Neural plasticity: a lifespan approach. Petit T, Ivy G (eds) Alan R Liss, New York

Steward O, Falk PM (1986) Protein-synthetic machinery at postsynaptic sites during synaptogenesis: a quantitative study of the association between polyribosomes and developing synapses. J Neurosci 6:412-423

Steward O, Vinsant SL (1983) The process of reinnervation in the dentate gyrus of the adult rat: a quantitative electron microscopic analysis of terminal proliferation and reactive synaptogenesis. J Comp Neurol 214:370-386

# GANGLIOSIDE TREATMENT OF EXPERIMENTAL BRAIN INJURY

ALFREDO GORIO, WISE YOUNG*, VINCENT DE CRESCITO*, ANTONELLA MANNAVOLA, and ANNA MARIA DI GIULIO

Department of Medical Pharmacology, University of Milano, Via Vanvitelli 32, 20129 Milano, Italy, and * Department of Neurosurgery, New York University Medical Center, School of Medicine, 550 First Avenue, New York, NY 10016

## INTRODUCTION

The investigation on the biological role of gangliosides in nervous system functions has been one of the fastest growing fields of neuroscience in the last five years. Such an interest probably derived from a series of reports suggesting an effect of these substances on the mechanisms of nervous system repair following a traumatic injury or chronic disorders (1).

Gangliosides are glycosphingolipids discovered some 50 years ago by Klenk ( 2,3,4 ). They are distinguished among one another by the different constitution and structure of the carbohydrate moieties linked to the ceramide hydrofobic portion of the molecule. The latter part is inserted in the lipid component of the outer leaflet of neuronal cell plasma membrane, while the hydrophilic carbohydrates are in contact with the

NATO ASI Series, Vol. H22
Neural Development and Regeneration
Edited by A. Gorio et al.

extracellular fluids ( 1 ). Such a distribution and the high concentration on cell surface have stimulated speculations on the role played by gangliosides in cellular functions, particularly during development ( 1 ). The biosynthesis and the overall fate of gangliosides are fairly well established. The molecule ceramidic portion is assembled in the endoplasmic reticulum, while the carbohydrates are step wise added in the Golgi apparatus. Cell fractionation experiments showed that Golgi derived vescicles might be the mean of ganglioside transport from the intracellular compartments to the cell surface ( 5,6 ). Recently, it has also been demonstrated that gangliosides are transported from the neuron cell body along the axon to the nerve terminal and viceversa , suggesting that the soma may be the only source of gangliosides in neurones (7).

Endogenous gangliosides may function as receptors for a variety of biological substances and toxins (1). Similar properties are also displayed by exogenous gangliosides upon incorporation into the host cell plasma membrane (1). Therefore the incorporated glycolipids may be capable of expressing biological properties by interacting with extracellular signals as normally occurs with the endogenous ones. On the other hand we are summarizing in this report a variety of evidences which suggest that exogenous gangliosides may be able of affecting the mechanisms of neuronal injury and repair by virtue of their interaction with the plasma membrane of the lesioned neurones.

## EXOGENOUS GANGLIOSIDES AND NEURONAL REGENERATION

Some twenty five - thirty years ago it was shown by Mc Ilwain and co-workers that naturally occurring substances were capable of restoring excytability of brain slices after intoxication or cold blockade ( 8, 9). Such crude extracts were rich in gangliosides (8,9). A direct evidence, that exogenous gangliosides could affect the mechanisms underlying neuronal differentiation, regeneration and repair in general, was supplied by the in vitro experiments utilizing primary neurons in culture or neuronal cell lines (1). The bathing media used in each specific condition were modified by adding various quantities of gangliosides, it was observed that such treatment enhanced neurite and synapse formation (1). The question whether the action of exogenously supplied gangliosides was direct or mediated by a specific growth factor was addressed using a cell line PC12 Pheochromocytoma, that requires Nerve Growth Factor (NGF) for differentiation (10). The results were strikingly clear:

1) Gangliosides enhanced neuritogenesis at very low doses, particularly in serum free conditions.

2) The effect was dependent upon the presence of NGF in the culture media. In other words, the absence of NGF from the bathing fluids prevented any neurite formation in spite of ganglioside addition.

3) The incubation of PC12 cells with gangliosides does not alter the properties and the amount of NGF binding.

In conclusion these data suggested that gangliosides affect the mechanisms regulating the processes of neuritogenesis by increasing the efficacy of the specific growth factor action (10). Perhaps the incorporation of gangliosides into the neuronal membrane causes changes in specific membrane microenvironments so that neurons may be more effectively responsive to the programs dictated by specific growth factors.

Such precise responses from the in vitro experiments reinforce the understandings and the interpretations of in vivo effects observed previously. The processes of neuronal sprouting was monitored during muscle reinnervation following either complete denervation caused by sciatic nerve crush or partial denervation caused by resection of one root constituting the sciatic nerve. The electrophysiological evaluation of the Extensor Digitorum Longus muscle reinnervation after sciatic nerve crush demonstrated that ganglioside treatment enhanced significantly the rate of sprouting of the regenerating axons until synaptic repression began (11). These data originally suggested that the action of gangliosides on the dynamics of sprouting was dependent upon a factor released by the denervated muscle (11). The partial denervation experiments showed that the extent of sprouting was also increased in addition to the rate (12).

These effects of gangliosides observed clearly in the peripheral nervous system are less clear in the CNS as far as is the data interpretation. In the case of CNS pathways lesions induced with selective neuritoxins, we have clearly shown that ganglioside treatment is capable of improving the restoration of the damaged pathways without affecting the primary degenerative process (13). Both serotoninergic and noradrenergic axons are reformed faster in the cortex than in case of saline treated animals. An early pretreatment with gangliosides seems to be crucial (14). In the following part of the paper the importance of the pretreatment paradigm for cns injuries will be evident. Such a regrowth stimulatory effect is also evident in the spinal cord after neonatal chemical lesion of the serotoninergic pathways (15). On the other hand there are clear indications that gangliosides do not promote outgrowth in an indiscriminate matter: the PC12 experience has shown that the neuritogenic effect requires NGF presence in the bathing medium and the motor axon sprouting effect requires denervation. These suggestions are strongly reinforced by the lack of ganglioside effect on cns hyperinnervation processes. In the case of new born animal lesions of the serotoninergic pathways, the slow reinnervation of the most distal regions is accompanied by the hyperinnervation of the most proximal regions. Ganglioside treatment reduces such an outgrowth (13,15), therefore acting in an opposite manner than in the cases indicated above. This effect is also observed in a different experimental condition. Noradrenaline is depleted almost permanently in the cortex of new born animals by an injection of 6-OHDA, 5-HT and DA fibers react to the deafferentation by hyperinnervating the frontal cortex. Ganglioside treatment fully prevent the reactive hyperinnervation by the 5-HT and DA fibers (13).

In conclusion, the effect of ganglioside treatment on either neuronal regeneration or axonal outgrowth in general is certainly more complex than some authors like to consider. The enhancement of axonal sprouting is certainly not a univocal response to ganglioside treatment.

## EXOGENOUS GANGLIOSIDES AND NEURONAL INJURY

One of the early and most important finding on ganglioside effects was reported a few years ago by Karpiak after entorhinal cortex lesion in rats (16). This experimental procedure causes denervation of the dendrite outer layer in the dentate gyrus of the hippocampus correlated with a behavioral deficit; both alterations gradually recover in 2-3 weeks (16). If the animals were treated with gangliosides the day before lesioning, both the same extent of denervation and the rate of reinnervation were unaffected by the treatment while the original behavioral deficit (48 hours after lesion) was greatly reduced (16,17). Such a quick effect could not be explained as due to sprouting or regeneration enhancement, since these processes take place much later. The authors suggested a protective effect of gangliosides, as if the treatment with these agents reduced the consequences of the lesion perhaps by reducing neuronal death.

This rapid effect cannot be attributed to the synergistic effect of gangliosides and trophic factors since they cannot be detected that soon after injury. On the other hand a direct effect of these agents on the cell membrane of injured must be born in mind. If hippocampal slices are subjected to a transient hypoxia-ischemia paradigm we observe a significant drop of Na-K ATPase activity and a mitochondria swelling probably due to Ca loading (18). When the experimental animals were pretreated with gangliosides for 3 days prior sacrifice and hippocampal slicing, both ATPase deactivation and mitochondrial Ca loading were fully prevented (18). These results strongly support the concept that some membrane microenvironment rearrangements occurring after ganglioside incorporation are responsible for the protective effect of these agents.

Cerebral ischemia is one of the latest experimental paradigms used for assessing ganglioside efficacy in the treatment of damaged brain, since a preliminary clinical report suggested a potential efficacy (19). Some experimental results are very encouraging, while others appeared only in proceedings of meetings deserve further examination. Permanent unilateral ligation of the common carotid artery in gerbils causes 52% mortality within 48 hours in saline treated animals (20). On the contrary GM1 treated gerbils showed a mortality reduced to 26%, a difference which is highly significant (20). Most likely the membrane mechanisms postulated above may be responsible of the effect. In search for membrane related events which could be responsible of the animal enhanced survival, we induced a permanent cerebral ischemia by occluding the middle cerebral artery (MCA) in the rat. The lesion area was examined histologically and the effects of the vascular injury monitored as alterations in the ionic distribution. It is well known that in the ischemic regions of the brain there is a large intracellular accumulation of Na and Ca with a concomitant loss of K and edema formation (21). The animals were treated with saline or with GM1 twentyfour hours and/or just before MCA occlusion, then the animals were sacrificed 24 later and the ions and water contents were examined in the lesioned areas as previously described in reference 21. No difference was found between GM1 ganglioside and saline treated groups of animals about the ionic alterations caused by MCA occlusion. However a very interesting result was obtained if the animals were pretreated for 3 days prior MCA occlusion and then kept alive for 7 days. Again no effect of GM1 treatment on the extent of edema formation and on both Na accumulation and K loss, but a highly significant protection on the calcium accumulation. The amount of calcium, which is loaded intracellularly in the main lesioned areas, gradually increases during the 7 days following the occlusion and reaches a level which can be 10 fold normal. In the animals pretreated with GM1 such Ca loading was maintained at a level usually found 24 hours after MCA occlusion.

In conclusion it is possible that pretreatment with GM1 may have prevented some membrane function deactivation and therefore reduce the enormous Ca accumulation normally found 7 days after MCA occlusion. These membrane and ionic mechanisms could be responsible of the protective effects of ganglioside treatment on the consequences of neuronal injury.

## REFERENCES


1. Gorio A. ( 1986 ), Ganglioside enhancement of neuronal differentiation, plasticity and repair. J. Clin. Neurobiol. 2:241-296
2. Klenk E. ( 1934 ), Uber die natur der phosphatide der Milz bei der Niemann-Pickschen krankheit. Z Physiol. Chem. 229: 151-156
3. Klenk E. ( 1935 ), Uber die nature der phosphatide und anderer lipoide des gehirns und der leber bei der Niemann-Pickschen krankheit, Z. Physiol. Chem. 235:24-36
4. Klenk E., ( 1939 ), Beitrage zur chemie der lipoidosen ,3. Mitt. Niemann-Pickschen krankheit und amaurotische idiotie. Z. Physiol. Chem. 282: 84-88
5. Caputto R., Caputto B.L., Domowicz M.S., and Kivatinitz S.C. ( 1987 ), Gangliosides: biosynthesis, transport and location in the plasma membrane. In: Gangliosides and modulation of neuronal functions ( ed. H. Rahman ). Springer-Verlag NATO ASI Series,251-258
6. Morre' D.J., Kartenbeck J., and Franke W. W. ( 1987 ), Membrane flow and interconversions among membranes. Biochem. Byophys. Acta 559: 71-152
7. Aquino D.A., Bisby M.A., and Ledeen R.W. (1987), Bidirectional transport of gangliosides, glycoproteins and neutral glycosphingolipids in the sensory neurones of rat sciatic nerve. Neuroscience, in press

8. Marks N. and Mc Ilwain H. (1959), Loss of excytability in isolated cerebral tissues, and its restorations by naturally occurring materials. Biochem. J. 73:401-410
9. Mc Ilwain H. (1961), Characterization of naturally occurring material which restore excitability to isolated cerebral tissue. Biochem. J., 90:442-448
10. Ferrari G., Fabris M. and Gorio A. ( 1983), Gangliosides enhance neurite outgrowth in PC12 cells, Dev. Brain Res. 8:215-221
11. Gorio A., Carmignoto G., Facci 1., and Finesso M. ( 1980), Motor nerve sprouting induced by ganglioside treatment. Possible implications for gan gliosides on neuronal growth. Brain Res. 197:236-241
12. Gorio A., Marini P., and Zanoni R. ( 1983), Muscle Reinnervation III. Motoneuron sprouting capacity, enhancement by exogenous gangliosides. Neuroscience,8:417-429
13. Jonsson G., Gorio A., Hallman H., Janigro D., Kojima K., Luthman J., and Zanoni R. (1984), Effect of GM1 ganglioside on developing and mature serotonin and noradrenaline neurones lesioned by selective neurotoxins. J. Neurosc. Res. 12: 459-475
14. Kojima H., Gorio A., Janigro D., and Jonsson G. (1984), GM1 ganglioside enhances regrowth of noradrenaline nerve terminals in rats cerebral cortex lesioned by the neurotoxin 6- Hydroxydopamine. Neuroscience, 13:1011-1022
15. Fusco M., Dona' M., Tessari F., Hallman H., Jonsson G., and Gorio A. (1986). GM1 ganglioside counteracts selective neurotoxin-induced lesion of developing serotonin neurons in the spinal cord. J. Neurosc. Res., 15:467-480
16. Karpiak S.E. (1983), Ganglioside treatment improves recovery of alternation behaviour after unilateral entorhinal cortex lesion. Exp. Neurol. 81:330-339
17. Gorio A. and Haber B., eds. (1984),Neurobiology of gangliosides. Alan R. Liss, New York
18. Bianchi R., Janigro D., Milan F., Giudici R., and Gorio A. (1986), "In vivo" treatment with GM1 prevents the rapid decay of ATPase activities and mitochondrial damage in hippocampal slices. Brain Research, 364:400-404
19. Bassi S., Albizzati M.G., Sbacchi M., Frattola L., Massarotti M. (1984). Double-blind evaluation of monosialoganglioside (GM1) therapy in stroke. J. Neurosc. Res. 12:493-498
20. Karpiak S.E., Li Y.S., Mahadik S.P. (1987), Gangliosides (GM1 and AGF2) reduce mortality due to ischemia: protection of membrane function. Stroke 18:184-187
21. Young W., Hadani M., Rappaport H., De Crescito V., Cornu P., and Flamm E.S. (1986), Tissue Na, K, and Ca changes in regional cerebral ischemia: their measurement and interpretation. CNS Trauma 3:215-234

# EFFECTS OF GANGLIOSIDES AND FIBROBLAST GROWTH FACTOR ON CENTRAL NEURONS IN CELL CULTURES OF RAT HIPPOCAMPUS AND CORTEX DURING DEVELOPMENT AND REGENERATION IN-VITRO

W. Seifert and F. Förster
Dept. of Neurobiology, Max-Planck-Institut f. biophys. Chem.
3400 Göttingen, W-Germany

## INTRODUCTION

Several biological functions of gangliosides are presently investigated in the mammalian nervous system. These include the possible involvement in cell-cell recognition and cell-substrate adhesion, the modulation of receptors and a functional role in synaptic transmission and synaptic plasticity (1,2,3,4). Finally the neurotrophic effects of gangliosides which have been studied mostly in cell culture systems during recent years might be of special importance also during in-vivo development and regeneration of the nervous system.

The first reports on a neurotrophic effect of exogenously added gangliosides were studies with neuroblastoma cells in culture. Thus we demonstrated in 1978/79 in our laboratory that bovine brain gangliosides induced neurite outgrowth and increased survival in serum-free medium for B104 cells, a neuronal cell line originated from rat brain (5). Similar effects for neurite outgrowth were later described for N2a neuroblastoma cells (6,7,8). Furthermore such a neurite-promoting effect of gangliosides was also demonstrated for primary cultures of dorsal root ganglia of the peripheral nervous system (7). Finally these studies were extended to investigate neurons from the central nervous system (9,10,11). The demonstration that gang-

NATO ASI Series, Vol. H22
Neural Development and Regeneration
Edited by A. Gorio et al.

liosides stimulated axonal sprouting and synaptogenesis following nerve injury in the PNS (12,13) generated great interest in clinical applications of gangliosides which contributed to the dynamic development of this area of research during recent years.

Another important development was the observation that fibroblast growth factor (FGF) may have a neurotrophic function for central neurons (14), - in addition to its well established proliferative function for cells of mesodermal origin, including endothelial cells and glial cells (15).
Studies in the laboratory of M. Sensenbrenner demonstrated the presence of FGF in neurons of the brain by immunohistochemical methods and the identity of the brain-derived "astroglial growth factor" (AGF) with FGF (16). Thus in addition to the recently established role of NGF as neurotrophic factor for cholinergic neurons in the CNS, the long known FGF may take a place as another important neurotrophic factor for central neurons such as the pyramidal neurons of cortex and hippocampus in the mammalian CNS.

Several years ago we established a serum - free cell culture system of predominantly pyramidal neurons from day 18 embryonic rat hippocampus, which is similar to the culture system described by M. Cowan's laboratory (17,18,19,20,21). This dissociated cell culture system of pyramidal neurons is used in our laboratory for developmental studies in-vitro, with special emphasis on glial-neuron trophic interactions and the functional role of both endogenous and exogenous gangliosides (22,9).

While this hippocampal cell culture system is useful for in-vitro studies on <u>development</u> of central neurons, we have established more recently another culture system which will serve as a model system for in-vitro studies of <u>regeneration</u>: this is a dense culture of cortex from newborn rats in which we have scratched a wound. This so-called "wound - culture" from the CNS allows us to study in a two-dimensional cell culture system regenerative processes which might otherwise occur in-vivo after lesions or injury to the brain. In both these systems we are investigating the effects of gangliosides and neurotrophic factors such as FGF on development and regeneration of central neurons.

METHODS

Cell cultures from rat hippocampus were prepared in serum-free hormone-supplemented medium as previously described (18,19,20). For the dissociated low-density cultures of hippocampal neurons, cells were taken from 18-day old rat embryos and plated at $2 \times 10^5$ cells/ml medium on polylysine coated coverslips. After the initial attachment phase in medium containing 5% horse serum and 5% fetal calf serum for 45 min, the coverslips were gently washed and placed into medium consisting of DMEM and hormone-supplement (insulin, transferrin, hydrocortison and triiodo-thyronine - as described in reference 18,19) and the appropriate additions of gangliosides or fibroblast growth factor. The final density of attached cells was $2\text{-}4 \times 10^4$ cells per $cm^2$.

High density cultures from rat cortex were prepared from newborn rats in a similar way, with the exception of a different hormone-mixture: N2-medium (J. Bottenstein and G. Sato, 1979) was used which seemed to improve longterm survival (I. Thorey, thesis 1987). These culture were used after 10 days for the "wound experiments" described in Fig. 3 and 4.

Identification of the cell types was done by immunofluorescence staining: anti-GFAP for astrocytes and anti-neurofilament for neurons. Cell survival was measured by fluorescence staining (F. Förster, unpublished) which in our hands is a much more reliable test than trypanblue exclusion. Individual gangliosides were obtained from Serolab, Munich. Fibroblast growth factor (FGF) was purchased from Sigma Co, Munich.

Observation of cells and neurites was done by phasecontrast

microscopy and by micro-cinematography. Neurite length in um per neuron was measured from phasecontrast photographs at appropriate magnifications. Routinely each experimental condition was determined in 3-5 independent experiments. Each experimental point consisted of 3 coverslips, and 4 different fields were quantitatively evaluated from each coverslip with a total cell count of approximately 400 cells per coverslip.

## RESULTS AND DISCUSSION

### 1. Effect of exogenous gangliosides on hippocampal neurons at low cell density in serum-free medium

As previously described (17,18) the neuronal cell culture system from embryonic rat hippocampus consists mostly of neuronal cells. Due to the developmental timing these cultures contain almost no granular neurons which develop postnatally and then form the cell layer of the dentate gyrus. They consist mainly of pyramidal neurons (glutamatergic) and to a lesser extent of basket neurons (gabanergic). In addition about 10% of the cells are astrocytes and less than 1% are other minor cell types such as oligodendrocytes and microglial cells. Therefore with about 90% neuronal cells of well described origin and developmental stage (about 24-48 hrs postmitotic), this neuronal cell culture system from the hippocampus can be considered for all practical purposes a relatively homogenous cell culture system, especially in view of the complexities of other systems from the central nervous system.

Due to the fact that these neurons have just become postmitotic and at the time of dissociation and plating onto culture dishes or coverslips have no processes, the outgrowth to neurites can be observed over the first 24 or 48 hrs. At low cell density individual cells and their neurite growth can be followed and measured by phasecontrast micro-photography and cinematography, as shown in Fig. 1.

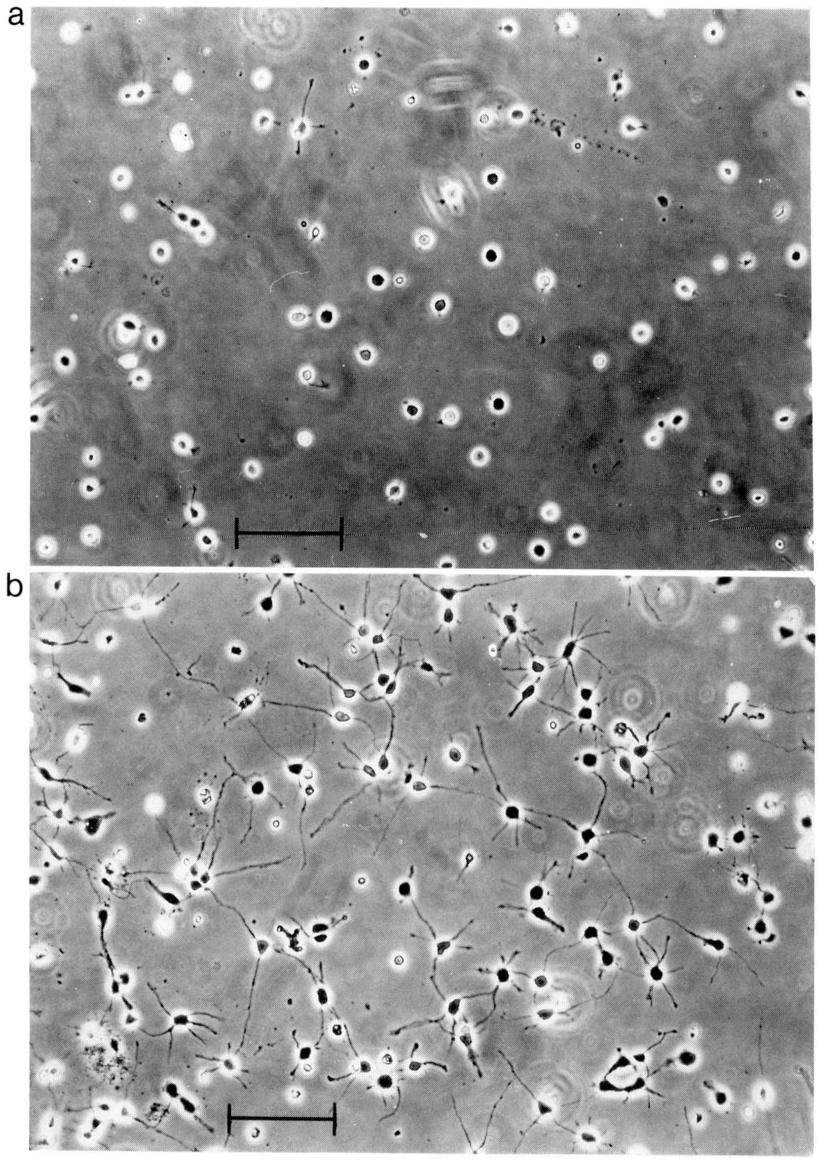


Fig. 1)

a) Phasecontrast photograph of hippocampal neurons 2 hrs after plating on polylysine-coated coverslips. Culture conditions as described in Methods. Only very short processes can be seen on some of the cells. Bar represents 100 μm.

b) The same culture of hippocampal neurons 24 hrs after plating. Extensive neurite outgrowth can be noticed. Most cells have developed two or more long processes. Bar represents 100 μm.

In this system we have previously studied the neurotrophic interaction of astrocytes and neurons and described a low-molecular weight neurotrophic factor (19,20). Further research in our laboratory demonstrated that there is also in addition a high-molecular weight factor in astrocyte-conditioned medium. As we have recently described (22), the low-molecular weight component has the survival activity and turned out to be pyruvate, as was also described in work from S. Varon's laboratory (23). The high-molecular weight component is responsible for the neurite-promoting activity and seems antigenically related to laminin (22).

In this communication we want to report results from our continued studies on the functional role of gangliosides in central neurons (4,5,9) with special emphasis on their neurotrophic potential. As already described in our first publication on this subject (5), exogenously added gangliosides are stably incorporated into the membranes of neuronal cells in culture with a kinetics which reaches a plateau after about 3 hrs. Therefore exogenous ganglioside can be used to mimick or promote biological functions of nerve cells which otherwise under conditions in-vivo might be triggered by the developmentally regulated appearance or disappearance of certain ganglioside species on the cell membrane.

As demonstrated in Fig. 2, exogenously added ganglioside may have two opposite effects on neurite outgrowth from hippocampal neurons, depending on the concentration used and on the individual ganglioside species. In this case we show as an example the effects of the ganglioside GT1b on neurite outgrowth.

At the concentration of $5 \times 10^{-5}$ M (50 μM) neurite outgrowth is completely inhibited. This effect is in itself not due to toxicity, since these cells are still alive as we could demonstrate in several survival tests (not shown here). A toxic effect is of course observed if we use higher concentrations: in this case cells detach from the dish and die. Also interesting is the observation that the neurons initially start growing out their processes in the presence of GT1b in the medium for up to about 6 hrs, - after that time they slowly retract them again.

Already at 10-fold lower concentration, i.e. at 5 μM GT1b, inhibition of neurite outgrowth is no longer observed. Thus the concentration range of the ganglioside is highly sensitive for the observed biological effect. Finally at very low concentrations - shown here for $1 \times 10^{-8}$ M (10 nM) - we have observed a significant stimulation of neurite outgrowth at 24 hrs. as compared to the control cultures (Fig. 2).

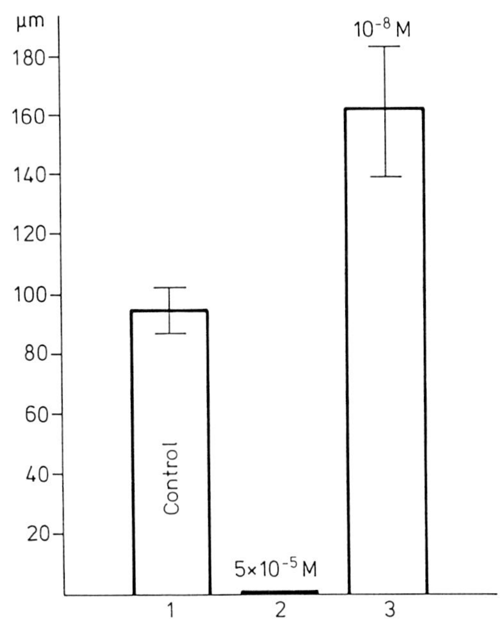


Fig. 2)

The effect of adding exogenous GT1b ganglioside for 24 hrs to a hippocampal cell culture as shown in Fig. 1. Neurite length is plotted in um per neuron, measured from magnifications of phasecontrast photographs as described in Methods. Bars represent the SEM of 3 independent experiments. Each experiment consisted of 3 coverslips with 4 different microscopic fields on each coverslip culture.

1) Control cultures with an average neurite length of 95 μm
2) Addition of GT1b at $5 \times 10^{-5}$ M: complete inhibition of neurite outgrowth.
3) Addition of GT1b at $1 \times 10^{-8}$ M: stimulation of neurite outgrowth with an average length of 160 μm.

Similar results as described here were obtained for other individual ganglioside species, in particular for GM1 and GD1a. But the dose-response curves for each individual ganglioside with respect to the specific biological effect are different. In general it seems that the polysialo-gangliosides like GT1b are more effective than the monosialo-ganglioside GM1, - both in terms of neurite-stimulation at low concentrations and in terms of neurite inhibition at high concentrations. The results of these studies will be described in more detail elsewhere (F. Förster and W. Seifert, in preparation). Finally it should be mentioned that the effects seem to be rather specific for molecules with a sialo-glycolipid structure such as gangliosides, since sialic acid and neutral glycolipids such as galactose-cerebroside had no effect at any concentration.

Our results tend to confirm previous observations that gangliosides at low concentrations may stimulate neurite outgrowth in different culture systems under restricted growth conditions.

In a study from Varon's laboratory a ganglioside effect on hippocampal neurons was noticed only at early times (11). These authors stressed the time-gain by gangliosides and measured as a parameter the percentage of neurite-bearing cells. In our study we can demonstrate a quantitative gain in absolute neurite length in presence of gangliosides even after 24 hrs in culture.

While these differences could also be due to culture conditions, we would like to emphasize the general conclusion from both studies that gangliosides at low concentrations may indeed effect the neurite outgrowth of cultured neurons from the CNS. At the same time it should be kept in mind that due to the presence of glial cells there are also neurotrophic factors in these culture systems. Therefore gangliosides may modulate the neurite outgrowth, but probably cannot substitute these neurotrophic factors. This at least has been conclusively demonstrated for the action of NGF on peripheral neurons.

Finally our studies demonstrate clearly a bimodal action of individual gangliosides on neurite outgrowth: while they stimulate neurite outgrowth at low concentrations they tend to inhibit neurite outgrowth at high concentrations.

## 2. Effects of gangliosides and fibroblast growth factor on high density nerve cell cultures from rat cortex in "wound experiments"

As already mentioned in the introduction we have developed in recent years a so-called "wound-culture system" which we consider a promising new model for studies of regeneration in a nerve cell culture system in-vitro. We like to think of this system as a two-dimensional model for the three-dimensional brain lesions which are commonly used for studies of regeneration. The obvious advantage of our system is the possibility of continued observation by micro-cinematography, the identification of all cell types by combining immunohistochemistry and autoradiography and the possibilities of manipulation by drugs, hormones and other substances such as gangliosides during the process of regeneration in an in-vitro system.

The culture system consists of nerve cells from rat cortex or hippocampus plated at high cell density and maintained for several days (1-2 weeks) in a serum-free, hormone-supplemented medium. Both neurons and glial cells are present under these conditions. Due to the long culture period, these dense culture can be considered to some extent a two-dimensional in-vitro system of the adult rat brain. Then a "wound" is scratched into the cell monolayer which in the phasecontrast microscope looks like an open "freeway". Such an example is shown in Fig. 3 where a) shows the phasecontrast photography at time 0 and b) is a view through the scanning microscope 24 hrs. later. This picture shows the outgrowing processes with the growth cones reaching out into the open space. The same 24 hr time point is shown in a phasecontrast photo in Fig. 4, a). Again neurite outgrowth and in addition individual cells migrating into the open "wound" can be noticed.

Routinely we observe our wound-experiments in phasecontrast microscopy and time-lapse cinematography and later identify the cell types of this same area by immunohistochemistry and autoradiography. Thus one can observe for example the different mobilities and activities of both neurons and astrocytes in this wound-paradigm.

With this wound-culture system we are now studying the effects of gangliosides and neurotrophic factors on such an "in-vitro-lesion". A more detailed description of these experiments will be described elsewhere (F. Förster and W. Seifert, in preparation). Here we like to demonstrate as an example the action of fibroblast growth factor in this system, as demonstrated in Figure 4, b). This is the same 24 hrs time point as shown in Fig. 4, a), but treated with 10 ng/ml FGF in the medium. The effect can be clearly seen: due to extensive neurite outgrowth and cell migration the open wound has been almost completely closed. While this is in agreement with the notion that FGF may act as a neurotrophic factor on central neurons (14), it demonstrates in addition in our "wound culture system" that FGF may actually be beneficial in a wound and therefore presumably also in an in-vivo lesion situation by stimulating regenerative processes.

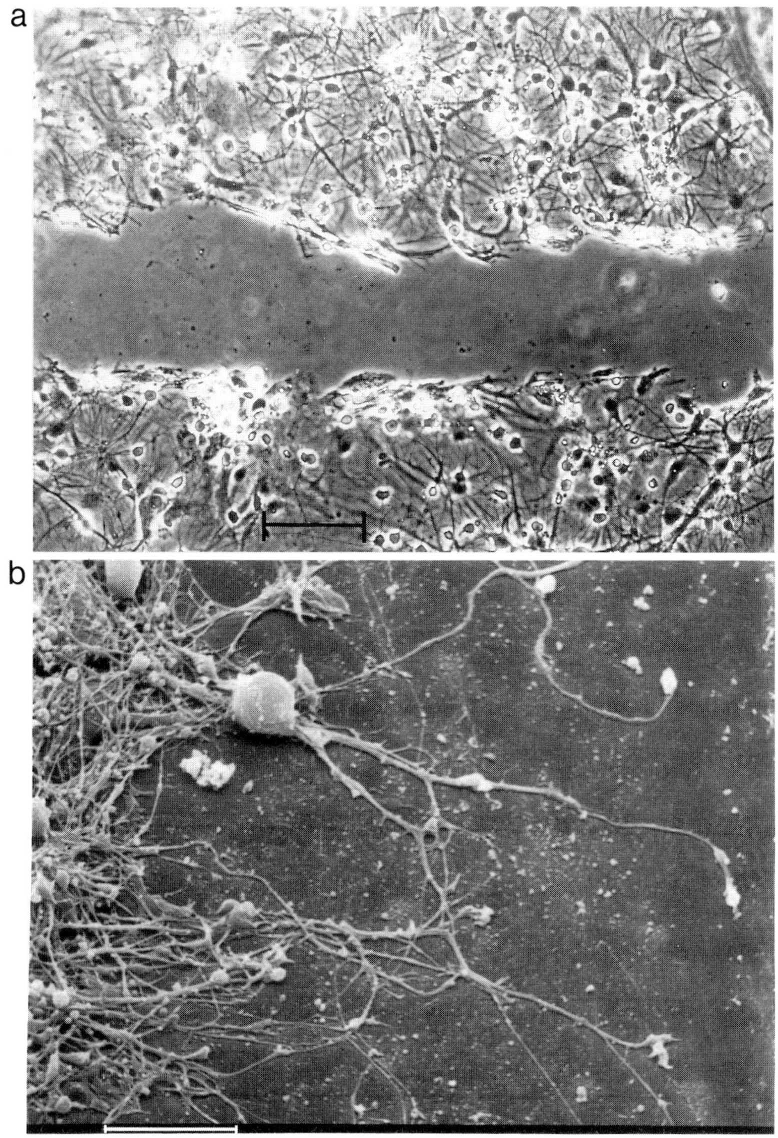

Fig. 3)

Phasecontrast photograph of "wound culture system" as described in Methods and Results. Dense cortex culture of newborn rats cultured in serum-free N2-containing medium for 10 days. Bar represents 10 µm.

a) at time 0 hr after scratching the wound into the culture

b) Scanning electronmicrograph taken at time 24 hrs after wounding. Long processes with growthcones are growing from the edge of the wound into the open space. Bar represents 10 µm.

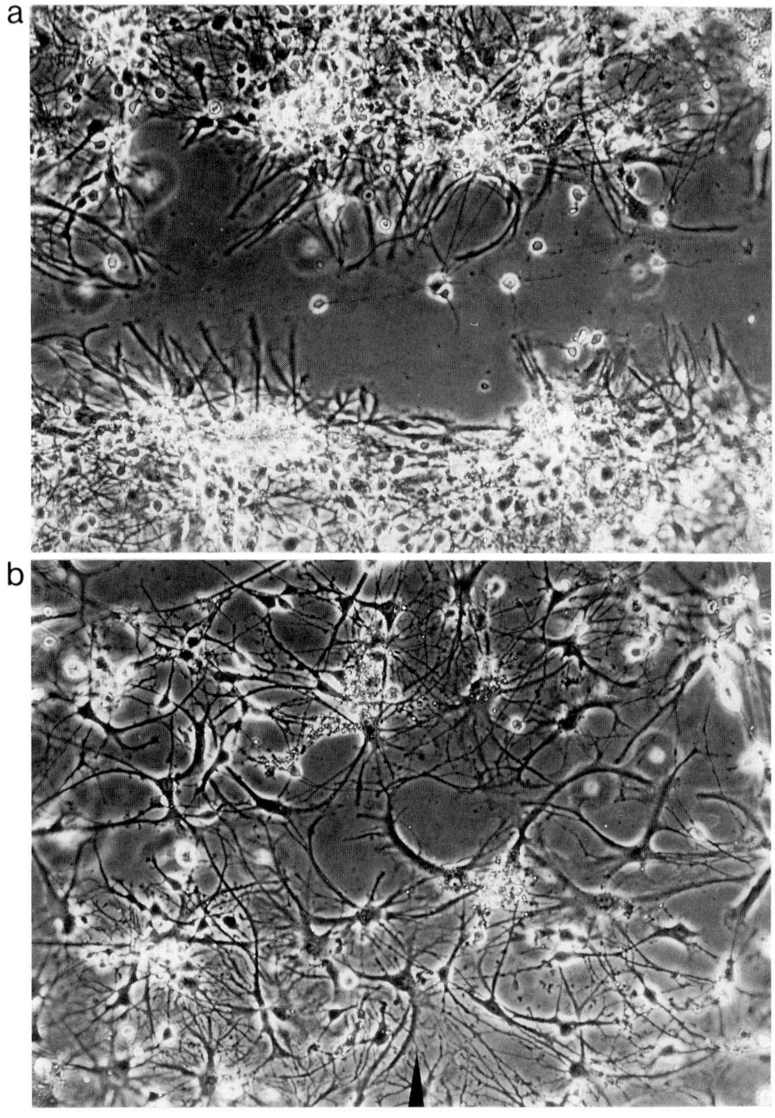

Fig. 4)

The same wound culture system as in Fig. 3a) at 24 hrs after wounding. Phasecontrast micrograph.

a) Control: no addition to medium. Notice outgrowing neurites and individual cells migrating into the wound.

b) Addition of 10 ng FGF/ml medium for 24 hrs: the wound is almost closed by extensive neurite outgrowth and glial cell migration.

## SUMMARY

We have studied the effects of gangliosides and neurotrophic factors in two different culture systems derived from the rat central nervous system:

1) in a dissociated cell culture system of hippocampal neurons at low cell density in serum-free medium
2) in a "wound culture system" prepared from cortical cultures at high cell density.

While the first system is useful for studies on development of central neurons, the second system is a new and promising two-dimensional cell culture model for studies on regeneration in the CNS following lesions or injury. In this system we have demonstrated a pronounced neurotrophic effect of FGF. With respect to the effects of exogenous gangliosides on central neurons we have shown a bimodal action on neurite outgrowth: individual gangliosides with somewhat different dose-response curves stimulate neurite outgrowth - measured as neurite length at 24 hrs - at low concentrations ($10^{-7}$ to $10^{-9}$ M), but inhibit neurite outgrowth at high concentrations ($10^{-5}$ to $10^{-4}$ M).

## ACKNOWLEDGEMENTS

We thank Barbara Scheufler for her excellent technical assistance, Dr. Irmgard Thorey for helpful discussions, and Claudia Jördening-Kalde for typing this manuscript.

## REFERENCES


1) Gorio A, Haber B (eds) (1985) Neurobiology of Gangliosides. Alan Liss Inc., New York
2) Tettamant G, Ledeen RW, Sandhoff K, Nagai Y, Toffano G (eds) (1986) Gangliosides and Neuronal Plasticity. Fidia Research Series Vol. 6. Liviana Press, Padova and Springer, Berlin Heidelberg New York
3) Rahmann H (ed) (1987) Gangliosides and Modulation of Neuronal Functions. NATO ASI Series H: Cell Biology, Vol. 7. Springer, Berlin Heidelberg New York
4) Seifert W, Hollmann M, Wieraszko A (1986) A functional role of ganglioside $GM_1$ in synaptic transmission and synaptic plasticity of the rat hippocampus. In: Matthies H (ed) Learning and Memory-Mechanisms of Information Storage in the Nervous System. Pergamon Press, Oxford, p 247
5) Morgan J, Seifert W (1979) Growth factors and gangliosides: a possible new perspective in neuronal growth control. J Supramol Struct 10:111-124
6) Dimpfel W, Moller W, Mengs U (1981) Ganglioside-induced neurite formation in cultured neuroblastoma cells. In: Rapport MM, Gorio A (eds) Gangliosides in Neurological and Neuromuscular Function, Development, and Repair. Raven, New York, pp 119-134
7) Roisen FJ, Bartfeld H, Nagele R, Yorke G (1981) Ganglioside stimulation of axonal sprouting in vitro. Science 214:577-578
8) Leon A, Facci L, Benvegnu D, Toffano G (1982) Morphological and biochemical effects of gangliosides in neuroblastoma cells. Dev Neurosci 5:108-114
9) Seifert W (1981) Gangliosides in Nerve Cell Cultures. In: Rapport M, Gorio A (eds) Gangliosides in Neurological and Neuromuscular Function, Development and Repair. Raven Press, New York
10) Massarelli R, Ferret B, Gorio A, Durano M, Dreyfus H (1985) The effect of exogenous gangliosides on neurons in culture: a morphometric analysis. Int J Dev Neuroscience 3:341-348
11) Skaper SD, Katoh-Semba R, Varon S (1985) $GM_1$ ganglioside accelerates neurite outgrowth from primary peripheral and central neurons under selected culture conditions. Dev Brain Res 23:19-26
12) Ceccarelli B, Aporti F, Finesso M (1976) Effects of brain gangliosides on functional recovery in experimental regeneration and reinnervation. In: Porcellati G, Ceccarelli B, Tettamanti G (eds) Ganglioside Function. Plenum. New York, pp 275-293
13) Gorio A, Carmignoto G, Facci L, Finesso M (1980) Motor nerve sprouting induced by ganglioside treatment. Possible implications for gangliosides on neuronal growth. Brain Res 197:236-241
14) Walicke P, Cowan WM, Meno N, Baird A, Guillemin R (1986) Fibroblast growth factor promotes survival of dissociated hippocampal neurons and enhances neurite extension. Proc Natl Acad Sci USA 83:3012-3016

15) Gospodarowicz D, Cheng J, Lui GM, Baird A, Bohlent P (1984) Isolation of brain fibroblast growth factor: identity with pituitary fibroblast growth factor. Proc Natl Acad Sci USA 81:6963-6967
16) Pettmann B, Gensburger C, Weibel M, Perraud F, Sensenbrenner M, Labourdette G (1987) Isolation of two astroglial growth factors from bovine brain; comparison with other growth factors; cellular localization. In: Althaus HH, Seifert W (eds) Glial-Neuronal Communication in Development and Regeneration. NATO ASI Series H: Cell Biology, Vol. 2. Springer, Berlin Heidelberg New York, pp 451-478
17) Seifert W, Ranscht B, Fink HJ, Förster F, Beckh S, Müller HW (1983) Development of hippocampal neurons in cell culture: a molecular approach. In: Seifert W (ed) Neurobiology of the Hippocampus. Academic Press, London, pp 109-135
18) Seifert W, Müller HW (1984) Neuron-glia interaction in mammalian brain: preparation and quantitative bioassay of a neurotrophic factor (NTF) from primary astrocytes. In: Barnes DW, Sirbasku DA, Sato GH (eds) Cell Culture Methods for Molecular and Cell Biology 4:67-77, Alan R. Liss, Inc., New York
19) Müller HW, Seifert W (1982) A neurotrophic factor (NTF) released from primary glial cultures supports survival and fibre outgrowth of cultured hippocampal neurons. J Neurosci Res 8:195-204
20) Müller HW, Beckh S, Seifert W (1984) Neurotrophic factor for central neurons. Proc Natl Acad Sci USA 81:1248-1252
21) Banker GA, Cowan WM (1977) Rat hippocampal neurons in dispersed cell culture. Brain Res 126:397-425
22) Beckh S, Müller HW, Seifert W (1987) Neurotrophic and neurite promoting activities in astroglial conditioned medium. In: Althaus HH, Seifert W (eds) Glial-Neuronal Communication in Development and Regeneration. NATO ASI Series H: Cell Biology, Vol. 2. Springer, Berlin Heidelberg New York, pp 385-406
23) Selak I, Skaper SD, Varon S (1985) Pyruvate participation in the low molecular weight trophic activity for central nervous system neurons in glia-conditioned media. J Neurosci 5:23-28

# PHOTOCHEMICALLY INDUCED VASCULAR THROMBOSIS (PHOTOTHROMBOSIS): CENTRAL NERVOUS SYSTEM CONSEQUENCES AND CLINICAL POSSIBILITIES

Brant D. Watson, W. Dalton Dietrich, Ricardo Prado, and Barth A. Green*
Cerebral Vascular Disease Research Center
Department of Neurology and Department of Neurological Surgery*
University of Miami School of Medicine
P. O. Box 016960
Miami, Florida 33101
USA

## INTRODUCTION

In central nervous system (CNS) injury induced by stroke, or by impact injury to the spinal cord (Balentine, 1985), vascular abnormalities leading to thrombosis or thromboembolism are often intimately involved in the expression of the clinical severity of the final disease state. However, in the interest of reproducibility, most animal models of "stroke" feature induction of cerebral ischemia by mechanical occlusion of brain arteries (Garcia, 1984; Pulsinelli and Brierley, 1979). The participation of thrombotic processes is thus obviated. In contrast, mechanical induction of experimental spinal cord injury is considered to facilitate rather realistic development of the manifestations seen clinically. Yet, exposure of the cord tissue prior to injury and disruption of the cord tissue at the time of injury complicate the reproducibility of the experiments (Koozekanani et al, 1976; Ford, 1983; Gale et al, 1985) and make it difficult to ascertain the contribution of vascular injury, whether direct or indirect, to the final outcome.

Recently the concept was formulated that the appearance of reactive oxygen-centered free radical species in the vascular network was a major accompaniment of tissue injury induced by hypertension or trauma in the CNS (Kontos, 1985), or by post-ischemic reperfusion in general (McCord, 1985). Although reperfusion injury mediated by oxygen radicals in brain is plausible, evidence for this process *in vivo* has been obtained only

NATO ASI Series, Vol. H22
Neural Development and Regeneration
Edited by A. Gorio et al.

infrequently (Watson et al, 1984; White et al, 1985; Mickel et al, 1987). Oxygen radical species are comprised of oxygen in different states of reduction (Fridovich, 1978; Del Maestro, 1980; Halliwell and Gutteridge, 1986), and include the superoxide anion radical, its dismutation product hydrogen peroxide, its protonated form the perhydroxyl radical, and the hydroxyl radical (the iron-catalyzed breakdown product of hydrogen peroxide). Reactions initiated especially by the latter two species are believed to initiate degradation of cell membranes by alterations of lipid and protein structure. The intermediary species thought to be responsible for these alterations are carbon-centered radicals (derived from lipid or protein molecules) which are thought to be capable of sustaining highly disruptive chain reactions leading to peroxidation of membrane constituents (Tappel, 1973; Freeman and Crapo, 1982; Slater, 1984; Sevanian and Hochstein, 1985). Although blood elements such as platelets (and perhaps neutrophils as well) respond to tissues injured by oxidant radicals, the extent of their capability to exacerbate tissue injury induced by mechanically initiated effects such as trauma, hypertension or reversible arterial occlusion leading to ischemia is not known and is being investigated actively. Similarly, although evidence that oxygen-centered radicals are formed also in the period following ischemia has stimulated great interest in the concept of reperfusion injury, the contribution of reactive blood cells to CNS tissue injury beyond that induced by ischemia also remains to be ascertained.

## NONINVASIVE INDUCTION OF CNS VASCULAR INJURY AND THROMBOSIS BY IN VIVO PHOTOCHEMISTRY

In recent years our group has developed reproducible models of brain and spinal cord infarction, based on the induction of thrombosis *in situ*, by combining the concept of tissue damage induced by peroxidation reactions with that of stimulated participation of blood elements, specifically platelets. In these models injury to the vascular endothelium is produced by a photochemical reaction following the absorption of light by an intravenously injected organic dye. Platelets respond so intensely to this stimulus that the physiological cascade of adherence, degranulation and aggregation is continued to the point of thrombotic occlusion (Watson et al, 1985). In earlier work by others, sodium fluorescein was used as the photosensitizing dye; when irradiated by blue light, pial vessels of the brain were occluded (Rosenblum and El Sabban, 1977; Povlishock et al, 1983). The initiation mechanism at that time was thought to be transfer of heat absorbed by the dye to the vascular endothelium, with resultant platelet occlusion.

By utilizing another dye, rose bengal (disodium tetraiodo-tetrachlorofluorescein), as the photosensitizer we have been able to decrease the blood concentration of injected dye (in comparison to fluorescein) by about 40 times, while extending the range of tissue damage to CNS regions at least 2 mm beneath the surface exposed to light. The great difference in potency between rose bengal and its fluorescein antecedent is explained by the internal heavy atom effect induced by the iodine atoms of rose bengal. The heavy atoms enhance the magnitude of spin-orbit interaction between the singlet (fluorescent) and metastable triplet (phosphorescent) quantum molecular states (Kasha, 1950). This results in efficient formation of the lowest triplet state following absorption of light into the singlet state manifold (Gandin et al, 1983). In contrast, as implied by its name, under ordinary conditions fluorescein very efficiently emits the absorbed light energy by fluorescence; triplet state formation is enhanced only at high concentrations. In either case the metastable triplet state sensitizes the formation of the first excited state of molecular oxygen, known as singlet oxygen, by transferring its excitation energy kinetically to molecular oxygen dissolved in the system (Foote, 1976). The quantum efficiency of singlet oxygen production from the rose bengal triplet state is generally taken as 100% (Gandin et al, 1983). Photochemistry based on this process of dye triplet state quenching by molecular oxygen is designated Type II.

Singlet oxygen is also metastable, but highly reactive with electron-donating molecules. Because singlet molecular oxygen has an unfilled orbital, it can accept an electron pair from a susceptible molecule, such as an unsaturated fatty acid, and peroxidize it directly. Photodynamic action is the name given to designate inactivation or alteration of biological systems by dye-sensitized photoperoxidation reactions of Type II (Spikes and Livingston, 1969). Singlet oxygen is not a free radical, and it will not initiate chain reaction processes typical of oxygen- or carbon-centered radicals. However, its potency for membrane destruction is undiminished. As has been shown, by means of endothelial protection afforded by singlet oxygen scavenger molecules, singlet oxygen is the principal agent of endothelial damage photochemically induced by fluorescein dyes (Hermann, 1983).

It should be emphasized that reactions sensitized by photochemical means do not require classical thermal processes for their induction, inasmuch as the major fraction of light energy absorbed by an efficient photosensitizing dye is transformed into singlet molecular oxygen by means of electronic-state (not thermal) transitions. On the other hand, if local heating effects in tissue are desired the required conditions are provided by the recently introduced concept of selective photothermolysis (Anderson and Parrish, 1983). Given a sufficiently short pulse of excitation light, heat will be dissipated in the immediate vicinity of a light-absorbing molecule or pigment, provided that the concentration of the specific molecule or pigment chromophore is sufficient to induce an relative increase in optical absorbance compared to the absorbance of the surrounding tissue. Under conditions of either continuous wave or long pulse excitation, such as in all our work with rose bengal, any absorbed heat will equilibrate with the bulk surroundings, thus obviating focal vascular injury by thermal effects.

## PHOTOCHEMICALLY INDUCED CORTICAL INFARCTION

In our early work, we induced cortical thrombotic stroke leading to reproducible brain infarction in rats by first injecting them intravenously with rose bengal solution to a final body concentration of 10 mg/kg, and irradiating their exposed skulls for 20 minutes with 0.18 watt/cm$^2$ of 560 nm light from an optically filtered xenon arc lamp (Watson et al, 1985; Dietrich et al, 1986). The translucence of the skull permitted approximately 70% of the excitation light to be transmitted to the cortical surface. The temperature in the region of the forming lesion was kept near 37$^o$ C by a fan system, in order to ensure that the photoinduced reaction was initiated by electronic-state transitions characteristic of Type II photochemistry and not by thermal effects. In later work (Dietrich et al, 1987a,b,c) addition of a supplementary fan enabled us to increase the irradiation system intensity to 0.58 watt/cm$^2$

and decrease the time required for lesion formation to 2 minutes; the temperature in the region of the forming lesion still remained in the physiological range. At 30 minutes following irradiation histopathologically observed alterations within the irradiated cortical region included thrombotic material within superficial and parenchymal vessels (Watson et al, 1985). Ultrastructural studies demonstrated that the thrombotic materal was composed of aggregating platelets (cf. Figs. 1 and 2) associated with damaged vascular endothelium (Watson et al, 1985; Dietrich et al, 1987a,b). Carbon black infusion as an indicator of vascular patency demonstrated a pale cortical region underlying the irradiated pial surface. Autoradiographic studies using $^{14}$C iodoantipyrine as an indicator of local cerebral blood flow showed that an ischemic focus surrounded by regions of moderate hyperemia was present at 30 minutes following irradiation (Dietrich et al, 1986). Thus, microvascular thrombosis leading to an acute decrease in perfusable cortical tissue is observed in this stroke model.

With time, the volume of nonperfusable cortical tissue seen increased acutely. The irradiated zone at 4 hours following irradiation contained a central zone in which the vessels contained stagnant blood.

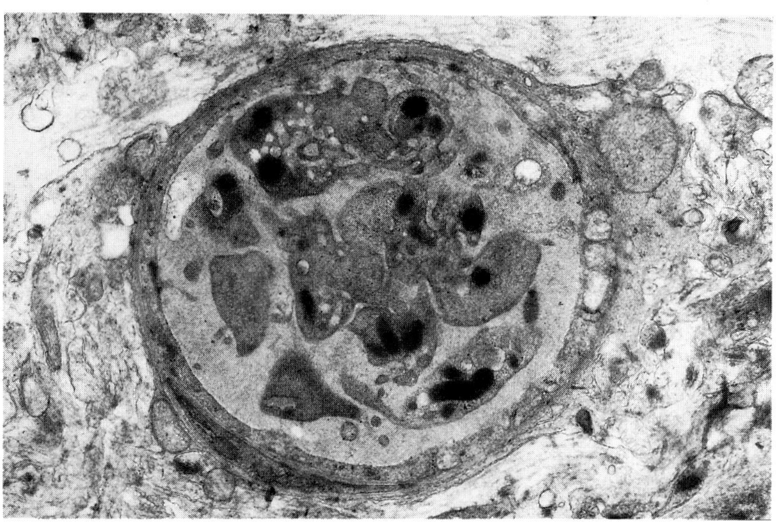

Fig. 1. Transmission electron micrograph of small cortical vessel from a rat intravenously injected with rose bengal dye and irradiated through the intact skull for 2 minutes with 0.58 watt/cm$^2$ of 560 nm green light from a filtered xenon arc lamp. The vessel lumen is filled with pseudopodic platelets in various stages of degranulation.

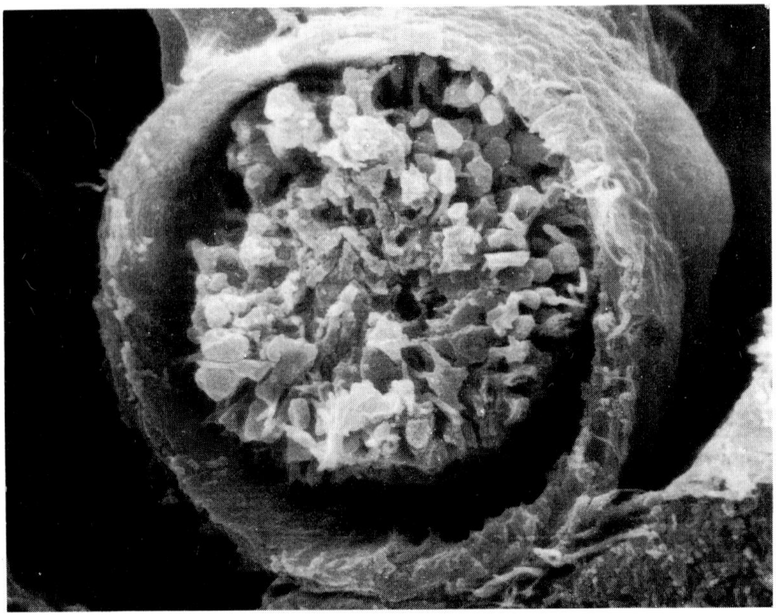

Fig. 2. Scanning electron micrograph of pial vessel from a rat injected with rose bengal, irradiated (as described in Fig. 1), and perfusion-fixed 2 minutes later. The lumen is completely packed with pseudopodic platelets. No fibrin strands are seen. X 4160. Reprinted with permission of the authors and the publisher (Dietrich et al., 1987b).

The peripheral zone of the lesion site appeared pale with few blood-filled vessels. Autoradiographic studies also demonstrated that the the area of severe hypoperfusion increased in size and the margins were no longer hyperemic (Dietrich et al, 1986). Cortical regions previously hyperemic (at 30 minutes) were now incorporated into the central ischemic zone. Photochemically induced cortical infarction is also associated with an acute breakdown of the blood-brain barrier to Evans blue and horseradish peroxidase (Dietrich et al, 1987c). These barrier alterations together with subsequent vasogenic edema likely contribute to the final pathological state. Rats which are studied histopathologically at more chronic survival periods demonstrate well demarcated cortical infarcts which are consistent in size and location. These experimental investigations therefore established that the photochemical model was thrombotic in nature and that the volume of cortical damage increased in size after cessation of irradiation.

PHOTOCHEMICAL INDUCTION OF SPINAL CORD INJURY

Spinal cord injury is associated with a complex series of pathological events which lead to membrane dysfunction at the neural and vascular levels following impact injury (Balentine, 1978 a,b). The vascular response is associated with endothelial damage, and consequent microvascular thrombosis (Goodman et al, 1979). Platelet-derived thromboxane $A_2$ ($TxA_2$), a known platelet aggregator and vasoconstrictor (Smith, 1980), may rise to levels which precipitate intravascular coagulation. Because the endothelial cells are damaged early in spinal cord injury (Goodman et al, 1979), $TxA_2$ may accumulate unimpeded by its counterpart prostacyclin ($PGI_2$), a known inhibitor of platelet aggregation with vasodilator properties, which is derived mainly from the endothelium (Smith, 1980). This alteration in the $PGI_2/TxA_2$ ratio has been observed following spinal cord injury (Hsu et al, 1985). Platelet aggregation and adhesion with fibrin formation in traumatic spinal cord injury occurs mainly in areas of endothelial breaks, or as a complex of thrombi covering larger areas of endothelial defects. This pro-aggregatory condition may contribute to the decrease in blood flow (ischemia) observed after experimental spinal cord injury.

It is evident that microvascular injury, whether due to impact trauma or to photochemical induction, may initiate thrombus formation or alterations in the blood-spinal cord barrier which significantly contribute to the ultimate outcome of the injury. A model of spinal cord injury based on the photochemical technique may afford an appropriate test system for the role played by the microcirculation in spinal cord injury. Initially, spinal cord infarction was engendered by injecting rats with 40 mg/kg rose bengal and irradiating the exposed vertebra at T8 for 40 minutes with the same filtered xenon arc lamp system used for inducing cortical infarction. The encasing bone structure was left entirely intact in order to ensure the noninvasive character of this approach. Transmission of the green excitation light through the bone was sufficient (50% through the T8 dorsal surface) to enable the photochemical reaction to take place. Seven days following photochemical injury, central hemorrhagic necrosis extending nearly through the entire cord thickness was observed (Watson et al, 1986). Paraplegia consistently resulted from this degree of injury.

With a modification of the irradiation parameters described above, spinal cord infarction could be induced more efficiently at reproducible degrees of severity. A train of high-powered pulses was produced by electromechanically gating the filtered xenon arc lamp run at its maximum ouput. A peak beam intensity at the focal point of 2.2 $watts/cm^2$ was achieved during the shutter open phase (37% duty cycle). This modification significantly reduced the time required to effect a complete lesion of the spinal cord. With this sytem four groups of rats underwent photoinduction times ranging from 30 seconds to 10 minutes. The longitudinal extent of the lesion at 30 minutes following a 10 minute irradiation period is shown in Fig. 3. Neurological and electrophysiological functions were assessed starting 1 week following irradiation and continuing for 8 weeks, at which time the animals were sacrificed for morphological evaluation. In rats irradiated for short periods (30 seconds or 1 minute) mild behavioral deficits were observed. In contrast, electrical conduction was suppressed acutely in both groups but recovered by 8 weeks to baseline or near baseline in the 30 second group but not in the 1 minute group. In rats irradiated for longer periods (5 or 10 minutes) severe behavioral and conduction abnormalities were detected at both the subacute and chronic testing periods. Although no significant difference in behavior was documented between the 5 and 10 minute groups acutely, the 5 minute rats demonstrated a significant improvement in behavior over time while the 10 minute group showed no improvement. A severe conduction block was present in both of these groups during the course of the study. Histopathological examination combined with morphometric measurements of lesion area in cross-section revealed 4 different degrees of spinal cord necrosis which correlated significantly with photoinduction times ($r= -0.86$, $p < 0.001$), and neurological scores ($r= -0.87$, $p < 0.001$) at 8 weeks (Prado et al, 1987).

Ultrastructural studies were carried out in rats irradiated for 5 minutes and immediately perfused transcardially (Prado et al, 1987). Vascular alterations at this early time period following irradiation were mainly restricted to the dorsal columns, dorsolateral fasciculus and lamina 1-5 of the central gray matter. Endothelial cells appeared swollen with sites of luminal discontinuity. A high frequency of luminal platelets exhibiting pseudopodia and degranulation, along with vascular congestion involving both surface and parenchymal vessels were observed. Pinocytotic vesicles lining both luminal and abluminal endothelial membranes were detected. Perivascular edema with astrocytic swelling was also a common occurrence. Neuronal cell bodies appeared relatively normal except for sites of perineuronal edema.

Given that four characteristic degrees of reproducible spinal cord infarction can be induced in the rat with the photochemical technique, we propose that mechanisms of lesion propagation may be studied systematically and that various therapeutic strategies, including fetal cell implantation, may be assessed accurately.

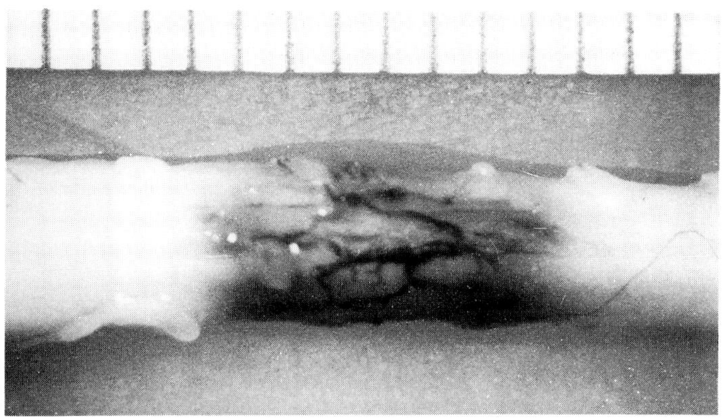

Fig. 3. Photograph of the spinal cord taken from a rat intravenously injected with rose bengal dye, subjected to 10 minutes of irradiation with a pulsed, high-intensity 560 nm green beam from filtered xenon arc lamp, and perfusion-fixed 30 minutes later. At the level of irradiation, Evans blue dye extravasation is shown extending slightly beyond the 4 mm cord segment irradiated. The scale at top is in millimeters.

## PHOTOSENSITIZED THROMBOSIS (PHOTOTHROMBOSIS) OF MAJOR ARTERIES

Recently, with the introduction of lasers as irradiation sources, we extended the range of the photochemical method to include occlusion of major arteries (Watson et al, 1987a,b). With an argon ion laser operating at 514.5 nm and an average power of 7.5 milliwatts, occlusion of the rat middle cerebral artery was observed within 4 minutes at incident intensities of 16 watts/cm$^2$, obtained by enveloping the 200 um arterial diameter with the focussed laser beam. The rat middle cerebral artery can also be occluded with a very low power (about 1 milliwatt) helium-neon laser operating at 543.5 nm by focussing the beam to an intensity of 10 watts/$cm^2$ (with crossed cylindrical lenses) onto the artery in a transverse line. The resulting thrombi are stable enough to facilitate studies of reperfusion injury in the middle cerebral artery territory (Nakayama et al, 1987; Dietrich et al, 1987d).

Larger arteries, such as the rat common carotid (about 800 - 1000 um) and femoral (700 - 900 um), also irradiated with the beam enveloping their diameters, require irradiation under water at much higher argon laser intensities (at least 160 watts/$cm^2$) in order to achieve their occlusion within times of several minutes (Watson et al, 1987a). Subsequently, in an effort to enhance the efficiency of the platelet response, the peak irradiation intensity was increased to approximately 300 watts/$cm^2$. By pulsing this beam at 200 Hz (in order to decrease the total energy required) during irradiation of the common carotid artery, it was discovered that platelet aggregates could be produced _in situ_. However, instead of facilitating occlusion, these aggregates embolized to the brain and induced multiple small foci of cerebral infarction (Futrell et al, 1987). No infarcts were seen in the brains of animals whose common carotid arteries were occluded photochemically. Thus, it appears from these observations that the photochemical technique can be used to study embolic stroke as well as thrombotic stroke.

During arterial irradiation an intense orange fluorescence is emitted, which is due to circulating rose bengal. Vasoconstriction, an early consequence of arterial irradiation, is followed by progressive diminution of fluorescence intensity and color bleaching. In the case of the middle cerebral artery, this continues until the irradiated segment appears colorless (Watson et al, 1987a,b). Examination of this segment by scanning electron microscopy revealed that the resultant white thrombus contains, for all practical purposes, only platelets and no associated fibrin (similar to Fig. 2). Thrombus formation in the larger arteries, however, is detected visually by the appearance of a reddish-brown clot and cessation of wall pulsations. The clot consists of islands of aggregated platelets interspersed among red blood cells and coagulum, which results from the high temperatures produced in the intensely irradiated vessel segment as the reaction proceeds in the narrowing lumen of these high-flow vessels (Fig. 4a). Irradiation at comparable laser intensities, in the absence of rose bengal, of the middle cerebral artery _in situ_ or the larger arteries under water yields

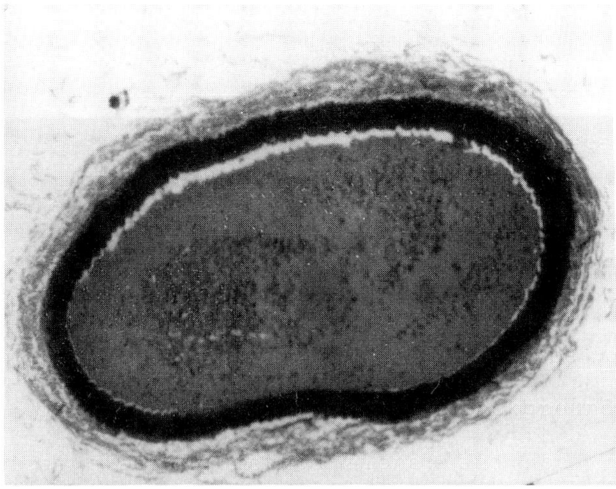

Fig. 4a. Light micrograph of thin plastic section of rat common carotid artery perfusion-fixed 30 minutes following photothrombotic occlusion. Photothrombosis was induced by the photochemical interaction between intravenously injected rose bengal dye (40 mg/kg body weight) and focussed 514.5 nm argon laser irradiation (160 watts/$cm^2$). The thrombus consists of coagulum mixed with islands of blood elements. Toluidine blue, X 280. Reprinted with permission of the authors and the publisher (Watson et al, 1987a).

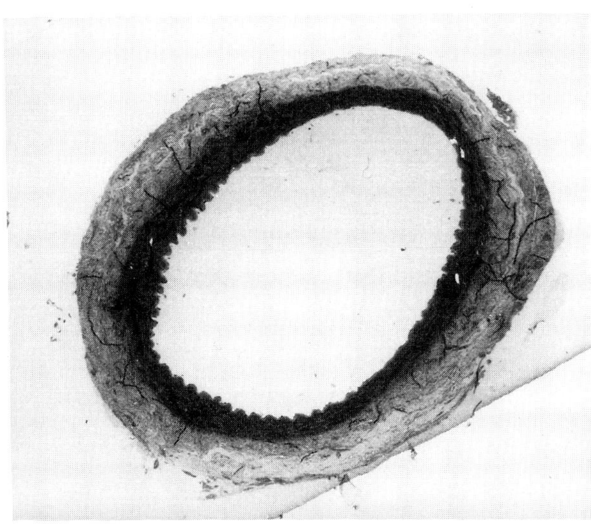

Fig. 4b. Light micrograph of thin plastic section of rat femoral artery perfusion-fixed 30 minutes following argon laser irradiation (as in Fig. 4a) in the absence of rose bengal infusion. Note the lack of luminal blood elements or signs of damage to wall elements. Toluidine blue, X 260.

temperature increases of less than 1$^{o}$ C. Consequently, no evidence at all of wall damage, let alone thrombosis, is observed (Fig. 4b).

These latter data illustrate the great difficulty of inducing clot formation by the technique of photocoagulation. Photocoagulation is based on transfer of thermal energy from photoirradiated erythrocytes to vascular endothelium in order to render the endothelium thrombogenic to the point of occlusion (Boergen et al, 1981). This process can be used in selected situations to occlude arteries much smaller than those we have utilized. The resultant thrombi are mixed in character and resemble those we have observed in the common carotid and femoral arteries. On the other hand, the dye-assisted photoirradiation technique affords such a great increase in occlusive efficiency that we have coined the term "photothrombosis" to designate this process and thereby distinguish it from photocoagulation. The reason that photothrombosis is so much more efficient than photocoagulation is that the endothelial damage expressed per quantum of light absorbed is much greater. In this case, the fraction of quantal energy of the irradiating beam that is absorbed by rose bengal appears in the form of electronic-state transitions. This energy is transferred (with a quantum efficiency of 76%; Gandin et al, 1983) directly to the lowest triplet state of rose bengal, and then to endothelial surface constituents by the sole photochemical product, singlet molecular oxygen. Singlet oxygen, produced with 100% efficiency from the oxygen-triplet state interaction, then destroys the nonthrombogenic character of the endothelial surface. Although thermal energy deposition in the irradiated vessel can certainly occur, it is not needed to initiate photothrombosis.

## CLINICAL SIGNIFICANCE AND APPLICATIONS OF THE PHOTOTHROMBOTIC TECHNIQUE

The appearance of unnecessary, unwanted blood vessels is a common feature of many difficult or intractable clinical conditions. The growth of neovasculature in the retina in late stage diabetes mellitus, or in the cornea following transplant rejection or denuding injury are representative of serious ophthalmic situations. The available method of treatment, photocoagulation, rarely yields a satisfactory clinical outcome owing to recanalization of the photocoagulated vessels or stimulation of new vessel growth by heat-induced inflammatory responses

(Mendelsohn et al, 1986). Similarly, although it is well known that treatment of arteriovenous malformations by mechanically induced blockade is still quite challenging, attempts to occlude the feeder arteries of these entangled vascular networks by photocoagulation have yet to be regarded as offering significant improvement in occlusive efficiency in the absence of mechanical contact (Watson et al, 1987).

The method of photothrombosis, however, does offer the possibility of advantageous clinical use in the elimination of undesired vasculature. For small vessels (less than 200 um in diameter) the fact that the photoinduced thrombus consists virtually entirely of aggregated platelets with little or no associated fibrin suggests that it should be resistant to natural thrombolytic processes involving tissue-type plasminogen activator (t-PA). Indeed, we have observed that lysis of photoinduced rat middle cerebral artery thrombi by recombinant t-PA is not possible without assistance from a vasodilator compound, such as nimodipine; even then, lysis is inconsistent (Watson et al, 1987b). Further, it is evident that photothrombosis can facilitate, with much less incident intensity and total energy deposited, occlusion of vessels which are far larger than can be treated with photocoagulation. Thus, damage to peripheral structures is minimized. Finally, inasmuch as intravenously injected rose bengal has been used extensively in past clinical assessments of liver function (Nordyke and Blahd, 1959; Pirotte, 1980), we conjecture that its toxicity may be sufficiently low to admit its use for the new purpose of photothrombosis.

Recently we have begun to assess the suitability of rose bengal-mediated photothrombosis for occlusion of corneal neovasculature. Permanent occlusion of these abnormal, free-standing vessels with argon laser irradiation alone has been vey difficult in practice (Cherry et al, 1973; Cherry and Garner, 1976; Marsh and Marshall, 1976; Marsh, 1982; Nirankari and Baer, 1986). Growth of new vessels into the corneas of rabbits was induced either by implantation of corneal sutures (Mendelsohn et al, 1987), or by corneal debridement and subsequent healing with vascularized conjunctiva-like tissue containing characteristic goblet cells (Huang et al, 1987). In the first case, secretion of lipid from the new vessels into the corneal stroma was observed (in rabbits fed a high-cholesterol diet), thus simulating the corneal condition known as lipid keratopathy. In the second case, intended to simulate a common response to direct corneal injury, it was hypothesized that retinoid compounds supplied to the conjunctival tissue by the neovasculature were responsible for inhibition of conjunctival transdifferentiation; i.e., transformation of conjunctiva-like tissue into the corneal phenotype. Therefore, occlusion of neovasculature in the first case should inhibit further corneal lipid deposition; while in the second, elimination of neovasculature in corneas healed with conjunctival tissue should facilitate expression of cornea-like characteristics such as increased clarity and surface smoothness.

Photothrombotic occlusion of the corneal new vessels (ranging in diameter from 30 um to 80 um) was achieved generally within 10 pulses of 514.5 nm argon laser light, 0.2 sec in duration. The effective laser power was 130 milliwatts and the focussed beam spot size, obtained at the output of a beam telescope interfaced to a fiber optic, was 63 um (Watson et al, 1987c). These parameters are very mild compared to those used in previous work utilizing photocoagulation for the same purpose (Mendelsohn et al, 1986); the intensity was nearly 10 times less while the total energy deposited was almost 30 times less (Mendelsohn et al, 1987). In the previous work on experimental lipid keratopathy, inflammation of the corneal tissue resulted from thermal damage to the corneal stroma induced by the high incident laser intensities. This had the effect of stimulating the growth of even more lipid-secreting vessels; thus the treated corneas contained more lipid (average 24%) than did the nontreated corneas. In contrast, the photothrombotic treatment did not induce an inflammatory response; accordingly, lipid deposition in the the treated corneas was attenuated by an average of 36% in comparison to untreated corneas. In the case of the rabbit corneas healed with conjunctiva-like tissue, corneal vessels treated by photothrombosis remained occluded for as long as 18 weeks, up to the time of sacrifice. Reductions in goblet cell density, and corneal clearing and enhancement of surface smoothness could be seen within 2 weeks, thus indicating transformation into the corneal phenotype (Huang et al, 1987).

## FURTHER DIRECTIONS AND APPLICATIONS

Currently, the chief application of photochemistry to clinical conditions concerns photosensitized destruction of tumor tissue.

Originally, it was observed that a mixture of compounds called hematoporphyrin derivative (HPD) was selectively taken up by tumors of many types (Dougherty, 1986). The active component was found to be a dihematoporphyrin ether (DHPE), which has recently come into use. There is no consensus yet on whether the mode of action of DHPE in tumor killing involves direct photodynamic destruction of tumor cells, primary or secondary collapse of tumor vasculature leading to ischemia-induced tumor death, or a combination of these features. Although it has been shown that HPD can sensitize the production of singlet oxygen (Weishaupt et al, 1976), endothelial breakdown and subsequent edema in the absence of thrombosis is apparently the dominant early mechanism of tumor destruction (Henderson et al, 1985). With a cranial irradiation procedure similar to ours (Watson et al, 1985) blood-brain barrier breakdown resulted from HPD photosensitization (Berenbaum et al, 1986); similar results were obtained by us recently (Dietrich et al, 1987c). Our preliminary experiments with DHPE as a potential photothrombotic agent in corneal neovasculature resulted in very efficient occlusion, but recanalization occurred within 10 days. Attempts to photothrombose the considerably larger rat middle cerebral artery were surprisingly negative, however; accumulation of reddish thrombotic material was observed but stabilization into an occlusive mass did not occur.

In light of the demonstrated capability of rose bengal to sensitize uniform thrombus formation, it appears that tumor vessel photothrombosis mediated by rose bengal should be investigated as a potentially reliable means of inducing tumor destruction, especially in the context of eye tumors. It is anticipated that many other uses for dye-assisted photothrombosis may be developed for those clinical situations in which photocoagulation is either impracticable or impossible.

## ACKNOWLEDGMENTS

The authors wish to thank Drs. Alan Mendelsohn, Andrew Huang, Scheffer Tseng, Nancy Futrell, Clark Millikan and Myron Ginsberg for their contributions to the development and application of the rose bengal-mediated photochemical technique. Dr. Dietrich is an Established Investigator of the American Heart Association. This work was supported by USPHS grants NS5820, NS23244, and EY05656.

REFERENCES

Balentine JD (1978a) Pathology of experimental spinal cord injury. 1. The necrotic lesion as a function of vascular injury. Lab Invest 39:236-253

Balentine JD (1978b) Pathology of experimental spinal cord injury. 2. Ultrastructure of axons and myelin. Lab Invest 39:254-266

Balentine JD (1985) Hypothesis in spinal cord trauma research. In: Becker DP, Povlishock JT (eds) Central Nervous System Trauma Status Report. NIH (NINCDS), Bethesda, pp 455-461

Berenbaum MC, Hall GW, Hoyes AD (1986) Cerebral photosensitization by haematoporphyrin derivative. Evidence for an endothelial site of action. Br J Cancer 53:81-89

Boergen KP, Birngruber R, Hillenkamp F (1981) Laser-induced endovascular thrombosis as a possibility of selective vascular closure. Ophthalmic Res 13:139-150

Cherry PMH, Faulkner JD, Shaver RP, Wise JB, Witter SL (1973) Argon laser treatment of corneal neovascularization. Ann Ophthalmol 5:911-920.

Cherry PMH, Garner A (1976) Corneal neovascularization treated with argon laser. Br J Ophthalmol 60:464-472.

Del Maestro RF (1980) An approach to free radicals in medicine and biology. Acta Physiol Scand (Suppl) 492:153-168

Dietrich WD, Ginsberg MD, Busto R, Watson BD (1986) Photochemically induced cortical infarction in the rat: 1. Time course of hemodynamic consequences. J Cerebr Blood Flow Metabol 6:184-194

Dietrich WD, Ginsberg MD, Busto R, Watson BD, Yoshida S (1987a) Vascular aspects and hemodynamic consequences of central nervous system injury. Central Nervous System Trauma 3:265-280

Dietrich WD, Watson BD, Busto R, Bethea JR, Scheinberg P, Ginsberg MD (1987b) Photochemically induced cerebral infarction: 1. Early microvascular alterations. Acta Neuropath (Berl) 72:315-325

Dietrich WD, Watson BD, Busto R, Bethea JR, Scheinberg P, Ginsberg MD (1987c) Photochemically induced cerebral infarction: 2. Edema and blood-brain barrier disruption. Acta Neuropath (Berl) 72:326-334

Dietrich WD, Nakayama H, Prado R, Watson BD, Halley M, Ginsberg MD (1987d) Middle cerebral artery thrombosis: microvascular consequences. J Cerebr Blood Flow Metabol 7:S601

Dougherty TJ (1985) Photodynamic therapy. Adv Exp Med Biol 193:313-328

Foote CS (1976) Photosensitized oxidation and singlet oxygen: consequences in biological systems. In: Pryor WA (ed) Free Radicals in Biology, Vol 2. New York, Academic Press, pp 85-134

Ford RWJ (1983) A reproducible spinal cord injury model in the cat. J Neurosurg 59:268-275

Freeman BA, Crapo JD (1982) Biology of disease. Free radicals and tissue injury. Lab Invest 47:412-426

Fridovich I (1978) The biology of oxygen radicals. Science 201:875-880

Futrell N, Watson BD, Dietrich WD, Prado R, Millikan C, Ginsberg MD (1987) A new model of embolic stroke in the rat from a photochemical nonocclusive carotid lesion. Ann Neurol 22:158

Gale K, Kerasidis H, Wrathall J (1985) Spinal cord contusion in the rat: behavioral analysis of functional neurologic impairment. Exp Neurol 88:123-134

Gandin E, Lion Y, Van de Vorst A (1983) Quantum yield of singlet oxygen production by xanthene derivatives. Photochem Photobiol 37:271-278

Garcia JH (1984) Experimental ischemic stroke: A review. Stroke 15:5-14
Goodman JH, Bingham WG, Hunt WE (1979) Platelet aggregation in experimental spinal cord injury. Arch Neurol 36:197-201
Halliwell B, Gutteridge JMC (1986) Oxygen free radicals and iron in relation to biology and medicine: some problems and concepts. Arch Biochem Biophys 246:501-514
Henderson BW, Waldow SM, Mang TS, Potter WR, Malone PB, Dougherty TJ (1985) Tumor destruction and kinetics of tumor cell death in two experimental mouse tumors following photodynamic therapy. Cancer Res 45:572-576
Hermann KS (1983) Platelet aggregation induced in the hamster cheek pouch by a photochemical process with excited fluorescein isothiocyanate-dextran. Microvasc Res 26:238-249
Hsu CY, Halushka PV, Hogan EL, Banik NL, Lee WA, Perot PL (1985) Alteration of thromboxane and prostacyclin levels in experimental spinal cord injury. Neurology 35:1003-1009
Huang AJW, Watson BD, Hernandez E, Tseng SCG (1987) Induction of conjunctival transdifferentiation by photothrombosis with rose bengal and argon laser. Invest Ophthalmol Vis Sci 28:159
Kasha M (1950) Characterization of electronic transitions in complex molecules. Faraday Soc Discuss 9:14-19
Koozekanani SH, Vise M, Hashemi RM, McGhee RB (1976) Possible mechanisms for observed pathophysiological variability in experimental spinal cord injury. J Neurosurg 44:429-434
Marsh RJ, Marshall J (1976) Treatment of lipid keratopathy with the argon laser. Br J Ophthalmol 66:127-135
Marsh RJ (1982) Lasering of lipid keratopathy. Trans Ophthalmol Soc UK 102:154-156
McCord JM (1985) Oxygen-derived free radicals in postischemic tissue injury. New Engl J Med 312:159-163
Mendelsohn AD, Stock EL, Lo GG, Schneck GL (1986) Laser photocoagulation of feeder vessels in lipid keratopathy. Ophthalmic Surg 17:502-508
Mendelsohn AD, Watson BD, Alfonso E, Lieb M, Mendelsohn G, Forster R, Dennis JJ (1987) Amelioration of experimental lipid keratopathy by photochemically induced thrombosis of feeder vessels. Arch Ophthalmol 105:983-988
Mickel HS, Vaishnav YN, Kempski O, von Lubitz D, Weiss JF, Feuerstein G (1987) Breathing 100% oxygen after global brain ischemia in Mongolian gerbils results in increased lipid peroxidation and increased mortality. Stroke 18:426-430
Nakayama H, Dietrich WD, Watson BD, Prado R, Busto R, Ginsberg MD (1987) Pharmacologically induced recirculation following experimental middle cerebral artery occlusion. J Cerebr Blood Flow Metabol 7:S23
Nirankari VS, Baer JC (1986) Corneal argon laser photocoagulation in penetrating keratoplasty. Ophthalomology 93:1304-1309
Nordyke RA, Blahd WH (1959) Blood disappearance of radioactive rose bengal - rapid simple test of liver function. JAMA 170:1159-1164
Pirotte J (1980) Study of $^{131}$I-rose bengal kinetics in normal man: a critical evaluation of a three-compartment model. Biomedicine 32:17-21
Povlishock JT, Rosenblum WI, Sholley MM, Wei E (1983) An ultrastructural analysis of endothelial change paralleling platelet aggregation in a light/dye model of microvascular insult. Am J Pathol 110:148-160
Prado RJ, Dietrich WD, Watson BD, Ginsberg MD, Green BA (to be published) Photochemically induced graded spinal cord injury: behavioral, electrophysiological, and morphological correlates. J Neurosurg

Pulsinelli WA, Brierley JB (1979) A new model of bilateral hemispheric ischemia in the unanesthetized rat. Stroke 10:267-272

Rosenblum WI, El-Sabban F (1977) Platelet aggregation in the cerebral microcirculation. Effect of aspirin and other agents. Stroke 40:320-328

Sevanian A, Hochstein P (1985) Mechanisms and consequences of lipid peroxidation in biological systems. Ann Rev Nutr 5:365-390

Slater TF (1984) Free radical mechanisms in tissue injury. Biochem J 222:1-15

Smith JB (1980) The prostanoids in hemostasis and thrombosis. Amer J Pathol 99:741

Spikes JD, Livingston R (1969) The molecular biology of photodynamic action: sensitized photoautoxidations in biological systems. Adv Rad Biol 3:29-121

Tappel AL (1973) Lipid peroxidation damage to cell components. Fed Proc 32:1870-1874

Watson BD, Busto R, Goldberg WJ, Santiso M, Yoshida S, Ginsberg MD (1984) Lipid peroxidation in vivo induced by reversible global ischemia in rat brain. J Neurochem 42:268-274

Watson BD, Dietrich WD, Busto R, Wachtel MS, Ginsberg MD (1985) Induction of reproducible brain infarction by photochemically initiated thrombosis. Ann Neurol 17:497-504

Watson BD, Prado R, Dietrich WD, Ginsberg MD, Green BA (1986) Photochemically induced spinal cord injury in the rat. Brain Res 367:296-300

Watson BD, Dietrich WD, Prado R, Ginsberg MD (1987a) Argon laser-induced arterial photothrombosis: characterization and possible application to therapy of arteriovenous malformations. J Neurosurg 66:748-754

Watson BD, Prado R, Dietrich WD, Busto R, Scheinberg P, Ginsberg MD (1987b) Mitigation of evolving cortical infarction in rats by recombinant tissue plasminogen activator following photochemically induced thrombosis. In: Raichle ME and Powers WJ (eds) Cerebrovascular Diseases - Fifteenth Princeton Conference. Raven Press, New York, pp 317-330

Watson BD, Huang AJW, Mendelsohn AD, Dietrich WD, Prado R, Tseng SCG (1987c) Rose bengal-induced photosensitized thrombosis of arteries: implications for ophthalmic photoradiation therapy. Lasers Surg Med 7:127

Weishaupt KR, Gomer CJ, Dougherty TJ (1976) Identification of singlet oxygen as the cytotoxic agent in photodynamic inactivation of a murine tumor. Cancer Res 36:2326-2329

White BC, Krause GS, Aust SD, Eyster GE (1985) Postischemic tissue injury by iron-mediated free radical lipid peroxidation. Ann Emerg Med 14:804-809

GRAFTED FETAL ASTROCYTES MIGRATE FROM HOST THORACIC SPINAL CORD TO LUMBAR CORD AND MEDULLA

William J. Goldberg and Jerald J. Bernstein
Laboratory of Central Nervous System Injury and Regeneration
VA Medical Center, Washington, DC, 20422 and Departments of Physiology and Neurosurgery, The George Washington University School of Medicine, Washington, DC, 20037, USA

## I. INTRODUCTION

Transplantation of fetal central nervous system [CNS] into adult host CNS ameliorated lesion-induced behavioral and learning deficits (Bernstein and Goldberg, 1987,1988b; Deckel et al, 1986; Dunnett et al, 1983a,b; Gage et al, 1986) and neuronal atrophy (Bregman et al, 1986; Sharp et al, 1986). Transplants were also efficacious in the treatment of Parkinson-like symptoms (Kamo et al, 1986; Sladek et al, 1987) produced by MPTP [1-methyl-4-phenyl-1,2,3,6-tetrahydropyridine] in monkeys and behavioral abnormalities resulting from chemical lesions of the nigrostriatal system in rats (Dunnett et al, 1983a; Dunnett et al, 1983b; Freed, 1983). The initial view of the mechanisms by which transplants affected the injured CNS focused on the formation of new neuronal circuits and release of transmitter substances by grafted neurons. It was recently demonstrated, however, that grafts of cultured astrocytes alone and transplants of Gelfoam removed from a wound cavity in the adult CNS were as efficacious in reversing a lesion-induced learning deficit as were grafts of fetal cerebral cortex (Kesslak et al, 1986). This is of interest since astrocytes in culture have been shown to produce a number of growth factors which support or enhance the survival and/or

NATO ASI Series, Vol. H22
Neural Development and Regeneration
Edited by A. Gorio et al.

sprouting of neurons in culture (Assouline et al, 1987). Given this new avenue of research, we felt it was of considerable importance to determine whether transplant derived astrocytes could migrate more than the 1-3 mm previously reported by other investigators (Jacque et al, 1986; Raisman et al, 1985). If migration on the order of centimeters rather than millimeters was possible, then a significant role for astrocyte-derived neurotrophic factors could be envisioned in the regeneration/repair process after CNS injury by transplantation of these cells.

Post transplantation migration of oligodendrocytes, astrocytes and neurons have been reported. Two groups have reported neuronal migration from xenografts placed in either adult rat (Wells et al, 1986) or newborn rat and mouse (Finsen et al, 1986) brain. Transplantation of fetal mesencephalon into host spinal cord resulted in migration of neuronal cell bodies for distances of up to 10 mm away from the transplantation site (Privat et al, 1986). When solid fragments of normal newborn olfactory bulb were transplanted into newborn Shiverer mouse brains significant myelination due to implanted oligodendrocytes was observed in the otherwise myelin-deficient Shiverer host brain (Lachapelle et al, 1983). Myelination in Shiverer mice was also observed following transplantation of normal neonatal cortex into the right lateral ventricle of the host (Friedman et al, 1986). Significant gliosis was observed in the corpus callosum of these animals which extended a considerable distance from the graft. The magnitude and extent of the gliosis could not be explained simply as a response to surgical trauma during the implantation procedure. Migration of transplanted astrocytes has been observed in xenografts of rabbit corpus callosum to newborn mouse thalamus (Jacque et al, 1986), homografts of newborn mouse cortex to 1 month old host lateral ventricle (Friedman et al, 1986) and in homografts of fetal rat hippocampi to adult hippocampus (Raisman et al, 1985). Migration occurred along nerve fiber bundles, along blood vessels and through the parenchyma. In this chapter we will review recent experiments from our laboratory using transplantation of fetal CNS prelabeled with Phaseolus vulgaris leucoagglutinin [PHAL] (Bernstein and Goldberg, 1988a; Goldberg and Bernstein, 1987,1988) with emphasis on the routes, extent and rate of migration of grafted astrocytes. PHAL is an excellent marker for transplanted cells because it is taken up by fetal cells but not by normal or reactive adult astrocytes (Gerfin and Sawchenko, 1984; Sawchenko and Gerfin, 1985). Adult neuronal cell bodies only take up PHAL when the lectin is iontophoresed. The specificity of the cells which are capable of taking up the lectin combined with the high specificity of the immunohistochemical detection system make for a powerful tool to follow the migration of grafted cells.

## II. Methods

Pressure-Injected Transplants (Goldberg and Bernstein,1987). Timed-pregnant Sprague-Dawley dams were anesthetized with 50 mg/kg pentobarbital and fetuses were removed by Caesarean section from one uterine horn on embryonic day 14 [E14]. The fetus was placed in 5 mM phosphate-buffered-saline containing 10 mM glucose [PBS-glucose]. The fetal cerebral cortex was dissected free, minced into 0.5 X 1.0mm pieces in PBS-glucose and placed in 2.0 ug/ml of PHAL in PBS-glucose for one hour. After rinsing 2 times in fresh PBS-glucose, the PHAL soaked pieces of fetal cerebral cortex were aspirated into a 30g needle attached to a 50 ul Hamilton syringe to produce a suspension of free cells and small clumps of undissociated tissue.

Hosts. Following laminectomy, a piece of PHAL soaked fetal cortex was pressure injected, subdurally, on the left side between the dorsal horn and column at the level of the sixth thoracic vertebrae [T6] of deeply anesthetized [pentobarbital, 50 mg/kg] host adult [300 gm] Sprague-Dawley male rats. After implantation, Gelfoam was placed over the exposed spinal cord and the wound closed. All hosts received a 0.1 ml [i.m.] injection of Longicil [Penicillin] postoperatively. Two adult rats were subdurally injected with PBS-glucose solution only at T6 to serve as sham operated controls and were sacrificed after 45 days. The implantation technique did not result in loss of experimental animal mobility, or cause bladder or defecation problems.

Tissue collection. Host rats were sacrificed 7,14,24,30 and 60 days after implantation. To collect the tissue, the rats were deeply anesthetized with pentobarbital [50 mg/kg] and perfused through the ascending aorta with 0.9% saline followed by formalin-acetic acid-alcohol. The spinal cord was exposed and the region containing the implant removed, dehydrated, infiltrated, embedded in 54$^{o}$C paraffin and sectioned at 8 um. The medulla and high cervical [C1] spinal cord were removed from the 60 day transplanted animals. In addition, cervical [C8] and lumbar [L5] spinal cord from all transplanted and sham operated animals were removed, prepared for paraffin embedding and sectioned at 8 um.

Gel Transplants (Bernstein and Goldberg, 1988a; Goldberg and Bernstein, 1988a). A laminectomy was performed as described previously (Bernstein and Goldberg, 1986) and above. However, after the dura was incised, the left dorsal column was blunt dissected [longitudinally] to make a pocket for the graft and disrupt the pia. The grafts were cell suspensions of 14 day gestation spinal cord grown for 14 days on collagen gels containing laminin (Bernstein and Goldberg, 1986). The gels were removed from the culture dish and sliced into 0.5 X 1.0 mm pieces which were placed in the pocket in the host dorsal column. The host was then closed as above.

Tissue Culture. Cultures of E14 fetal rat spinal cord were prepared by isolating several spinal cords under an operating microscope and removing the leptomeninges. The spinal cords were dissected free and placed in modified DMEM supplemented with an acid stable neuron survival factor isolated from horse serum (Kaufman et al, 1983). The spinal cords were then dissociated into single cells by gentle trituration. The cell suspension was plated at a density of 1,500-2,000 cells/mm$^2$ on collagen gels containing 5 ug/ml laminin (Bernstein and Goldberg, 1986).

Tissue collection. Host rats were sacrificed 1,2 and 3 months after implantation. To collect the tissue, the rats were deeply anesthetized with pentobarbital [50 mg/Kg] and perfused through the ascending aorta with 0.9% saline followed by formalin-acetic acid-alcohol (Cammer et al, 1985). The spinal cord and medulla were exposed and processed as above.

PHAL-GFAP Double Labeling (Goldberg and Bernstein, 1987,1988). The paraffin was removed from 8 um sections with three 5 minute xylene baths. The tissue was rehydrated in a graded series of alcohols followed by a rinse in 0.05 M phosphate buffered saline. After a 30 minute blocking step in PBS containing 5% sheep serum, the sections were incubated overnight at $4^{o}C$ with combined antisera to GFAP [Rabbit anti-GFAP] and PHAL [Goat anti-PHAL] diluted [1:600 each] in PBS containing 0.25% lambda carageenan, 0.25% Triton X-100, 1% sheep serum and 0.1% bovine serum albumin. The sections were rinsed 4 x 5 minutes in PBS containing 1% sheep serum [PBS-serum] and then incubated for 30 minutes with combined sheep antisera to goat IgG [fluorescein conjugated] and rabbit IgG [rhodamine conjugated] diluted 1:50 in PBS-serum. After rinsing 4 times in PBS-serum the FITC fluorescence was intensified by incubating the sections in FITC-conjugated goat anti-mouse IgG diluted 1:50 in PBS-serum. Sections for double labeling experiments were rinsed 4 times in PBS and coverslipped with Technicon mounting medium. FITC- and RITC-specific fluorescences were observed using an Olympus BH-2 microscope with epifluorescence attachment and appropriate excitation and emission filters. For excitation of FITC and RITC barrier filters with cutoffs of 455 nm [EY455] and 515 nm [EO515] were used, respectively, to reduce non-specific excitation. Emission crossover was eliminated through the use of a 515-525 nm bandpass filter [G520] for FITC and a 610 nm barrier filter [R610] for RITC; these filters provided non-overlapping windows for FITC and RITC fluorescence. Photographic records were made of the 2 fluorescent markers.

Controls. Negative staining controls [pre-immune serum instead of primary antibody or elimination of primary antibody] and cross-fluorescence controls [sections reacted with rabbit anti-GFAP and then incubated with FITC-conjugated sheep anti rabbit IgG [SAR] and observed under RITC optics or incubated with RITC-conjugated SAR and observed under FITC optics] were performed. Positive controls were performed by incubating sections previously reacted with GFAP antiserum and FITC-conjugated SAR with rabbit peroxidase-anti-peroxidase complex [PAP] diluted 1:50 in PBS followed by a 20 minute incubation with diaminobenzidine [DAB] to produce a brown immunoprecipitate. Sections used for positive controls were coverslipped with 1:1 glycerol:PBS for fluorescence photography; coverslipping with Technicon mounting medium resulted in loss of peroxidase activity.

## III. RESULTS

For the first 2 weeks post transplantation there was very little migration of transplanted astrocytes regardless of whether the transplanted material was cultured spinal cord cells grown on collagen gels or pressure injected pieces of fetal cortex. At 14 days post implantation [DPI] of pressure-injected fetal cortex at T6 PHAL-GFAP positive astrocytes were only observed within an 0.1 mm zone surrounding the implantation site. At 24,30 and 60 DPI transplant derived astrocytes were observed on the pial surface, surrounding parenchymal blood vessels and lying within the parenchyma of the dorsal columns of the host thoracic spinal cord [Figure 1]. Parallel chains of double labeled astrocytes were observed 3.5 mm caudal to the transplantation site [Figure 2].

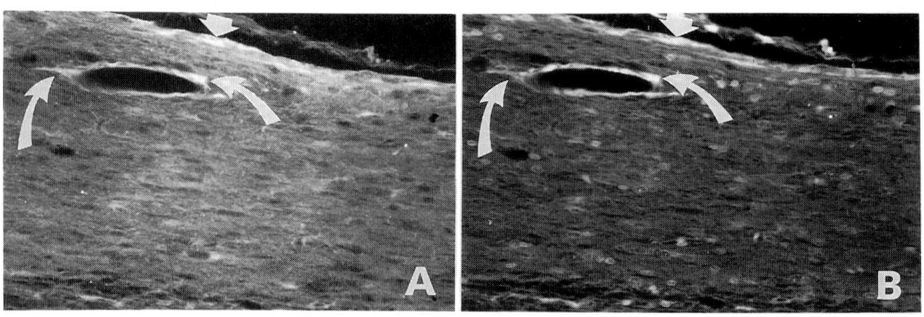


Figure 1. Host spinal cord (24 DPI) labeled for PHAL (FITC) in A and for GFAP (RITC) in B. Double labeled transplant derived astrocytes are observed surrounding blood vessels (curved arrows) and on the pial surface (arrowheads).

At 60 DPI PHAL positive astrocytes were found in the dorsal columns of the host lumbar [L5] and cervical [C1] spinal cord, a distance of at least 3.5 cm from the implantation site at T6.

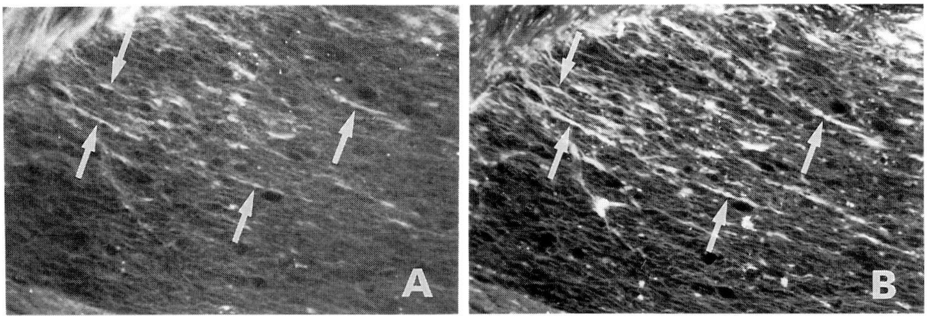


Figure 2. Host thoracic dorsal column (60 DPI; 3.5 mm caudal to the implantation site) labeled for PHAL (FITC) in A and for GFAP (RITC) in B. Parallel chains of double labeled transplant derived astrocytes (arrows) are observed.

Subtracting the 14 day period of little or no migration there was a calculated migration rate of ca. 0.76 mm/day. Penetration of transplanted astrocytes into the gray matter of the host thoracic spinal cord was limited to approximately 0.1 mm at this time. Five 0.15 mm width zones, located 0.0, 0.5, 1.0, 1.5 and 2.0 mm from the edge of the transplant, were selected for calculations of the frequencies of PHAL-GFAP and GFAP-only labeled astrocytes [Figure 3].

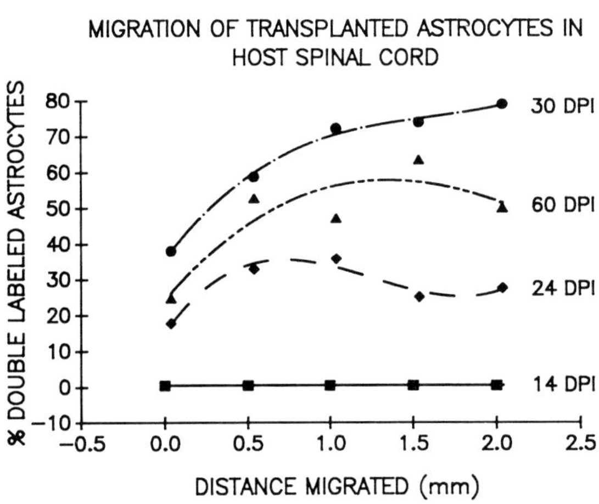


Figure 3. Third order polynomial regression lines for distances migrated by transplanted astrocytes.

When cultured fetal spinal cord cells were implanted [gel transplant] PHAL-GFAP positive astrocytes were observed in a wedge shaped region in the left dorsal column of host T6 spinal cord [transplantation site] at 30 DPI. No PHAL positive astrocytes were observed in the contralateral dorsal column, within either dorsal horn, or on the pial surface. PHAL-GFAP positive astrocytes were observed in host cervical spinal cord at the C8-T1 interface, a distance of 19-20 mm from the transplantation site. These cells were located in a wedge shaped region in the dorsal column and along the pial surface. No penetration into host gray matter was observed. After 60 DPI PHAL positive astrocytes were observed bilaterally in host thoracic spinal cord; the density of transplant derived astrocytes was greater ipsilateral to the transplantation site. PHAL positive astrocytes were also observed bilaterally on the pial surface. Transplant derived astrocytes were confined to a wedge shaped region in the ipsilateral dorsal column in cervical spinal cord [Figure 4]. A small

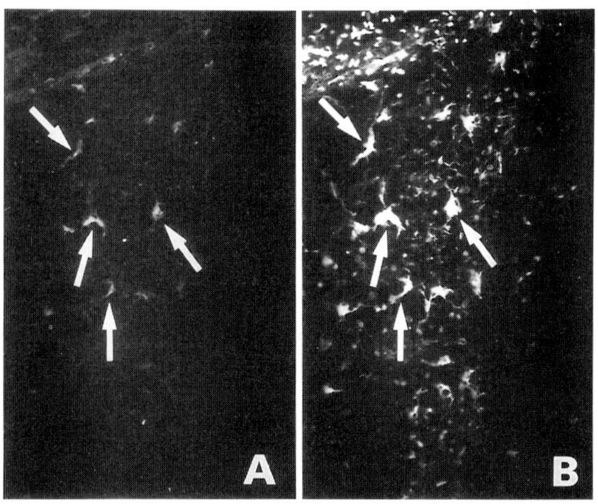


Figure 4. Cervical spinal cord (60 DPI gel transplant) labeled for PHAL (FITC) in A and for GFAP (RITC) in B. Transplant derived double labeled astrocytes (arrows) are confined to a wedge shaped shaped region of the ipsilateral dorsal column. PHAL and GFAP are distributed differently within migrated astrocytes.

number of PHAL-GFAP positive astrocytes were observed on the pial surface. At 90 DPI transplant derived astrocytes were observed bilaterally in nucleus gracilis [lower medulla] and along the pial surface [Figure 5]. The density of PHAL labeled astrocytes was greater ipsilateral to the transplant. Transplant derived astrocytes migrated a distance of ca. 5.5 cm to reach nucleus gracilis in 90 days. Taking into account the 14 day delay in the onset of migration, a migration rate of 0.72 mm/day was calculated. Transplant derived astrocytes were not observed in medulla or on the pial surface 0.25 mm rostral to nucleus gracilis at 90 days [Figure 6].

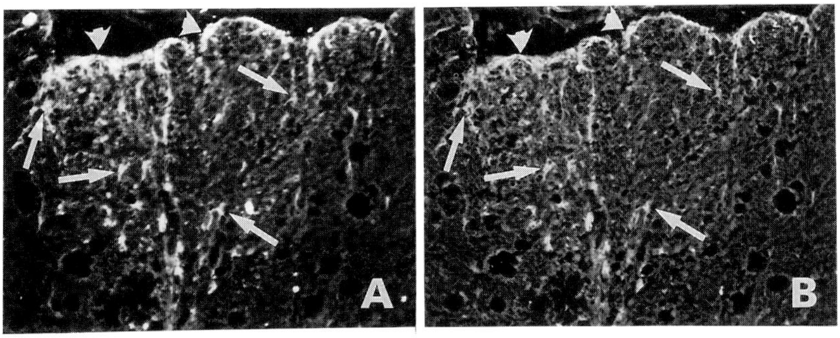


Figure 5. Lower medulla (90 DPI gel transplant) labeled for PHAL (FITC) in A and for GFAP (RITC) in B. Double-labeled transplant-derived astrocytes are located bilaterally in the nucleus gracilis (arrows) and on the pial surface (arrowheads).

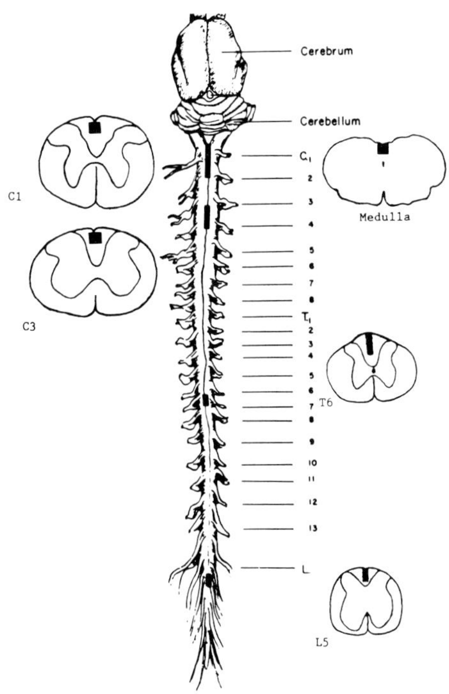


Figure 6. Astrocytic migration within the spinal cord after T6 homografts. Areas containing migrated astrocytes are indicated by black bars.

## IV. Discussion

These data demonstrate that transplant derived astrocytes initiate migration after a 14 day delay period and travel along normal, degenerated and partially degenerated nerve fiber bundles, along blood vessels, within the spaces of Virchow-Robins, and along pial surfaces regardless of the source of the fetal transplant material, the method of implantation or the site of implantation. This 14 day delay period also occurs in xenografts of rabbit cortex to mouse thalamus (Jacque et al, 1986). Overall migration rates of 0.72-0.76 mm/day are calculated based on migrations of 3.5 and 5.5 cm in 60 and 90 days, respectively. Migration along fiber bundles and blood vessels is known to occur in transplants of fetal to adult hippocampus (Raisman et al, 1985). The 3.5-5.5 cm migrated by grafted astrocytes in these experiments is an order of magnitude longer than the 1-3 mm described previously. Differences in the age of the donor material may affect the ability of transplanted cells to migrate. In our studies 14 day gestation [E14] fetal cortex or spinal cord homografts were used whereas Jacque et al (1986) utilized xenografts of neonatal rabbit corpus callosum to host neonatal mouse brain and Raisman et al (1985) used homografts of E16-P1 hippocampus. In addition, prelabeling of transplant material with PHAL may have greater resolution than with tritiated thymidine (Raisman et al, 1985). More PHAL is taken up by individual cells and it is distributed over a greater portion of the cells. Thus, loss of signal due to cell divisions is less of a problem. The 0.5 $mm^2$ pieces of transplanted collagen gel each contain about 875 cells, approximately 260 of which are astrocytes. If these 260 astrocytes are evenly distributed over the 7 cm of lumbar to cervical spinal cord we would expect a density of 4 astrocytes/mm, assuming that all the astrocytes migrate in a straight line. However, an 8 um section may contain 15 or more astrocytes spread throughout the dorsal columns at 2 months post implantation, indicating that a significant number of cell divisions have occurred. Signal washout is compensated for by addition of an extra step in the immunohistochemical procedure. Incubation of the tissue sections with FITC-conjugated goat anti-mouse results in a second FITC fluorochrome binding to the tissue-bound FITC-conjugated sheep anti-goat. The resulting increase in the FITC signal makes it possible to detect the presence of PHAL at later time periods [60-90 days] post implantation.

It becomes clear that many of the fetal or neonatal cells transplanted do not remain at the transplantation site and may migrate long distances. Migration along parallel nerve fibers, blood vessels and pial surfaces appears to be more facile than migration through the parenchyma. Release of neurotrophic substances by migrated astrocytes may well be involved in the neuronal sparing observed following transplantation (Bregman and Reier, 1986; Sharp and Gomez, 1986). These factors may be released at some distance from the "target" cells and be delivered via retrograde transport or may exert local effects in the immediate surroundidng tissue. Such factors may also be involved in promoting host- and transplant-derived neuronal sprouting (Assouline et al, 1987) which may lead to the formation new neuronal circuits or repair of damaged ones. 21 days following a lesion at C3 there is a significant deficit in hind-limb placement which is ameliorated by transplantation of fetal spinal cord at the time of lesion (Bernstein and Goldberg, 1987,1988b). The distance from the lesion/transplantation site to nucleus gracilis, the first relay nucleus in the dorsal column-medial lemniscal system, is less than 1 cm. Taking into account the 14 day delay in the initiation of migration and a migration rate of 0.76 mm/day, transplanted astrocytes could have reached the nucleus gracilis and exerted their trophic effects locally at 21 days post implantation. The calculated migration rates are estimates of the average migration such that there are likely to be some migrating astrocytes arriving at nucleus gracilis "ahead of schedule". At 90 days the nucleus gracilis represents the point of furthest migration. There is no reason to expect that migration has ceased after 90 days however. At the present time we have no data on how far astrocytes are capable of migrating. While the role of new synaptic connections involving transplanted neurons in affecting lesion-induced behavioral and learning deficits cannot be ruled out, a role for migrating astrocytes and oligodendrocytes must now be considered.

**Acknowledgements**

This work was supported by the Veterans Administration. The authors thank Ms. J. Chang, Ms. L. Yao and Ms. V. Williams for their technical assistance.

**References**

Assouline JG, Bosch P, Lim R, Kim IS, Jensen R, Pantazis NJ (1987) Rat astrocytes and Schwann cells in culture synthesize nerve growth factor-like neurite-promoting factors. Dev Brain Res 31:103-118.

Bernstein JJ, Goldberg WJ (1986) Transplantation of cultured fetal spinal cord grafts, grown on a histocompatible sub trate, into adult spinal cord. Brain Res 377:403-408.

Bernstein JJ, Goldberg WJ (1987) Fetal spinal cord homografts ameliorate the severity of lesion induced hind limb behavioral deficits. Exp Neurol (in press)

Bernstein JJ, Goldberg WJ (1988a) Cultured fetal spinal cord astrocytes migrate into adult host lumbar and cervical spinal cord as well as medulla following transplantation into thoracic spinal cord. In: Norenberg MD, Hertz L, Schousboe A (eds) The Biochemical Pathology of Astrocytes (in press)

Bernstein JJ and Goldberg WJ (1988b) Fetal spinal cord homografts reduce expected hind limb deficits from spinal cervical fasiculus gracilis lesion. In: Gorio A, Haber B, Perez-Polo R (eds) Cellular and Molecular Aspects of Regeneration, Springer-Verlag, New York, (in press)

Bregman BS, Reier P (1986) Neural Tissue transplants rescue axotomized rubrospinal cells from retrograde death. J Comp Neurol 244:86-95.

Cammer W, Sacchi R, Sapirstein V (1985) Immunocytochemical localization of carbonic anhydrase in the spinal cords of normal and mutant (Shiverer) adult mice with comparisons among fixation methods. J Histochem Cytochem 33:45-54.

Deckel A, Moran T, Robinson R (1986) Behavior recovery following Kainic acid lesions and fetal implants of the striatum occurs independent of dopaminergic mechanisms. Brain Res 363: 383-385.

Dunnett SB, Bjorklund A, Schmidt RH, Stenevi U, Iversen SD (1983a) Intracerebral grafting of neuronal cell suspensions IV. Behavioural recovery in rats with unilateral 6-OHDA lesions following implantation of nigral cell suspensions in different forebrain sites. Acta Physiol Scand Supp 522:29-37.

Dunnett SB, Bjorklund A, Schmidt RH, Stenevi U, Iversen SD (1983b) Intracerebral grafting of neuronal cell suspensions. V. Behavioural recovery in rats with bilateral 6-OHDA lesions following implantation of nigral cell suspensions. Acta Physiol Scand Supp 522:39-47.

Finsen B, Zimmer J (1986) Timm staining of hippocampal nerve cell bodies in the Kyoto rat. A cell marker in allo- and xeno-

grafting of rat and mouse brain tissue, revealing neuronal migration. Dev Brain Res 29:51-59.
Freed WJ (1983) Functional brain tissue transplantation: Reversal of lesion-induced rotation by intraventricular substantia nigra and adrenal medulla grafts, with a note on intracranial retinal grafts. Biol Psychiat 18:1205-1267.
Friedman E, Nilaver G, Carmel P, Perlow M, Spatz L, Latov N (1986) Myelination by transplanted fetal and neonatal oligodendrocytes in a dysmyelinating mutant. Brain Res 378:142-146.
Gage FH, Bjorklund A (1986) Cholinergic septal grafts into the hippocampal formation improve spatial learning and memory in aged rats by an atropine-sensitive mechanism. J Neurosci 6: 2837-2847.
Gerfin C, Sawchenko P (1984) An anterograde neuroanatomical tracing method that shows the detailed morphology of neurons their axons and terminals: Immunohistochemical localization of an axonally transported plant lectin Phaseolus vulgaris leucoagglutinin. Brain Res 290:219-238
Goldberg WJ and Bernstein JJ (1987) Transplant derived astrocytes migrate into host lumbar and cervical spinal cord after implantation of E14 fetal cerebral cortex into adult thoracic spinal cord. J Neurosci Res 17:(in press)
Goldberg WJ and Bernstein JJ (1988) Migration of cultured fetal spinal cord astrocytes into adult host cervical cord and medulla following transplantation into thoracic spinal cord. J Neurosci Res (in press).
Jacque CM, Suard IM, Collins VP, Raoul MM (1986) Interspecies identification of astrocytes after intracerebral transplantation. Dev Neurosci 8:142-149.
Kamo H, Kim SU, McGeer PL, Shin DH (1986) Functional recovery in a rat model of Parkinson's disease following transplantation of cultured human sympathetic neurons. Brain Res 397: 372-376.
Kaufman LM, Barrett JN (1983): Serum factor supporting long-term survival of rat central neurons in culture. Science 220:1394-1396.
Kesslak JP, Nieto-Sampedro M, Globus J, Cotman CW (1986) Transplants of purified astrocytes promote behavioral recovery after frontal cortex ablation. Exp Neurol 92:377-390.
Lachapelle F, Gumpel M, Baulac M, Jacque C, Duc P, Baumann N (1983) Transplantation of CNS fragments into the brain of shiverer mutant mice: Extensive myelination by implanted oligodendrocytes. I. Immunohistochemical studies. Dev Neurosci 6: 325-334.
Privat A, Mansour H, Pavy A, Geffard M, Sandillon F (1986) Transplantation of dissociated foetal serotonin neurons into the transected spinal cord of adult rats. Neurosci Lett 66:61- 66.
Raisman G, Lawrence JM, Zhou C-F, Lindsay RM (1985) Some neuronal, glial and vascular interactions which occur when developing hippocampal primordia are incorporated into adult host hippocampi. In: Bjorklund A, Stenevi U (ed) Neural Grafting in the Mammalian CNS, Elsevier Press, Amsterdam, pp 125-150.
Sawchenko P, Gerfin C (1985) Plant lectins and bacterial toxins as tools for tracing neuronal connections. Trends Neurosci 8:378-384.

Sharp FR, Gonzalez MF (1986) Fetal cortical transplants ameliorate thalamic atrophy ipsilateral to neonatal frontal cortex lesions. Neurosci lett 71:247-251.

Sladek JR, Redmond DE, Collier TJ, Haber SN, Elsworth JD, Deutch AY, Roth RH (1987) Transplantation of fetal dopamine neurons in primate brain reverses MPTP induced parkinsonism. In: Seil FJ, Herbert E, Carlson BM (ed) Neural Regeneration, Elsevier Press, Amsterdam, pp 309-323.

Wells J, Vietje BP, Wells DG, Boucher M, Bodony RP (1986) Xenografts of brain cells labeled in cell suspensions show growth and differentiation in septo-hippocampal transplants. Brain Res 383:333-338.

# T H E M E IV

# NEURONAL ENDOCRINE-IMMUNE INTERACTIONS

# Theme IV - INTRODUCTION

Neuroimmunomodulation has its roots in work done in clinical psychology, where anecdotal clinical findings suggested that there were levels of interaction between the nervous system and the immune system that were not understood. Also, interest in the autoimmune phenomena expressed in EAE, led to the concept that perturbations of the "priviledged status" of the nervous system might be associated with the immunogenic properties of certain peptides present in the nervous system.

In the fifties and sixties, tumor growth studies with rats showed that behavioral experiences and conditioning of animals has profound effects on tumor growth. However, it is in the last decade that neuroimmunomodulation has experienced explosive growth due to the development of well defined conditions for the growth in culture of neural cells, the isolation of well defined neural growth factor substances and lymphokines and the application of hybridoma and recombinant DNA technology. It is now accepted that so called lymphokines are not restricted in their targets to lymphoid cells but also play a role in glial activation and proliferation and the neuronal growth factors, like NGF, and neurotransmitters and neuromodulators can act on lymphoid cells. Receptors for developmental factors, like NGF, and for neuroendocrine hormones and psychoactive peptides have been demonstrated for selected populations of lymphoid cells. The following chapters speak to the evidence for these interactions. What is not known yet, is the mixed role of these substances in development and disease but it is increasingly clear that this interdisciplinary area of research will yield answers of an integrated nature that will be physiologically relevant to our understanding of organismic function and dysfunction.

In the work here discussed, particular attention is focussed on the innervation of lymphoid organs and the neuroendocrine control of lymphoid function. Also, the effects of lymphokines on glial cells are discussed. It is demonstrated that NGF is not restricted in its range of action to CNS and CNS neurons where it acts to allow cell survival and induce neurite elongation in a typical pleiotropic response but that, as it does for immature chromaffin cells of the adrenal, it can have mitogenic effects on some lymphoid cells where the presence of receptors to NGF has also been demonstrated.

# THE SOURCE AND DISTRIBUTION OF AUTONOMIC NERVOUS SYSTEM NERVES AND RECEPTORS WITHIN THE THYMUS GLAND

KAREN BULLOCH, TRICIA RADOJCIC, AND LESLIE TOLLEFSON

Karen Bulloch Ph.D., Director
Neuroimmune Physiology Laboratory
Helicon Foundation
4622 Santa Fe St.
San Diego, California 92109

## ABSTRACT

The thymus gland has a rich autonomic nervous system innervation consisting of both cholinergic and adrenergic nerve fibers. Based on retrograde transport studies the ANS cholinergic nerves are derived from nucleus retrofacial, nucleus ambiguus and two distinct regions of the spinal cord (C1-C4). More recent double-labelled retrograde transport studies have revealed distinct innervation patterns for the thymus as opposed to the adjacent tissues. Adrenergic innervation of the thymus originates from the stellate ganglion, superior cervical ganglion, and other small ganglia of the rostal sympathetic chain. Neuropharmacological studies have demonstrated receptive fields for this ANS innervation. Adrenergic and cholinergic receptors have been identified on subsets of T lymphocytes as well as other lymphoid cells. There is evidence that cholinergic and adrenergic agonists and antagonists modulate immune function and may factor into immune cell development. This neuroanatomical and neuropharmacological data offers some of the best evidence for neuroimmune interaction and opens the way to elucidating the role of autonomic circuitry.

The scientific approach to immunology has undergone many transformations during the past hundred years, as new information and technical achievements have changed our way of thinking about the immune system and how it functions. During the early 1900's the immune system was viewed as an integrated part of the body's vegetative physiology, subject to regulation by the autonomic

NATO ASI Series, Vol. H22
Neural Development and Regeneration
Edited by A. Gorio et al.

nervous system (ANS) (Kuntz, 1953; Korneva et al., 1985; Belak, 1941).. More modern molecular approaches have directed scientific thinking away from this concept and have not taken into consideration the integration of the immune system into the physiology of the body. Although these approaches have yielded a wealth of information about the molecular biology of the immune system, they do not address questions such as why there are similarities in surface antigens, humoral mediators, and regulatory mechanisms within the nervous and immune systems. In view of these unanswered questions, it becomes advantageous to re-examine the immune system within the context of a system subject to some type of homeostatic monitoring and governing by the ANS.

In order to scientifically establish the basis for a significant relationship between the nervous and immune system, it is important to demonstrate ANS regulation and monitoring of the immune system via a complete neurophysiological communication loop. There are three fundamental criteria that establish the existence of such a regulatory loop. First, the existence of efferent, humoral or anatomical pathways from the brain to these peripheral tissues and organs. Second, that these pathways affect the development and/or function of a given system. Third, that some mechanism of afferents, humoral and/or anatomical, send information back t the nervous system indicating that the efferent message was received and carried out. This feedback loop would in turn complete the circuitry by terminating or enhancing the initial signal.

Although the fundamental requirements that would demonstrate the existence of a neuroimmune physiological circuit have by no means been totally satisfied by experimental evidence, there is now a great deal of new data that supports its existence. The representation of the ANS fibers within the lymphoid tissue and organs of vertebrates offers perhaps the best documentation for the existence of regulatory pathways between the nervous and immune systems. Furthermore, the nature of this innervation strongly suggests that the role of these nerves within the lymphoid tissues encompasses the development, maintenance, and, in part, the function of the immune system. Additional support for the efficacy of this ANS innervation is provided by the existence of receptors for adrenergic and cholinergic neurotransmitters on membranes of both immature and mature cells of the immune system.

The major focus of this review will be to examine the neuroanatomical and neuropharmacological components of the regulatory loop between one of the primary immune organs, the thymus, and the ANS. This overview will serve as a model for considering ways in which autonomic regulation can affect different aspects of immune system development and function.

## Neuroanatomy of the Thymus

The thymus is the primary organ of the immune system. This lympho-epithelial gland not only provides the specialized microenvironment that educates T-lymphocytes but also produces factors that modulate both hypothalamic and immune functions (Besedovsky & Sorkin, 1977; Pierpaoli & Besevodovsky, 1975).

In birds a large part of this gland contains neurally

derived tissues. Le Douarin (1974), using chick quail chimeras, showed that the support cells of the thymus are derived from neural crest, whereas Hammond's studies (1954) indicated that the third epibranchial placode contributes to thymic development. Although it is not clear if the mammalian thymus has a similar origin, such an origin would explain, in part, some of the molecular similarities between the thymus and the brain.

The innervation of the thymus by the ANS occurs during the early phases of the gland's development preceding both its differentiation and the immigration of pre-T cells. Nerve fibers from the vagus enter the primordium and are distributed to areas that define the future cortico-medullary boundary (Bulloch, 1985; Bulloch & Pomerantz, 1984; Hammar 1935). After vagal fibers have been distributed within the thymus, the parenchymal cells develop into the structural pattern of the adult gland and precursors of T-lymphocytes begin to enter the gland. As the thymus descends from its cervical location, the thymic branch of the vagus nerve continues to develop complex nerve nets at the cortico-medullary boundary.

During the perinatal and prepubescent periods, other ANS nerves penetrate the parenchyma of the thymus. The nerves which supply the thymus of the adult mouse are derived from the vagus, the phrenic, and the recurrent laryngeal nerves, as well as from the stellate and other small ganglia of the thoracic sympathetic chain (Fig. 1) (Bulloch & Pomerantz, 1984). Despite minor differences, the innervation pattern of the mouse thymus is comparable to that reported for other species (Bulloch, 1985).

Initially, the horseradish peroxidase (HRP) retrograde

transport method was used to identify the neuronal sources of thymic innervation. These studies revealed that the thymuses of rats and mice are innervated by neurons whose cell bodies lie in the brainstem's nucleus ambiguus and the nucleus retrofacial and in three distinct columns in the cervical spinal cord, C1-C4 (Bulloch & Moore, 1981), as well as in the nodose and superior cervical ganglia (Bulloch et al., 1984). Experiments carried out in the chick yielded similar findings in the brainstem and spinal cord (Bulloch, 1987).

As neuroanatomical techniques became more sophisticated there was speculation that the results of some of these earlier studies might have been due to diffusion of HRP into the surrounding tissues (Nance et al., 1986). However, re-examination of this problem utilizing a new, more sensitive double-labelling retrograde transport technique clearly showed that the original studies did reflect a true representation of thymic innervation (Figs. 2 & 3). Briefly the results of these experiments showed that when equivalent doses of HRP or Fluoro-gold were injected into the thymus, and the esophagus or adjacent musculature, each of the tissues had distinct labelling patterns in the spinal cord and brainstem. Some neurons did demonstrate both labels within the neuronal perikaryon but it was unclear if this was due to diffusion onto adjacent tissue, lymphatic drainage and subsequent uptake by the non-injected tissue, or to the existence of axonal collaterals innervating each of the injected tissues (Bulloch & Tollefson, 1987; Bulloch & Tollefson, manuscript in prep.).

The function of ANS innervation in the thymus gland is just beginning to be understood. The distribution of the nerve fibers and the time of their appearance suggests several possible roles for the nervous system in the development of the thymus gland and in the regulation of its function. An analysis of the innervation of the dysgenic thymus of the nude (nu/nu) mutant mouse and of syngeneic embryonic thymus transplanted under the kidney capsule of nude mice supports a role for innervation in the development of this gland (Fig. 4) (Bulloch et al., 1987; Bulloch & Pomerantz, 1984; Hammar, 1935).

Although the ANS innervation of the thymus has been the focus of this review, it is now recognized that the ANS innervates every known tissue and organ of the immune system (Bulloch, 1985). What makes this ANS innervation unique is that the distribution of the fibers to these tissues and organs differs with respect to the representation of neurotransmitters and their appearance developmentally. Such anatomical studies have begun to provide valuable information for developing new strategies to further our understanding of the function of these nerves within the tissues and how they may operate as part of neurophysiological communication loops.

## Neurotransmitter Receptors on Thymus-Derived Lymphocyte

The presence of nerve terminals within the thymus is only meaningful if there are recipients for neurotransmitter signal inputs. Thus the demonstration of functional neuroreceptors on thymocytes and mature lymphocytes would offer additional confirmation of the existence of a complete neurophysiological communication loop. It is now clear that several such receptor types do in fact, exist on lymphoid cells, among which are those responsive to acetylcholine (or cholinergic input) and those responsive to the catecholamines, norepinephrine and epinephrine (or adrenergic input). A classification of these receptors and their known function with regard to immune cells will be presented as an overview of the magnitude of their representation within the immune system.

a. Adrenergic Receptors

On the basis of their differential responsiveness to adrenergic agonists, the adrenergic receptors can be divided into several subtypes namely, alpha-1, alpha-2 and beta-1, beta-2. The beta 1 & 2 subtypes are reported to activate adenylate cyclase production of cyclic AMP, whereas, stimulation of alpha-2 receptors inhibits this effect. On the other hand, the alpha-1 subclass regulates phosphotidylionositol turnover as well as the activation of calcium ionic flux. Both alpha and beta classes of adrenergic receptors have been characterized on human and mouse lymphocytes (Titinchi & Clark, 1984; Sanders & Munson, 1985).

The studies that relate to the distribution and function of adrenergic receptors predominate among those studies which characterize the incidence of neuroreceptors on T-cells. The presence of adrenergic receptors was initially characterized on mixed populations of lymphoid cells. More recent attempts at seperating the cells by effector function and maturational state have not revealed that all adrenergic receptors are uniformly distributed on lymphocytes. For example, an increase in beta receptor density is observed during the maturational sequence of the thymocyte to the circulating T-cell (Pochet & Delespesse, 1983; Van de Griend et al., 1983). Further differences are noted between T and B-cells, where the T-cell expresses two fold fewer beta receptors than B-cells (Landemann et al., 1984; Pochet & Delespesse, 1983).

These data would imply an adrenergic component in the regulation of the immune response. More recently, studies carried out on mouse cloned lymphoid cell lines as well as purified human T cells have demonstrated differential receptor distribution with respect to the functional subset. Human and mouse T suppressor, T cytolytic, and T helper cells showed a progressive decline in receptor number as well as in adenylate cyclase responsiveness to stimulation by beta adrenergic agonists (Landemann et al., 1984; Kahn et al., 1985a; Kahn et al., 1985b; Kahn et al., 1984). In the cloned lines beta receptor-mediated increases in intracellular cyclic AMP did not enhance either suppressor cell function or T helper cell secretion of IL2, although histamine was able to affect both these functions (Kahn et al., 1985a). The degree of coupling to adenylate cyclase is not always directly correlated with the beta adrenergic receptor number on the surface of lymphoid cells. Murine thymocytes, for example, show increased cyclic AMP accumulation in response to adrenergic agonist stimulation. On the other hand T and B cells (which bear a greater number of beta adrenergic receptors than do thymocytes) show reduced cyclic AMP accumulation after receptor activation (Pochet & Delespesse, 1983; Bach, 1975; Niaudet et al., 1976).

Adrenergic control of T-cells and thymocytes may have a wide variety of effects on the development of the immune system and the execution of its function. For instance, in the thymus, adrenergic fibers are localized in discrete areas, primarily in association with the vascular supply. Low numbers of highly reactive beta receptors on thymocytes imply a specialized type of neuro-immune interaction in the maturation of the fully immunocompetent T-cell. On the other hand in the spleen, there is a rich network of adrenergic fibers associated with lymphoid follicles. This fact, coupled with: 1. the overall increase in beta receptors on mature lymphocytes over thymocytes 2. the differences in receptor number among different classes of lymphocytes, and 3. the alterations in cyclic AMP responsiveness to adrenergic agonists strongly suggests an adrenergic involvment in the maintenence and regulation of discrete immune function.

More direct evidence for ANS control of T-cell immune function is provided by studies which demonstrate adrenergic control of immune cell proliferation. In these studies adrenergic agonists were shown to induce proliferation of thymocytes (Morgan et al., 1984), yet inhibit the mitogen stimulated mature T-cell proliferation. Feldman et al. (1986) postulated the latter effect might be caused by an adrenergic-induced decrease in IL2 receptors.

Several other functions of mixed populations of lymphocytes have been shown to be affected by adrenergic receptor activation They include the beta-mediated decrease of sterol synthesis (Krone et al., 1984) and natural killer activity (Hellstrand et al., 1985) as well as alpha-1 and beta-2 influences in the regulation of the antibody response (Sanders & Munson, 1985). In human monocytes, complement synthesis is stimulated by alpha-1 receptor mechanisms (Lapin & Whaley, 1982). However, the adrenergic influences on T-cell contributions to these functions have yet to be defined.

b. Cholinergic Receptors

Like the adrenergic sympathetic nerves, the cholinergic parasympathetic nerves are differentially distributed among the lymphoid tissues. Acetylcholine and its agonists stimulate the nicotinic and muscarinic classes of cholinergic neuroreceptors. These receptors, like those for catecholamine neurotransmitters are functionally distinct. Nicotinic receptors have been reported to control ion channel gating, while the muscarinic receptors are linked to cyclic-GMP production. Both types of receptors have been reported on rat lymphocyte and thymocyte cell membranes (Maslinski et al., 1980; Morgan et al., 1984). Nicotinic receptors are also expressed by rabbit thymocytes (Ueno et al., 1980) whereas muscarinic receptors have been characterized on human (Laskowska-Bozek et al., 1986; Bidart et al., 1983; Zalcman et al., 1981), rat (Grabczewska et al., 1985; Krzystyniak et al., 1982; Maslinski et al., 1980) and mouse lymphocytes (Atweh et al., 1984; Strom et al., 1981). The muscarinic receptors also show a differential distribution pattern among the lymphocyte population. T-cells bear significantly greater numbers of receptors than do B-cells (Strom et al., 1981). Furthermore, like the beta adrenergic receptor, T-cell maturation within the thymus may be associated with a concomitant increase in muscarinic receptor number (Maslinski et al., 1986).

Although the functional consequences of these distribution patterns remain to be clarified, there is some indication that one role of these receptors might be to regulate cytotoxic T-cell function (Strom et al., 1981). Other proposed functions include cholinergic neuroregulation of both thymocyte (Morgan et al., 1984) and mature T-cell (Strom et al., 1981; Richman & Arnason, 1975) proliferation and T-cell membrane depolarization (Shapiro & Strom, 1980). Additional work must be completed on cholinergic receptor distribution on T cell subsets before parasympathetic ANS control of immune function can be effectively clarified.

## SUMMARY

The anatomical and neuropharmacological evidence presented in this review suggests that the ANS regulates the development and function of the immune system. The study of the interaction between the nervous and immune systems is still evolving as a discipline with many questions unanswered. Part of the problem lies in our incomplete understanding of the anatomy of the central and peripheral ANS as well as the fundamental tenets governing ANS regulated homeostasis. Nevertheless, our knowledge of the neuroanatomy of the thymus and other immune system organs and tissues has grown considerably and provides a basis on which to evaluate the physiology of neuroimmune interaction.

ACKNOWLEDGEMENTS: This work was supported by grant N0001485k0528 of the Office of Naval Resources and a grant from the Joan B. Kroc Foundation of Psychoneuroimmunology. A debt of gratitude is owed to Dr. Melvin Cohn of the Salk Institute and Theodore Melnechuk of the Helicon Foundation for their editorial comments and professional advice in the preparation of this manuscript.

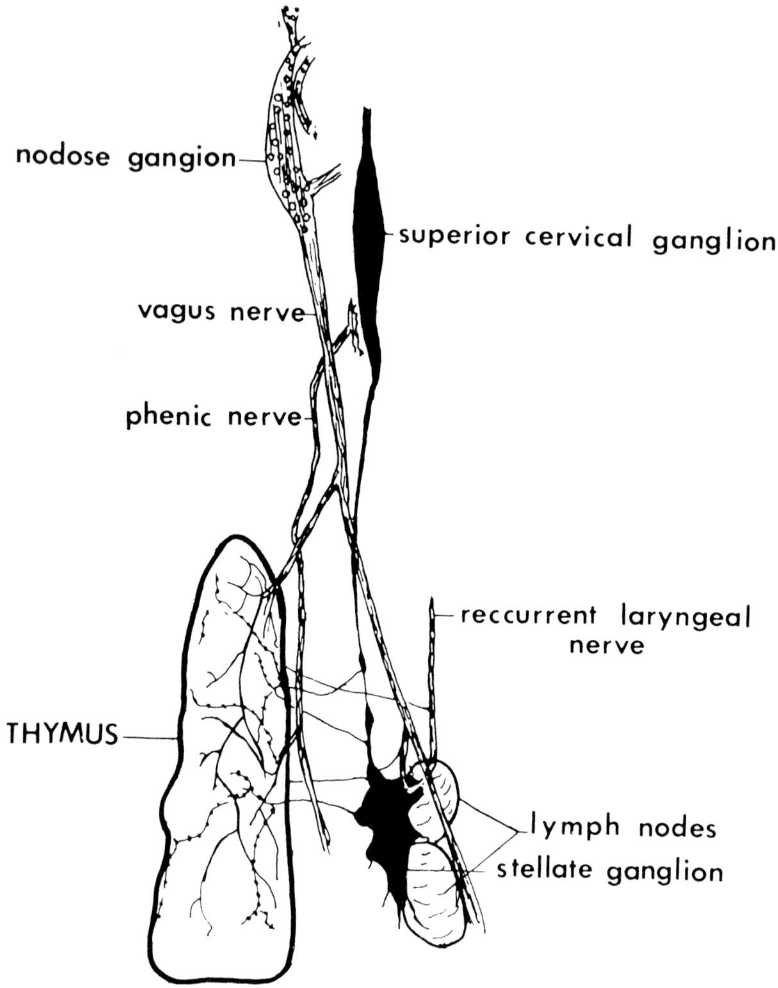


1

Figure 1. Schematic representation of the innervation of the thymus gland.

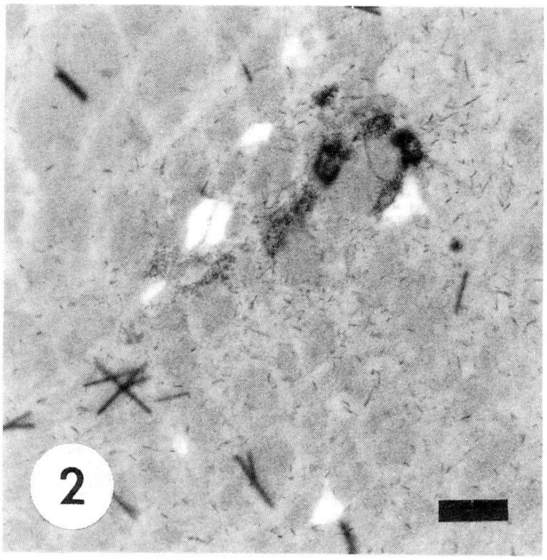

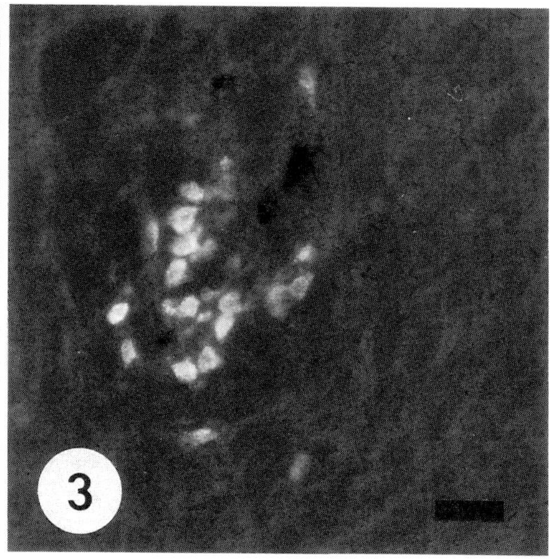

Figure 2. Labelled cells in medial aspects of nucleus retrofacial of the mouse following Fluora-gold injections into the thymus and HRP into the esophagus. Marker bar=50 um.

Figure 3. Labelled cells in caudal aspects of nucleus retrofacial of the mouse following Fluora-gold injections into the thymus and HRP into the esophagus. Marker bar=50 um.

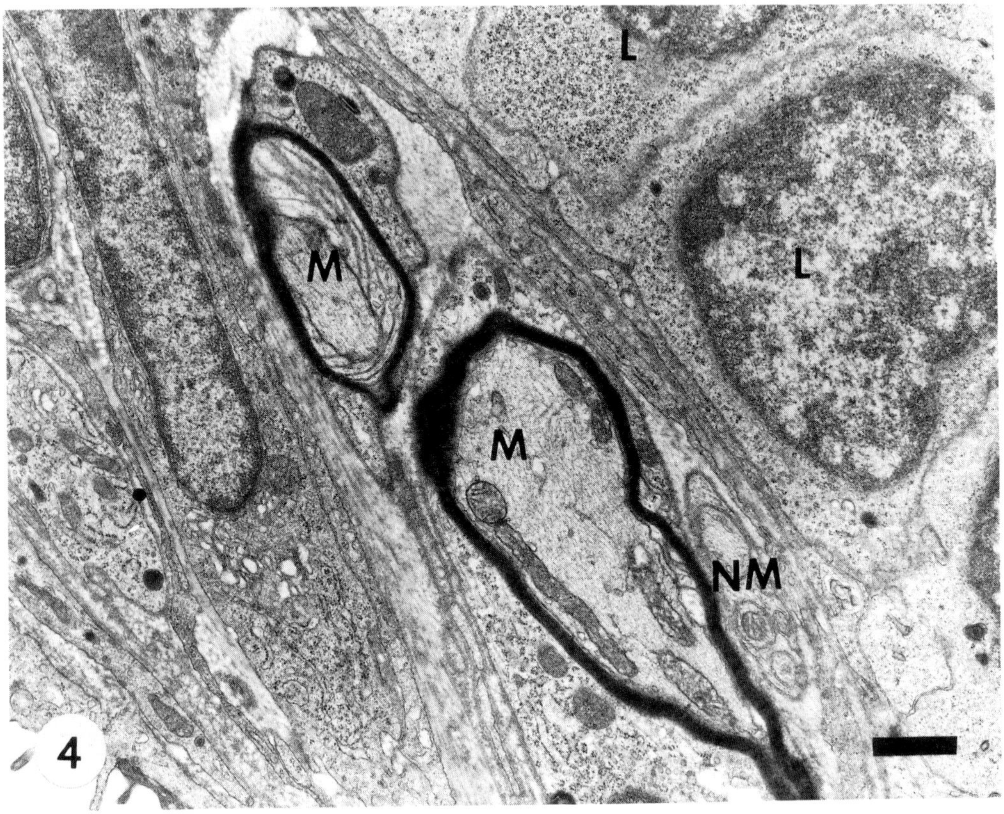


Figure 4. Electron micrograph showing the the penetration of myelinated (M) and non-myelinated neuronal processes (NM) into the parenchyma of thymic tissue transplanted under the kidney capsule of a nude mouse. Note the small lymphocyte directly adjacent to the nerve fibers. L=lymphocyte Marker bar=2 um.

## References


Atweh SF, Grayhack JJ, Richman DP (1984) A cholinergic receptor site on murine lymphocytes with novel binding characteristics. Life Sciences 35:2459-2469

Bach MA (1975) Differences in cyclic AMP changes after stimulation by prostaglandins and isoproterenol in lymphocyte subpopulations. J of Clin Invest 55:1074-1081

Belak S (1941) Ztschr. Immunitatsforsch. u. exper. Therap. 100:264-292

Besedovsky HO, Sorkin E (1977) The role of the thymus in programming of neuroendocrine functions. J Clin Exp Immunol 27:1-12

Bidart JM, Moingeon PH, Bohuon C (1983) Muscarinic cholinergic receptors on circulating human lymphocytes: evidence for a particulate binding site. Res Comm in Chem Path and Pharm 39:169-172

Blalock JE (1984) The immune system as a sensory organ. J Immunol 132:1067-1070

Bulloch K (1987) A comparative study of the autonomic nervous system innervation of the thymus in the mouse and chicken. Int J of Neurosci in press

Bulloch K (1985) Neuroanatomy of Lymphoid Tissues in Neural Modulation of Immunity Eds. Guillemin R, Cohn M, and Melnechuk T 111-141

Bulloch K, Cullen MR, Schwartz RH, Longo DL (1987) Development of innervation within syngeneic thymus tissue transplanted under the kidney capsule of the nude mouse: a light and ultrastructual microscopic study. J Neurosci Res 18:1-12

Bulloch K, Moore RY (1981) Innervation of the thymus gland by brain stem and spinal cord in mouse and rat. Amer J Anat 162:157-166

Bulloch K, Pomerantz W (1984) Autonomic nervous system innervation of thymic-related lymphoid tissue in wild type and nude mice. J of Comp Neurol 228:57-68

Bulloch K, Roth E, Cullen MR (1984) Nodose and superior cervical ganglia projections to the rat thymus gland. Soc Neurosci Abst 10:723

Bulloch K, Tollefson L (1987) Double-labelling retrograde transport in the mouse thymus and adjacent tissue. Soc for Neurosci Abst in press

Feldman RD, Hunninghake GW, McArdle WL (1986) Beta adrenergic receptor agonists downregulate IL2 receptors in human lymphocytes. Clin Res 34

Grabczewska E, Maslinski W, Ryzewski J (1985) Muscarinic receptors of rat lymphocytes- differences in young and old animals. Acta Physiologica Polska 36:276-280

Hall NR, Goldstein AL (1984) Immunomodulating Agents: Properties and Mechanisms. Marcel Dekker N.Y. 533-563

Hammar JA (1935) Konstitutionsanatomische Studien uber die Neurotiscerung des Menschenembryos IV Uber die innervationsverhaltnisse der inkretorgone und der thymus bis den 4. Fotalmonat. Z Mikrosk Anat 38:253-293

Hammond WS (1954) Origin of thymus in the chick embryo. J Morphol 95:501-522

Hellstrand K, Hermodsson S, Strannegard O (1985) Evidence for beta adrenoreceptor-mediated regulation of human natural killer cells. J of Immunol 134:4095-4099

Kahn MM, Melmon KL, Fathman CG, Hertel-Wulff B, Strober S (1985a) The effects of autocoids on cloned murine lymphoid cells: modulation of IL2 secretion and the activity of natural suppressor cells. J of Immunol 134:4100-4106

Kahn MM, Sansoni P, Silverman ED, Engleman EG, Melmon KL (1985) Beta adrenergic receptors on human suppressor helper and cytolytic lymphocytes. Biochem Pharm 35:1137-1142

Kahn MM, Sansoni P, Engleman E, Melmon KL (1984b) Distribution of beta adrenergic receptors in human T cell subsets. Proceedings of the Western Pharmacological Society 27:349-351

Korneva EA, Klimenko VM, Schkhinek EK (1985) Neurohumoral Maintenance of Immunity. Univ of Chicago Press

Krone W, Earl U, Muller-Wieland D, Greten H (1984) Stimulation of beta-2 adrenergic receptors suppresses sterol synthesis in human mononuclear leukocytes. Biochimica et Biophysica Acta 804:137-140

Krzystyniak K, Ryzewski J, Maslinski W (1982) Cholinergic receptors of rat lymphocytes during adjuvant polyarthritis. Biochimica et Biophysica Acta 691:341-344

Kuntz A (1953) The Autonomic Nervous System. Lea & Febiger Philedelphia 462-476

Landemann RMA, Burgisser E, Wesp M, Buhler T. (1984) Beta adrenergic receptors are different in subpopulations of human circulating lymphocytes. J of Receptor Res 4:37-50

Lapin D, Whaley K (1982) Adrenergic receptors on monocytes modulate complement component synthesis. J Clin Exp Immunol 47:606-612

Laskowska-Bozek H, Grabczewska E, Maslinski W, Ryzewski J, Filipowicz-Sosnowska A Sadowska-Wroblewska M (1986) Expression of muscarinic cholinergic receptors on lymphocytes during rheumatoid arthritis. Int J Tiss Reac 7:475-483

Le Douarin NM (1974) Origin of thymus in the chick embryo. Dev Biol 41:162-184

Maslinski W (1986) Appearance of muscarinic cholinergic receptors on mature thymocytes make them sensetive for cholinergic stimulation. Second International Workshop on Neuroimmunomodulation 33

Maslinski W, Grabczewska E, Ryzeswski J (1980) Acetylcholine receptors of rat lymphocytes. Biochimica et Biophysica Acta 633:269-273

Morgan J, Wigham CG, Perris AD (1984) The promotion of mitosis in cultured thymic lymphocytes by acetylcholine and catecholamines. J of Pharmacy and Pharmacol 36:511-515

Nance DM, Hopkins DA, Bieger D (1986) Re-examination of the innervation of the thymus gland in mice and rats. Soc for Neurosciences Abst 12:1064

Niaudet P, Beaurain G, Bach MA (1976) Differences in effect of isoproterenol stimulation on levels of cyclic AMP in human B and T lymphocytes. Eur J of Immunol 6:834-836

Pierpaoli W, Besedovsky HO (1975) Experimental analysis of the migration and differentiation of neuroblasts of the autonomic nervous system and of mesenchymal derivations using a biological cell marking technique. J Clin Exp Immunol 20:323-338

Pochet R, Delespesse G (1983) Beta adrenoceptors display different efficiency on lymphocyte subpopulations. Biochem Pharm 32:1651-1655

Richman DP, Arnason BGW (1979) Nicotinic acetylcholine receptor: evidence for a functionally distinct receptor on human lymphocytes. Proc Natl Acad Sci USA 76:4632-4635

Sanders VM, Munson AE (1985) Norepinephrine and the antibody response. Pharm Reviews :229-248

Shapiro HM, Strom TB (1980) Electrophysiology of T lymphocyte cholinergic receptors. Proceedings of the Natiuonal Academy of Sciences 77:4317-4321

Strom TB, Lane MA, George K (1981) The parallel time dependent bimodal change in lymphocyte cholinergic binding activity and cholinergic influence upon lymphocyte-mediated cytotoxicity after lymphocyte activation. J of Immunol 127:705-710

Titinchi S, Clark B (1984) Alpha-2 adrenoceptors inhuman lymphocytes: direct characterization by [3H]yohimbine binding. Biochem and Biophys Res Commun 121:1-7

Ueno S, Wada K, Takahashi M, Tarui S (1980) Acetylcholine receptor in rabbit thymus: antigenic similarity between acetylcholine receptors of muscle and thymus. Clin Exp Immunol 42:463-469

Van de Griend RJ, Astoldi A, Wyerman P, Van Dorn R, Roos D. (1983) Low beta adrenergic receptor concentration on human thymocytes. J Clin Exp Immunol 53:53-60

Zalcman SJ, Neckers LM, Kaayalp O, Wyatt RJ (1981) Muscarinic cholinergic binding sites on intact human lymphocytes. Life Sciences 29:69-73

# NEUROENDOCRINE FUNCTIONS IN LYMPHOID TISSUES

Ruth Hogue Angeletti, Ren-Yu Xu, Eva Ling, Jiang Qian
Neuropathology
University of Pennsylvania
Philadelphia, Pennsylvania 19104-6079
USA

## INTRODUCTION

The acidic protein chromogranin A has recently been detected in cells within immune tissues using immunohistochemical and immunoblotting analysis (Angeletti and Hickey, 1985). Although other neural and endocrine peptides have also been identified or found to have effects within these tissues (Plotnikoff et al., 1985; Smith et al., 1986; Wybran, 1985), the identification of chromogranin A has somewhat different implications. Individual neuropeptides such as enkephalins, endorphins, vasoactive intestinal peptide, are found in neuronal and endocrine vesicles only in tissue locations appropriate to their functions. Chromogranin A, however, is a pan-neuroendocrine marker protein, found in endocrine and some neurosecretory vesicles, but not in exocrine vesicles (Fischer-Colbrie et al., 1985; Lloyd and Wilson, 1983; O'Conner, 1983).

Two hypotheses were offered to explain the presence of chromogranin A in these new locations in the immune system. First, chromogranin A could be present within well known lymphoid cells. Alternatively, true neuroendocrine cells, as yet unidentified, may exist within tissues of immunological importance. Several experimental approaches may be taken in order to distinguish between these two hypotheses. The presence of other neuropeptides in immune tissues may be examined and compared to distribution of chromogranin A. Furthermore, chromogranin A containing cells may be isolated from spleen and lymph node, and then characterized with respect to immunological and cell biological markers. Finally, purified lymphoid cell populations and tumor cell lines representing defined lymphoid cell types may be analyzed for the presence or absence of chromogranin A and other neuroendocrine markers and functions.

NATO ASI Series, Vol. H22
Neural Development and Regeneration
Edited by A. Gorio et al.

## FUNCTIONS OF CHROMOGRANIN A

Chromogranin A is an enigmatic protein whose function has remained elusive to the examination of many investigators (Banks and Helle, 1965; Smith and Kirshner, 1967; Smith and Winkler, 1967). Our studies using chromogranin A as a marker have suggested new aspects of neural-endocrine-immune interactions. A limitation on the interpretation of our data is that the function of chromogranin A is still unknown. Several functions have been proposed for this molecule, based on its tissue location in secretory vesicles and some preliminary studies. Chromogranin A may be a protein which binds or sequesters catecholamines or ATP found in the vesicles. It could be a hormone or prohormone. The structure of the cDNA for chromogranin A has been elucidated, but yielded no significant homologies to previously identified proteins which might provide some clue to its function (Iacangelo et al., 1986). Experimental results had indicated that chromogranin A is a calcium binding protein (Felicitas and Gratzen, 1986). Two calcium binding sequences were indeed identified. The predicted amino acid sequence also contained eight sets of paired basic residues. These types of sequences are commonly found in proteins from which biologically active peptides have been cleaved. A relevant observation has been made by investigators in another field. The 49-residue peptide pancreastatin, which strongly inhibits insulin secretion from islet cells (Tatemoto et al., 1986), was found to have 70% of its structure identical to a region within the chromogranin A sequence (Eiden, 1987). These observations suggest that chromogranin A may release peptides involved in regulating endocrine secretion.

## PROBES FOR NEUROENDOCRINE FUNCTION

Assays for defined neuroendocrine functions will be critical to confirm our observations, and to help discriminate among hypotheses. The hallmark molecules of neuroendocrine cells are: biologically active peptides, the enzymes responsible for processing the peptide precursors, and chromogranin A. The active peptides secreted by neuroendocrine cells are themselves of interest in the immune system. However, these peptides are usually restricted to a very few cells. Each type of neuroendocrine cell possesses a different set from among the known peptides. The common feature related to these peptides in neuroendocrine cells is the presence of the enzymes required to release them from their precursor polypeptides and process them to their mature form. The dibasic peptidase cleaves them (Loh et al., 1985; Parish et al., 1986), and a carboxypeptidase trims away the excess amino acids (Fricker et al., 1986). The alpha-amidating enzyme may further modify them. These enzymes should be universal endocrine marker proteins. Interleukins and lymphokines, proteins secreted by lymphoid cells, are not processed in this manner.

We chose the endocrine carboxypeptidase as the broader spectrum marker for neuroendocrine cells (Fricker et al., 1986). As noted above, this enzyme is involved in processing polypeptide precursors in a way characteristic of neuroendocrine cells, but not of lymphoid cells. The cDNA for this protein has recently been cloned and sequenced. Fricker and coworkers (1986) found that its structure is highly homologous to all other known carboxypeptidases, but possesses amino terminal and carboxy terminal extensions found only in this form. Again, several peptides corresponding to these sequences were synthesized and used as antigens. An effective antibody was made against SF24 [SERKEEEKEELMEWWKMMSETLNF], the carboxy terminal peptide. As expected, this antibody detected all endocrine cells tested and most neurons as well.

Antibodies against natural bovine chromogranin A have been shown to be effective probes of neuroendocrine cells, but one could question that they detect proteins which contaminate our preparations. Therefore, unambiguous, defined probes for chromogranin A have been constructed. Several synthetic peptides corresponding to amino acid sequences predicted by the cDNA sequence for chromogranin A were prepared and used as antigens. The most effective was the peptide PL26 [PEDQELESLSAIEAELEK-VAHQLEEL], which is three amino acid residues removed from the carboxy terminus of the protein (Iacangelo et al., 1986). This antibody performs identically to chromogranin A in immunohistochemical and immunoblotting experiments.

## CHROMOGRANIN A AND ENDOCRINE CARBOXYPEPTIDASE IMMUNOHISTOCHEMISTRY

These two antisera, PL26 and SF24, were compared in their immunohistochemical staining in immune tissues. Since the endocrine carboxypeptidase (SF24) is a marker for neuroendocrine processing, and chromogranin A is a marker for a yet undefined neuroendocrine function, we

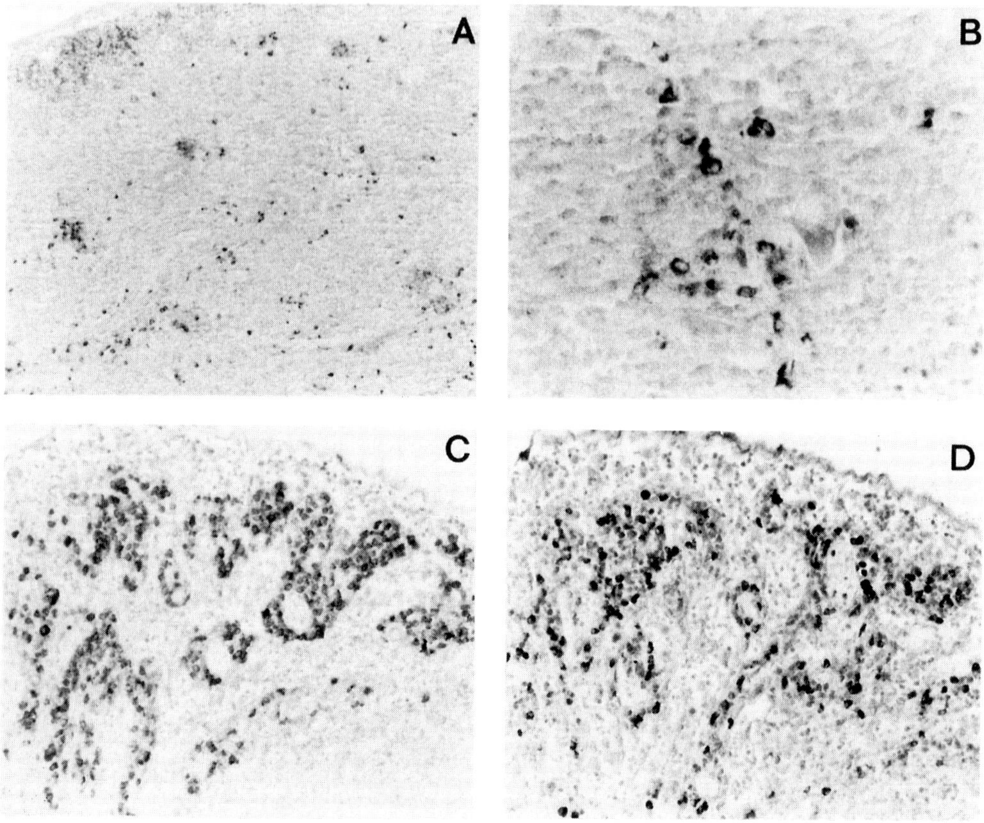


Figure 1. Immunohistochemistry of immune tissues with antibodies specific for chromogranin A and endocrine carboxypeptidase. A. Endocrine carboxypeptidase (SF24) staining of Lewis rat spleen using the PAP procedure. B. The same as in A, at higher magnification. Note that the antibody detects mononuclear cells. C. Anti-chromogranin A (PL26) staining of Lewis rat lymph node. D. Lewis rat lymph node stained with antibody to endocrine carboxypeptidase (SF24).

expect these two antibodies to be overlapping, but not coextensive in localization. In spleen, the PL26 antibody detects scattered, intensely positive cells. In studies reported elsewhere, dense chromogranin A containing cells have been purified from spleen, and appear to be a unique cell type (Angeletti and Hickey, 1987). The SF24 antibody reveals far more positive cells in spleen than the PL26 antibody (Figure 1A and 1B). Since SF24 is a marker for an enzyme involved in neuroendocrine type processing, this distribution may reflect not only the existence of neuroendocrine type cells, but also the more extensive presence of neuroendocrine peptides in normal lymphoid and accessory cells. For example, macrophages have been found to produce proopiomelanocortin (Smith et al., 1986; Wybran, 1985), and both macrophages and mast cells produce preproenkephalin (Martin et al., 1987). Furthermore, it has been found that T helper cells activated by concanavalin A begin to produce preproenkephalin (Zurawski et al., 1986).

A similar staining pattern prevails within the lamina propria of the gut, a tissue of immunological importance. The PL26 antibody detects a few scattered cells within the lamina propria. The SF24 antibody, however, reveals a large number of positive cells. Several investigators have detected neuroendocrine type cells in this tissue by silver staining and electron microscopic observations (Aubock and Ratzenhofer, 1982; Matsuo et al., 1976; Masson, 1932; Stachura et al., 1981). However, the number of the cells observed was small, more consistent with the number of PL26-positive cells which we have observed. Experiments are now being performed to see if the more abundant SF-24 positive cells represent tissue mast cells or another defined cell type.

Figure 1 (C and D) also shows a comparison of the immunohistochemical staining of these two antibodies in Lewis rat lymph node. In this tissue, both antibodies detect large, mononuclear cells in similar numbers, mostly in the medullary cord region. These cells are frequently found in the area of lymphatic sinuses. The staining observed does not correspond to the known distribution of specific lymphoid cells. The lymph node is poor in most of the granulated cells, such as mast cells and natural killer cells. Therefore, the staining in this location does not represent the major granulated lymphoid or circulating cell types. For this reason, lymph nodes may be an interesting source from which to isolate chromogranin A containing cells.

## TUMOR CELL LINES

One approach to identifying chromogranin A containing lymphoid cells is to employ tumor cell lines which maintain the properties of the primary cells from which they were derived. Cell lines were selected from the American Type Culture Collection to represent a variety of cell types. The immunohistochemical distribution of chromogranin A positive cells described above is not consistent with its presence in B lymphocytes. Nonetheless, a B type lymphoma was tested, and was indeed found to be negative with the PL26 antibody. Similarly, chromogranin A positive cells are not sufficiently abundant in lymphoid tissues to be among the granulated accessory cells, such as macrophages. Two macrophage-like cell lines (TIB 67 and TIB 68) were examined by immunoblotting techniques with PL26 and SF24 antibodies. Both cell lines clearly appeared to have the SF24 marker protein. However, only one (TIB 69) had clear-cut reactivity with the PL26 antibody. The presence of chromogranin A in macrophages is not consistent with many other observations. Since transformed cells may have properties not found in natural cells, pure macrophages derived from cultures of bone marrow will be analyzed.

Promyelocytes are precursors in the granulocytic series of bone marrow cell development. They possess large, dense-cored vesicles and morphologically resemble the chromogranin A containing mononuclear cells which we have isolated from spleen (Angeletti and Hickey, 1987). However, when a pure population of bone marrow derived promyelocytes was examined, they were found to lack chromogranin A. The HL-60 cell line, derived from a human promyelocytic leukemia, was examined for the presence of the natural PL26 and SF24 antigens. As seen in Figure 2, HL-60 cells are very rich in the endocrine carboxypeptidase, but do not possess chromogranin A. Thus, promyelocytes may have neuroendocrine type processing. It will be interesting to study whether induced differentiation of HL-60 cells will change this phenotype.

Studies of large granular lymphocytes (Henkart et al., 1985; Millard et al., 1984) have been conducted together with Pierre Henkart. It was found that both normal and transformed large granular lymphocytes contain both chromogranin A and the endocrine carboxypeptidase. For the tumor cell line, it was also shown that the granules within the cell contain chromogranin A.

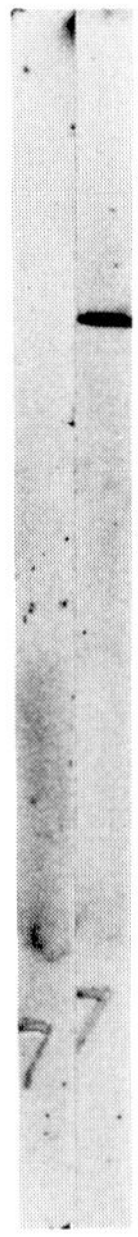


Figure 2. Immunoblots of HL-60 human promyelocytes. The left strip was incubated with antiserum to chromogranin A (PL26). The right strip was incubated with antibody to endocrine carboxypeptidase (SF24). Detection was accomplished with alkaline phosphatase linked secondary antibodies.

DISCUSSION

We have presented a partial, ongoing analysis of neuroendocrine functions in immune tissues. Two hypotheses had been presented as consistent with the presence of chromogranin A, a pan-neuroendocrine marker. It may result that both of these hypotheses are correct. For example, of the known granulated lymphoid cell types, macrophages, mast cells, and promyelocytes do not appear to possess chromogranin A. However, large granular lymphocytes (Henkart et al., 1984) do contain chromogranin A in their vesicles. They also contain the endocrine carboxypeptidase. This protein is used in processing of neuropeptides, which have been detected in a number of lymphoid cells. Finding this enzyme in the LGL cells suggested that these cells produce some neuropeptides as well as perforin and other lytic functions. Although chromogranin A is not found in the other known cells analyzed, the carboxypeptidase is. This observation is consistent with the more widespread occurrence of neuropeptides in lymphoid cells than heretofore suggested.

Chromogranin A has also been found in cells which do not fit into predefined functions. Our laboratory has purified a chromogranin A containing cell from spleen which is phenotypically a novel cell type. A cell line from bone marrow stroma, which produces a B cell growth factor, has been isolated by Hunt et al. (1987). These cells also do not conform to a known cell type, have large dense cored vesicles, and contain chromogranin A. Another cell upon which we will focus is chromogranin A containing cell in lymph node. Because of the absence of other granulated cell types, it is possible that these cells are also candidates to be a novel cell. Future investigations will complete this familial analysis of neuroendocrine relationships in lymphoreticular systems, and explore the role of chromogranin A in these tissues.

## REFERENCES

Angeletti RA Hogue (1986) Chromogranins and neuroendocrine secretion. Editorial. Lab Investigations 55:387-390

Angeletti RH, Hickey WF (1985) A neuroendocrine marker in tissues of the immune system. Science 230:89-84

Aubock L, Ratzenhofer M (1982) "Extraepithelial enterochromaffin cell-nerve fibre complexes" in the normal human apendix, and in neurogenic appendicopathy. J Pathol 136:217-226

Banks P, Helle K (1965) The release of protein from the stimulated adrenal medulla. Biochem J 97:40c

Eiden LE (1987) Is chromogranin a prohormone? Nature 325:301

Felicitas UR and Gratzen M (1986) Chromogranins, widespread in endocrine and nervous tissue, bind calcium. FEBS Letters 195:327-330

Fischer-Colbrie R, Lassmann H, Hagn C, Winkler H (1985) Immunological studies on the distribution of chromogranin A and B in endocrine and nervous tissues. Neuroscience 16:547-555

Fricker LD, Evans CJ, Esch FS, Herbert E (1986) Cloning and sequence analysis of cDNA for bovine carboxypeptidase. Nature 323:461-464

Henkart PA, PJ Millard, Reynolds and Henkart MP (1984) Cytolytic activity of purified cytoplasmic granules from cytotoxic rat large granular lymphocyte tumors. J Exper Med 160:75-93

Hunt P, Robertson D, Weiss D, Resnick D, Lee F, Witte ON (1987) A single bone marrow-derived stromal cell type supports the in vitro growth of early lymphoid and myeloid cells. Cell 48:997-1007

Iacangelo A, Affalter HU, Eiden LE, Herbet E, Grimes M (1986) Bovine chromogranin A sequence and distribution of its messenger RNA in endocrine tissues. Nature 323:82-86

Lloyd RV, Wilson BS (1983) Specific endocrine tissue marker defined by a monoclonal antibody. Science 222:628-630

Loh YP, Parish DC, Tutya (1985) Purification and characterization of a paired basic residue specific pro-opioonelancartein processing enzyme for bovine pituitary intermediate lobe secretory vesicles. J Biol Chem 260:7194-7205

Martin J, Prystowsky MB, Angeletti RA Hogue (1987) Preproenkephalin mRNA in T cells, macrophages and mast cells. J Neurosci Res, in press

Matsuo Y, Seki A, Fukuda S (1976) Neuro-endocrine cells in the lamina propria of rat stomach. In: Fujita T (ed.) Endocrine gut and pancreas, Elsevier Publishing, Amsterdam, pp. 159-165

Masson P (1932) Neural proliferations in the vermiform appendix. In: Penfield W (ed.) Cytology and cellular pathology of the nervous system, vol III, ch XXV

Millard PJ, Henkard MP, Reynolds CW and Henkart PA (1984) Purification and properties of cytoplasmic granules from cytotoxic rat LGL tumors. J Immunol 132:3197-3204

Nolan JA, Trojanowski JQ, Angeletti RH (1985) Neurons and neuroendocrine cells contain chromogranin: detection of the molecule in normal bovine tissues by immunochemical and immunohistochemical methods. J Histochem Cytochem 33:791-798

O'Conner DT, Burton D, Deftos LJ (1983) Chomogranin A: immunohistology reveals its universal occurance in normal polypeptide producing endocrine glands. Life Sci 33:1657-1663

Parish DC, Tuteja R, Altstein M, Gainer H, Loh YP (1986) Purification and Characterization of a paired basic residue-specific prohormone-converting enzyme from bovine pituitary neural lobe secretory vesicles. J Biol Chem 261:14392-14397

Plotnikoff NP, Murgo AJ, Miller GC, Corder CN, Faith RE (1985) Enkephalins: immunomodulators. Fed Proc 44:118-122

Smith AD, Winkler H (1967) Purification and properties of an acidic protein from chromaffin granules of bovine adrenal medulla. Biochem J 103:483

Smith EM, Morrill AC, Meyer WJ III, Blalock JE (1986) Corticotropin releasing factor induction of leukocyte-derived immunoreactive ACTH and endorphins. Nature 321:881-881

Smith WJ, Kirshner N (1967) A specific soluble protein from the catecholamine storage vesicle of bovine adrenal medulla. Mol Pharm 3:52

Strachura J, Krause WJ, Ivey, KJ (1981) Ultrastructure of endocrine-like cells in lamina propria of human gastric mucosa. Gut 22:534

Tatemoto K, Efecdic S, Mutt V, G Makk, Feistner GJ, Barchas JD (1986) Pancreastatin, a novel pancreatic peptide that inhibits insulin secretion. Nature 324:476-478

Whitlock CA, Tidmarsh GF, Muller-Sieburg C, Weissman IL (1987) Bone marrow stromal cell lines with lymphopotetic activity express high levels of a pre-B neoplasma associated molecule. Cell 48:1009-1021

Wybran J, Appelboom T, Famey JP, Govaerts A (1979) Suggestive evidence for receptors for morphine and methionine-enkephalin on normal human blood T lymphocytes. J Immunol 123:1068-1070

Zurawski G, Benedik M, Kamb BJ, Abrams JS, Zurawski Lee FD (1986) Activation of mouse T-helper cells induces abundant preproenkephalin mRNA synthesis. Science 232:772-775.

# INTERACTIONS BETWEEN THYMOSINS AND NEUROENDOCRINE CIRCUITS

Nicholas R.S. Hall
Maureen P. O'Grady
Robert C. Steiner
Allan L. Goldstein
Department of Biochemistry
George Washington University
School of Health Sciences
2300 Eye Street, N.W.
Washington, D.C. 20037
USA

## INTRODUCTION:

Neuroanatomical and chemical pathways linking the brain with the immune system are now well documented. Coupled with evidence that one's emotional state can be correlated with an altered level of immune responsiveness, these chemical and neuroanatomical pathways have been regarded as constituting a potential conduit by which the CNS is able to influence the cells and tissues of the immune system. However, a growing body of evidence indicates that the flow of information is not simply unidirectional, but that products of the immune system are capable of modulating several brain mediated events (Hall, et al, 1985). These products include complement proteins, (Schupf, et al., 1983), Interleukin 1 (IL-1) (Krueger, et al., 1984), interferon (Abrams, et al., 1985) as well as thymosin peptides. Table 1 summarizes the CNS mediated activities that these immunotransmitters have been found to exert.

Although all of these CNS mediated biological activities can be interpreted as contributing to host defense against pathogens, one category can be viewed as constituting a potential feedback circuit whereby the immune system may be able to regulate it's own functioning via the release of immunomodulatory pituitary hormones. Evidence that this does occur will be discussed in this chapter.

## PITUITARY-ADRENAL AXIS.

Glucocorticoids have been found to exert well documented effects upon a number of cell types that comprise the immune system (Claman, 1975). Unfortunately, the

NATO ASI Series, Vol. H22
Neural Development and Regeneration
Edited by A. Gorio et al.

majority of studies have utilized pharmacologic doses or forms of steroid not native to the species being studied- i.e. dexamethasone or hydrocortisone in murine models. Based upon the results of these studies, there is a widely held belief that glucocorticoids inhibit the immune system. However, careful scrutiny of the literature reveals that this class of steroid is capable of exerting biphasic effects. Stimulation of lymphoid cell growth and proliferation occurs at low concentrations (Ambrose, 1964) while inhibition of these measures occurs only at high concentrations of the steroid. (See Hall and Goldstein, 1984).

TABLE 1

IMMUNOTRANSMITTERS THAT ARE PRODUCED BY THE IMMUNE SYSTEM AND ARE ACTIVE IN THE BRAIN

| MOLECULE | BRAIN MEDIATED ACTIVITY |
|---|---|
| Thymosin $\beta_4$ | Stimulates hypothalamic-pituitary gonadal axis |
| Thymosin $\alpha_1$ | Stimulates hypothalamic-pituitary adrenal axis |
| Thymosin F5 | Stimulates hypothalamic-pituitary adrenal axis |
| Lymphokines | Decrease hypothalamic norepinephrine |
| Lymphokines | Stimulate glial cells |
| Interleukin 1 | Stimulates hypothalamic-thermo regulatory centers |
| Interleukin 1 | Stimulates slow wave sleep |
| C3a | Modulates feeding behavior at level of hypothalamus |
| ACTH | (Neural and Pituitary peptide also produced by lymphocytes) |
| $\beta$-Endorphin | (Neural and pituitary peptide also produced by lymphocytes) |
| Interferon | Induces lethargy and depression |

Consequently, activation of the hypothalamic-pituitary axis has the potential to effect biphasic changes upon the immune system. At least two immune system products have been found to be capable of activating this hormonal system - a hydrophobic component of a partially purified bovine thymic extract called Thymosin fraction-5 (TF-5) and IL-1. Stimulation of steroidogenesis by TF-5 has now been documented in several species including cynomologous monkeys, rats, mice and humans. (Healy, et al., 1983; McGillis, et al., 1985; Dumonde, et al., 1982).

We first reported this effect using prepubertal, female macaque monkeys that had a chronically implanted catheter in the femoral vein (Healy, et al., 1983). This was secured by the use of a mobile harness and tether assembly that enabled he animals to freely move about their cage. Several treatment conditions were evaluated. These included TF-5 and the purified component peptides, thymosin alpha 1 and thymosin beta 4. Two control treatments were incorporated into the design: one group received saline vehicle while another was treated with bovine serum albumin (BSA). The latter treatment was included in order to control for the potential immunogenicity of the bovine TF-5.

The results of this study revealed that TF-5 stimulated a significant elevation in adrenocorticotropin hormone (ACTH) and cortisol in a dose and time dependent manner. Peak levels of ACTH were detected at 30 minutes following TF-5 injection while cortisol levels were still rising at 90 minutes. Correlated with the change in ACTH levels was a concommitant rise in plasma beta-endorphin. Neither thymosin alpha 1 nor beta 4 was effective in stimulating ACTH or cortisol using this model. Furthermore, none of the treatments was found to stimulate either luteinizing hormone (LH), follicle stimulating hormone (FSH), prolactin, growth hormone or thyroid stimulating hormone under these conditions. Although direct stimulation of adrenal fasciculata cells could not be ruled out, the initial release of ACTH followed by that of cortisol strongly suggested that TF-5 was exerting its effects at the level of either the brain and/or the anterior pituitary gland. Each of these possibilities was considered in subsequent studies.

A direct effect at the level of the adrenal gland was initially ruled out by incubating TF-5 with isolated adrenal fasciculata cells (Vahouny, et al., 1983). During this study, we also evaluated the effects of the purified component peptides of TF-5 as well as lymphokine containing supernatant fluid generated from concanavalin (Con-A) stimulated spleen cells. No changes in either corticosterone or cyclic-AMP were detected during these studies. The possibility that TF-5 might act synergistically with ACTH was evaluated by adding it at various concentrations to a sub-optimal amount of ACTH. However, the amount of corticosterone and cyclic-AMP released did not differ from that released by the ACTH alone.

We next explored the possibility that thymosin might be capable of activating the circuit at the level of the brain and/or pituitary gland. Using rats that had guide cannulas chronically implanted in the calvarium overlying the hypothalamus, TF-5 was injected into this diencephalic region (Hall, et al., 1982). To control for leakage out of the brain into the general circulation, TF-5 was also injected intraperitoneally (ip) into a separate group of rats. Additional control procedures included an implanted, but non-injected control group and a group that received kidney fraction 5 instead of TF-5. The kidney preparation was prepared in a manner identical to TF-5 except that the kidney and not the thymus was used as the substrate. Rats receiving hypothalamic injections of TF-5 had a significant elevation of adrenal weight. No other treatment resulted in any effect upon the adrenals. There was also no change in the weights of either the testes or thyroid gland.

As a result of these findings, we recently conducted an experiment designed to evaluate the possibility that TF-5 might effect changes in brain levels of biogenic amines that have been correlated with stress induced activation of the hypothalamic-pituitary-adrenal axis (Dunn and Hall, 1987). The concentrations of the catecholamines, norepinephrine and dopamine, the indoleamine, serotonin and their major metabolities were measured in order to evaluate fluctuations in the absolute levels of these neurotransmitters as well as of their turnover rate. Each of these was assessed in prefrontal cortex, septum, caudate-putamen, hypothalamus and brain stem, however, no changes were detected following the injection of corticogenic doses of TF-5. Consequently, it was concluded that the corticogenic effects of TF-5 are most likely mediated at a site other than the brain.

Although these data do not rule out completely a CNS site of action, the most parsimonious interpretation of the data is that TF-5 exerts its effects via a direct action at the level of the pituitary gland. Thus, the increase in adrenal weight that was observed in rats that received intrahypothalamic injections of TF-5 was probably due to leakage from the brain into the pituitary gland. In vitro studies support this interpretation. Two model systems have been used to evaluate the potential of TF-5 to directly stimulate ACTH and beta-endorphin release from the pituitary: coincubation of thymosin peptides with normal rat pituitary cells and with neoplastic cell lines. Both models reveal that TF-5 is able to act at this level. A dose dependent increase in ACTH has been measured following incubation of normal rat anterior pituitary cells with TF-5. A similar response has also been found following the incubation of TF-5 with AtT-20 cells, an ACTH and beta-endorphin secreting mouse tumor cell line (Farah, et al., 1987).

Thymosin alpha-one has been found to be incapable of stimulating ACTH or beta-endorphin from cultured pituitary cells. However, it has been found capable of activating the pituitary-adrenal axis following injection into the lateral cerebroventricle of chronically cannulated mice. In one particular experiment, male mice were fitted with a polyethylene guide tube that was surgically implanted into the calvarium overlying the lateral ventricle (Hall, et. al, 1982). Following a two week recovery period, groups of mice received injections or either thymosin alpha 1, thymosin beta 4 or the saline vehicle. A fourth group remained uninjected. On the day of the experiment, each animal received 1 ug of the peptide. Three hours later, the mice were sacrificed and trunk blood was collected and frozen for subsequent determination of corticosterone levels. As can be seen in Table 2, mice receiving thymosin alpha 1 had significantly elevated levels of corticosterone while thymosin beta 4 and saline-treated mice did not differ from the uninjected control animals. Thus, while thymosin alpha 1 is ineffective in directly stimulating ACTH release from cultured pituitary cells, it was capable of activating corticogenesis when injected directly into the brain. The physiological significance of this observation is not clear since it is unlikely that the peptide is capable of crossing the blood-brain-barrier. However, unpublished observations made in this laboratory (McGillis, et al.) strongly suggest that the peptide may be produced in the brain. Sub-fractionation of homogenized brain revealed that the highest concentrations of this peptide were located in the synaptosomal fraction and at levels comparable to peptides such as bombesin and VIP that are known to be produced in the brain. Other studies have revealed that the greatest amount of immunoreactive thymosin alpha 1 is to be found in the hypothalamus (Hall, et al., 1982), which regulates corticotropin releasing factor (CRF) release.

## PITUITARY-GONADAL AXIS

During the early part of this century, evidence was collected suggesting that the thymus gland was a reproductive tissue. A review of these data as well as the clinical use of thymic extracts to treat reproductive disorders was published by Anderson (1932). Throughout the intervening decades, evidence that thymic extracts were capable of altering the pituitary-gonadal axis was reported. (See Hall and Goldstein, 1983).

These studies have been extended with recent evidence that a component of TF-5 is capable of stimulating LH release as well as prolactin and growth hormone release. The stimulation of LH is most likely mediated directly at the level of the hypothalamus via the release of luteinizing hormone releasing hormone (LHRH). This site of action was earlier suggested as that for several other thymic extracts (Weinstein, 1978; Deschaux, et al., 1979) and was later found to be true for thymosin beta-4 which was found to stimulate LHRH from superfused medial basal hypothalamus (Rebar, et al., 1981). Using an *in vivo* model, it was found that this same peptide was capable of stimulating LH release following its injection into the lateral ventricle of chronically cannulated mice (Table 2).

TABLE 2

THYMOSIN ALPHA 1 AND BETA 4 STIMULATE CORTICOSTERONE AND LH RELEASE FOLLOWING INTRACEREBROVENTRICULAR INJECTION INTO MICE

| TREATMENT | CORTICOSTERONE (ng/ml ± SEM) | LH (ng/ml ± SEM) |
|---|---|---|
| Noninjected | 118.8 ± 31.3 | 0.89 ± 0.45 |
| Saline | 92.2 ± 13.2 | 0.42 ± 0.07 |
| $T\beta_4$ (1 $\mu$g) | 82.6 ± 19.6 | 2.82 ± 0.75[a] |
| $T\alpha_1$ (1 $\mu$g) | 225.9 ± 57.5[b] | 0.34 ± 0.75 |

[a]$p < 0.01$ vs saline
[b]$p < 0.02$ vs saline

Prolactin is another hormone capable of exerting biological effects upon the reproductive axis. Thus far, TF-5 has been found to be active in stimulating the release of this peptide from both the GH-3 tumor cell line as well as from normal rat pituitary cells (Spangelo, et al., 1987a: 1987b). In addition growth hormone is also stimulated in these assay systems. Recent data indicate that the biologically active component of TF-5 responsible for stimulating prolactin and growth hormone release is different from that which causes ACTH and beta-endorphin release (unpublished observation).

## DISCUSSION

The evidence described above indicates that components of the immune system may be capable of activating a number of neuroendocrine circuits. Furthermore, each of the hormones that is subsequently released has been found to be capable of modulating the course of the immune response. Thus, in addition to the direct effects of thymosin peptides upon the immune system, these peptides also have the potential to indirectly regulate the immune system via a number of neuroendocrine pathways. Whether this constitutes an important physiological process is too speculative to conclude based upon the existing data. Nonetheless, several theoretical schemes have been proposed to explain the biological significance of such pathways.

One hypothesis is that immune system products, such as thymosins, that are capable of activating neuroendocrine circuits comprise a feedback loop in order to maintain homeostasis within the immune system compartment. In the case of the pituitary-adrenal axis, it has been proposed that the feedback is inhibitory in nature and that it represents a mechanism by which the immune system down regulates itself toward the end of an immune response. This was proposed by Besedovsky and Sorkin (1977) to account for the significant rise in corticosterone that was observed to occur at about the time of peak antibody titers. Other evidence revealed that during the course of an immune response, electrical, morphological and neurochemical changes occur. Collectively, these data strongly suggest that a signal from the immune system was responsible for these changes (Besedovsky, et al., 1983:1985).

The original explanation for the rise in corticosterone was that it constituted a form of lateral inhibition that resulted in the down regulation of lymphocytes with a relatively high density of glucocorticoid receptors. These happen to be the less mature thymocytes at a stage prior to their sensitization to an antigen. As these cells undergo differentiation, they lose their steroid sensitivity. Consequently, those lymphocytes actively involved in producing lymphokines would be relatively resistant to the inhibitory effects of the glucocorticoids. Inhibition of those cells with weak or no affinity for the antigen would result in fine tuning of the immune response. A precedent for this type of model is lateral inhibition whereby collateral projections from axons inhibit adjacent sensory cells thereby fine tuning the subsequent response. The release of glucocorticoids is presumably triggered by a component peptide of TF-5 as well as by IL-1. Thus, the signal that ultimately activates this immunomodulatory hormonal circuit is provided by the immune system compartment itself.

An alternative hypothesis is that the release of glucocorticoids does not occur for the purpose of regulating the immune system. Instead, it results from the requirement of the host for additional energy substrates which would be expected following exposure to an antigen - a source of energy for the cells of the immune system as well as for the tissue repair processes that might be required. An effect of the glucocorticoids upon the immune system might be regarded as an aberration, possibly with deleterious effects. It is noteworthy that several lines of evidence suggest that the immune system has the capability of overcoming steroid induced immunosuppression. Historically, the thymus has long been regarded as an anti-stress organ working in opposition to the adrenal glands (Martin, 1976). There is also evidence that lymphocytes have the ability to convert glucocorticoids to non-immunosuppressive forms (Berliner and Dougherty, 1961), as well as evidence that immune system products may be capable of blocking the binding of steroids to their receptors in lymphocytes (see Hall and Goldstein, 1983). Consequently, some of the same factors that are capable of inducing glucocorticoid release may be able to protect the immune system from potential adverse effects of the elevated steroids.

It is unlikely that the hormonal pathways that are activated by immune system products constitute major immunoregulatory circuits since many of them have well characterized functions within other physiological systems, However, in situations whereby the immunocompetence of the host may be partly compromised, the impact of additional hormonal influences may be enough to alter the outcome following exposure to a disease causing pathogen. The same is true when considering the impact of emotional state upon the immune responsiveness of the host. While certain of the hormonal systems that have well characterized effects upon lymphocyte function can be influenced by emotional distress, there are numerous regulatory circuits within the immune system compartment itself so that a tremendous buffering ability appears to exist. Nonetheless, even a small effect may be important under well defined circumstances warranting a better understanding of immunoregulatory hormonal circuits and how they might be influenced by products of the immune system. Finally, one has to ponder the possibility that diseases that were once considered to involve a primary aberration of an endocrine circuit may instead reflect an aberration of the immune system. Thus, a better understanding of the biodirectional pathways that link the brain with the immune system is clearly warranted.

REFERENCES


Abrams, P.G., McClamrock, E. and Foon, K.A. (1985) Evening administration of alpha-interferon. N. Engl. J. Med. 312:443.

Ambrose, C.T. (1964) The requirement for hydrocortisone in antibody-forming tissue cultivated in serum-free medium. J. Exp. Med. 119:1027-1049.

Anderson, D.H., (1932) The relationship between the thymus and reproduction. Physiol. Rev. 12:1-22.

Berliner, D.L. and Dougherty, T.F. (1969) Hepatic and extraheptic regulation of corticosteroids. Pharmacol. Rev. 13:329-359.

Besedovsky, H O and Sorkin, E (1977) Network of immune-neuroendocrine interactions. Clin. Exp. Immunol. 27:1-12.

Besedovsky, H.O., del Ray, A.E. and Sorkin, E. (1985) Immune -neuroendocrine interactions, J. Immunol. 135 (Suppl.): 750s-754s.

Besedovsky, H.O., Del Ray, A.,Sorkin, E., Da Prada, M., Burri, R. and Honegger, C. (1983) The immune response evokes changes in brain noradrenergic neurons. Science 221:564-565 (1983).

Claman, H.N. (1975) How corticosteroids work. J. Allergy Clin. Immunol. 55:145-151.

Deschuax, P., Massaengo, B., and Fontages, R. (1979) Endocrine interaction of the thymus with the hypophysis, adrenals and testes: effects of two thymic extracts. Thymus 1:95-108.

Dumonde, D.C., Pulley, M.S., Hamblin, A.S., Singh, A.K., Southcott, B.M., O'Connell, D., Paradinas, F.J., Robinson, M.G.R., Rigby, C.C., den Hollander, F., Schuurs, A., Verheul, H., and van Vliet, E., (1982) Short term and long term administration of lymphoblastoid cell line lymphokine (LCL-LK) to patients with advanced cancers. In: (A.L. Goldstein and M.A. Chirigos, eds.) Lymphokines and Thymic Hormones: Their Potential Utilization In Cancer Therapeutics, pp. 301-318. Raven Press, New York.

Dunn, A.J., and Hall, N.R., (in press) Thymic extracts and lymphokine-containing supernatant fluids stimulate the pituitary-adrenal axis, but not cerebral catecholamine or idoleamine metabolism, Brain, Behavior and Immunity.

Farah, J.M., Hall, N.R., Bishop, J.F., Goldstein, A.L. and O'Donohue, T.L., (in press) Thymosin fraction 5 stimulates secretion of immunoreactive beta-endorphin in mouse corticotrophic tumor cells. J. Neuroscience Research.

Hall, N.R., McGillis, J.P., Spangelo, B.L., Palaszynski, E., Moody, T. and Goldstein, A.L., (1982) Evidence for a neuroendocrine-thymus axis mediated by thymosin polypeptides. Dev. Immunology 17:853-860.

Hall, N.R. and Goldstein, A.L., (1984) Endocrine regulation of host immunity, In: (Fenichel, R.L. and Chirigos, M.A., eds.) Immune Modulation Agents and Their Mechanisms., Marcel Dekker, New York, p.533-563.

Hall, N.R., McGillis, J.P., Spangelo, B.L., and Goldstein, A.L., (1985) Evidence that the thymosins and other biological response modifiers can function as neuroactive immunotransmitters. J. Immunology 135:806s-811s.

Healy, D.L., Hodgen, G.D., Schultz, H.M., Chrousos, G.P., Louriaux, D.L., Hall, N.R., and Goldstein, A.L., (1983) The thymus-adrenal connection: thymosin has corticotropin-releasing activity in primates. Science 222:1353-1356.

Krueger, J., Dinerello, C., Wolff, M., Chedid, L. and Walker, J., (1984) Sleep-promoting effects of endogenous pyrogen (Interleukin 1). Am. J. Physiol. 246:R994.

Martin, C.R. (1976) Textbook of Endocrine Physiology. Williams and Wilkin, Baltimore.

McGillis, J.P., Hall, N.R., Vahouny, G.V., and Goldstein, A.L., (1985) Thymosin fraction 5 causes increased serum corticosterone in rodents <u>in vitro</u>. J. Immunol. 134:3952-3955.

Rebar, R.W., Miyake, A., Low, T.L.K. and Goldstein, A.L., (1981) Thymosin stimulates secretion of luteinizing hormone-releasing factor. Science 214: 669-671.

Schupf, N., Williams, C.A., Hugh, T.E., and Cox, J. (1983) Psychopharmacological activity of anaphylatoxin C3a in rat hypothalamus. J. Neuroimmunol. 5:305-316.

Spangelo, B.L., Hall, N.R., Dunn, A.J., and Goldstein, A.L. (1987a) Thymosin fraction 5 stimulates the release of prolactin from cultured GH3 cells. Life Sciences 40. 283-288.

Spangelo, B.L., Judd, A.M., Ross, P.C., Login, I.S., Jarvis, W.D., Badamchian, M., Goldstein, A.L. and MacLeod, R.M., (in press b) Thymosin fraction 5 stimulates prolactin and growth hormone release from anterior pituitary cells <u>in vitro</u>. Endocrinology.

Vahouny, G.V., Kyeyune-Nyombi, E., McGillis, J.P., Tare, N.S., Huang, K.Y., Tombes, R., Goldstein, A.L., and Hall, N.R., (1983) Thymosin peptides and lymphokines do not directly stimulate adrenal corticoteroid production *in vitro*. J. Immunol. 130:791-794.

Weinstein, Y. (1978) Impairment of the hypothalamus-pituitary-ovarian axis of the athymic "nude" mouse. Mech. Aging Dev. 8:13-68.

ACKNOWLEDGEMENTS

Research reviewed in this chapter was supported by a grant from the National Institutes of Health (NS21210) and a contract from the Office of Naval Research (N00014-84-K-0300). N.R.S.H. is supported by NIMH Research Scientist Development Award (MH00648).

# NERVE GROWTH FACTOR AND THE IMMUNE SYSTEM

L. W. Thorpe, B. Morgan, C. Beck, K. Werrbach-Perez and J.R. Perez-Polo
Department of Human Biological Chemistry and Genetics
University of Texas Medical Branch
Galveston, Texas, 77550

Evidence from both in vitro and in vivo studies would support the hypothesis that there is a bidirectional flow of information between the immune system and the nervous system. The efferent limb of this neuro-immunoregulatory circuit involves signals from both the central (CNS) and peripheral (PNS) nervous systems (Besedovsky et al, 1977; Besedovsky et al, 1983; Besedovsky et al, 1985). These signals, soluble neurochemical messengers, are released into the microenvironment of lymphoid tissues by nerve fibers or taken up from the circulation (Besedovsky et al, 1985; Bulloch, 1985; Livent et al, 1985; Roszman et al, 1985). These messengers, neurotransmitters and neuropeptides, influence the integrity of neuronal function and the functional regulation of the immune system. These neurosubstances have also been shown to modify diverse immunologic parameters by receptor mediated mechanisms (Goetzl et al, 1985; Roszman et al, 1985; Coffey & Djeu, 1986). Specific receptors for neuropeptides and neurotransmitters have been demonstrated on immune cells of diverse origin including lymphocytes, macrophages, NK cells, neutrophils and mast cells (Arrenbrecht, 1974; Hazum et al, 1979; Richman et al, 1979; Johnson & Gordon, 1980; Maslinski et al, 1980; Danek et al, 1983; Mehrishi & Miles, 1983; Abrass et al, 1985; Koff & Dunegan, 1985; Ruff et al, 1985; Shanahan et al, 1985; Coffey & Djeu, 1986; ). The presence of these receptors would suggest that there is a physiologic and, perhaps, a pathologic role for neurosubstances in the immune system. Detailed in vitro studies have demonstrated that a variety of these neuronal messengers can modulate cell cycle events either through the enhancement or the inhibition of the blastogenic response of cultured lymphocytes (Johnson et al, 1981; Gilman et al, 1982; Payan et al, 1983; Slauson et al, 1984; O'Dorisio et al, 1985; Payan & Goetzl, 1985; Simon et al, 1985). Extrapolation of the in vitro results, would suggest that similar

NATO ASI Series, Vol. H22
Neural Development and Regeneration
Edited by A. Gorio et al.

regulatory activities occur in vivo since immune tissues are continually exposed to these factors and the in vitro effects take place at physiologic concentrations of the ligands.

Nerve growth factor (NGF) is a well characterized neurotrophic protein found throughout the CNS and PNS. Early studies of NGF demonstrated that it has a critical role in the development and survival of sympathetic and sensory neurons (Yankner & Shooter, 1982; Levi-Montalcini, 1983; Perez-Polo & Haber, 1983). Recently, it has been shown that NGF is implicated in the development and maintenance of cholinergic neurons of the basal forebrain and striatal regions of the brain (Korsching et al, 1985; Mobley et al, 1985; Taniuchi et al, 1986). Among the biological activities of NGF is the potential for induction of mitogenesis of embryonic neural crest cells and adrenal chromaffin cells (Lillien & Claude, 1985; Bernd, 1986). Binding of NGF to specific cell surface receptors (NGFR) is obligatory for NGF actions(Yankner & Shooter, 1982; Perez-Polo & Haber, 1983). NGFR have been demonstrated on neuronal cells of the CNS and PNS and several cell lines of neuronal origin (Yankner & Shooter, 1982; Lyons et al, 1983; Stach & Perez-Polo, 1987; Marchetti & Perez-Polo, 1987). There are two kinds of NGF binding activities; a high affinity receptor with an equilibrium dissociation constant, $K_d$, in the $10^{-11}$ M range, and a low affinity receptor with a $K_d$ of $10^{-9}$ M, with the low affinity receptor being the predominant species (Lyons et al, 1983; Yankner & Shooter, 1982; Stach & Perez-Polo, 1987).

NGF has been shown to act on non-neuronal tissues as a modulator of immune and inflammatory reactivity (Table 1). The first report of an immune and inflammatory effect of NGF was a report by Aloe and Levi-Montalcini (1977) which showed that systemic treatment of neonatal rats with NGF resulted in widespread accumulation of mast cells in subepidermal areas and other tissues. Subsequent in vitro studies demonstrated that NGF activates putative receptor mediated noncytotoxic degranulation and histamine release from rat peritoneal mast cells (Bruni et al, 1982; Mazurek et al, 1986; Pearce & Thompson, 1986). NGF also functions in vitro and in vivo as a chemoattractant for human polymorphonuclear neutrophils (PMN) at concentrations similar to those which evoke in vitro neurite outgrowth from human neuroblastoma and PC12 cells (Gee et al, 1983; Boyle et al, 1985). In light of the association of mast cells, PMN, and vasoactive amines with the inflammatory response,

TABLE 1

NGF EFFECTS ON THE CELLS AND FUNCTION OF THE IMMUNE SYSTEM

| | |
|---|---|
| Tissue Accumulation of Mast Cells | Aloe and Levi-Montalcini, 1977 |
| Mast Cell Degranulation | Bruni et al, 1982<br>Mazurek et al, 1986<br>Pearce & Thompson, 1986 |
| In vitro Neutrophil Chemotaxis | Gee et al, 1983 |
| In vivo Neutrophil Chemotaxis | Boyle et al, 1985 |
| Anti-inflammation | Banks et al, 1984 |
| T Cell Dependent Antibody Synthesis | Manning et al, 1985 |
| NGFR on Lymphocytes & Accessory Cells | Thorpe et al, 1987 |
| Lymphoproliferation | Thorpe & Perez-Polo, 1987 |
| Upregulation of Lymphocyte IL2-R | Thorpe et al, 1987 |

there is an apparently contradictory report demonstrating that when NGF is given locally, or systemically, it acts as a potent anti-inflammatory agent, preventing carageenin induced hindpaw edema (Banks et al, 1984). This contradiction has not been resolved. However, there is sufficient data to suggest that NGF has some role in the early cellular events associated with the acute inflammatory response.

While exploring the possible mechanisms of NGF protection of guanethidine-induced neuronal injury, Manning and co-workers examined the effects of NGF on the modulation of several in vitro and in vivo immune parameters (Manning et al, 1985). They observed that NGF, at higher concentrations (10 ug/ml), caused a slight, but significant, augmentation of murine mixed lymphocyte reactivity. In addition, treatment of young rats with NGF prior to and after immunization with sheep red blood cells resulted in an augmentation of T-dependent antibody synthesis as measured by the plaque forming cell assay. These findings were highly suggestive of a modulatory effect of NGF on both cellular mediated and humoral immunity. Subsequently, receptors for NGF (NGFR) have been demonstrated on human and rat lymphocytes and macrophages (Thorpe et al, 1987; Marchetti et al, in preparation) The presence of NGFR on macrophages has also been observed by Heumann and co-workers (R. Heumann, personal communication).

Visualization of binding of NGF to rat splenic mononuclear (MC) and human peripheral blood mononuclear cells (PBMC) was detected by immunofluorescence using NGF with heterologous anti-NGF as well as NGFR specific monoclonal antibodies. NGFR positive cells comprised approximately 25-50 percent of the mononuclear cells and peripheral blood mononuclear cells. To determine if NGFR positive cells were expressed on selected lymphocyte populations, rat MC were doubly stained for NGFR using IgG-192 (Chandler et al, 1984) and monoclonals (McMasters & Williams, 1979; Brideau et al, 1980; Sternberg et al, 1986; White et al, 1986) which distinguish T cells (OX 19), T cell subsets (W3/25, OX 8), and Ia positive (OX 4) B cells. These studies revealed that NGFR were found on a variable percentage of both the T cell and B cell population (Thorpe et al, unpublished). In addition, it appeared that within the T lymphocytes, the majority of the NGFR positive cells were phenotypically T suppressor/cytotoxic cells (OX 8); while only a small percentage of T helper cells (W3/25) were NGFR positive. Although these results are of a preliminary nature, they suggest that NGFR are selectively expressed on a yet undefined population of T and B lymphocytes. This is not unique to NGF. Beta-adrenergic and substance P receptors are selectively distributed among specific lymphocyte cell population subsets (Landmann et al, 1984; Payan et al, 1985). In addition, Simon, et al, (1986) have reported that stimulation of human lymphocytes in culture with angiotensin II selectively stimulates DNA synthesis in OKT-8 positive cells, the human T-suppressor/cytotoxic cell. Thus, NGF positive immunocytes may be a functionally distinct population that is reactive to the modulatory effects of NGF.

NGF binding studies of unfractionated MC and PBMC revealed a relatively rapid, saturable and reversible binding of NGF to solubilized membranes (Thorpe et al, 1987; Marchetti et al, in preparation). Scatchard analysis of binding data for rat MC NGFR showed an equilibrium dissociation constant of $10^{-9}$ M, consistent with the existence of a single low affinity binding site (Thorpe et al, 1987). Scatchard analysis of human PBMC gave a biphasic binding curve with Kd's of $10^{-11}$ and $10^{-9}$ M, consistent with the existence of both high and low affinity receptors on human cells (Marchetti et al, in preparation). Molecular weights of the NGFR on MC were determined by SDS-PAGE analysis of IgG-192 immunoprecipitated NGFR. Two molecular species of approximately 190 and 125 kilodaltons (KDa) were found (Thorpe et al, 1987). Molecular weight determination of solubilized PBMC NGFR followed by lentil-lectin chromatography and SDS-PAGE, revealed two proteins with molecular weights of 133 and 100 KDa.

In vitro culture studies have demonstrated that lymphocytes and/or accessory cells are targets of NGF, presumably through receptor-mediated mechanisms. The addition of NGF to cultures of rat MC resulted in the stimulation of blastogenic activity both in the presence and absence of T and B cell mitogens (Thorpe & Perez-Polo, In Press). In the absence of mitogen NGF stimulated DNA synthesis in MC as measured by tritiated thymidine uptake after 96 hours in culture. Significant increases in thymidine incorporation in a dose dependent fashion were noted at NGF concentrations of 0.1-10 ug/ml, corresponding to molar concentrations of 3.7-370 nM. The minimal effective concentration of NGF was 3.7 nM, similar to the level of NGF required for occupancy of half the binding sites on unfractionated rat splenic MC. The highest level of stimulation was observed at 10 ug/ml. In addition, the response of splenic MC to mitogenic stimulation was also significantly augmented in the presence of NGF. In the presence of mitogen, the lymphoproliferative response was dependent on the concentration of the mitogen and the concentration of NGF. For the T cell mitogen concanavalin A (Con A), the highest levels of NGF stimulation of DNA synthesis were observed at suboptimal concentrations of the mitogen (Fig 1).

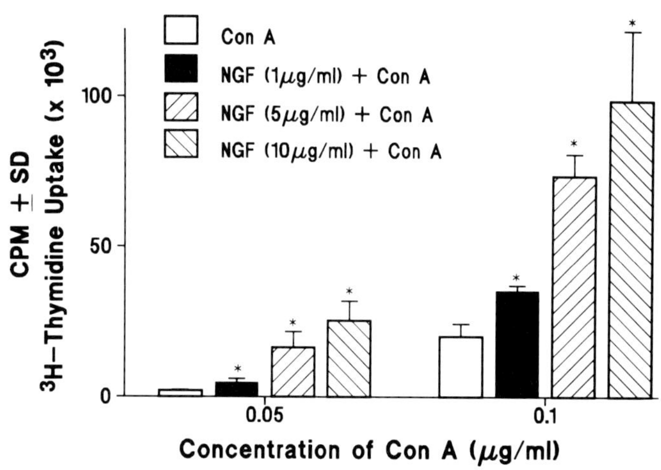


Figure 1 Enhancement of the response of rat spleen MC to NGF at suboptimal concentrations of the T cell mitogen Con A. Augmentation by NGF was dose-dependent and significantly higher than mitogen alone at all concentrations.

Similar findings of a dose dependent NGF augmentation were observed for another T-cell mitogen, phytohemagglutinin. Additionally, there was potentiation by NGF of the B-cell proliferative response in the presence of the mitogen lipopolysaccaride (LPS) in a dose dependent way. Unlike the T-cell mitogen studies, where the optimal responses were seen at suboptimal mitogen concentrations, NGF potentiation of LPS stimulated cells took place over a broad range of mitogen concentrations. In experiments designed to examine the effects of serum on the NGF induced proliferative response a serum free media, Ventrex HU-1, was used. When splenic cells were cultured in Ventrex and ConA, NGF augmented the ConA response. Here the response to NGF was again significant at suboptimal concentrations of mitogen whereas the optimal NGF effect took place at lower NGF concentrations, in the 0.1-1 ug/ml range, in sharp contrast to the previous results of maximal stimulation at 10 ug/ml of NGF obtained in the presence of serum. Previous studies have shown that NGF binds to serum components (Perez-Polo et al, 1980). Therefore, the high concentration of NGF needed for maximal NGF effects on rat splenic cell proliferation in serum containing media might be due to interference by serum factors.

Mitogens are polyclonal activators of immune cells. A better in vitro correlate of the in vivo immune response to antigenic challenge is that of the mixed lymphocyte response (MLR). The study by Manning and her colleagues (1985) found no increased MLR activity by NGF in rat mixed lymphocyte cultures (MLC) at concentrations of 0.05-1 ug/ml. However, in mouse MLC, an increased stimulation by NGF was noted in cultures with 10 ug/ml NGF. Preliminary results of rat mixed lymphocyte cultures stimulated with NGF have demonstrated that NGF also potentiates rat MLC reactivity and that this augmentation by NGF was only seen at concentrations of 10 ug/ml NGF (Fig. 2). In contrast to the mitogen studies, here NGF at concentrations of 1 ug/ml, or less, had no effect on the MLR. The NGF potentiation of the proliferative response is not restricted to differentiated lymphocytes. Thymocytes from young rats also responded in culture to NGF in the presence of Con A (Fig. 3). However, there was no effect on thymidine uptake by thymocytes cultured with NGF in the absence of mitogen (Thorpe, unpublished).

The mechanisms of action of NGF effects on the proliferation of MC and the mitogen stimulated lymphocytes and thymocytes is not known. Lymphocyte mitogenesis is the result of a complex series of interactions

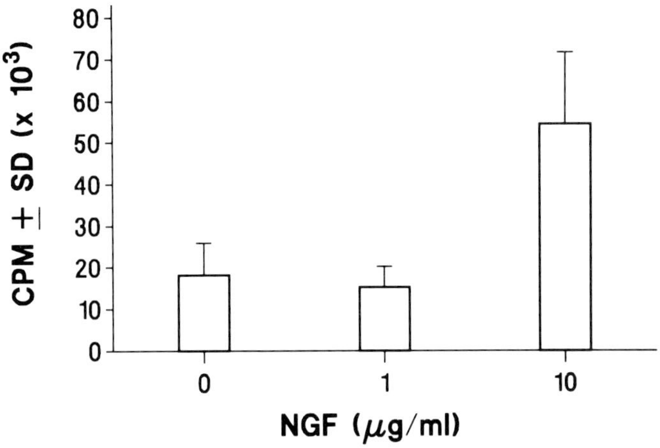


Figure 2. Effect of NGF (10 ug/ml) on the MLR response of rat one-way mixed lymphocyte cultures (Lewis vs irradiated BN).

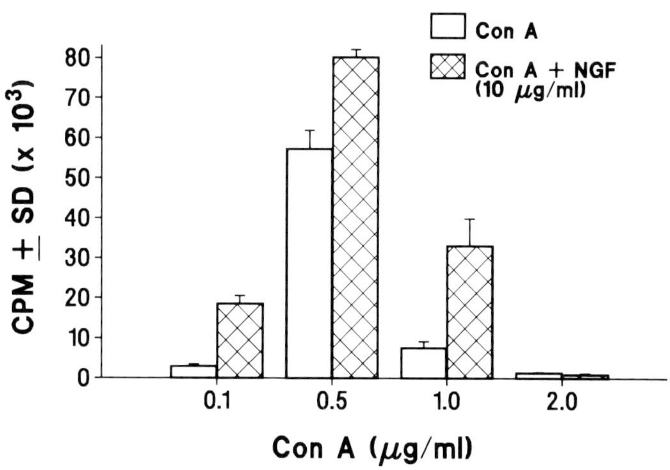


Figure 3. NGF enhancement of proliferation of thymocytes in the presence of Con A. NGF (10 ug/ml) significantly potentiated the response to mitogen through a defined range of Con A concentration.

involving direct lymphocyte and macrophage cell mediated interactions and their response to monokines and lymphokines (Cantrell & Smith, 1984).

Since lymphoproliferation occurs in response to a number of different cellular interactions, the role of the different NGFR positive cell types (lymphocytes and macrophages) in the NGF induced blastogenic response is not obvious. An early event obligatory to the activation of the cell cycle of lymphocytes is the stimulation of interleukin 2 (IL-2) synthesis and the upregulation of IL-2 receptors (IL2-R). In the absence of antigen or mitogen stimulation, NGF increased the expression of IL2-R on cultured human PBMC (Thorpe et al, in press). The upregulation of receptors was observed after approximately 72 hours in culture and preceded the increase in DNA synthesis observed after 96 hours of culture. Similar IL2-R modulation by thymic hormones has been reported by Sztein et al (1986). The cellular events associated with the IL2-R induction by NGF are unknown.

These results provide evidence for an immunomodulatory role for the NGF protein. The results of the NGF treatment in vivo suggest that NGF-immune interactions are not limited to in vitro parameters. The role of NGF in immune homeostasis remains unknown. Within the PNS, NGF is intimately associated with the sympathetic innervation of various organs (Shelton & Reichardt, 1984). In vitro, catecholamines and steroids can induce NGF synthesis by cultured cells (Perez-Polo et al, 1977; Furukawa et al, 1986). A number of studies have described the immunoregulatory properties of the sympathetic nervous system (SNS) (Besedovksy et al, 1979; del Rey et al, 1981; Johnson et al, 1981; Livnet et al, 1985; Miles et al, 1985). Bulloch (1985) has reviewed the innervation of the thymus and the various lymphoid organs by the autonomic nervous system and has shown that these tissues are extensively innervated by sympathetic nerve fibers. The modulatory effects of the SNS on immune function and the effects of NGF on SNS innervation in development would suggest that NGF might play a role as a neuropeptide signal from the SNS to cells within the lymphoid microenvironment. In addition, NGF has been shown to stimulate the pituitary-adrenal axis (Otten et al, 1979). The influence of the hypothalamic-pituitary-adrenal axis on immune function is well established (Besedovsky et al, 1983; Besedovsky et al, 1985). Again these latter findings suggest a route by which NGF might interact with the immune system. The availability of NGF to cells, both immune and neuronal, throughout the various organ systems would seem to in some way implicate NGF as an active participant in the conversation among the cells of the nervous and immune system (Perez-Polo et al, in press). The spectrum of messages regulating neuro-immune function are just beginning to be perceived. Here, we would suggest that the NGF protein is also involved.

Acknowledgements This research was supported by grants from the Office of Naval Research and the National Institute of Health. Thanks to D. Masters for manuscript preparation.

## References

Abrass CK, O'Connor SW, Scarpace PJ, Abrass IB (1985) Characterization of the beta-adrenergic receptor of the rat peritoneal macrophage. J Immunol 135:1338-1341.

Aloe L, Levi-Montalcini R (1977) Mast cells increase in tissues of neonatal rats injected with nerve growth factor. Brain Res 133: 358-366.

Arrenbrecht S (1974) Specific binding of growth hormone to thymocytes. Nature 252:255-257.

Banks BEC, Vernon CA, Warner JA (1984) Nerve growth factor has anti-inflammatory activity in the rat hindpaw oedema test. Neuroscience Letters 47:41-45.

Bernd P (1986) Characterization of nerve growth factor binding to cultured neural crest cells: Evidence of an early developmental form of the NGF receptor. Dev. Biol. 115:415-424.

Besedovsky H, Sorkin E (1977) Network of immune-neuroendocrine interactions. Clin Exp Immunol 27:1-1.

Besedovsky HO, del Rey AE, Sorkin E (1983) What do the immune system and the brain know about each other? Immunol Today 4:342-346.

Besedovsky HO, del Rey AE, Sorkin E, Da Prada M, Keller HH (1979) Immunoregulation mediated by the sympathetic nervous system. Cell Immunol 48:346-355.

Besedovsky HO, del Rey AE, Sorkin E (1985) Immune-neuroendocrine interactions. J Immunol 135:750s-754s.

Besedovsky HO, del Rey A, Sorkin E, Lotz W, Schwulera U (1985) Lymphoid cells produce an immunoregulatory glucocorticoid increasing factor (GIF) acting through the pituitary gland. Clin Exp Immunol 59:622-628.

Boyle MDP, Lawman MJP, Gee AP, Young M (1985) Nerve growth factor: a chemotactic factor for polymorphonuclear leukocytes in vivo. J Immunol 134:564-568.

Brideau RJ, Carter PB, McMaster WR, Mason DW, Williams AF (1980) Two subsets of rat T lymphocytes defined with mononlonal antibodies. Eur J Immunol 10:609-615.

Bruni A, Bigon E, Boarato E, Mietto L, Leon A, Toffano G (1982) Interactions between nerve growth factor and lysophosphatidylserine on rat peritoneal mast cells. Febs Letters 138:190-192.

Bulloch K (1985) Neuroanatomy of lymphoid tissues. In Guillemin R, Cohen M, Melnuchuk T (eds) Neural Modulation of Immunity, Raven Press, New York, pp 110-141.

Cantrell DA, Smith KA (1984) The interleukin-2 T-cell system: A new cell growth model. Science 224:1312-1316.
Chandler CE, Parsons LM, Hosang M, Shooter EM (1984) A monoclonal antibody modulates the interaction of nerve growth factor with PC12. J. Biol Chem 259:6882-6889.
Coffey RG, Djeu JY (1986) Endocrine receptors on lymphocytes: Integration of endocrine and immune systems. In Conn PM (ed) The Receptors vol IV, Academic Press, New York, pp 379-423.
Danek A, O'Dorisio MS, O'Dorisio TM, George JM (1983) Specific binding sites for vasoactive intestinal polypeptide on nonadherent peripheral blood lymphocytes. J. of Immunol 131:1173-1177.
del Rey A, Besedovsky HO, Sorkin E, Da Prada M, Arrenbrech S (1981) Immunoregulation mediated by the sympathetic nervous system II. Cell Immunol 63:329-334.
Furukawa Y, Furukawa S, Satoyoshi E, Hayashi K (1986) Catacholamines induce an increase in nerve growth factor content in the medium of mouse L-M cells. J. Biol Chem 261:6039-6047.
Gee AP, Boyle MDP, Munger KL, Lawman MJP, Young M (1983) Nerve growth factor: Stimulation of polymorphonuclear leukocyte chemotaxis in vitro. Proc Natl Acad Sci (USA) 80:7215-7218.
Gilman SC, Schwartz JM, Milner RJ, Bloom FE, Feldman JD (1982) Beta-endorphin enhances lymphocyte proliferation responses. Proc Natl Acad Sci (USA) 797:4226-4230.
Goetzl EJ, Chernov, T, Renold F, Payan DG (1985) Neuropeptide regulation of the expression of immediate hypersensitivity. J Immunol 135: 802s-805s.
Hazum E, Chang KJ, Cuatrecasas P (1979) Specific nonopiate receptors for Beta-endorphin. Science 205:1033-1035.
Ignatius MJ, Chandler CR, Shooter EM (1985) Nerve growth factor-treated neurite-bearing PC12 cells continue to synthesize DNA. J Neurosci 5:343-351.
Johnson DL, Gordon MA (1980) Characteristics of adrenergic binding sites associated with murine lymphocytes isolated from spleen. J Immunopharmacol 2:435-452.
Johnson DL, Ashmore RC, Gordon MA (1981) Effects of beta-adrenergic agents on the murine lymphocyte response to mitogen stimulation. J Immunopharmacol 3:205-219.
Koff WC, Dunegan MA (1985) Modulation of macrophage-mediated tumoricidal activity by neuropeptides and neurohormones. J Immunol 135:350-354.
Korsching S, Auburger G, Scott J, Thoenen H (1985) Levels of nerve growth factor and its mRNA in the central nervous system of the rat correlate with cholinergic innervation. The EMBO Journal 4:1389-1393.
Landmann RMA, Burgisser E, Wesp M, Buhler FR (1984) Beta-adrenergic receptors are different in subpopulations of human circulating lymphocytes. J Receptor Res 4:37-50.
Levi-Montalcini R (1983) The nerve growth factor-target cells interactions: a model system for the study of directed axonal growth and regeneration. In Haber B, Perez-Polo JR, Hashim G, Guiffrida-Stella AM (eds) Nervous system regeneration 19 vol. 4 Alan Liss New York, pp 3-22.
Lillien LE, Claude P (1985) Nerve growth factor is a mitogen for cultured chromaffin cells. Nature 317:632-634.
Livnet S, Felten SY, Carlson SL, Bellinger DL, Felten DL (1985) Involvement of peripheral and central catacholane systems in neural-immune interactions. J. Neuroimmunol 10:5-30.

Lyons CR, Stach RW, Perez-Polo JR (1983) Binding constants of isolated NGF-receptors from different species. Biochem Biophys Res Commun 115:368-374.

Manning PT, Russell JH, Simmons B, Johnson Jr EM (1985) Protection from guanethidine-induced neuronal destruction by nerve growth factor: Effects of NGF on immune function. Brain Res 340:61-69.

Marchetti D, Perez-Polo JR (1987) Nerve growth factor receptors in human neuroblastoma cells. J of Neurochem 49:475-486.

Marchetti D, Thorpe LW, Perez-Polo JR (in preparation) Demonstration of NGF receptor present on human peripheral blood leukocytes.

Maslinski W, Grabczewska E, Ryzeski J (1980) Acetylcholine receptors on rat lymphocytes. Biochem Biophy Acta 633:269-273.

McMasters WR, Williams AF (1979) Identification of Ia glycoproteins in rat thymus and purification from rat spleen. Eur J Immunol 9:426-433.

Mehrishi JN, Mills IH (1983) Opiate receptors on lymphocytes and platelets in man. Clin Immunol Immunopathol 27:240-249.

Miles K, Chelmicka-Schoor E, Atweh S, Otten G, Arnason BGW (1985) Sympathetic ablation alters lymphocytic membrane properties. J Immunol 135:797s-801s.

Mobley WC, Rutkowski JL, Tennekown GI, Beuchanan KR, Johnson MV (1985) Choline acetyltransferase activity in the striatum of neonatal rats increased by nerve growth factor. Science 229:284-287.

O'Dorisio MS, Wood CL, O'Dorisio TM (1985) Vasoactive intestinal peptide and neuropeptide modulation of the immune response. J Immunol 135: 792s-796s.

Otten J, Baumann JB, Girard J (1979) Stimulation of the pituitary-adrenocortical axis by nerve growth factor. Nature 282:413-414.

Payan DG, Goetzl EJ (1985) Modulation of lymphocyte function by sensory neuropeptides. J Immunol 135:783s-786s.

Payan DG, Brewster DR, Goetzl EJ (1983) Specific stimulation of human T lymphocytes by substance P. J Immunol 131:1613-1615.

Payan DG, Brewster DR, Missirian-Bastian A, Goetzl EJ (1985) Sustance P recognition by a subset of human T lymphocytes. J Clin Invest 74:1532-1539.

Perez-Polo JR, Hall K, Livingston K, Westlund K (1977) Steroid induction of nerve growth factor synthesis in cell culture. Life Sci 21:1535-1544.

Perez-Polo JR, Beck C, Blum M (1980) Biochemical correlates of behavior: What is a neurochemist to measure. In Baxter C, Melnechuk T (eds) Prespectives in Schizophrenia Research, Raven Press, NY, pp-237-246.

Perez-Polo JR, Haber B (1983) Neuronotrophic interactions. In Rosenberg RN (ed) The Clinical neurosciences, Neurobiology vol 5. Churchill-Livingston New York, pp 37-51.

Perez-Polo JR, Beck C, Marchetti D, Morgan B, Thorpe L, Werrbach-Perez K (1987) Role of NGF receptors in intercellular communications. In Benzi G (ed) Proceedings of the Second ISM Congress, John Libbey Eurotext Ltd, Montrouge France, in press.

Richman DP, Arnason BGW (1979) Nicotinic acetylcholine receptor: Evidence for a functinally distinct receptor on human lymphocytes. Proc Natl Acad Sci USA 76:4632-4635.

Roszman TH, Jackson JC, Cross RL, Titus MJ, Markesbery WR, Brooks WH (1985) Neuroanatomic and neurotransmitter influences on immune function. J Immunol 135:769s-772s.

Ruff MR, Pert CB, Weber RJ, Wahl LM, Wahl SM, Paul SM (1985) Benzodiazepine receptor-mediated chemotaxis of human monocytes. Science 229:1281-1283.

Shanahan F, Denburg JA, Fox J, Bienstock J, Befus D (1985) Mast cell heterogeneity: effects of neuroenteric peptides on histamine release. J Immunol 135:1331-1337.

Shelton DL, Reichardt LF (1984) Expression of the Beta-nerve growth factor gene correlates with the density of sympathetic innervation in effector organs. Proc Natl Acad Sci USA 81:7951-7955.

Simon MR, Engel DE, Weinstock JV (1986) Angiotensin II suppression of human mononuclear cell reactivity is associated with enhanced OKT8+ lymphocyte thymidine incorporation. J Immunopharmacol 8:289-297.

Simon MR, Engel DE, Weinstock JR, Roi LD (1985) The effect of angiotensin II on human mononuclear cell reactivity: Suppression of PHA-P-induced thymidine incorporation. Immunol Invest 14:389-400.

Slauson DO, Walker C, Kristensen F, Wang Y, de Weck AL (1984) Mechanisms of serotonin-induced lymphocyte proliferation inhibition. Cell Immunol. 84:240-252.

Stach RW, Perez-Polo JR (1987) Binding of nerve growth factor to its receptor. J Neurosci Res 17:1-10.

Sternberg EM, Trial J, Parker CW (1986) Effect of serotonin on murine macrophages: Suppression of Ia expression by serotonin and its reversal by 5 $HT_2$ serotonergic receptor antagonists. J Immunol 137:276-282.

Sztein MB, Serrate SA, Goldstein AL (1986) Modulation of interleukin-2 receptor expression on normal human lymphocytes by thymic hormones. Proc Natl Acad Sci USA 83:6107-6111.

Taniuchi M, Schweitzer JB, Johnson EM Jr (1986) Nerve growth factor receptor molecules in rat brain. Proc Natl Acad Sci (USA) 83:1950-1954.

Thorpe LW, Perez-Polo JR (1987) The influence of nerve growth factor on the in vitro proliferative response of rat spleen lymphocytes. J Neurosci Res in press.

Thorpe LW, Werrbach-Perez K, Perez-Polo JR (1987) Effects of nerve growth factor on the expression of interleukin-2 receptors on cultured human lymphocytes. Ann NY Acad Sci in press.

Thorpe LW, Stach RW, Hashim GA, Marchetti D, Perez-Polo JR (1987) Receptors for nerve growth factor on rat splenic mononuclear cells. J Neurosci Res 17:128-134.

Waldmann TA (1986) The structure function and expression of interleukin-2 receptors on normal and malignant lymphocytes. Science 232:727-732.

White RAH, Mason DW, Williams AF, Galfre G, Milstein C (1978) T-lymphocyte heterogeneity in the rat: Separation of functional subpopulations using a monoclonal antibody. J Exp Med 148:664-672.

Yankner BA, Shooter EM (1982) The biology and mechanism of action of nerve growth factor. Ann Rev Biochem 51:845-868.

# Evidence for Lymphoid Cell Participation in Neuroendocrine Pathways

Richard A. Franklin
Keith W. Kelley
Laboratory of Immunophysiology
162 ASL
1207 W. Gregory
University of Illinois
Urbana, IL 61801

*Introduction* For many years, the immune system was thought to be subject only to internal regulation by subsets of lymphoid cells and their products, such as antibodies and cytokines. It is now apparent that there is also extrinsic regulation of the immune system, and the nervous and endocrine systems are intimately involved in this regulation. It is also clear that lymphocytes serve a sensory role, and after perturbation may be capable of relaying this signal to the nervous system, thus forming a reciprocal link between the immune and nervous systems (1).

The finding that the immune and neuroendocrine systems communicate with each other is not unexpected. Jerne (2) noted analogies between the immune and nervous systems thirteen years ago. Both systems serve sensory roles. In addition, both the

NATO ASI Series, Vol. H22
Neural Development and Regeneration.
Edited by A. Gorio et al.

immune and the nervous systems exhibit memory, tolerance (habituation), and are able to receive, transmit and process large amounts of information. Jerne even suggested that these phenotypic analogies might have arisen from similarities in sets of genes that govern expression and regulation of both systems. Indeed, a number of new findings have shown that both the immune and nervous systems senthesize some of the same peptides and receptors that were once thought to be exclusive to the other system. This paper briefly highlights some of these recent findings and provides new information on pro-opiomelanocortin (POMC) gene expression in lymphoid cells.

*Brain lesions and immune reactivity* The studies of Roszman et al. (3) examined the effects of brain lesioning on immune reactivity. Electrolytic lesions in the anterior hypothalamus suppressed, while lesions in the amygdala and hippocampus augmented, a variety of immune responses when compared to both control-lesioned and normal animals. Renoux and his co-workers found that partial ablation of the left fronto-parietal cerebral cortex decreased the number of spleen cells and mitogen-induced T cell proliferative responses, while symmetric lesions of the right neo-cortex caused an opposite effect (4). These results not only showed that the brain modulates some immune responses, but that a certain degree of lateralization may also exist.

*Mental illness and immune responses* Immunologic abnormalities have been described in patients suffering from mental illnesses, such as schizophrenia. Toorey (5) found that schizophrenia patients had significantly higher IgA concentrations in cerebral spinal fluid than controls. Similarly, new evidence suggest that there may be an immunologic basis for dementia in both Alzheimer's and Down's patients (6). A preliminary report by Jersild (7) found a higher incidence of two particular major histocompatibility antigens, HLA antigens A28 and 35, in schizophrenia patients than found in normal controls. Lymphocyte dysfunctions are also found in people with major depressive disorders (8,9).

*Innervation of the immune system and neurotransmitters* A neural link between the neuroendocrine and immune systems is well documented. Felton et al. (10) described noradrenergic innervation of the thymus, spleen, lymph nodes, bone marrow and gut-associated lymphoid tissue. There is a loss of sympathetic innervation in the spleen of aged rats and this loss is associated with reduced T cell responses in aged animals (11). In the thymus, most of the noradrenergic fibers end in the cortical parenchyma near lymphoid cells. Bulloch and Moore (12) also found neural projections to the thymus that arise from the nucleus ambiguus.

Lymphoid cells have many of the receptors needed to respond to neurotransmitters. $\beta$-adrenergic receptors are found on lymphocytes (13), particularly rapidly dividing T cells (14), and these receptors are capable of being down-regulated by appropriate agonists (14). In addition, Besedovsky et al. (15) reported that levels of norepinephrine in the spleen decrease during the course of an immune response, and these findings have been recently confirmed by Lionat et al (16). Thorpe (17) described the presence of nerve growth factor receptor (NGF-R) on lymphoid cells. A role for serotonin in regulation of the immune response has been described by Jackson et al. (18). These authors found that the *in vivo* administration of serotonin, or its precursor 5-hydroxytryptophan (5-HTP), decreased both the IgM and IgG primary antibody response. These authors also found that the *in vivo* administration of para-chlorophenylalanine, a compound that interferes with serotonin synthesis, markedly enhanced the antibody response. Acetylcholine activity is found in the thymus (19), and acetylcholine receptors are found on lymphocytes (20). This leads to the possibility of dual sympathetic-parasympathetic control, not unlike control of the heart, which also functions independently of the brain.

*Pituitary hormones and the immune response* Hormones produced by the pituitary gland have a number of effects on the immune system. Growth hormone and prolactin both appear to be immunopotentiators (reviewed by Berczi (21)). For example, reconstitution of thymic structure and architecture, as well as T cell proliferative responses and IL-2 synthesis, occur in aged rats after they have been implanted with pituitary tumor cells that secrete both prolactin and growth hormone (22). These findings suggest that the endocrine environment may play an important role in the normal thymic atrophy and decline in T cell responses of aged subjects. In addition to this observation, growth hormone enhances the antibody response in both hypophysectomized and pituitary dwarf mice (23) and prolactin is important for the homing of lymphoid cells to the mammary gland (24). Thyroid hormones released in response to pituitary TSH are also known to affect lymphoid tissue. Young mice treated with $T_3$ have elevated serum levels of thymulin, as well as the number of thymulin-containing cells in their thymus glands (25). In addition, TSH augments antibody synthesis (26).

Perhaps the best documented effect of pituitary hormones on the immune response is that of ACTH acting via the adrenal gland. In this system, ACTH is produced in the pituitary by the processing of POMC and is released into the blood where it acts on the adrenal to augment both the production and release of glucocorticoids from adrenal cortical cells. Glucocorticoids then act on the lymphoid cells of the immune system where they have a variety of actions, most of which are immunosuppressive.

These examples highlight a number of studies carried out on the influences of pituitary hormones on immune functions. For a complete review see Berczi (27).

*Communication between the neuroendocrine and immune systems is not unidirectional* Not only have pituitary hormones been shown to affect lymphocyte responsiveness, but lymphokines and monokines have been shown to affect pituitary cells. Besedovsky et al. (28) described a biological role for a product in the supernatants of Con A-stimulated lymphocytes that increases the release of ACTH (termed glucocorticoid-increasing factor). IL-1 releases ACTH *in vivo* (29) and from a transformed pituitary cell line (30), but it is without effect on normal pituitary cells *in vitro* (31). Therefore, perhaps another factor induced by IL-1 *in vivo* is needed to stimulate ACTH release from the pituitary gland. Hepatocyte-stimulating factor is derived from monocytes and is a more potent releasor of ACTH than corticotropin releasing factor on transformed pituitary cells (30).

Lymphokines not only affect ACTH release from pituitary cells, but they have many other properties as well. Interleukin-1 plays a role in inducing slow wave sleep (32) and fever induction (33), and $\alpha$-MSH may be a natural antagonist of IL-1 (34). A lymphokine known as neuroleukin, a product of lectin-stimulated T-cells, supports the survival of cultured sensory neurons that are insensitive to nerve growth factor (35). Neuroleukin has also been suggested to play a role in immunoglobulin secretion (36).

Interferon has a number of actions on the neuroendocrine system. Interferon augments uptake of iodine by thyroid cells, causes an induction of melanin synthesis in melanoma cells, is a antagonist of insulin action, and is able to bind opiate receptors and excite neurons (37). One particular interferon that is produced by T-lymphocytes, known as interferon-$\gamma$, augments Ia expression by astrocytes in the brain (38). Peptides produced by lymphoid tissues also affects neuroendocrine tissue. Thymosin fraction 5 stimulates the release of prolactin from a pituitary cell line (39) and increases serum corticosterone in rodents (40).

Since both the immune and neuroendocrine systems function as sensory systems and communication appears to exist between these two systems, it is logical that these two systems might share some of the peptides that are used in this communication network, as implied by Jerne. Recent evidence strongly suggests that this is the case (1).

*Peptides and receptors shared by the neuroendocrine and immune system* A transformed pituitary cell line (AtT-20) is now known to constitutively express IL-2 receptors (41), but it is unknown whether these are high or low affinity or whether normal pituitary cells also express IL-2 receptors. Production of pro-opiomelanocortin (POMC) by these cells is regulated by IL-1 and IL-2 (42). Interleukin-1 is also produced by glial cells in the brain (43).

Lymphoid cells are now known to secrete many of the peptides that were once thought to be used exclusively by the neuroendocrine system. Evidence for production of pituitary hormones, such as POMC and its products (44-48), thyroid stimulating hormone (49), human chorionic gonadotropin (50), somatostatin (51), vasoactive intestinal peptide (52,53), growth hormone (54), prolactin (54,55) and preproenkephlin (56) has been presented. In addition, vasoactive intestinal peptide (10), oxytocin, vasopressin and neurophysin (57,58) have been found in the thymus and met-enkephalin, cholecystokinin and neurotensin have been detected in the spleen (10). In many cases, lymphoid cells did not constitutively produce the hormone, but had to be activated to display this activity.

*Evidence for a lymphoid-adrenal axis* Blalock and co-workers found that murine splenocytes infected with Newcastle disease virus (NDV) stained positively with antibodies to ACTH (45), which suggested that lymphoid cells can synthesize and secrete ACTH. Non-infected cells did not produce irACTH, which suggested that the ACTH-like peptide was synthesized *de novo*. When this irACTH was affinity purified from supernatants of infected splenocytes, it was shown to be similar to pituitary-derived ACTH on the basis of bioactivity, molecular weight, and retention time on reverse phase high pressure liquid chromotograpy (1,45). However, it remained unknown whether the ACTH was derived from the prohormone POMC, as is known to occur in the pituitary gland.

*POMC expression in NDV-infected murine splenocytes* Our laboratory has established the molecular foundation for this lymphoid-adrenal axis by showing that the irACTH found in the cytoplasm of lymphoid cells can be derived from the processing of POMC (48). POMC RNA has also been found in nonactivated macrophages (46,47). In our study, total cellular and poly(A)+ RNA were isolated from NDV-infected and non-infected murine splenocytes. Total cellular RNA was isolated from a murine pituitary cell line that secretes ACTH, murine liver and murine splenocytes that were or were not exposed to 10 hemagglutination units of NDV. Poly(A)+ RNA was isolated from AtT-20 cells and murine splenocytes that were or were not exposed to NDV. This RNA was hybridized under high stringency conditions with the plasmid pMKSU16, which contains an insert comprising the entire coding sequence of the murine POMC gene (59). These results showed positive hybridization of the plasmid containing the POMC insert to total and poly(A)+ RNA from both AtT-20 and NDV-infected murine splenocyte RNA. The plasmid did not hybridize to either total or poly(A)+ RNA from uninfected murine splenocytes or total RNA from liver tissue (48).

The POMC insert was not originally purified from the plasmid since the parent plasmid (pBR322) did not hybridize with RNA from infected splenocytes or AtT-20 cells. However, these findings were extended by carrying out identical experiments with the restricted POMC insert. Results of these experiments were identical (60) to those experiments in which the entire plasmid was used. Northern blot analysis showed that poly(A)+ RNA was similar in size to poly(A)+ RNA isolated from AtT-20 cells (48), suggesting that POMC protein derived from the pituitary and virus infected-lymphoid cells is quite similar, if not identical. These results further suggested that the irACTH observed by Smith and Blalock was derived from a system that has been well described in pituitary cells.

*Regulation of POMC expression* Smith and co-workers also described the presence of irACTH and β-endorphin in the supernatants of leukocytes stimulated with corticotropin releasing factor (CRF) (61). This irACTH was augmented by co-treatment of leukocytes with arginine vasopressin and was suppressed by dexamethasone. These results suggested that production of ACTH by the immune system was under some of the same control systems as the anterior pituitary gland. We now have preliminary evidence which extends these findings by showing that CRF can induce the appearance of POMC RNA in lymphoid cells.

*POMC expression by CRF-treated lymphocytes* To test the hypothesis that CRF treatment of murine splenocytes leads to an augmentation of POMC RNA, total cellular RNA from AtT-20 cells and liver tissue and cytoplasmic RNA from CRF-treated and untreated murine splenocytes were hybridized under the conditions described previously to the probe containing the entire coding sequence of the murine POMC gene (pMSKU16) (59). Dot blots of RNA from the AtT-20 and CRF-treated splenocytes showed positive hybridization to this probe, whereas dot blots of RNA from liver tissue and untreated splenocytes showed only minor hybridization (Figure 1). When the coding region for the POMC molecule was restricted from the plasmid, identical results were obtained when probed against an identical blot (Figure 2). Initial studies with Northern blots indicate that the hybridizing RNA is similar in size to POMC RNA obtained from the ACTH-secreting, AtT-20 pituitary cell line.

*Possible regulation of POMC expression by serum factors* We now offer preliminary evidence for the possibility of another regulator of POMC synthesis in lymphoid cells. In initial experiments, we found that background hybridization varied among lots of fetal calf serum. For these reasons, a serum-free system was developed to culture lymphoid cells. Although there are a number of unknown factors in serum, one serum component that varies greatly from lot to lot is serotonin (62). Serotonin has also been implicated in the regulation of the secretion of POMC-derived peptides in the intermediate pituitary (63,64) and in non-mammalian species that lack direct inhibitory hypothalamic control (65).

We have initiated studies on the effects of serotonin on POMC synthesis. Initial results are shown in Figures 1 and 2. When cells were cultured in the absence of serum and also incubated with serotonin, there appeared to be an increase in the level of RNA encoding for POMC over that found in control

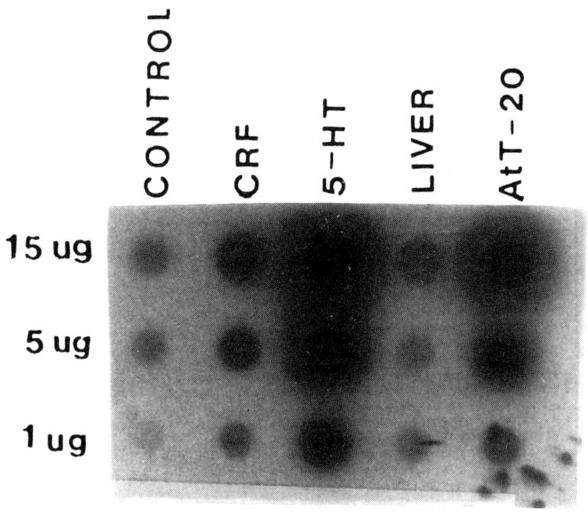


*Figure 1* Dot blot hybridization of cytoplasmic RNA isolated from murine splenocytes that were untreated or exposed to 50nM CRF or 50nM serotonin for 18 hr and total cellular RNA isolated from murine liver and AtT-20 pituitary cells. Done at high stringency to a plasmid containing the coding sequences for the murine POMC gene (48).

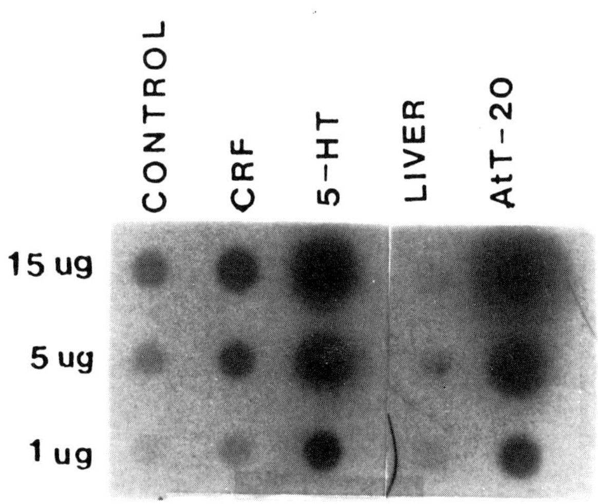


*Figure 2* Dot blot hybridization of cytoplasmic RNA isolated from murine splenocytes that were untreated or exposed to 50nM CRF or 50nM serotonin for 18 hr and total cellular RNA isolated from murine liver and AtT-20 pituitary cells. Done at high stringency to a restricted POMC cDNA probe (48).

cells. These initial studies, if confirmed, raise many interesting questions. If the regulation of lymphocytes is similar to that of the intermediate pituitary and anterior pituitary lobes, perhaps products of POMC processing differ with the form of immunologic stimulus.

*Conclusions* These data suggest that products of the neuroendocrine system can modulate the immune system and that products produced by cells of the immune system can regulate neuroendocrine activities. In addition, the findings that many receptors and hormones are shared by these two systems suggests there is a biochemical and molecular foundation for bi-directional communication between these systems. Future work in our laboratory is directed at confirming these preliminary results and further elucidating the molecular mechanisms involved in the interaction between the immune and neuroendocrine systems.

*Address correspondence to Keith W. Kelley, 162 ASL, 1207 W. Gregory Drive, University of Illinois, Urbana IL 61801.* *This research was supported by grants to Keith W. Kelley from the National Institutes of Health (AG06246-01), U.S Department of Agriculture (86-CRCR-1-2003) and Moorman Manufacturing Company.*

1) Blalock JE, Smith EM (1985) A complete regulatory loop between the immune and neuroendocrine systems Fed Proc 44:108-111
2) Jerne NK (1974) Towards a network theory of the immune system. Ann Immunol (Paris) 125C:373-387
3) Roszman TL, Jackson JC, Cross RJ, Titus MJ, Markesbery WR, Brooks WH (1985) Neuroanatomic and neurotransmitter influences on immune function J Immunol 135:769s-772s
4) Renoux G, Biziere K, Renoux M, Guillaumin J-M, Degenne D (1983) A balanced brain asymmetry modulates T cell-mediated events J Neuroimmunol 5:227-238
5) Torrey EF (1977) CSF better than serum in study of immunology in mental patients Clin Psychiatr News 5
6) Singh VK, Fudenberg HH, Brown FR (1987) Immunologic dysfunction: Simultaneous study of Alzheimer's and older Down's patients Mech Ageing Devel 37:257-264
7) Jersild C (1976) Lect., 1st int. symp. immunol. components schizophrenia Galvaston, Texas
8) Schleifer SJ, Keller SE, Siris SG Davis KL,Stien M (1985) Depression and Immunity Arch Gen Psychiatry 42:129-133
9) Schleifer SJ, Keller SE, Meyerson AT, Raskin MJ, Davis KL, Stien M (1984) Lymphocyte function in major depressive disorder Arch Gen Psychiatry 41:484-486
10) Felton DL, Felton SY, Carlson SL, Olschowka JA, Livnat S (1985) Noradrenergic and peptidergic innervation of lymphoid tissue J Immunol 135:755s-765s
11) Felton SY, Bellinger DL, Collier TJ, Coleman PD, Felton DL (1987) Decreased sympahetic innervation of spleen in aged Fischer 344 rats Neurobiol Aging 8:159-165
12) Bulloch K, Moore RY (1980) Nucleus ambiguus projections to the thymus gland: Possible pathways for regulation of the immune response and the neuroendocrine network Anat Rec 196:25A
13) Bourne HR, Lichtenstein LM, Melmon KL, Henney CS, Weinstien Y, Shearer GM (1974) Modulation of inflammation and immunity by cAMP Science 184:19-28
14) Westly HJ, Kelley KW (1987) Down-regulation of glucocorticoid and β-adrenergic receptors on lectin-stimulated splenocytes Proc Soc Exp Med 185:211-218.
15) Besedovsky HO, del Ray A, Sorkin E, Da Prada M, Keller HH (1979) Immunoregulation mediated by the sympathetic nervous system Cell Immuno 48:346-355
16) Livnat S, Felton SY, Carlson SL, Bellinger DL, Felton DL (1985) Involvement of peripheral and central catecholamine systems in neural-immune interactions J Neuroimmunol 10:5-30
17) Thorpe LW, Stach RW, Hashim HD, Marchetti D, Perez-Polo JR (1987) Receptors for nerve growth factor on rat spleen mononuclear cells J Neurosci Res 17:128-134
18) Jackson JC, Cross RJ, Walker RF, Brooks WH, Markesbery WH, Roszman TL (1984) Neuroimmunomodulation: Influence of serotonin on the immune response Immunology 54:505-512
19) Engel WK, Trotter JL, McFarlin DE, McIntosh CL (1977) Thymic epithelial cell contains acetylcholine receptor Lancet 1:1310-1311

20) Singh U (1979) Effect of catecholamines on lymphopoiesis in fetal mouse thymic explants J Anat 129:279-292
21) Berczi I (1986) The influence of the pituitary-adrenal axis on the immune system In: Berczi I (ed) Pituitary Function and Immunity. CRC Press, Boca Raton, Florida. pp 49-132
22) Kelley KW, Brief S, Westly HJ, Novakofski J, Bechtel PJ, Simon J, Walker EB (1986) $GH_3$ pituitary adenoma cells can reverse thymic aging in rats Proc Natl Acad Sci (USA) 83:5663-5667
23) Ahlqvist J (1976) Endocrine influences on lymphatic organs, immune responses, inflammation and autoimmunity Acta Endocrinol (Copenhagen) suppl 206
24) Klareskog L, Forsum U, Peterson PA (1980) Hormonal regulation of expression of Ia antigens on mammary gland epithelium Eur J Immunol 10:958-963
25) Savino W, Wolf B, Aratan-Spire S, Dardenne M (1984) Thymic hormone containing cells. IV. Fluctuations in thyroid hormone levels *in vivo* can modulate the secretion of thymulin by the epithelial cells of the young mouse thymus Clin Exp Immunol 55:629-635
26) Kruger TE, Blalock JE (1986) Cellular requirements for thyrotropin enhancement of *in vitro* antibody production J Immunol 137:197-200
27) Berczi I (ed) (1986) Pituitary Function and Immunity. CRC Press, Boca Raton, Florida.
28) Besedovsky HO, del Ray A, Sorkin E, Lotz W, Schwular U (1985) Lymphoid cells produce an immunoregulatory glucocorticoid increasing factor (GIF) acting through the pituitary gland Clin Exp Immunol 59:622-628
29) Besedovsky HO, del Ray A, Sorkin E, Dinarello CA (1986) Immunoregulatory feedback between interleukin-1 and glucocorticoid hormones Science 233:652-654
30) Woloski BMRNJ, Smith EM, Meyer III WJ, Fuller GM, Blalock JE (1985) Corticotropin releasing activity of monokines Science 230:1035-1037
31) Uehara A, Gillis S, Arimura A (1987) Effects of interleukin-1 on hormone release from normal rat pituitary cells in primary culture Neuroendocrin 45:343-347
32) Krueger JM, Walter J, Dinarello CA, Wolfe M, Chedid L (1984) Sleep-promoting effects of endogenous pyrogen (interleukin-1) Am J Physiol 246:R994
33) Fontana A, Weber E, Dayer JM (1984) Synthesis of interleukin-1/endogenous pyrogen in the brain of endotoxin-treated mice: A step in fever induction? J Immunol 133:1696-1698
34) Cannon JG, Tatro JB, Reichlin S, Dinarello CA (1986) $\alpha$ Melanocyte stimulating hormone inhibits immunostimulatory actions of interleukin-1 J Immunol 137:2232-2236
35) Gurney ME, Heinrich SP, Lee MR, Hsiang-shu Y (1986) Molecular cloning and expression of neuroleukin, a neurotropic factor for spinal and sensory neurons Science 234:566-574.
36) Gurney ME, Apatoff BR, Spear GT, Baumel MJ, Antel JP, Brown-Bania M, Reder AT (1986) Neuroleukin: A lymphokine product of lectin stimulated T-cells Science 234:574-581

37) Blalock JE (1984) Relationships between neuroendocrine hormones and lymphokines Lymphokines 9:1-13
38) Hirsch MR Wietzerbin Y, Pierres M, Goridis C (1983) Expression of Ia antigen by cultured astrocytes treated with γ-interferon Neurosci Lett 41:204-210
39) Spangelo BL, Hall NR, Dunn AJ, Goldstein AL (1987) Thymosin fraction 5 stimulates the release of prolactin from cultured $GH_3$ cells Life Sci 40:283-288
40) McGillis JP, Hall NR, Vahouny GV, Goldstein AL (1985) Thymosin fraction 5 causes increased serum corticosterone in rodents *in vivo* J Immunol 134:3952-3955
41) Brown SL, Smith LR, Blalock JE (1987) Interleukin-1 and interleukin-2 modulate the expression of pro-opiomelanocortin mRNA in the pituitary Fed Proc 46:925
42) Smith LR, Brown SL, Blalock JE (1987) Pituitary cell expression of interleukin-2 receptors and regulation of pro-opiomelanocortin by interleukin-2 Fed Proc 46:925
43) Fontana A, Kristensen F, Dubs R, Gemsa D, Weber E (1982) Production of prostaglandin E and interleukin 1-like factor by cultured astrocytes and C-6 glioma cells J Immunol 129:2413-2419
44) Blalock JE (1984) The immune system as a sensory organ J Immunol 132:1067-1070
45) Smith EM, Blalock JE (1981) Human lymphocyte production of corticotropin and endorphin like substances: association with leukocyte interferon Proc Natl Acad Sci (USA) 75:7530-7534
46) Lolait SJ, Lim ATW, Toh BH, Funder JW (1984) Immunoreactive β-endorphin in a subpopulation of mouse spleen macrophages J Clin Invest 75:277-280
47) Lolait SJ, Clements JA, Markwick AJ, Cheng C, McNally, Smith AI, Funder JW (1986) Pro-opiomelanocortin messenger ribonucleic acid and post-translational processing of beta endorphin in spleen macrophages J Clin Invest 77:1776-1779
48) Westly HJ, Kleiss AJ, Kelley KW, Wong PKY, Yuen PH (1986) Newcastle disease virus-infected splenocytes express the pro-opiomelanocortin gene. J Exp Med 163:1589-1594
49) Smith EM, Phan M, Kruger TE, Coppenhaver DH, Blalock JE (1983) Human lymphocyte production of immunoreactive thyrotropin Proc Natl Acad Sci (USA) 80:6010-6013
50) Harbour-McMenamin D, Smith EM, Blalock JE (1986) Production of immunoreactive chorionic gonadotropin during mixed lymphocyte reactions: A possible selective mechanism for genetic diversity Proc Natl Acad Sci (USA) 83:6834-6838
51) Lygren I, Revhaug P, Barhol PG, Giercksky KE, Jenssen TG (1984) Vasoactive intestinal peptide and somatostatin in leukocytes Scand J Clin Lab Invest 44:347-351
52) O'Dorisio MS, Wood CL, O'Dorisio TM (1985) Vasoactive intestinal peptide and neuropeptide modulation of the immune response J Immunol 135:792s-796s
53) Giachetti A, Goth A, Said SA (1978) Vasoactive intestinal polypeptide (VIP) in rabbit platlets and rat mast cells Fed Proc 37:657
54) Heistand PC, Mekler P, Nordmann R, Grieder A, Perminongkol C (1986) Prolactin as a modulator of lymphocyte responsiveness

provides a possible mechanism of action for cyclosporin. Proc Natl Acad Sci (USA) 83:2599-2603
55) Montgomery DW, Russell DH, Buckley AR, Zukoski CF (1987) Concanavalin A (Con A)-stimulated lymphocytes produce a prolactin (PRL)-like mitogen for Nb2 node lymphoma cells Fed Proc 46:529
56) Zurawski G, Benedik M, Kamb BJ, Abrams JS, Zurawski SM, Lee FD (1986) Activation of mouse T-helper cells induces abundant preproenkephalin mRNA synthesis Science 232:772-775
57) Geenen V, Legros J-J, Franchimont P, Baudrihaye M, Defresne M-P, Boniver J (1986) The neuroendocrine thymus: Coexistence of oxytocin and neurophysin in the human thymus Science 232:508-511
58) Markwick AJ, Lolait SJ, Funder JW (1986) Immunoreactive arginine vasopressin in the rat thymus Endocrinol 119:1690-1696
59) Uhler M, Herbert E (1983) Complete amino acid sequence of mouse pro-opiomelanocortin derived from the nucleotide sequence of pro-opiomelanocortin cDNA J Biol Chem 258:257-261
60) Westly HJ, Kleiss AJ, Kelley KW, Wong PKY, Yuen PH (1987) The postulated lymphoid-adrenal axis: A molecular approach In: Neuroimmunomodulation. New York Academy of Sciences, New York (in press)
61) Smith EM, Morrill AC, Meyer III WJ, Blalock JE (1986) Corticotropin releasing factor induction of leukocyte-derived immunoreactive ACTH and endorphins Nature 321:881-882
62) Hyclone Laboratories, Inc. (1985) Serotonin: A biologically active hormone *in vivo* and in cell culture Art to Science Vol 4 No 2:5
61) Kraicer J, Morris AR (1976) *In vitro* release of ACTH from dispersed rat pars intermedia cells. II. Effect of neurotransmitter substances Neuroendocrinol 21:175-192
62) Randel JCR, Moor BC, Kraicer J (1983) Differential control of the release of pro-opiomelanocortin-derived peptides from the pars intermedia of the rat pituitary Neuroendocrinol 37:131-140
63) Olivereau M, Olivereau J-M, Aimar C (1980) Responses of MSH and prolactin cells to 5-hydroxytryptophan (5-HTP) in amphibians and teleosts Cell Tiss Res 207:377-385

# IMMUNE SYSTEM GROWTH FACTOR MODULATION OF NEONATAL OLIGODENDROCYTE GROWTH *IN VITRO*.

R.P. Saneto[*], A. Altman[†], R.L. Knobler[§] and J. de Vellis[*]

*Department of Anatomy and Psychiatry, UCLA School of Medicine, Mental Retardation Research Center, Laboratory of Biomedical and Environmental Sciences, University of California, Los Angeles, CA 90024; †Scripps Clinic and Research Foundation, La Jolla, CA 92037; §Department of Neurology, Thomas Jefferson Medical College, Philadelphia, PA 19107

## INTRODUCTION

Traditionally, the immune system and central nervous system (CNS) have been thought to be distinct and non-interactive compartments. The blood-brain barrier formed via the tight junctions of the CNS capillary endothelia appears to exclude most immune system peptides and cell types from the CNS under normal conditions. However, the finding of shared ligand-receptor interactions between these two systems has radically changed this non-interacting concept.

Immune system peptides are synthesized by and interact with CNS cell types. The monokine interleukin 1 (IL-1) is secreted by activated cultured astrocytes (Fontana et al., 1982) and microglia (Giulian and Baker, 1986). In addition, IL-1 is an autocrine mitogen for cultured astrocytes (Giulian and Lachman, 1985). The lymphokine interleukin 3 can stimulate the *in vitro* proliferation of microglia (Giulian and Baker, 1986) while a factor secreted from the transformed human T-cell line Mo, can induce growth of cultured oligodendrocytes (Benveniste et al., 1985). Implied but not verifed, is the presence of corresponding receptors for these ligands, which would be required for specific ligand induced physiological function.

Recently, we demonstrated that interleukin 2 (IL-2) could inhibit the proliferation of isolated neonatal rat oligodendrocyte progenitor cells *in vitro* (Saneto et al., 1986). This ligand induced inhibition was receptor mediated (Saneto et al., 1986; Saneto et al., 1987), suggesting the possibility of direct communication between the immune and CNS.

NATO ASI Series, Vol. H22
Neural Development and Regeneration.
Edited by A. Gorio et al.

## OLIGODENDROCYTE PROGENITOR CELL PROLIFERATION

Primary mixed glia cultures initiated from 1-2 day postnatal rat cerebral cortices yield a bedlayer of flat polygonal cells, overlaid by phase-dark process-bearing cells (McCarthy and de Vellis, 1980). Once isolated, greater than 95% of process-bearing cells can be induced in a chemically defined medium to express ultrastructural, biochemical and immunological characteristics of oligodendrocytes (Saneto and de Vellis, 1985). Recently, we developed a serumless, chemically defined medium (ODM) that reproducibly induces cell proliferation (Fig. 1). In the presence of transferrin (500 ng/ml), insulin (5 μg/ml) and basic fibroblast growth factor (5 ng/ml) a 3-5 fold increase in cell number occurs over a 5 day period (Saneto and de Vellis, 1985). Autoradiography indicated that greater than 90% of the culture was undergoing {$^3$H}thymidine incorporation and culture purity was routinely immunocytochemically 95-98% positive for the oligodendrocyte marker glycerol phosphate dehydrogenase (Leveille et al., 1980). Hence, we have named the proliferating cell type, cultured in ODM, oligodendrocyte progenitor cell. The milieu of ODM induces proliferation and a cell capable of regulated oligodendrocyte phenotypic expression. Upon isolation, the maturation marker galactocerebroside (GC) represents approximately 50-60% of the total population of cells. The remainder of the culture was found to be A2B5 positive, a marker for bipotential cells that in the presence of serum-free medium become GC positive oligodendrocytes (Raff et al., 1983). With time in culture, the intensity of GC expression per cell and the number of cells expressing GC can be influenced by extrinsic factors (Bologa et al., 1987; Saneto and de Vellis, 1985; Saneto et al., 1987). However, with time in culture greater than 90% of the culture can become positive for GC suggesting that these cells are proliferating oligodendrocytes (unpublished data).

## IMMUNOMODULATION OF OLIGODENDROCYTE PROGENITOR CELL PROLIFERATION

The lymphokine IL-2, synthesized and secreted by activated T-helper cells (Morgan et al., 1976), regulates the growth of both T-cells and B-cells (Smith, 1980; Zubler et al., 1984). To exert its growth promoting activity, IL-2 must interact with a high affinity receptor (Robb et al., 1981) and the receptor-ligand complex subsequently internalized (Weissman et al., 1986). Although resting T or B cells do not express IL-2 receptors,

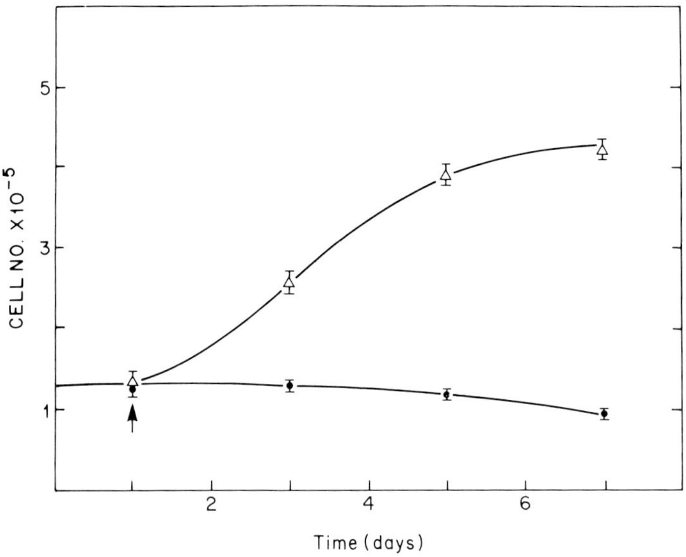


Fig. 1. Growth curve of isolated oligodendrocytes. Cells were grown in either serum-supplemented medium (●) or ODM (Δ). Data represent cell numbers per well, values are the mean of six wells $\pm$ SEM. Arrow indicates when ODM was added to cultures.

once exposed to antigen or mitogen these cells rapidly express IL-2 receptors and become responsive to IL-2. Leonard et al., (1982) have demonstrated that the monoclonal antibody TAC specifically binds to one subunit of the IL-2 receptor.

Both homogeneous affinity purified and recombinant IL-2 identically inhibited {$^3$H}thymidine incorporation into oligodendrocyte progenitor cells in a dose-responsive manner (Fig. 2). This inhibitory activity of IL-2 was found when added to either cultures freshly seeded or in log-phase growth (Fig. 3) with specificity of IL-2 activity immunoprecipitable with monospecific antibodies against IL-2 (Saneto et al., 1986).

The possible need for a progenitor cell IL-2 receptor became evident with studies dealing with changes of cell number with IL-2 exposure. Although IL-2 inihibited cell proliferation (Fig. 4), the inclusion of IL-1 was necessary to observe IL-2 effects on cell number. After initial exposure to IL-2, restimulation with IL-2 had no effect on thymidine incorporation, even after 72 hr of additional culture growth without IL-2 present (Fig.5 ). Upon continued IL-2 exposure to cultures, there was no decrease in cell number over control cultures. To examine the rationale

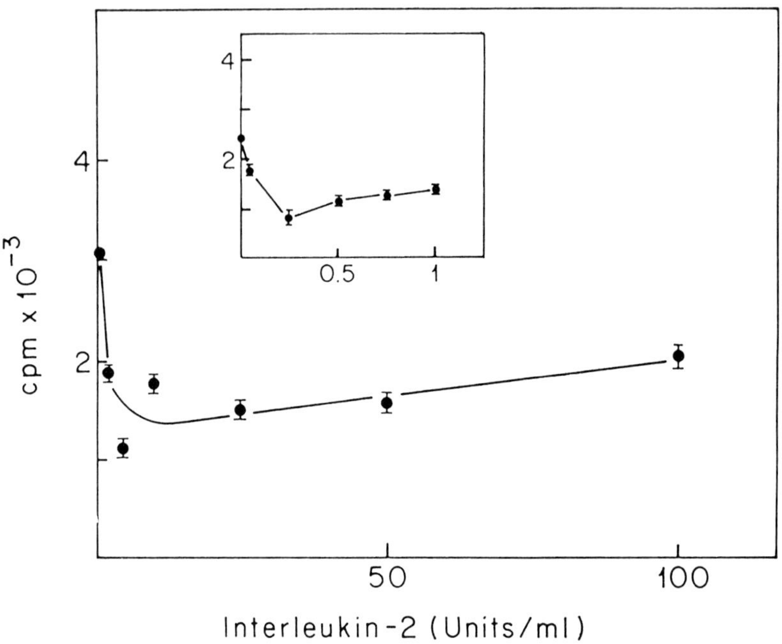


Fig. 2. Dose-response curve of {$^{3}$H}thymidine incorporation into oligodendrocyte progenitor cells as a response to IL-2. Oligodendrocyte progenitor cells were isolated and cultured for 24 hr in ODM containing various amounts of either affinity-purified IL-2 or recombinant IL-2. Radiolabel was added 2 hr before termination of the experiment. Cultures were processed and assayed for radioactivity as described (Saneto et al., 1986). (Inset) Data derived from low concentrations of IL-2. Both graphs represent three experiments, and data points are means of triplicate trials $\pm$ SD.

for conflicting data of thymidine incorporation and cell number, we investigated whether IL-2 receptors might modulate cell growth. Upon isolation, greater than 90% of progenitor cells expressed TAC receptors (Fig. 6). However, after exposure to IL-2 for 48 hr the immunocytochemical detection of the TAC receptor was lost and did not reappear over a 72 hr culture period (Saneto et al., 1986). During receptor down-regulation, IL-2 had no inhibitory effect on thymidine incorporation (Fig. 5). However, if IL-1 was added to the cultures after TAC receptor down-regulation, both IL-2 responsiveness and TAC receptor staining were induced (Saneto et al., 1987). Furthermore, in the presence of IL-1, IL-2 inhibited cell number increases, collaborating the {$^{3}$H}thymidine incorporation data (Fig. 2). Added by itself, IL-1 had no effect on thymidine incorporation or growth of oligodendrocyte progenitor cells. Although we can not rule out the possibility of a TAC reacting epitope regulated by IL-1 serendipitously, the data indicate

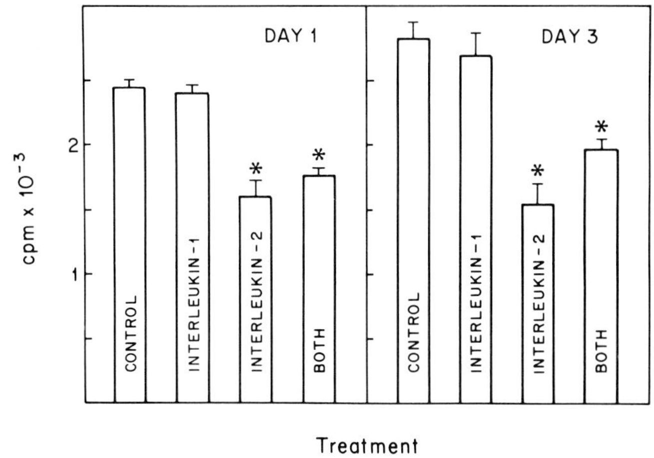


Fig. 3. IL-2 inhibition of {$^3$H}thymidine incorporation into oligodendrocyte progenitor cells. Radiolabel was added 2 hr before termination of the experiment and assayed for radioactivity as previously described (Saneto et al., 1986). Treatments are added at either the initial medium change to defined medium (day 1) or at the next medium change (day 3). IL-2 was used at 5 units per ml, and IL-1 was used at 3 units per ml:cpm represent the mean of triplicate experiments. *significant at $P < 0.01$.

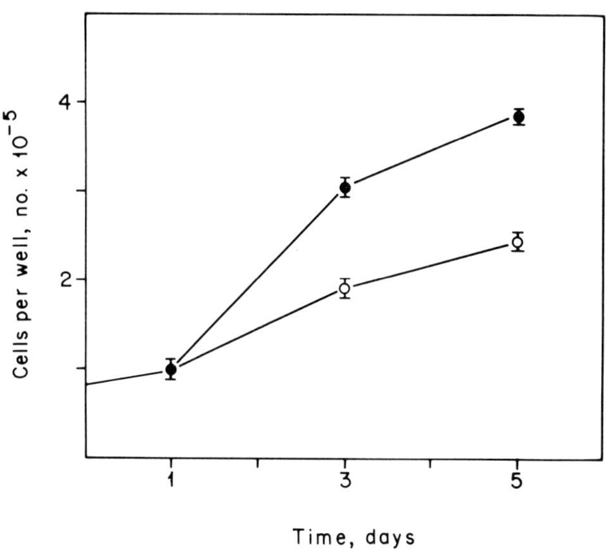


Fig. 4. Growth curve of isolated oligodendrocyte progenitor cells as a response to IL-1 combined with IL-2. Progenitor cells were isolated and cultured in ODM with (o) or without (•) IL-1 (3 U/ml) and IL-2 (2 U/ml). Data points represent the cell number per well; values are means of six wells ± SEM. This is representative of triplicate experiments.

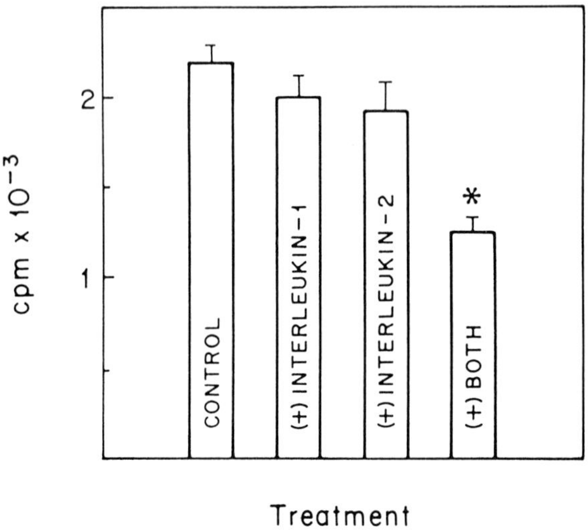


Fig. 5. IL-1 modulation of IL-2 inhibition of {$^3$H}thymidine incorporation into oligodendrocyte progenitor cells after previous IL-2 exposure. Oligodendrocyte progenitor cells are isolated and seeded as described (Saneto et al. 1986). Cultures were exposed to IL-2 (5 U/ml) for 48 hr. Subsequently cultures were washed 3 x with basal medium, then ODM was added with or without IL-1, IL-2, or both together. {$^3$H}Thymidine incorporation are the mean of triplicate experiments. *Significant at $P < 0.005$

that TAC receptor expression is regulated by IL-1 and IL-2. Furthermore, the inhibitory activity of IL-2 seems to be regulated by TAC receptor expression suggesting it to be the IL-2 receptor on oligodendrocyte progenitor cells.

Upon isolation, oligodendrocyte progenitor cells were found to express TAC receptors (Fig. 6). Greater than 90% of the culture was found TAC positive. We feel that the TAC receptor is likely induced in mixed glial culture and is not constitutively expressed by progenitor cells. After down-regulation by IL-2, the TAC receptor is not up-regulated once the ligand is removed. In isolated culture, IL-1 can up-regulate the TAC receptor. Cultured astrocytes can secrete IL-1 (Fontana et al., 1982) and are the likely source of TAC receptor induction in mixed glial culture.

The TAC receptor found on oligodendrocyte progenitor cells is likely distinct from the corresponding receptor found on T cells. Immunocytochemical precipitation of the TAC receptor from progenitor cells revealed a 70-75,000 dalton protein under reducing gel conditions (Fig. 7). The TAC receptor on both human and rat T cells has been described as a 50-55,000 dalton glycoprotein under the same conditions (Leonard et al., 1984;

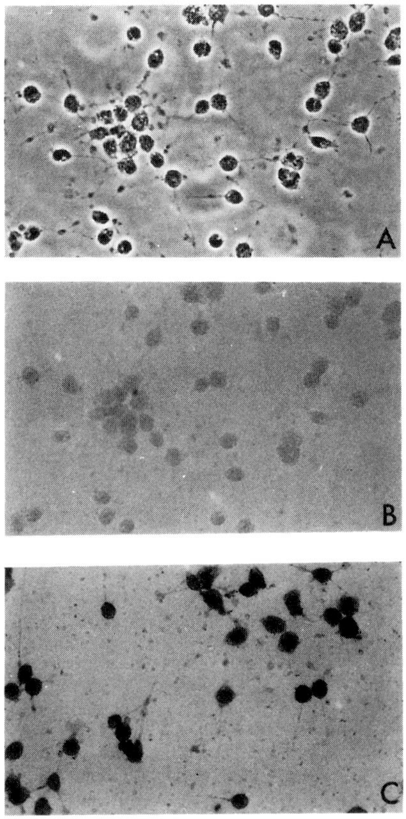

Fig. 6. Immunocytochemical staining of purified isolated oligodendrocyte progenitor cells with anti-TAC monoclonal antibody. Micrographs are either (A) phase-contrast or (B,C) bright field photographs of the avidin-biotin complex, with glucose oxidase staining of progenitor cells after 24 hr in culture. (B) Micrograph of oligodendrocytes stained with control sera. (C) Sister culture stained with anti-TAC (1:5000). (x330)

Kohda et al., 1986). In addition, IL-2 does not up-regulate the TAC receptor as found in T cells (Reem and Yeh, 1984). Furthermore, exposure to IL-2 rapidly down-regulated its receptor on progenitor cells whereas down-regulation occurs over a much longer time span on T cells (DeFreitas et al., 1986); a process independent of receptor-saturating concentrations of IL-2 (Contrell and Smith, 1983). However, IL-2 inhibitory activity at pM amounts and IL-1 modulation of receptor expression indicate similarity between the T cell and oligodendrocyte progenitor cell IL-2 receptor.

## CONCLUSION

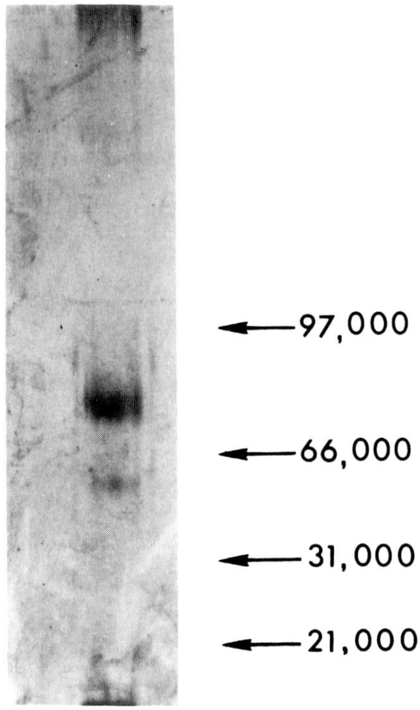


Fig. 7. Immunoprecipitation of TAC antigen. Approximately $10^9$ oligodendrocyte progenitor cells were grown in ODM, washed 2x with basal medium and solubilized in 2 ml extraction buffer (10 mM Tris, pH 7.4, 0.15 M NaCl, 100 µg ml$^{-1}$ phenylmethylsulphenyl fluoride, 0.5% NP-40) for 45 min on ice. Cell homogenates were centrifuged in a microfuge to remove debris and supernatant exposed to protein A-Sepharose at 4$^o$C for 2 hr with gentle shaking. After centrifugation, antibody was added for 18 hr at 4$^o$C with agitation, the protein A-Sepharose solution was added for an additional 18 hr with agitation. Pelleted beads were washed 3x with extraction buffer and transfered to SDS sample buffer and heated to 100 $^o$C for 5 min. Samples were then electrophoresed using a 10% polyacrylamide gel under reducing conditions and gel silver stained for protein.

The data presented indicate that IL-2 can inhibit the proliferation of oligodendrocyte progenitor cells grown in a serumless, chemically defined medium. IL-2 was found to have activity in the pM range on oligodendrocyte progenitor cells while having no activity on astrocyte type I cells. The inhibitory activity of IL-2 was dependent on the expression of a 70-75,000 dalton receptor that was immunocytochemically TAC positive. This TAC receptor was down-regulated by exposure to IL-2 and up-regulated by IL-1. IL-2 had no inhibitory activity detected by thymidine incorporation when this receptor, detected by immunocytochemical staining with the antibody

TAC, was not expressed.

The specific interaction of IL-2 with its receptor inducing inhibition of oligodendrocyte progenitor cell growth, suggests potential immunoregulation of CNS physiology. For example, the autoimmune disease multiple sclerosis (MS) has a characteristic depletion of oligodendrocytes in areas of pathological lesions (Andrews, 1972). The speculative extrapolation of cell culture data suggests that lymphokines and monokines can affect the proliferative potential of oligodendrocyte progenitor cells and hence, may partially account for the paucity of oligodendrocytes found in a MS lesion. Monokines, lymphokines, T cells and TAC antibody reacting cells are found within MS lesions (Hofman et al., 1986) indicating the possible validity of our speculation. These data might explain the limited remyelination found in some autoimmune diseases, which may be a function of whether oligodendrocytes can proliferate in respect to astrocytic gliosis.

## ACKNOWLEDGEMENTS

This work was supported by National Institutes of Health Grants HD 06576, CA35299 and AM35411;Department of Energy Contract DE-AC03-76-00012:Basic Research Support Grant from the University of California, Los Angeles, School of Medicine;a Leukemia Society Scholarship to A.A.; and Teacher Investigator Development Award NS00961 to R.L.K.

## REFERENCES

Fontana AB, Kristensen F, Dubs R, Gemsa D, Weber E (1982) Production of prostaglandin E and interleukin 1-like factor by cultured astrocytes and C6 glioma cells. J Immunol 129;2413-2419.

Giulian D, Baker TJ (1986) Characterization of ameboid microglia isolated from developing mammalian brain. J Neurosci 6:2163-2178.

Giulian D, Lachman LB (1985) Interleukin 1 stimulates astroglial proliferation after brain injury. Science 228:497-499.

Benveniste, EN, Merrill JE, Kaufman SE, Golde DW, Gassen JC (1985) Purification and characterization of a human T-lymphocyte-derived glial growth-promoting factor. Proc Natl Acad Sci (USA) 82:3939-3934.

Saneto RP, Altman A, Knobler RL, Johnson HM, de Vellis J (1986) Interleukin 2 mediates the inhibition of oligodendrocyte progenitor cell proliferation in vitro. Proc Natl Acad Sci (USA) 83:9221-9225.

Saneto RP, Chiapelli F, de Vellis J (1987) Interleukin 2 inhibition of oligodendrocyte progenitor cell proliferation depends on expression of the TAC receptor. J Neurosci (in press)

McCarthy KD, de Vellis J (1980) Preparation of separate astroglial and oligodendroglial cell cultures from rat cerebral tissues. J Cell Biol 85: 890-902.

Saneto RP, de Vellis J (1985) Characterization of cultured rat oligodendrocytes proliferating in a serum-free chemically defined medium. Proc Natl Acad Sci (USA) 82:3509-3513.

Bologa L, Cole R, Chiappelli F, Saneto RP, de Vellis J (1987) Serum contains inducers and inhibitors of oligodendrocyte differentiation. (in preparation)

Morgan DA, Fuscetti FW, Gallo RC (1976) Selective in vitro growth of T-lymphocytes from normal human bone marrow. Science 193:1007-1008.

Smith KA (1980) T cell growth factor. Immunol Rev 51:337-357.

Zubler RH, Lowenthal JW, Erard F, Hashimoto N, Devos R, MacDonald HR (1984) Activated B cells express receptors for and proliferate in response to pure interleukin 2. J Exp Med 160:1170-1183.

Robb RJ, Munch A, Smith KA (1981) T cell growth factor receptors. J Exp Med 154:1455-1474.

Weissman AM, Harford JB, Svetlik PB, Leonard WL, Depper JM, Waldmann TA, Greene WC, Klausner RD (1986) Only high affinity receptors for interleukin 2 mediated internalization of ligand. Proc Natl Acad Sci (USA) 83:1463-1466.

Leorard WL, Depper JM, Uchiyama T, Smith KA, Waldmann TA, Greene WC (1982) A monoclonal antibody that appears to recognize the receptor for human T cell growth factor:partial characterization of the receptor. Nature 300:626-631.

Kohda H, Toshimitsu U, Yuasa H, Yamaki T, Osawa H, Diamanstein T, Yodai J. Kikuchi K (1986) Construction of rat-mouse T cell hybridomas that express regulatable rat interleukin 2 receptor. J Immunol 137:1557-1563.

Reem GH, Yeh N-H (1984) Interleukin 2 regulates expression of its receptor and synthesis of gamma interferon by human T lymphocytes. Science 225:429-430.

DeFreitas EC, Sandberg-Wollheim M, Schonely K, Boufal M, Koprowski H (1986) Regulation of interleukin 2 receptors on T cells from multiple sclerosis patients. Proc Natl Acad Sci (USA) 83:2637-2641.

Contrell D, Smith KA (1983) Transient expression of interleukin 2 receptors. Consequences for T-cell growth. J Exp Med 158:1895-1911.

Andrews JM (1972) The ultrastructural neuropathology of multiple sclerosis. In: Hall VE (ed): Multiple Sclerosis UCLA Forum in Medical Sciences. Academic Press, New York, pp 23-49.

Hofman FM, von Hanwehn RI, Dinarello CA, Mizel SB, Hinton D, Merrill JE (1986) Immunoregulatory molecules and IL 2 receptors identified in multiple sclerosis brain. J Immunol 136:3239-3245.

# POSTER ABSTRACTS

# AN INVESTIGATION OF THE ROLE OF PHOSPHATIDYL IONOSITOL TURNOVER IN THE REGENERATING RABBIT PERIPHERAL NERVE TRUNK.

D.R. Archer and W.G. McLean
Department of Pharmacology and Therapeutics,
P.O. Box 147,
Liverpool, L69 3BX,
U.K.

In recent years phosphoinositide metabolism has been implicated in the control of a variety of cellular processes including cell proliferation. The receptor mediated hydrolysis of phosphatidyl inositol, 4,5-bisphosphate produces two second messengers, diacylglycerol and inositol trisphosphate both of which appear to be important in controlling cell growth (Michell, 1982). In the experiments described here we have investigated the role of phosphatidyl inositol turnover during regeneration of the rabbit vagus nerve. The effect of Nerve Growth Factor (NGF) was also studied in this system in order to investigate the role NGF may play in nerve regeneration.

Male New Zealand White rabbits were anaesthetised with a combination of fentanyl, fluanisone and diazepam. One cervical vagus nerve was surgically exposed and crushed with silk thread 40 mm from the nodose ganglion. Seventeen days later, nerve pieces were taken containing the most distal 20mm of the regenerating fibres. An equivalent nerve piece, the same distance from the nodose ganglion, was taken from the contralateral control nerve. Each nerve piece was split in two, desheathed, and incubated with 7.5µCi tritiated inositol in Krebs-Ringer bicarbonate (pH 7.4) for two hours. The preparations were washed twice to remove excess inositol and then incubated in buffer containing 10 mmol/l lithium chloride for one hour. For the final hour-long incubation, 0.1 µmol/l 2.5S NGF was added to one of the two samples from both the control and regenerating nerves. The incubation was terminated by adding TCA. Two fractions were extracted from each sample; a water soluble fraction containing the inositol phosphates and a fraction containing the lipids in the preparation. The water soluble fraction was applied to Dowex anion exchange resin to separate the inositol and the inositol phosphates. The radioactivity in the lipid fraction and in each 2ml fraction eluted from the anion exchange columns was determined by liquid scintillation counting.

The activity within the phosphatidyl inositol cycle was assessed by combining the radioactivity in the fractions associated with inositol mono-, bis- and trisphosphates. The mean radioactivity in inositol phosphates significantly

NATO ASI Series, Vol. H22
Neural Development and Regeneration
Edited by A. Gorio et al.

increased in the regenerating nerve segment (6321 dpm (range 3396-14474)) compared to that in control nerves (3487 dpm (range 2079-5660)), n=7, $p < 0.02$ Wilcoxon rank test. The radioactivity incorporated into inositol phospholipids did not differ significantly in the regenerating nerves (57100 dpm (range 30856-71676)) from that in the control nerves (48554 dpm (range 33018-95074)). The addition of NGF to the final incubation did not cause any significant change from the preparations without NGF for either the activity within the inositol phosphate cycle or the incorporation of tritiated inositol into inositol phospholipids.

Despite an increase in the incorporation of inositol into phospholipids in the nodose ganglion of rengerating rabbit vagus nerves (Archer and McLean 1987), this was not associated with any alteration in phosphatidyl inositol turnover. The increased activity in the phosphatidyl inositol cycle found in this report in regenerating nerves was associated with that part of the preparation which contained the growing axons. A fast axonally transported protein induced during regeneration, is a component of neuronal growth cones (Skene et al, 1986). This protein is likely to be phosphoprotein B50 which has also been reported in growth cones isolated from foetal rat brain (De Graan et al, 1985). It is known that phosphoprotein B50 is a substrate for protein kinase C (Zwiers et al, 1980) and it has been suggested that it plays a role in the modulation of the receptor mediated hydrolysis of phosphoinositides (De Graan et al, 1985). Although this evidence points towards a role for phosphoinositide metabolism in axon regeneration, our preparation also includes many supporting cells which may be involved in a degenerative/regenerative response involving activation of this cycle. Further work is required to determine the exact location of the changes we have described. The present experiments provide no evidence for a role of NGF in the production of these responses.

Archer DR, McLean WG (1987) An investigation of the role of phosphatidyl inositol hydrolysis in regenerating rabbit peripheral nerve. Neurosci Lett Suppl 29:S34.

De Graan PNE, Van Hoof COM, Tilly BC, Oestreicher AB, Schotman P, Gispen WH (1985) Phosphoprotein B-50 in nerve growth cones from fetal rat brain. Neurosci Lett 61:235-241

Michell RH (1982) Inositol lipid metabolism in dividing and differentiating cells. Cell Calcium 3:429-440.

Skene JHP, Jacobson RD, Snipes GJ, McGuire CB, Norden JJ, Freeman JA (1986) A protein associated with axon growth (GAP-43) is a major component of growth cone membranes. Science 233:783-786.

Zwiers H, Schotman P, Gispen WH (1980) Purification and some characteristics of an ACTH-sensitive protein kinase and its substrate kinase in rat brain membranes. J Neurochem 34:1689-1699.

# EFFECT OF EGF ON THE LABELING OF VARIOUS RNA SPECIES AND OF PROTEINS FROM SUBCELLULAR FRACTIONS IN PRIMARY RAT ASTROGLIAL CELL CULTURES.

R. Avola, D.F. Condorelli, L. Turpeenoja, M. Renis, N. Ragusa, F. Ingrao, S. Reale and A.M. Giuffrida Stella.
Institute of Biochemistry, Faculty of Medicine, University of Catania, 95125 Catania, Italy.

The ability of epidermal growth factor (EGF) to stimulate cell growth, proliferation and differentiation has been shown for a variety of cell types. Rat cerebral astrocytes bind high amounts of EGF and are responsive to the mitogenic stimulation of EGF when cultured in serum-free medium (1).

The addition of EGF to primary rat astroglial cell cultures, maintained in serum-free basal medium supplemented with BSA, significantly stimulated the incorporation of labeled precursors into DNA and RNA (2).

In the present study, the effect of EGF on the labeling of the various RNA species and of proteins from subcellular fractions in primary rat astroglial cell cultures was investigated. Cell cultures, prepared as previously described (3), were grown for 14 days *in vitro* in serum supplemented medium. Before addition of EGF (10 ng/ml medium) cell cultures were maintained in serum free-medium (DMEM), supplemented with BSA, for a starvation period of 24 hours. For RNA labeling experiments, [5,6-$^3$H]uridine (5uCi/ml) was added to cells treated with EGF for 6 hours and to control cells; the

NATO ASI Series, Vol. H22
Neural Development and Regeneration
Edited by A. Gorio et al.

incubation was continued for 2 hours. For protein labeling, $[^3H]$amino acid mixture (10 uCi/ml) was added to cells treated with EGF for 2 hours and to control cells; the incubation was continued for 4 hours. Total RNA was extracted by phenol method and the poly(A)$^-$ RNA and the poly(A)$^+$ mRNA were separated by oligo-(dT)-cellulose (4).

The incorporation of $[^3H]$amino acids into glial proteins, was measured in the following subcellular fractions: mitochondria, microsomes, soluble fractions and nuclei. From purified nuclei, the histones and non-histone proteins (NHP) were prepared as previously described (5).

The results indicate a stimulatory effect of EGF on the labeling of the various RNA species and of proteins from all the subcellular fractions examined.

The addition of EGF to astroglial cell cultures increased histone labeling, while total NHP labeling was less modified, except for some proteins with Mw approximately 95,000-83,000 and 44,000 daltons, which were significantly more labeled in EGF treated cells than in controls.

The higher labeling of histones may be correlated with the increased DNA synthesis produced by EGF (2), and the higher labeling of proteins with the increased synthesis of the various RNA species in EGF treated cells. It is probable that EGF stimulates the ability of ribosomes to bind mRNA, leading to an increased protein synthesis.

From these results it seems that EGF treatment may modulate some of the molecular events correlated with the regulation of gene expression in astroglial cells.

Acknowledgments:

Accomplished by financial supports of MPI and CNR Italy.

References:

1) Simpson DC, Morrison R, de Vellis J, Herschman HR (1982) Epidermal growth factor binding and mitogen activity on purified populations of cells from central nervous system. J Neurosci Res 8:453-462

2) Avola R, Condorelli DF, Surrentino S, Turpeenoja L, Costa A, Giuffrida Stella AM (1987) Effect of epidermal growth factor and insulin on DNA and RNA labeling in primary rat astroglial cell cultures. J Neurosci Res (submitted).

3) Avola R, Serra I, Curti D, Lombardo B, Renis M, Condorelli D, Giuffrida AM (1986) Nuclear and mitochondrial DNA synthesis and energy metabolism in primary rat glial cell cultures. Neurochem Res 11:789-8ØØ.

4) Serra I, Cupello A, Gadaleta MN, Viola M, Ragonese P, Giuffrida AM (1983) Labeling of RNA in young and adult rat brain: evidence for different RNA processing. Neurochem Res 8:433-447

5) Serra I, Avola R, Condorelli DF, Surrentino S, Renis M, Kamiyama M, Hashim GA, Giuffrida AM (1986) Acetylation and phosphorylation of histones and non-histone chromosomal proteins in neuronal and glial nuclei purified from cerebral hemispheres of developing rat brain. J Neurochem 46:1881-1887

# MYELIN TREATED MACROPHAGES RELEASE MITOGEN FOR SCHWANN CELLS

R.R.Baichwal, J.W.Bigbee and G.H.DeVries
Department of Biochemistry and Molecular Biophysics
Box 614, MCV Station
Virginia Commonwealth University
Richmond VA 23298

Schwann cell (SC) proliferation is a prominent feature of Wallerian degeneration, however the signal for this response is not yet known. Interruption of cellular contact between SCs (1) or SC and axolemma (2) have been proposed as possible stimuli for SC mitosis. A possible involvement of the myelin sheath has been suggested by Salzer and Bunge (3). Finally, the role of macrophages (macs) has been implicated by Beuche and Friede (4) who correlate SC division with mac phagocytosis of myelin debris. We have previously shown that cultured SCs prepared from sciatic nerves of two day old rat pups proliferate in response to an exogenously added rat CNS myelin- (MEF) and axolemma-enriched fraction (AEF) (5). We are studying the role of macs in mediating the mitogenic response of cultured SCs to MEF using cultured rat peritoneal macs. We have shown that conditioned medium (CM) from rat peritoneal macs which have phagocytosed rat CNS MEF is mitogenic to SCs.

Phagocytosis of the MEF by cultured peritoneal macs has been confirmed by electron microscopy. Time course for the production of the mitogenic CM by macs incubated with MEF was studied. Mac cultures were incubated either alone or in the presence of 200ug protein/ml of rat MEF for time periods varying from 8 to 48 hours. Following incubation, the CM was filtered and added to SC cultures after diluting 1:1 with incubation medium. The proliferation of SCs was measured by autoradiography as previously described (6). The mitogenicity of the CMs increased with increasing time periods of incubation with a maximum response at 48h. CMs from mac cultures incubated with increasing amounts of MEF for 48h showed a dose dependent increase in mitogenicity to SCs. The production of the mitogenic CM was found to be specific to myelin membranes, as the addition of an AEF did not stimulate the production of a mitogenic CM nor did incubation with rat

NATO ASI Series, Vol. H22
Neural Development and Regeneration.
Edited by A. Gorio et al.

liver microsomes, polystyrene beads or lipopolysaccharide. The production of the mitogenic CM is not species restricted, as MEFs from rat, bovine and human CNS and PNS produce a CM mitogenic for rat cultured SCs . CM obtained by the addition of PNS MEFs is 2-3 times less mitogenic than the CNS MEF supernatants. The mitogenic factor(s) present in the mac CM is sensitive to heat and trypsin treatment suggesting that it may be a polypeptide. The mitogenicity of the CM is decreased by 60% when mac cultures are treated with 7mM ammonium chloride, an inhibitor of lysosomal activity. Whether the mitogenic factor is an intrinsic part of the myelin membrane or is synthesized by the macs has not yet been determined. The mitogenic factor does not appear to be IL-1 because, commercially available IL-1 is not mitogenic for cultured SCs. Our observation that MEF and not AEF CM is mitogenic to SCs supports our previous findings that two distinct mitogenic signals exist in fractionated nervous tissue. We propose that SC proliferation in Wallerian degeneration, may be due to a soluble mitogenic factor released by the macs involved in the removal of myelin debris. [Supported by NS 15408 and NS 10821 (Javits Neuroscience Grant)].

1. Crang AJ, Blakemore WF (1986) Observations on Wallerian Degeneration in explant cultures of cat sciatic nerve. J Neurocytol 15:471-482
2. Pellegrino RG, Politis MJ, Ritchie JM, Spencer PS (1986) Events in degenerating cat peripheral nerve : induction of Schwann cell S phase and its relation to nerve fibre degeneration. J Neurocytol 15:17-28
3. Salzer JL, Bunge RP (1980) Studies of Schwann cell proliferation: I. An analysis in tissue culture of proliferation during development, Wallerian Degeneration and direct injury. J Cell Biol 84:739-752
4. Beuche W, Friede, RL (1984) The role of non-resident cells in Wallerian degeneration. J Neurocytol 13:767-796
5. Yoshino JE, Dinneen MP, Lewis BL, Meader-Woodruff JH, DeVries GH (1984) Differential proliferative responses of cultured Schwann cells to axolemma- and myelin-enriched fractions. I. Biochemical Studies. J Cell Biol 99:2309-2313
6. Baichwal RR, Yan L, Bosler A, DeVries GH (to be published) An automated method for autoradiographic analysis of cultured Schwann cells. J Neurosci Methods

# COMPARATIVE STRUCTURAL FEATURES OF NERVE GROWTH FACTOR AND ITS RECEPTOR

C. Beck, K. Werrbach-Perez, M. Blum, K. Hubner and J.R. Perez-Polo.
Department of Human Biological Chemistry and Genetics
University of Texas Medical Branch
Galveston, Texas, 77550

INTRODUCTION: The nerve growth factor protein, NGF, is a subunit containing protein that plays a central role during developmental events associated with neuronal cell death, neurite extension and synapse formation in peripheral neurons of sensory and sympathetic ganglia. Also, NGF has been shown to allow recuperative and regenerative events for some central and peripheral neuronal structures. Lastly, it has been demonstrated that NGF has mitogenic effects on neural crest precursor cells and on cells of the immune system although the role of NGF in the development of the immune system is not known. It is known, however, that in all instances where NGF effects have been demonstrated, the NGF effect is initiated by binding of the NGF beta subunit in a specific and saturable fashion to cell surface NGF receptors, NGFR. In order to better understand the mechanism of action of NGF, we have studied structural features of the NGF molecule and its receptor derived from different cell types and species.

NGF: Although similar in many respects, there are also important differences in the subunit composition of the NGF molecules isolated from different species. In spite of consistent amino acid and DNA sequence homologies among all beta NGF molecules these different NGF forms express different epitopes as judged by antisera crossreaction

NATO ASI Series, Vol. H22
Neural Development and Regeneration
Edited by A. Gorio et al.

determinations and are highly specific in assembling with alpha and gamma subunits.

| SPECIES | TISSUE | ALPHA | BETA | GAMMA |
|---|---|---|---|---|
| Snake | Venom | - | + | + |
| Mouse | Submaxillary Gland | + | + | + |
| Rat | Submaxillary Gland | + | + | ? |
| Guinea Pig | Prostate | ? | + | - |
| Bovine | Seminal vesicle | ? | + | - |
| Human | Placenta | + | + | - |

Beta NGF of murine origin is equally active on chick, rat, mouse or human NGF responsive neurons. Murine and human beta NGF can displace each other from human neuroblastoma cells. Beta NGF isolated from human term placenta has an amino acid composition, isoelectric point and molecular weight that is very similar to its murine counterpart. Also, tryptic digests of murine beta NGF generated with pepsin and analyzed by SDS PAGE would suggest that these two proteins are very similar. These findings are in keeping with available DNA sequence data.

NGFR: For sympathetic and sensory ganglia, NGFR binding exhibits two equilibrium dissociation constants of $10^{-9}$ and $10^{-11}$M. Rat and human lymphocytes as well as rat astrocytes, on the other hand, display only receptors for NGF with a Kd of $10^{-9}$M. SDS-PAGE analysis of cell surface $^{125}$Iodinated proteins following immunoprecipitation with MC192 would suggest that lymphocytes have NGFR with strong similarities to its neuronal counterpart. For PC12 we find an 207 KDa and an 63 KDa NGFR whereas on rat lymphocytes we find an 178 KDa and 119 KDa molecular species of NGFR.

CONCLUSIONS: These studies would suggest that there are structural similarities in the NGF and the NGFR present in different tissues. Given the different effects of NGF in these tissues, defining these differences might help us to understand the biological significance of the interactions between NGFR, NGF and the second messengers acting in these NGF responsive cells. Supported in part by NINCDS Grant NS 18708.

# FETAL SPINAL CORD HOMOGRAFTS REDUCE EXPECTED HIND LIMB DEFICITS FROM SPINAL CERVICAL FASICULUS GRACILIS LESION

Jerald J. Bernstein and William J. Goldberg
Laboratory of Central Nervous System Injury and Regeneration, VA Medical Center, Washington, DC, 20422, USA; Departments of Neurosurgery and Physiology, George Washington University

Dorsal column (DC) lesion at T13 resulted in a reorganization of the synaptic circuitry in the rat DC-lemniscal system and somatomotor cortex. This lesion resulted in hind limb slips from a platform that appear 60-120 days after the lesion[1]. The present study explored the ability of fetal spinal cord grafts into C3 fasiculus gracilis (FG; similar to a T13 DC lesion) to influence hind limb performance.

Ten adult Sprague-Dawley rats were placed on a schedule of 23-h off and 1-h on water schedule and preoperatively trained to traverse a narrow platform for water. Criterion was 10 trials completed in 15-s for two consecutive days. Hind and fore limb performance was ranked for slips, recovery and manner of traverse. The animal numbers were coded, laminectomy performed at C3 and the FG aspirated. Five randomly chosen subjects had two, one mm segments of E14 spinal cord placed in the aspiration pocket. Coded lesion-alone and lesion-grafted animals were tested at 21,30,45,60 and 90 days later until criterion or for 4 days.

Ranked scores were statistically analyzed from coded data by a non-parametric Friedman two-way analysis of variance *a priori* and the Mann-Whitney U test *a posteriori* (Fig.). Hind limb performance of lesion alone (ANOVA $X^2$=13.04, df=5; $p<0.05$) and lesion-graft groups (ANOVA $X^2$=11.82, df=5; $p<0.05$) showed that the C3 fetal grafts significantly decreased ($p<0.05$) the effect of spinal shock due to the lesion-alone by reduced severity of hind limb deficit at 21 days and significantly

NATO ASI Series, Vol. H22
Neural Development and Regeneration
Edited by A. Gorio et al.

($p<0.05$) decreased the expected foot slips and limb recovery expected at 90 days. There were no deficits in fore limb performance (ANOVAs $p>0.05$).

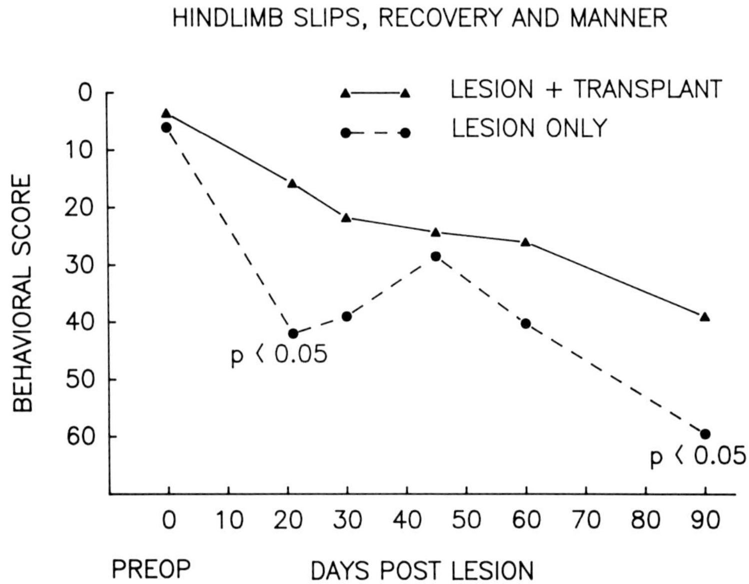


There were statistically significant ANOVAS for the lesion only ($X^2=13.04$, df=5; $p<0.05$) and lesion-transplant groups ($X^2=11.82$, df=5; $p<0.05$). Differences between groups was analyzed with the Mann-Whitney U test. There were significant differences ($p<0.05$) at 21 and 90 days.

There were a few small caliber nerve fibers in the FG at the level of C1. For this reason the graft induced decreased severity of deficit appeared to be due to the trophic and tropic aspects of the transplant. It has recently been shown that graft derived astrocytes migrate into the nucleus gracilis of the medulla after T6 spinal implantation[2]. These migrated astrocytes may be part of the mechanism for the reduction of the hind limb deficit.

[1]Bernstein JJ., Ganchrow D, Wells M (1983) Nervous System Regeneration, (Giuffrida-Stella A et al eds.), Alan R. Liss, NY 135-149.
[2]Goldberg W, Bernstein JJ (1987) Transplant derived astrocytes migrate into host lumbar and cervical spinal cord after implantation of E14 fetal cerebral cortex into adult thoracic spinal cord. J Neurosci Res 17: (in press).

# THE TEMPORAL RELATION BETWEEN A CORNEAL NEURONOTROPHIC FACTOR AND CORNEAL NERVE REGENERATION

Kwan Y. Chan
Department of Ophthalmology
University of Washington
Seattle, WA 98195
U.S.A.

Epithelial neuronotrophic factor (ENF) is a protein secreted specifically by cultured corneal and conjunctival epithelial cells of rabbit (1,2). It is absent in corneal fibroblasts and endothelial cells (1), or epithelial cells of the lens, retina, skin, and kidney (2). ENF acts selectively on cultured sensory neurons (trigeminal and dorsal root ganglia) by both prolonging their survival and inducing neurite outgrowth (1,2). It has no effect on sympathetic neurons. ENF also stimulates protein synthesis in cultured trigeminal neurons, such as glycoproteins (independent of sprouting) and proline-labeled proteins (neurite-dependent), including collagens that are deposited extracellularly (3). The newly-synthesized proteins are increasingly distributed to both the particulate (somata) and neurite fractions with time. Indirect evidence suggests that ENF is not NGF, collagen, fibronectin, laminin or certain glycosaminoglycans (4). Presumably, ENF belongs to a class of endogenous trophic factors that are secreted by tissues to initiate and maintain proper innervation by neurons.

A comparative study on neonatal and adult rabbits has shown that neonatal corneal epithelial cells secrete more ENF than the adult counterpart (2). In addition, neonatal trigeminal neurons are more responsive to ENF than the adult neurons. It is conceivable that ENF may play a role in the development of corneal nerves. In this study the role of ENF in corneal nerve regeneration in the adult was investigated.

A model of heptanol-induced epithelial wounding was utilized to remove completely a circular area of corneal epithelium (4 mm diameter) including all the intraepithelial nerves. In this model, natural wound closure was completed after 2 days (effected by epithelial cell migration). Regeneration of the epithelial multilayers occurred after 3-4 days. By 1 wk after wounding, the epithelium was normal in thickness.

Wounded and unwounded (control) corneas were excised weekly during 4 wks and placed in organ culture to collect ENF that was secreted from the epithelium. A neuronal bioassay based on neurite outgrowth of neonatal

NATO ASI Series, Vol. H22
Neural Development and Regeneration
Edited by A. Gorio et al.

trigeminal neurons was utilized to quantify ENF. The ratios of total ENF released per wounded cornea to that per control cornea were 1.4, 2.4 ($p < 0.05$), 2.1 and 1.2, respectively, at 1, 2, 3 and 4 wks.

The gold chloride impregnation technique was utilized to visualize corneal nerves and monitor nerve regeneration. Morphometry was undertaken to determine corneal neural density at 0, 1.5 (both inside the wounded area) and 3 mm (outside the wound) radial distance from the center. In the control epithelium, neural density was highest at the center and gradually decreased towards the periphery. In the wounded corneas, the intraepithelial nerve arborizations were absent after 1 wk, being replaced by parallel-running, wound-oriented neurites. This contributed to a transient increase in neural density at the wound periphery (98% greater than the control). At 2 wks, the first sign of regeneration of permanent nerves was observed, with a simultaneous decline in the wound-oriented neurites. The neural density inside the wounded area was 64-88% less than the control. Beginning at 3 wks, the wound-oriented neurites were completely absent, while the permanent nerve arborizations appeared normal and typical. The normal pattern of centripetal increase of neural density was restored, but numerically the densities were 34-47% less than the control. Thus, corneal nerves were partially regenerated 3 wks after wounding.

In conclusion, a surge in ENF secretion occurred 2 wks after wound-induced denervation of the corneal epithelium, preceding the subsequent nerve regeneration by 1 wk. It was unlikely that this increased trophic activity in the corneal epithelium was related causally to epithelial cell migration during wound closure, epithelial mitosis during epithelial regeneration or the appearance of the transient, wound-oriented neurites. The results suggest that ENF may mediate corneal nerve regeneration. (Supported by EY04538 from NIH.)

(1) Chan KY, Haschke RH (1982) Exp Eye Res 35:137-156
(2) Chan KY, Haschke RH (1985) Exp Eye Res 41:687-699
(3) Chan KY, Haschke RH, Kapoor R (1986) Trans Am Soc Neurochem 17:309
(4) Chan KY, Haschke RH (1981) J Neurosci 1:1155-1162

# SLOW AXONAL TRANSPORT IN NERVE FROM MICE WITH A GENETIC MYELIN DEFICIENCY (TREMBLER)

S. Kint de Waegh, S. Brady
Department of Cell Biology
University of Texas Health Science Center at Dallas
5323 Harry Hines Boulevard
Dallas, Texas 75235
U.S.A.

In a myelinated nerve, there is a relation between axonal diameter and the size of its myelin sheath: the larger the diameter of the axon, the thicker the myelin sheath. When the axonal diameter increases above 1 micron during development or regeneration, myelin formation in surrounding Schwann cells is triggered. However, recent studies suggest that the relation between axon and Schwann cell is more complex. In experiments involving sciatic nerve grafts between the normal and the myelin deficient mutant Trembler mice, Schwann cells were shown to locally influence the morphology and the diameter of axons (A.Aguayo 1977). Axonal diameter is dependent on its cytoskeleton and the cytoskeletal proteins are moving along the axon with the slow components of axonal transport. When slow axonal transport of the cytoskeletal protein decreases, as during regeneration for instance, one observes that the reduction in transport correlates with the decrease in axonal diameter. This has been quantified by Hoffman et al. for the neurofilament protein (Hoffman 1986). We are using the Trembler mouse as an experimental model to analyze the local effect of poorly myelinating Schwann cells on the slow axonal transport of the cytoskeleton.

To study the slow axonal transport, 0.3 mci of $^{35}$S-methionine is injected in the dorsal root ganglion (DRG) of normal control C57BL/6N mice and Trembler mice. Three to 14 days after the injection, the mice are decapitated and the sciatic nerve is removed, frozen and cut in consecutive segments of 1.5 mm each. The distribution of labeled cytoskeletal proteins is then analyzed using SDS gel electrophoresis, fluorography and liquid scintillation counting. Studies in the sciatic nerve of normal mouse have shown that the rates for slow component A (SCa) and

NATO ASI Series, Vol. H22
Neural Development and Regeneration
Edited by A. Gorio et al.

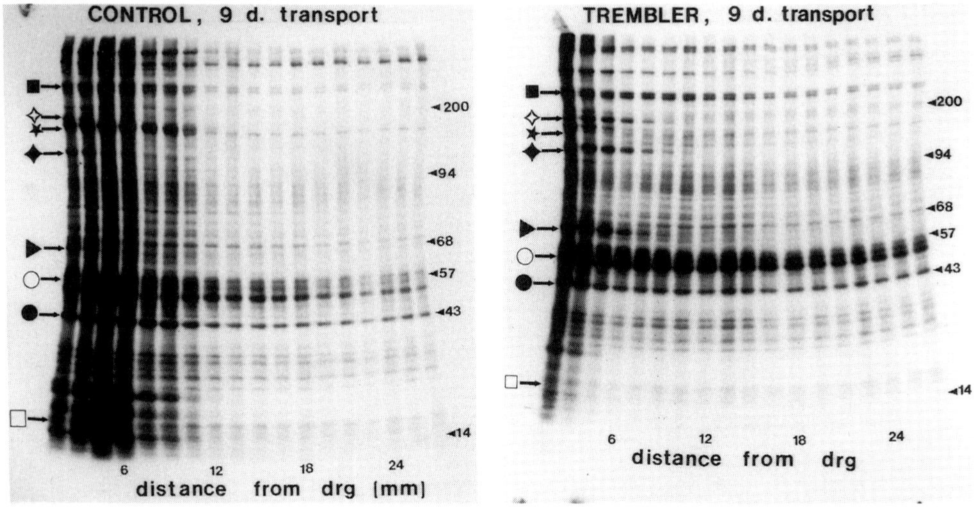


Fig. 1: Fluorographs of transported labeled proteins 9 days after injection of $^{35}$S-methionine. Consecutive 1.5 mm segments of sciatic nerve from normal and Trembler mice were analyzed by SDS gel electrophoresis. Gels were exposed to obtain similar density of the actin bands in the two fluorographs. Marker proteins are indicated as follows: (■)spectrin, (✧) NF200, (✶) clathrin, (✦)NF145, (►)NF68, (o) tubulin, (●) actin, (□)calmodulin.

slow component B (SCb) are similar to those previously measured in spinal motor axons in the rat (McOuarrie 1986). The radiolabeled tubulin peak moves into the nerve at the rate of 1.64 mm/day. Neurofilament triplet (NFT) is transported slightly slower at 1.36 mm/day. Marker proteins for SCb of axonal transport also show two different velocities; spectrin and clathrin peaks are moving along the axon at a rate of 3.55 mm/day and calmodulin and actin are slightly slower at 3.0 mm/day. Fluorographs of transported proteins from Trembler and normal mice are compared for similar experimental conditions to analyze the influence of poor myelination on the slow axonal transport (Fig. 1). Comparison indicates the existence of qualitative variations. In the Trembler mouse, the relative amount of tubulin seems greater than the normal mouse. There is also a change in the proportion of tubulin transported with SCa and SCb. In Trembler mice, more tubulin is carried with SCa and neurofilaments are comparatively more heavily labeled. By contrast, the relative amount of clathrin in SCb seems reduced. Initial results suggest that there may be differences in rate as well as in composition between normal and Trembler mice. The differences noted in slow axonal transport between normal and myelin deficient Trembler mice reinforce the hypothesis that there is a complex local relation between the Schwann cells and the axon.

---

Aguayo A (1977) Abnormal myelination in transplanted Trembler mouse Schwann cells. Nature 265:73-75

Hoffman PN, Thompson GW, Griffin JW, Price DL (1985) Changes in neurofilament transport coincide temporally with alterations in the caliber of axons in regenerating motor fibers. J Cell Biol 101:1332-1340

McQuarrie IG, Brady ST, Lasek RJ (1986) Diversity of axonal transport of structural proteins: Major differences between optic and spinal axons in the rat J. Neuroscience 6(6):1593-1605

# BEHAVIOURAL AND IMMUNOLOGICAL CHANGES IN THE AGING RAT

P. Foresta, O. Ghirardi, C. Albertoni, M.T. Ramacci, L. Angelucci*

Sigma Tau Biological Research Laboratories

00040 Pomezia

Italy

Main features of the aging process in the rat are marked changes in immunological activities and in behavioural performances.

Both of them can be attributed to a progressive loss of integration within the brain and between the brain on one hand and the neuroendocrine and immunological systems on the other.

The aim of the present investigation was to ascertain the parallelism of these changes through a compared evaluation of behavioural and immunological parameters occurring at various stages in the course of aging in populations kept in the same environmental and chronological settings from birth to death.

Male Sprague Dawley rats (Charles River) were used for the behavioural study at 4,14 and 23 months of age and for immunological responsiveness evaluation at 2,5,16 and 28 months of age.

The behavioural study (swimming activity in ten minute periods for nine consecutive days) showed a progressive phenomenon of passiveness, proportional in intensity to degree of aging (Tab. 1) and not due to aging related muscular inability; in fact natatory activity in the first session was exactly the same in all animal age-groups.

The immunological study using the delayed type hypersensitivity test (DTH, subcutaneous injection of BCG vaccine, followed 11 days later by inoculation of 20 ug PPD in middle line of the ear) demonstrated a decrease in responsiveness as a function of age (Tab. 2).

---

* Dept. of Pharmacology II, "La Sapienza" University of Rome, Italy

NATO ASI Series, Vol. H22
Neural Development and Regeneration
Edited by A. Gorio et al.

This was in agreement with a concomitant decrease in blood and spleen lymphocytes (Tab. 2).

**Table 1. Number of movements (crossings of photocell beam) in the first 5 min of each session. Mean ± S.E.M.**

| Age in months | Sessions 1 | 3 | 5 | 7 | 9 |
|---|---|---|---|---|---|
| 4 (n=10) | 108±3 | 104±5 | 118±4 | 102±4 | 91±11 |
| 14 (n=9) | 106±4 | 106±5 | 90±8°° | 82±5°° | 81±7 |
| 23 (n=10) | 104±3 | 77±9°° | 66±9°°° | 64±6°°° | 58±7°° |

Student's "t" test vs. 4-month old rats; °° and °°°: p = .01 and .001, respectively.

**Tab. 2. DTH response and cell counts in rats at various ages. Mean ± S.E.M.**

| Age in months | DTH Ear thickness ($\Delta$ mm) | BLOOD WBCx$10^3$ | Lymphocytes % | Neutrophils % | SPLEEN n° cells x$10^7$ |
|---|---|---|---|---|---|
| 2 (n=10) | 0.72±0.15 | 22.8±1.7 | 81.9±1.8 | 13.9±1.3 | 65.8±6.5 |
| 5 (n=15) | 1.10±0.08 | 24.7±2.2 | 78.0±1.2 | 17.0±1.2 | 61.8±3.0 |
| 16 (n=14) | 0.60±0.12°° | 19.3±1.8 | 68.7±2.7°° | 26.0±2.5 | 57.4±4.4 |
| 28 (n=5) | 0.48±0.20° | 13.5±1.1°° | 50.2±5.8°° | 43.2±5.9° | 39.6±5.2° |

Dunnett test vs. 5-month old rats; ° and °°: p= .05 and .01, respectively.

We interpret the change in behavioural response as indicating a different emotional reaction during repeated exposures to the same ambient conditions in rats at different ages.

According to Williams (1971), number of movements in such situation is inversely proportional to emotional activation (stress). On one side, reduced behavioural adaptation capacity may be attributed to the loss of hippocampal control, occurring with aging (Angelucci 1986), on these behavioural and endocrine parameters which are largely related to the hippocampus function.

On the other side reduced function of the immune system in the aged rat is due to the decline of thymus function, namely reduced production of thymic hormones.

According to this, the DTH reaction, a typical manifestation of cellular immune competence mediated by T cells, shows a reduction with increasing age.

Considerable experimental evidence has ascertained interconnections and mutual influences between the thymus and the neuroendocrine system, particularly the hypothalamo-pituitary-adrenocortical axis (Fabris 1981).

The intricate connections in the psychoneuroendocrinoimmunological activity at the basis of the changes in behaviour and immunological responsiveness in aging, make necessary the use of a multi-disciplinary approach for the proper understanding of our experimental results.

## REFERENCES

Williams D I (1971) Maze exploration in the rat under different levels of illumination. Anim Behav 19: 365-367

Angelucci L, Ghirardi O, Patacchioli FR, Ramacci MT (1986) Disinhibition of the hypothalamo - pituitary - adrenocortical axis as a marker of brain aging in the rat: a model for the study of anti-aging agents. Clin Neuropharmacol 9: 104-106

Fabris N, Piantanelli L (1981) In: Adelman R, Roth J (eds) Hormones and aging. CRC Press, Palm Beach

# MORPHOLOGICAL AND BIOCHEMICAL EFFECTS ON STRIATAL ASTROCYTES AFTER CO-CULTIVATION WITH SUBSTANTIA NIGRA NEURONS IN PRIMARY CELL CULTURE

E. Hansson[1] and L. Rönnbäck[1, 2]
Institute of Neurobiology[1]
and Dept. of Neurology[2]
University of Göteborg
P.O.B. 33 031
S-400 33 Göteborg
Sweden

Summary: A co-cultivation system was developed with neuron-enriched primary cell cultures from substantia nigra, grown 1 mm apart from astroglial primary cell cultures from striatum. The astrocytes went through a morphological differentiation with extension of processes after co-cultivation. The astrocytes also showed a higher active uptake of $^{3}$H-L-glutamate and a slightly increased glutamine synthetase (GS) activity after co-cultivation, compared to controls.

Astrocytes constitute a large volume of the brain (Pope, 1978) Due to their anatomical proximity to neurons and the synaptic regions, the cells might be involved in neuronal metabolic events. Several reports on transmitter-induced biochemical effects on astrocytes, and on active membrane properties of these cells, have appeared recently. They act as $K^+$-buffers (Kuffler and Nicholls, 1966), participate in uptake and metabolism of amino acid transmitters (Hertz and Schousboe, 1980; Hansson, 1986a), and bear receptors for various neurotransmitters and neuromodulators (van Calker and Hamprecht, 1980; Hansson, 1987). Consequently, it could be suggested that the cells play an important role for the functions of neurons. Cell culture technique has the advantage that one cell type can be enriched, and in primary cell cultures from newborn rat most of the cells stain positively for glial fibrillary acidic protein (GFAp) and S-100 (Hansson et al., 1984). However, their degree of differentiation is not as high as in the adult brain and could be due to growth in the absence of neurons. One way to increase the differentiation of the astrocytes in culture would be to co-cultivate astroglial cultures with neuronal cultures. The cells should grow in the near vicinity of each

NATO ASI Series, Vol. H22
Neural Development and Regeneration
Edited by A. Gorio et al.

other, while remaining physically separated and allowing humoral transfer. This study reports on a technique for co-cultivation of astrocytes from striatum and neurons from substantia nigra where morphological and biochemical effects on the astrocytes are described.

Cultivation of astroglial primary cell cultures from newborn rat striatum was done according to Hansson and co-workers (1984).

Cultivation of neuronal primary cell cultures from 15-17-day fetal rat Substantia nigra was done according to Hansson (1986c), with some modifications. The cell medium was changed after 1 and 6 days. At 6 days, the cultures were treated with cytosine arabinoside to curtail astrocytic growth, and only 10% (v/v) fetal calf-serum was used instead of 20%.

Ten days after seeding, the substantia nigra cultures were placed above 3-day old striatum cultures. The co-cultivation procedure has been described recently (Hansson, 1986 b,c).

Uptake of $^{3}$H-L-glutamate and the glutamine synthetase assay were done according to Hansson (1986d).

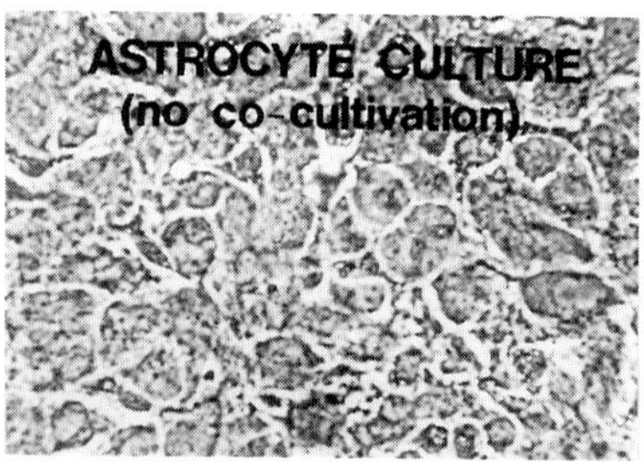


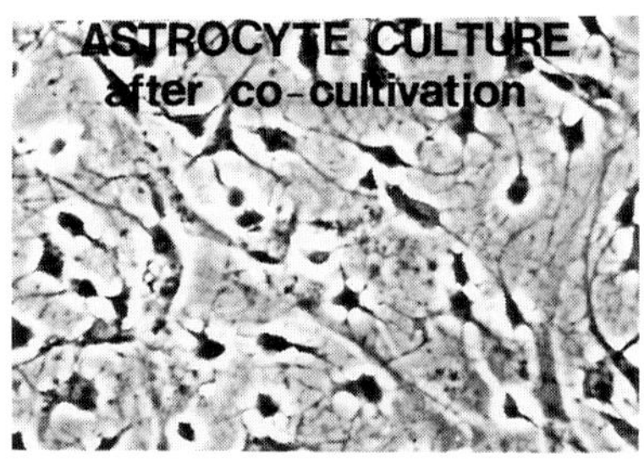


Fig. 1 a) Striatal astrocytes in primary cell culture. No co-cultivation. There are few or no visible processes.

b) Striatal astrocytes after co-cultivation with substantia nigra neurons. The astrocytes are polygonal and spindle-shaped with long branching processes.

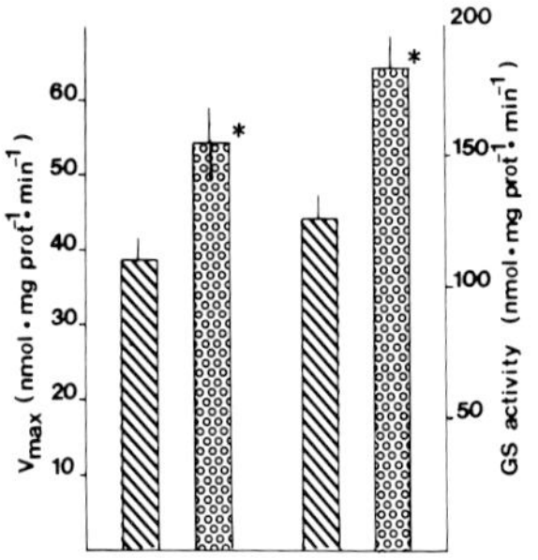


Fig. 2 $^{3}$H-glutamate uptake represented as $V_{max}$ (nmol· mg prot$^{-1}$· min$^{-1}$) and glutamine synthetase activity (nmol· mg prot$^{-1}$·min$^{-1}$) in striatal astrocytes after co-cultivation with substantia nigra neurons.
▧ = control
* $p<0.05$, Student's t-test

Most of the cells in the striatal primary cell culture from newborn rat have previously been characterized as being astrocytes, as they stain positively for glial-fibrillary acidic protein (GFAp) and S-100 (Hansson et al., 1984). No neurons have been detected in these cultures. In the primary cultures from embryonic rats, the majority of cells stained with antibodies against the neuron-specific enolase (NSE) and were thus considered neurons (Hansson, 1986c). When the neuron-containing cultures had grown 1 mm apart from the astrocyte culture for one week, the astrocytes adopted a differentiated appearance from a morphological point of view with extension of long processes, and a more spindle-shaped appearance compared to controls (Fig. 1). The $^{3}$H-glutamate uptake and glutamine synthetase activity increased also in the astrocyte cultures, suggesting a biochemical differentiation (Fig. 2). The influence of neurons in one brain region on astrocytes in another region constituting a natural projection area for the neuronal pathways in a co-cultivation system, emphasizes the possibility of restoring _in situ_ some of the direct interactions which may occur between cells _in vivo_.

This study received support from the Swedish Medical Research Council (project Nos. 12X-06812, 12P-7308), from Åke Wiberg's and Magnus Bergvall's Foundations.

Hansson E (1986a) Primary astroglial cultures. A biochemical and functional evaluation. Neurochem Res 11:759-767

Hansson E (1986b) Co-cultivation of astroglial and neuronal primary cultures from rat brain. Brain Res 366:159-168

Hansson E (1986c) Co-cultivation of astroglial enriched cultures from striatum and neuronal containing cultures from substantia nigra. Life Sciences 39:269-277

Hansson E (1986d) Primary cultures from defined brain areas. III. Effects of seeding time on $^{3}$H-L-glutamate transport and glutamine synthetase activity. Dev Brain Res 24:203-209

Hansson E (1987) Astroglia from defined brain regions as studied with primary cultures. In: Kerkut GA, Phillis JW (eds) Progress in Neurobiology. Pergamon Press, Oxford, in press

Hansson E, Rönnbäck L, Persson LI, Lowenthal A, Noppe M, Alling C, Karlsson B (1984) Cellular composition of primary cultures from cerebral cortex, striatum, hippocampus, brain stem and cerebellum. Brain Res 300:9-18

Hertz L, Schousboe A (1980) Interactions between neurons and astrocytes in the turnover of GABA and glutamate. Brain Res Bull 5: Suppl 2:389-395

Kuffler SW, Nicholls JG (1966) The physiology in neuroglial cells. Ergebn Physiol Biol Chem Exp Pharmakol 57:1-90

Pope A (1978) Neuroglia: quantitative aspects. In: Schoffeniels E, Franck G, Tower DB, Hertz L (eds) Dynamic properties of glia cells. Pergamon Press, Oxford, p 13

van Calker D, Hamprecht B (1980) Effects of neurohormones on glial cells. In: Fedoroff S, Hertz L (eds) Advances in cellular neurobiology, vol. I Academic Press, New York, p 31

# NERVE GROWTH FACTOR-MEDIATED INDUCTION OF CHOLINE ACETYLTRANSFERASE IN FETAL AND NEONATAL RAT SEPTAL CHOLINERGIC NEURONS IN ORGANOTYPIC CULTURE.

Hiroshi Hatanaka
Nobuyuki Takei
Hiroko Tsukui
Department of Neuroscience
Mitsubishi-Kasei Institute of Life Sciences
11 Minamiooya, Machida-shi
Tokyo 194,
Japan

Nerve growth factor (NGF) is thought to be synthesized in the hippocampus and neocortex regions in CNS and to be transported retrogradely to basal forebrain cholinergic neurons which have sufficient NGF binding sites (Korsching et al.; 1985). The dissociated cultured cells from fetal rat septum have NGF-responsible choline acetyltransferase (ChAT) activities (Hefti et al.; 1985). In addition to the septal cells, we have previously reported that NGF-mediated induction of ChAT activities occurred in the dissociated cultured cells from fetal rat amygdala and striatum among the tested six different cholinergic areas in CNS (Hatanaka, Tsukui; 1986). In the present study, we examined the effect of NGF on the organotypic cultured septal pieces from fetal and neonatal rats.

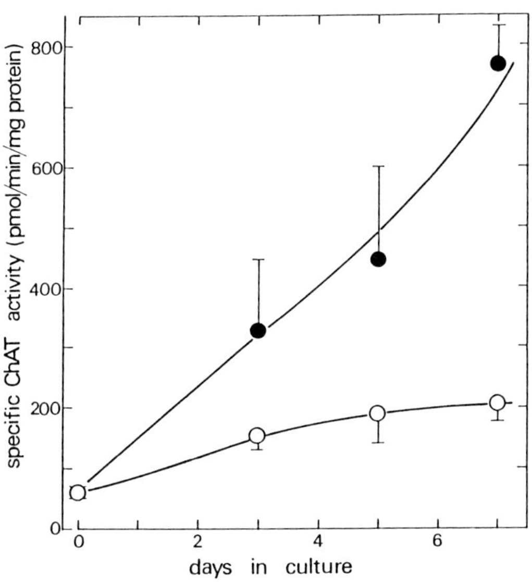


Fig. 1. Culture time-dependent increase of ChAT activities in organotypic E17 septal culture by NGF. Culture was done as described in the legend to Table 1. Closed and open circles represent with and without NGF (100ng/ml), respectively. Values were means±S.D. (n=4).

Fig. 1 shows the culture time-dependent change of ChAT activities in the organotypic cultured E17 septal pieces. The ChAT activities in cultures without NGF gradually increased. The activities with NGF increased remarkably. The activities relative to the culture without NGF at 7 days in culture was 370%. This induction was completely abolished by the addition of specific antibodies to NGF. And also, the addition of the

NATO ASI Series, Vol. H22
Neural Development and Regeneration
Edited by A. Gorio et al.

Table 1. Effects of NGF on ChAT activities of organotypic septal culture obtained from E17-P7 rats.

| rat age | NGF addition | organotypic culture | sliced culture | monolayer culture |
|---|---|---|---|---|
| | | specific ChAT activities in | | |
| | | (pmol/min/mg protein) | | |
| E17 | none | 154 ± 32 | | 115 ± 8 |
| | NGF | 411 ± 104 | | 321 ± 38 |
| E19 | none | 213 ± 13 | | 73.7 ± 14.6 |
| | NGF | 582 ± 59 | | 120 ± 16 |
| E22 | none | 189 ± 41 | 87.7 ± 32.6 | |
| | NGF | 585 ± 302 | 321 ± 177 | |
| P1 | none | | 86.9 ± 60.0 | |
| | NGF | | 367 ± 90 | |
| P3 | none | 64.5 ± 12.6 | | |
| | NGF | 154 ± 68 | | |
| P7 | none | 8.3 ± 2.4 | | |
| | NGF | 21.8 ± 9.1 | | |

The septum was dissected out from Wistar rats (E17-P7) and were cut into small pieces of ca 1mm$^3$. Alternatively, sliced pieces were also used after the 0.4mm slicing. Monolayer culture was done as described previously (Hatanaka, Tsukui; 1986). Several pieces were placed on polyethylenimine-coated 24-well plates. After the 24hr in culture by using sera-containing medium, medium was changed to serum-free TIP/DF medium (Hatanaka, 1981). NGF was added at 100ng/ml. ChAT activities were determined by the previous method after the cell disruption by sonication. Protein was determined by Lowrey et al. Values were means±S.D. (n=4).

antibodies to the culture without NGF decreased by a 22%, meaning that the synthesis of a low amount of endogenous NGF in the culture occurred. The organotypic cultures of E17 amygdala and striatum were also carried out as the same manner as septum. NGF could induce the ChAT activities in the both cultures, though at low level induction. Table 1 represents the effect of NGF on ChAT activities in septal organotypic cultures prepared from the different ages of rats. The cultivation was possible until P7 postnatal rats in this study. The ChAT activities in cultures without NGF and also the NGF-responses among the pieces obtained from embryonic rats. Even at P7 septal pieces in culture, NGF was found to increase the ChAT activity. However, the ChAT activities in the postnatal rat decreased. These results suggest that NGF might have the ability to affect the cholinergic property of the septal neurons from postnatal rats.

Hatänaka H (1981) Nerve growth factor-mediated stimulation of tyrosine hydroxylase activity in a clonal rat pheochromocytoma cell line. Brain Res., **222**: 225-233.

Hatanaka H, Tsukui H (1986) Differential effects of nerve growth factor and glioma-conditioned medium on neurons cultured from various regions of fetal rat central nervous system. Develop. Brain Res., **30**: 47-56.

Hefti F, Hartikka J, Eckenstein F, Gnahn H, Heumann R, Schwab M (1985) Nerve growth factor increases choline acetyltransferase but not survival or fiber outgrowth of cultured fetal septal cholinergic neurons. Neurosci., **14**: 55-68.

Korsching S, Auburger G, Heumann R, Scott J, Thoenen H (1985) Levels of nerve growth factor and its mRNA in the central nervous system of the rat correlate with cholinergic innervation. EMBO J., **4**: 1389-1393.

# THE DEVELOPMENTAL EXPRESSION OF GLIAL SPECIFIC mRNAS IN CULTURED RAT BRAIN CELLS IDENTIFIED BY IN SITU HYBRIDIZATION

E. Holmes, G. Hermanson, R. Cole, and J. deVellis
Departments of Anatomy, UCLA School of Medicine; Molecular Biology Institute; Mental Retardation Research Center; and Laboratory of Biomedical and Environmental Sciences, UCLA, LA, CA.

## Introduction

The differentiation of glial cells in brain and in tissue culture preparations has been extensively analysed through the visualization of cell specific marker antigens by immunocytochemical techniques (see Kim, 1985). The technique of in situ hybridization, while complementing immunohistochemistry, provides an advantage by allowing for the detection of mRNAs at the single cell level which reflects the activation of genes necessary for the differentiation of specific cell types. As cDNAs encoding glial fibrillary acidic protein (GFAP), (Lewis and Cowan, 1985), a known astrocyte marker, and myelin basic protein (MBP), (de Ferra *et al.*, 1985), a known oligodendrocyte marker, have been made available to our laboratory, it is now possible to study the expression of those mRNAs in glial cell cultures. The developmental appearance of GFAP and MBP mRNA in primary cultures of newborn rat brain by in situ hybridization is described.

## Materials and Methods

Preparation of probes: The 1.1kb GFAP insert in pUC9 and the 380 base-pair MBP insert in pBR322 were excised and recloned into pTZ18 and pTZ19 T7 polymerase riboprobe vectors (Pharmacia) in opposite orientations to obtain sense and anti-sense RNA probes upon transcription of 1 µg of the linearized vector. High specific activity, $10^9$ CPM/µg of RNA synthesized, $^{35}$S-labeled RNA probes were transcribed and purified as specified by Promega Biotec, Inc. (Madison, WI). The concentration of probe used in each 5 µl reaction was 0.3 µg/ml/kb complexity.

Preparation of cells: Primary cultures of dissociated brain cells were prepared from 1-2 day postnatal cerebral cortices as described (McCarthy and deVellis, 1980) and plated directly on acid-cleaned glass slides that had been treated with 5µg/ml poly-D-lysine. The cultures were plated at a intial density of 12 X $10^6$ cells in 150-mm petri dishes and harvested after 8, 12, 14, and 19 days in culture. The cells were fixed and stored as described (Kumar *et al.*, 1986).

Pretreatment and hybridization of cells: Rehydrated slides were pretreated and hybridized overnight at 52°C, the slides were then treated with RNase A as described (Cox *et al.*, 1984) followed by washes in 2 liters with 3 changes of 2XSSC and 50% formamide at 50°C for 18 hours ending with a final 30 min. wash of 0.1XSSC . Dehydration and autoradiographic procedures were done as described (Kumar *et al.*, 1986).

NATO ASI Series, Vol. H22
Neural Development and Regeneration
Edited by A. Gorio et al.

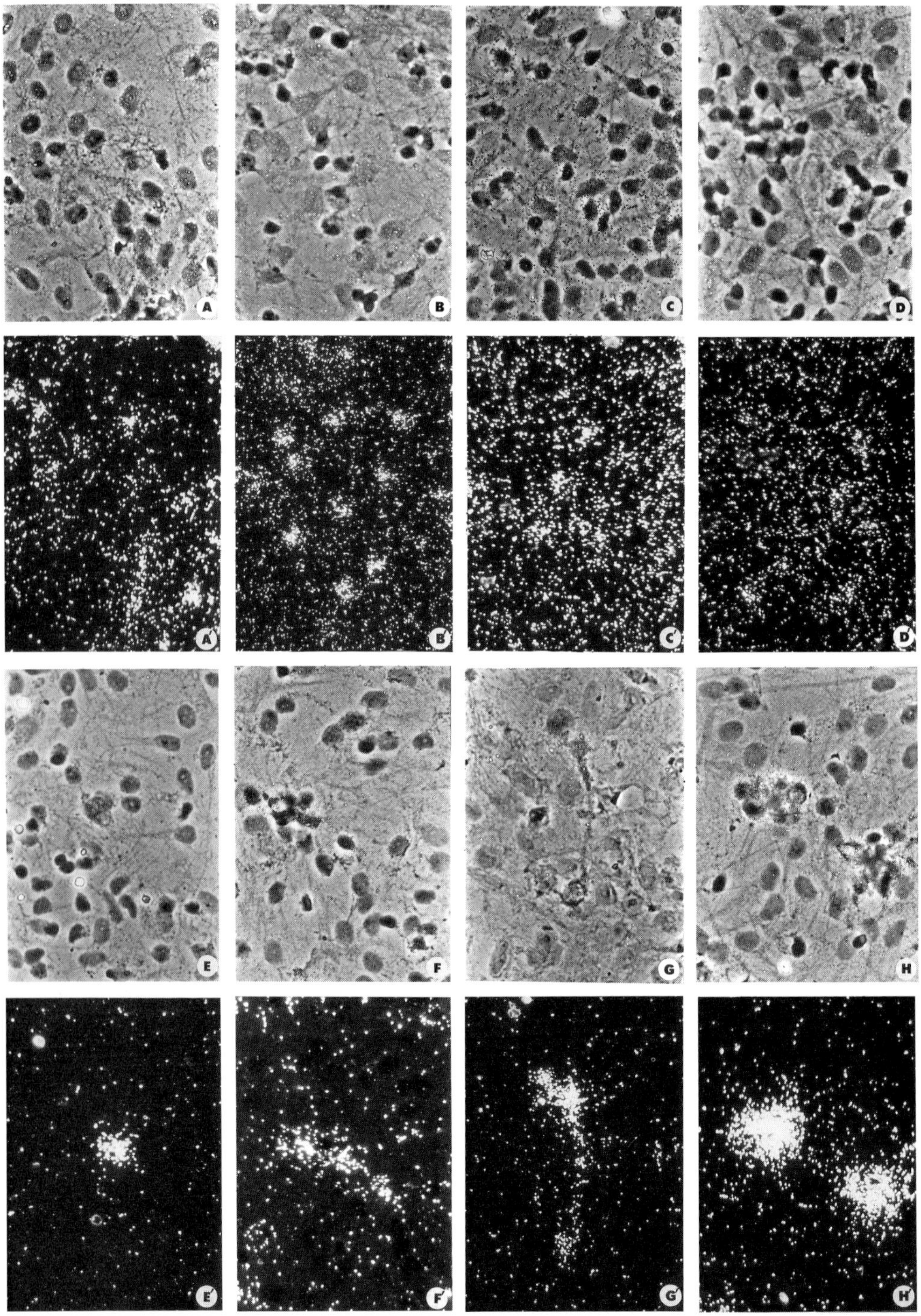

Figure 1. Pairs of phase contrast and dark field photographs are indicated by a letter and its prime, respectively. A - D show hybridization with the GFAP riboprobe and E - H show hybridization with the MBP riboprobe. A and E are 8 day cultures, B and F are 12 day cultures, C and G are 14 day cultures, and lastly, D and H are 19 day cultures.

### Results and Discussion

Preliminary studies to verify the specificity of the riboprobes was performed on slot blots of crude RNA extracts from 31 day old rat brain and from confluent cultures of astrocytes (data not shown). The sense probe for both GFAP and MBP did not hybridize to either rat brain or astrocyte RNA whereas both anti-sense probes hybridized with an abundant signal to rat brain RNA. The GFAP RNA probe, but not the MBP RNA probe, hybridized strongly to the astrocyte RNA. In our culture system, primary cultures of newborn rat brain stratify into a population of flat polygonal cells, astrocytes, covered by another population of phase-dark process-bearing cells. If the latter are switched to oligodendrocyte defined medium (ODM), the cells express many oligodendroglial markers, whereas if the cells are maintained in serum, one-third of the cells express GFAP (Saneto and deVellis, 1985).

The expression of GFAP and MBP mRNA in mixed glial cultures grown in serum correlate with these immunocytochemical characterizations. In Figure 1, pairs of phase contrast and dark field photographs for each detected mRNA species are presented for the 4 time points 8, 12, 14, and 19 days. GFAP mRNA expression increases through day 12 and thereafter seems to plateau although cell density increases over time. This data mirrors that seen in mouse (Lewis and Cowan, 1985). The astrocyte bed layer is predominantly labeled as are some phase-dark cells. The expression of MBP mRNA exhibits a strikingly different pattern. Very few cells in the entire hybridized area were positive at day 8. Approximately a 20-fold increase in the number of MBP mRNA positive cells occurred by day 12 and 14. Cellular processes increased and were heavily labeled as seen in Figure 1, G and G'. By 19 days in culture, large clumps of cells dominated the culture and were intensely labeled with grains. Hybridization with the sense probes was equal to emulsion background. Future work includes extending the time course, adding probes to other glial markers to the analysis, and correlating the expression of mRNAs with immunocytochemistry to glial cell markers.

### References


Cox K, DeLeon D, Angerer L, Angerer, R (1984) Detection of mRNA in sea urchin embryos by in situ hybridization using asymmetric probes. Dev Biol 101:485-502

deFerra F, Engh H, Hudson L, Kamholz J, Puckett C, Molineaux S, Lazzarini R (1985) Alternative splicing accounts for the four forms of myelin basic protein. Cell 43,721-727

Kim S (1985) Antigen expression by glial cells grown in culture. J of Neuroimmunol 8:255-282

Kumar S, Holmes E, Scully S, Birren B, Wilson R, deVellis J (1986) The hormonal regulation of gene expression of glial markers. J of Neurosci Res 16:251-264

Lewis S, Cowan N (1985) Temporal expression of mouse GFAP mRNA studied by a rapid in situ hybridization procedure. J of Neurochem 45:913-919

McCarthy K, deVellis J (1980) Preparation of separated astroglial and oligodendroglial cell cultures from rat cerebral tissue. J Cell Biol 85:890-902

Saneto R, deVellis J (1985) Characterization of cultured rat oligodendrocytes proliferating in a serum-free, chemically defined medium. PNAS 82:3509-3513

# INFLUENCE OF NEUROTROPHIC FACTORS ON THE PHOSPHORYLATION OF EXTRACELLULAR PROTEINS

Anke-Peggy Holtorf, Klaus Unsicker, Hans-Dieter Hofmann*
Institut für Anatomie und Zellbiologie
Philipps Universität Marburg
Robert Koch Straße 6
D-3550 Marburg / FRG

Extracts from bovine seminal vesicles have been shown to contain two neurotrophic factors (NTFs), nerve growth factor (NGF) and seminal vesicle derived growth factor (SVNF, Hofmann and Unsicker, 1982 and 1987). Both polypeptide factors address the same spectrum of target cells and are indistinguishable with regard to their biological effects. Their molecular properties, however, are clearly different, and there is some evidence that they exert their trophic effects via different biochemical mechanisms. Here, we present evidence for the dependence of an extracellular phosphoprotein on the synergistic action of NGF and SVNF.

PC12 pheochromocytoma cells were incubated with $^{32}P\text{-}PO_4^{3-}$ (1mCi/ml of phosphate free DME-medium) in the presence or absence of the NTFs. Extracellular proteins were precipitated with trichloroacetic acid, analysed by SDS-gelelectrophoresis, and phosphorylated proteins were identified autoradiographically.

If an SVNF containing fraction of bovine vesicle extract was added to PC12 cultures, a phosphorylated extracellular protein with an apparent molecular weight of 65kD (PEP65) was observed after 15 minutes. PEP65 could not be detected by standard protein staining procedures with Coomassie blue or silver. It is phosphorylated and released maximally within the first hour, but still appears after 24 hours of continuous stimulation.

No radioactivity was bound to proteins of cell-free medium or PC12 conditioned medium incubated with the SVNF fraction and $^{32}$P-phosphate, or if the cells were incubated with the SVNF fraction and $\gamma$-$^{32}$P-ATP. Therefore, we assume that the protein is released into the medium after being phosphorylated intracellularly. It is unclear, however, whether its release or its phosphorylation or both its phosphorylation and its release is enhanced by SVNF.

*Max-Planck-Institut für Hirnforschung, Deutschordenstr. 46, 6000 Frankfurt/Main - FRG

NATO ASI Series, Vol. H22
Neural Development and Regeneration
Edited by A. Gorio et al.

Several cell types were screened for PEP65. It was neither secreted by dorsal root or sympathetic ganglion cells or adrenal chromaffine cells nor by C6-glioma cells, but could be produced by several neuroblastoma cell lines in a comparable manner as described for PC12.

NGF, EGF, and the ciliary neuronotrophic factor CNTF did not elicit comparable effects. Although PEP65 was consistently seen after stimulation of PC12 cells with the SVNF containing fraction of the seminal vesicle from A 1.5m Biogel column, it was not induced by the electrophoretically purified protein. NGF (0.5 - 100ng/ml), however, restored the PEP65 inducing activity, when applied together with the purified SVNF.

Analysis of the phosphate binding sites by hydrolysis and 2-D-high voltage thin layer chromatography clarified, that PEP65 is exclusively phosphorylated at serine residues.

(supported by the Deutsche Forschungsgemeinschaft. SFB 215/A6)

Literature:

Hofmann H.-D., Unsicker K (1982) The seminal vesicle of the bull: A new and very rich source of nerve growth factor. Eur.J.Biochem. 128:421-426

Hofmann H.-D., Unsicker K (1987) Characterization and partial purification of a novel neuronotrophic factor from bovine vesicle. J.Neurochem., in press

# ASTROCYTE BINDING OF EPIDERMAL GROWTH FACTOR

K. Huff
Division of Neurology, Childrens Hospital of Los Angeles
University of Southern California School of Medicine
4650 Sunset Boulevard
Los Angeles, California 90027 USA

Astrocytes proliferate as a part of normal brain development; in many disease states such as infection, stroke, and trauma; and in neoplastic transformation forming a glioma. The signals involved in controlling and regulating these proliferation responses of the astrocyte are still not completely characterized. Epidermal Growth Factor (EGF) is a mitogen for many target cell types including astrocytes and is found in the nervous system immunohistologically(1). It is also transcribed from a highly conserved base sequence involved in specification of nervous system ontogenic cell lineage and is a ligand for a receptor which is the proto-oncogene highly expressed in gliomas. We have studied the response of astrocytes to EGF in primary tissue culture and presently report data concerning the transduction of this mitogenic signal through binding studies using 125-Iodine radiolabelled EGF.

Cells were purified by the method of McCarthy and de Vellis (2), producing 95% polygonal GFAP-positive cells which clearly showed an increase in autoradiographic grains and DNA incorporation of 3-H thymidine after 24 hours EGF treatment at 2 ng/ml following a 48 hour incubation in serum free media. Immunofluorescent staining of bound EGF seemed to indicate a cell surface location on the polygonal cells for the binding sites. Binding of EGF by a fibroblast cell line C3H 10T1/2 and cultured meningeal cells was less than by the purified astrocytes, also making the possibility unlikely of meningeal fibroblast contamination being the major source of our binding. Binding of EGF by the astrocytes was saturable reaching a maximum after 45 minutes and was specific and not competed by Nerve Growth Factor (NGF), Fibroblast Growth Factor (FGF), Insulin, Multiplication Stimulating Factor II (MSA), or thyroid hormone. A Scatchard analysis of binding data yielded a single high affinity binding site with a dissociation constant (Kd) of 2.0 X 10-9. Binding was similar whether the cells were grown on plastic or glass sub-

NATO ASI Series, Vol. H22
Neural Development and Regeneration
Edited by A. Gorio et al.

strates although it was less when the cells were scraped into suspension. Binding was increased in the presence of the lectins phytohemagglutinin, wheat germ, and concanavalin A; decreased in the presence of vicia villosa; and abolished by tunicamycin. Reduction in temperature during the assay reduced the binding affinity of EGF.

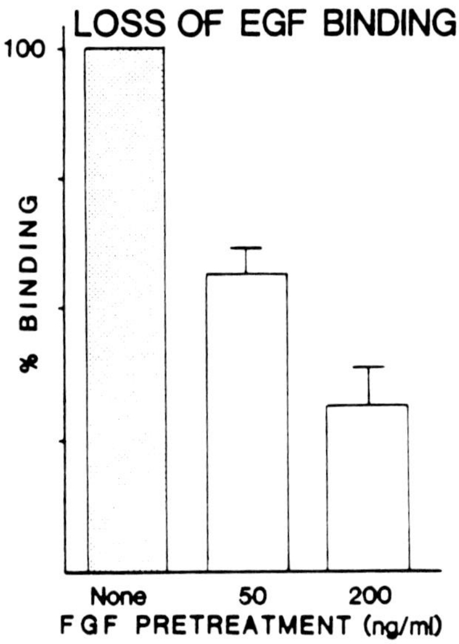


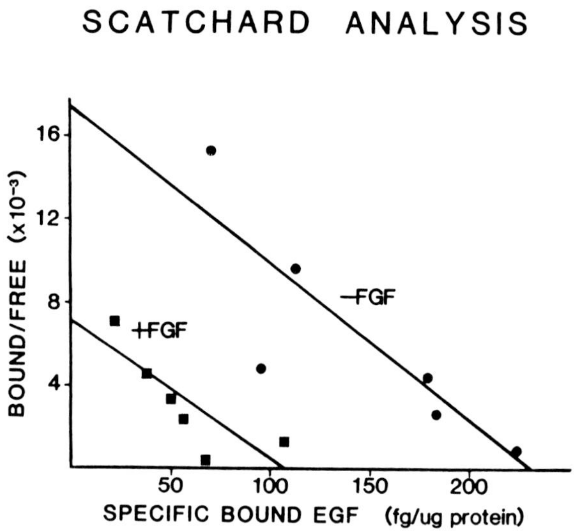


When the cultured astrocytes were pretreated with FGF for 18 hours, a 70% reduction in EGF binding was observed. This pretreatment inhibition was FGF dose dependent and FGF specific, not duplicated by NGF, Insulin, MSA, thyroid hormone, or dexamethasone. A Scatchard analysis of binding after FGF pretreatment indicated a loss in number of binding sites rather than a change in affinity.

Our data suggests specific saturable cell surface tranducers for EGF on astrocytes. The affinity of binding is high but temperature dependent, and the site may be glycosylated with N-acetyl glucosamine and galactosamine. An inhibition of the astrocyte's response to EGF produced by FGF pretreatment may be modulated through a heterologous down regulation of the number of EGF binding sites perhaps by cointernalization and processing of nearby surface receptors. FGF may serve as an off switch for the EGF mitogenic signal.

1.Fallon JH, Seroogy KB (1984) Epidermal Growth Factor Immunoreactive Material in the Central Nervous System. Science 224: 1107-1109
2.McCarthy K, deVellis J(1980) Preparation of Astroglial and Oligodendroglial Cultures from Rat Cerebral Tissue J Cell Bio 85:890-902

# SCHWANN CELLS PROLIFERATE IN RESPONSE TO NON-MYELINATED AXONS

P.W.Mason and G.H.DeVries
Department of Biochemistry and Molecular Biophysics
Box 614, MCV Station
Virginia Commonwealth University
Richmond VA 23298

During development of the PNS, Schwann cells (SC) proliferate in response to growing axons. In vitro studies (1) have confirmed that the axolemma is a powerful mitogen for SC, however only axons that were glial ensheathed, or those destined to become ensheathed, were used as a stimulus. The axons of granule cells (GC) of the cerebellum provide a unique opportunity to study the axonal mitogenic stimulus for unlike most axons of the CNS and PNS they lack glial ensheathment.

SCs were isolated by the method of Brockes et.al. (2) from 2 day old rat pups. GCs were isolated from 8 day old rat cerebella as described by Annunziata et.al. (3). The GCs were maintained separately in culture for 8 days after which time SCs were added and cocultured for an additional 72 hours with 3H-thymidine being added for the last 24 hours. SCs were identified morphologically and immunologically using the SC-specific antibody, 217C (4,5). 3H-Thymidine incorporation was determined by autoradiography. Cocultured SCs had a labeling index of 9.5% compared to 0.3% when cultured alone.

To examine this mitogenic signal, isolated GC membrane were introduced to SC cultures at concentrations of 5 to 300ug of protein/ml and incubated for 72 hours, with the addition of 3H-thymidine for the last 24 hours. 3H-Thymidine incorporation was determined by the cell harvester assay system and expressed as % of control. A dose response curve of the GC membrane showed a sigmoidal 3H-thymidine incorporation

NATO ASI Series, Vol. H22
Neural Development and Regeneration
Edited by A. Gorio et al.

by SCs reaching a maximum of a 21 fold increase over background at a concentration of 200ug of protein/ml. Glial growth factor and forskolin, a non-specific mitogen for SCs, showed a maximum stimulation 146 fold over background.

Preliminary studies on the biochemical properties of the mitogenic factor revealed that it was heat and trypsin sensitive. Heating the membrane to 100C for 10 min. completely abolished the response and trypsin treatment reduced the incorporation to only 7% of control. These experiments indicate that the mitogenic signal might, in part be a protein. The addition of a lysosomal inhibitor, $NH_4Cl$, at a concentration of 9mM produced no inhibition of $^3H$ thymidine incorporation indicating that the mitogenic signal does not need to undergo lysosomal processing to elicit its mitogenic effect.

Our results indicate that both GC membrane fragments and intact cells can induce normally quiescent SC to proliferate. Although further work is needed to determine if the signals are related, these studies suggest that the state of glial ensheathment of an axon does not dictate the mitogenic potential of the membrane.

[Supported by NS15408 and NS10821 (Javits Neuroscience Grant)]

1. DeVries GH, Salzer JL, Bunge RP (1982) Axolemma-enriched fractions isolated from PNS and CNS are mitogenic for cultured Schwann cells. Dev Brain Res 3:295-299

2. Brockes JP, Fields KL, Raff MC (1979) Studies on cultured rat Schwann cells. I. Establishment of purified populations from from cultures of peripheral nerve. Brain Res 165:105-118.

3. Annunziata P, Regan C, Balazs R (1983) Development of Cerebellar Cells in Neuron-Enriched Cultures: Cell Surface Proteins. Dev Brain Res 8:261-273

4. Peng WW, Bressler JP, Tiffany-Castiglioni E, De Vellis J (1982) Science 215:1102-1104

5. Fields KL, Dammerman M (1985) A Monoclonal Antibody Equivalent to Anti-Rat Neural Antigen-1 as a Marker for Schwann Cells. Neuroscience 15:877-885

# EFFECTS OF NERVE GROWTH FACTOR AND MONOSIALOGANGLIOSIDE GM1 ON FOREBRAIN CHOLINERGIC NEURONES

D. Maysinger, L. Garofalo and A.C. Cuello
Department of Pharmacology and Therapeutics
McGill University
3655 Drummond Street
Montreal H3G 1Y6
Canada

The relevance of cortical cholinergic innervation has attracted great interest since severe losses of choline acetyltransferase (ChAT) enzymatic activity and cell loss in the nucleus basalis of Meynert were demonstrated in the cerebral cortex of patients with Alzheimer's disease (Coyle et al. 1983, Collerton 1986). In rats with unilateral cortical lesion specific biochemical and morphological retrograde changes occur in the nucleus basalis magnocellularis (NBM). Thirty days following devascularizing lesion of the cortex choline acetyl transferase (ChAT) activity in the NBM decreased significantly from control values while no significant change was noted in the neurochemical marker for GABAergic function glutamic acid decarboxylase (GAD). Cholinergic neurones of the basal forebrain stained immunocytochemically for ChAT appear shrunken in this animal model. Morphological parameters obtained using an image analyser (Cambridge instruments, Quantimet 920) showed that there was a significant decrease in the cross sectional area of the nucleus basalis neurones in devascularized animals as compared to controls. As well, the number of neuronal processes appeared to be remarkably decreased in the NBM of vehicle treated rats (Figure 1a). However, chronic administration of monosialoganglioside GM1, nerve growth factor (NGF) or a combination of both prevented these morphological (Figure 1b) and biochemical (Figure 1c) retrograde degenerative changes. GM1 and NGF were administered via osmotic mini pumps (Alzet2001,5 mg/kg/day of GM1 and 80 ug/animal/week of NGF). For morphological studies, free floating sections obtained as previously described by Cuello et al., 1986) were stained for ChAT immunoreactive sites using a rat monoclonal antibodies against ChAT (Eckenstein et al., 1982).

The presented data lend support to the concept that trophic factors such as GM1, NGF and perhaps other as yet unidentified factors can protect against retrograde subcortical degeneration. The mechanism by which gangliosides bring about these protective effects upon cholinergic neurones is still

NATO ASI Series, Vol. H22
Neural Development and Regeneration
Edited by A. Gorio et al.

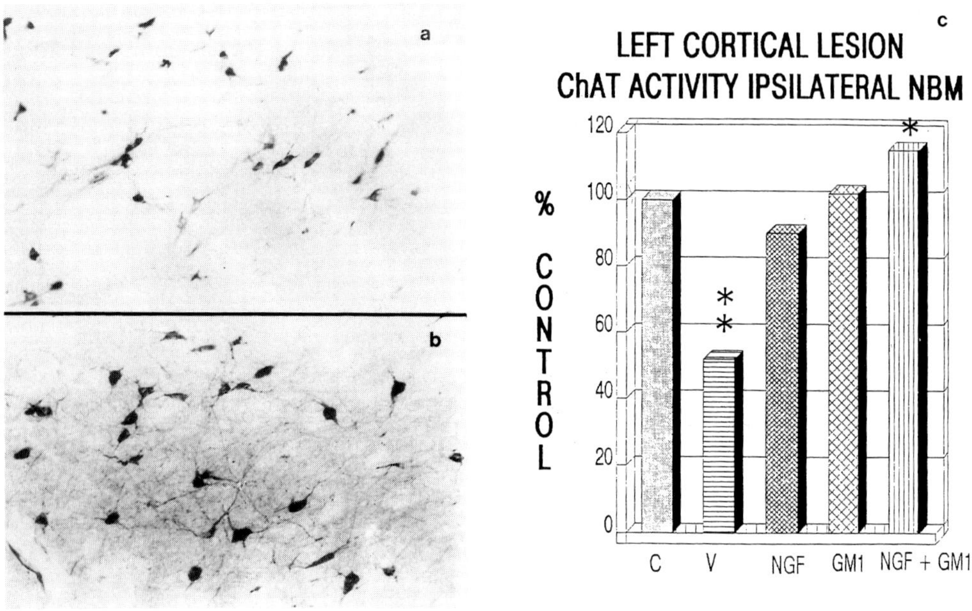


Figure 1. The effect of NGF and GM1 on morphological (a, b) and biochemical changes (c) of retrograde degeneration in the NBM. a) ChAT immunoreactive neurones in the NBM of lesioned animals indicating shrinkage of somata b) ChAT positive neurones in the NBM of lesioned rats treated with a combination of NGF + GM1 for 7 days. c) ChAT enzymatic activity in the NBM of control (C, n=6) and lesioned rats treated with vehicle (V, n=6), NGF (n=6), GM1 (n=6) or NGF + GM1 (n=6).

unclear but the cooperativity found in our studies by the simultaneous administration of GM1 and NGF are suggestive of gangliosides as modulators of membrane functions thereby facilitating the NGF response.

## References


Coyle JT, Price DL, DeLong MR (1983) Alzheimer's disease: A disorder of cortical Cholinergic Innervation. Science 219:1184-1190.

Collerton D (1986) Cholinergic function and intellectual decline in Alzheimer's disease. Neuroscience 19: 1-28.

Cuello AC, Stephens PH, Tagari PD, Sofroniew MV, Pearson RCA (1986) Retrograde changes in the nucleus basalis of the rat caused by cortical damage are prevented by exogenous ganglioside GM1. Brain Research 376: 373-377.

Eckenstein F, Thoenen H (1982) Production of specific antisera and monoclonal antibodies in choline acetyltransferase. Characterization and use for identification of cholinergic neurones. EMBO J 1: 363-368.

# MODULATION OF NEURITE GROWTH BY GABA IN CELL CULTURE

A. Michler und J.R. Wolff
Department of Anatomy
University of Göttingen
Kreuzbergring 36
3400 Göttingen
FRG

The role of -aminobutyric acid (GABA) as an inhibitory transmitter of the central nervous system has been documented by a great number of studies. At least two classes of receptors seem to be involved in mediating the response to GABA. The $GABA_A$ receptor is sensitive to bicuculline and appears to be associated with a chloride channel while the $GABA_B$ receptor specifically binds (-)baclofen which leads to a change in calcium ion permeability of the membrane (Dunlap, 1984). Apart from its transmitter function GABA seems to influence the morphogenesis of neurons which includes changes in ultrastructural composition and facilitation of synaptogenesis (De Feudis and Mandel, 1981). In the present study the influence of GABA on neurite growth of chick tectal neurons and its interaction with supplements of the medium was investigated.

Dissociated tectum cells from 6 day embryonic chicken were plated either in serum-free N2 or serum supplemented medium (SSM). GABA at concentrations ranging from $10^{-8}$M up to $10^{-3}$M was added to the cultures 24 h after plating. Nerve growth factor (NGF; 20 ng/ml), potassium (24.5 mM final concentration) and calcium (1.36 mM final concentration) were added immediately at the time of plating. After 3 days the effect of different medium components on neurite extension was assayed by screening fixed cell cultures in an inverted Zeiss microscope. The number of neurites and somata

NATO ASI Series, Vol. H22
Neural Development and Regeneration
Edited by A. Gorio et al.

crossing defined lines in the visual field of the microscope was counted and the quotient of number of neurites (N) versus number of somata (S) determined.

In SSM tectal neurons had only short more or less unbranched processes. When GABA ($10^{-3}$M) was present in these cultures neurite outgrowth was strongly stimulated and the quotient N/S raised by a factor of about 2 as compared to controls. In N2 medium a different morphology of neurons was observed compared to those grown in SSM. In the defined medium they had numerous long and branched processes. In the presence of GABA ($10^{-3}$M) a quite unexpected effect was seen, e.g. neurite growth was suppressed resulting in a less dense neuronal network. The inhibiting effect of GABA in N2 medium was dose dependent.

When NGF was added to N2 medium it had no effect on neurite growth alone but in combination with GABA the inhibitory influence was abolished. In the presence of positive ions like potassium or calcium neurite elongation was stimulated in N2 medium. This effect was most pronounced in the case of calcium ions. Concomittant presence of GABA and potassium slightly decreased N/S values which were, however, not smaller than controls grown in N2 medium alone. In contrast, when GABA was added to high calcium medium an increase in N/S values could be observed, which even exceeded those obtained in N2 medium and N2 medium plus calcium.

It is concluded that the opposite effects of GABA on neurite growth may depend on the environment the cells are grown in. Depending on the type of medium used a particular set of GABA receptors may be expressed on tectal cells which influence neurite elongation in different ways. The involvement of $GABA_B$ receptors and hence Ca-channels in this regulation will further be investigated.

DeFeudis FV, Mandel P (eds) (1981) Amino Acid Neurotransmitters. Adv Biochem Psychopharmacol vol 29. Raven Press New York

Dunlap K (1984) Functional and pharmacological differences between two types of GABA receptor on embryonic chick sensory neurons. Neurosci Lett 47: 265-270

# EFFECTS OF AN ALPHA-2 ADRENERGIC RECEPTOR AGONIST IN SPINAL RATS

N.E. Naftchi, R.Lehrer, and J.A.Sleis
Department of Rehabilitation Medicine
New York University Medical Center
400 East 34th street
New York, N.Y.

It is now several decades that diverse surgical and pharmacological treatments have been employed to prevent and/or ameliorate the sensory motor deficits which ensue an injury to the spinal cord. The restoration of impaired histological and physiologic parameters by compounds which are membrane stabilizers, antiinflammatory, and antioxidant , and which increase the regional blood flow such as methylprednisolone sodium succinate, naloxone, hypothalamic thyrotropic releasing hormone, and epsilonaminocaproic acid suggest that the changes seen after trauma may be secondary to a marked membrane disorganization and dysfunction. The changes in the phospholipid-dependent, membrane bound enzyme monoamine oxidase and the formation of microglobules and noncellular material on the endothelial lining are early signs of membrane pathology (1). After the transection of spinal cord, axoplasmic transport continues to the lesion site, resulting in the accumulation of serotonin (5-hydroxytryptamine), and norepinephrine above the lesion in the spinal cord and brain stem (2) and a loss of the biogenic amines from the distal portion of the spinal cord (3). In contrast to monoaminergic descending pathways, SP-containing fibers in the spinal cord represent ascending spinal tracts; SP accumulates below the lesion level (4). Therefore, after chordotomy, the axons of descending and ascending neurons from the cells of origin to the site of the lesion remain biologically and functionally viable. Spasticity and episodic hypertensive crisis (autonomic dysreflexia) are caused by noxious stimuli arising from afferent somatic and visceral inputs; these stimuli are conducted by the spinal cord below the level of the lesion(5).

The adrenergic system is a major descending pathway. The bulbospinal projections of the noradrenergic system, and those of the serotonergic and dopaminergic systems, project to the same or different regions of the spinal cord (6). Therefore, the alpha-2 adrenergic agonist, clonidine was chosen for our studies because it might also affect serotonin and dopamine containing neurons through the intimate interconnections of their circuitry in the spinal cord (6) and because clonidine has a high degree of selec-

NATO ASI Series, Vol. H22
Neural Development and Regeneration
Edited by A. Gorio et al.

tivity for the alpha-2 adrenergic receptors in the CNS (7).

## METHODS

Rats were decapitated and the spinal cord tissue was dissected quickly. A longitudinal section centered at the transection site and 1 cm above and below the lesion as well as other specimens rostral and caudal to this section were frozen immediately in a container of isopentane immersed in liquid nitrogen. After freeze drying and condensing with formaldehyde vapor at 80°C, according to the technique of Falk and Hillarp, the specimens were embedded in paraffin wax and sectioned at 7-10 um in thickness.

## RESULTS and CONCLUSION

None of the control animals, some followed as long as 3½ months after spinal cord transection, exhibited any coordinated movements. These animals went through flexor withdrawal of the hind limbs followed by extensor spasms. They dragged their hind limbs with plantar surface facing upward and the dorsal surface touching the ground. Within one week to 12 days, the biogenic amines, NE and 5-HT, disappeared from the caudal stump and began accumulating rostrally. This is most likely due to loss of negative feedback between the cells in the brain stem and the specific receptors for these monoamines in the spinal cord, i.e. the loss of receptor activation. Alternatively, it may result from the curtailment of end-product feed-back inhibition or both mechanisms.

In contrast to the random spasticity observed in untreated control rats, some of the rats treated with alpha-2 receptor agonist, clonidine, developed a "normal" mode of locomotion; the movements in the hind limbs were deliberate and coordinated with those of the front limbs. Furthermore, the plantar surfaces of the hind limbs were placed properly for the purpose of weight bearing and participation in appropiate locomotion. Among many treated rats, four walked "normally". The main motor function that these "normal" walking rats lacked consistently was the inability to raise their tail above the trunk or stand on their hind limbs without holding to the wall of the track (5 feet long x 1½ feet wide x 1 foot high) with either one or the other forelimb. The major problem with the other treated rats that did not ambulate properly was development of kyphoscoleosis or lordosis due to insipient osteoporosis resulting from significant loss of bone mineral and matrix which starts almost immediately after spinal cord transection (8) and is exacerbated by sedative effect of clonidine which extends the immobilization period of the animals. Another adverse side effect suffered by these animals was peripheral neuropathy due to lying on one side over extended periods of time. Electrostimulation of the tail in the treated rats also resulted in vocalization and vocalization after discharge. Histofluorescence studies of the treated rats not only showed little accumulation of monoaminergic fluorescence above the lesion but they also exhibited reappearance of yellowgreen (5-hydroxytryptamine) and green (norepinephrine) fluorescence in the sections of the spinal cord below the level of transection. These observations indicate a reactivation of the descending monoaminergic pathways involved in locomotion and the reestablishment of the ascending nociceptive pathways due to treatment with an alpha-2 adrenoceptor agonist.

## REFERENCES


1) Naftchi NE (1982) Prevention of damage in acute spinal cord injury by peptides and pharmacological agents. Peptides 3:235-247.
2) Naftchi NE, Kirschner A, Demeny M, Viau AT (1981) Alterations in Norepinephrine, Serotonin, c-AMP, and transsynaptic induction of Tyrosine Hydroxylase after spinal cord transection in the rat. Neurochem Res 6:1205-1215.
3) Anden NE, Haggendal J, Magnusson T, Rosengrin E (1964) The time course of disappearance of norepinephrine and 5-hydroxytryptamine in the spinal cord after transection. Acta Physiol Scand 62:115-118.
4) Naftchi NE, Abrahams S, St.Paul HM, Lowman EW, Schlosser W (1978) Localization and changes of substance P in spinal cord of paraplegic cats. Brain Res 153:507-513.
5) Naftchi NE, Demeny M, Lowman EW, Tuckman J (1978) Hypertensive crisis in quadriplegic patients:changes in cardiac output, blood volume, serum dopamine-beta-hydroxylase activity and arterial prostaglandin $pge_2$. Circulation 57:336-341.
6) Naftchi NE (1982) Functional restoration of the traumatically injured spinal cord in cats by clonidine. Science 217:1042-1044.
7) U'Prichard DC, Bechtel WD, Rouot B, Snyder SH, (1979) Mol Pharmacol 16:46.
8) Naftchi NE (1985) Alterations of Neuroendocrine functions in spinal cord injury. Peptides 6:85-94.

# INDUCTION OF THE 68/72 kDa HEAT-STRESS PROTEIN IN HYDROGEN PEROXIDE TOXICITY

R. N. Nishimura[1], B. E. Dwyer[1], R. Cole[2], J. de Vellis[2]
Departments of Neurology[1] and Anatomy[2]
UCLA
RNRC 4231
Los Angeles, California 90024-1769
USA

The heat shock or stress proteins (HSPs) are synthesized by most mammalian cells in response to hyperthermia and other noxious stimuli (1). Since this response is thought to be a protective reaction by the stressed cell, it has raised much interest, particularly the induction of the 68/72 kDa HSP since this protein is not synthesized constitutively by most cells. In the mammalian nervous system the synthesis of the 68/72 kDa HSP has been induced by trauma, hypoxia-ischemia and heat shock. Capillary endothelial cells and retinal neurons are among cell types suspected of synthesizing these proteins but in most studies the cellular origin has gone undetermined. In-vitro, purified rat glial cells (2) and cortical neurons synthesize the 68/72 kDa HSP (3) in response to heating (45°C) but the data suggest that compared to glia, the neuronal response is attenuated. In these experiments we have studied induction of the 68/72 kDa HSP in response to $H_2O_2$.

Purified astrocytes were prepared by the method of McCarthy and de Vellis (4). Primary cultures were separated from oligodendrocytes by shaking the flasks. Prior to addition of the $H_2O_2$ all feeding medium was changed to Dulbecco's modified essential medium/Ham's F-12, 1:1, at 37°C. Final concentrations of $H_2O_2$ were 2, 4, and 6 µM. Controls were untreated. Cultures were exposed to $H_2O_2$ in DMEM/F-12 medium for 1 hour only. Radioactive labeling with $^{35}$S-methionine was performed in methionine deficient medium (30 µCi/ml) at 37°C from 2-4 and 4-6 hours after $H_2O_2$ exposure. The cultures were processed by successive washes with ice-cold PBS, 0.1M, pH 7.4, then treated with 10% TCA supplemented with 0.1% methionine and then washed with PBS again. Cells were then scraped from the flasks and homogenized in 0.1% SDS and heated 3 minutes at 100°C. Samples were then examined by SDS protein electrophoresis as per Laemmli (5).

Our results (figure 1) show the time and dose response to $H_2O_2$.

NATO ASI Series, Vol. H22
Neural Development and Regeneration
Edited by A. Gorio et al.

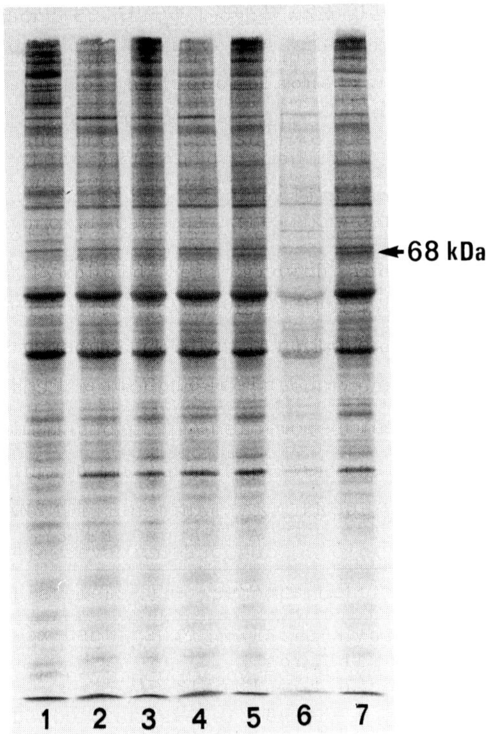


Figure 1. 12.5% polyacrylamide gel of $H_2O_2$ treated astrocytes. See text for explanation.

Lane 1 is the control. Lanes 2 and 3 show the response to 2 µM $H_2O_2$ at 2-4 and 4-6 hours respectively; lanes 4 and 5, 4 µM $H_2O_2$ at 4-6 and 4-6 hours respectively; and lanes 6 and 7, 6 µM $H_2O_2$ at 2-4 and 4-6 hours respectively. Equal numbers of counts were added to each lane except lane 6 where considerable numbers of cells were lost due to the toxicity of $H_2O_2$. These results show that the greater the concentration of $H_2O_2$ the more pronounced the induction of the 68/72 kDa HSP. At the earlier time points the response is much less than later. In contrast to Burdon (6) these results are in accordance with Love et al (7) who found that large doses of 50 mM or pretreatment with 1 mM then 50 mM $H_2O_2$ induced HSP mRNA transcription in Drosophila melanogaster. In view of the present findings it is possible that the induction of HSP 68/72 in ischemia and anoxia and trauma may be partially regulated by oxidative stress similar to $H_2O_2$ toxicity. If the response is protective to the affected cells then therapy aimed at inducing or prolonging this response may be beneficial to cell survival.

1. Subjeck JR, Thung-Tai S (1986) Stress proteins systems of mammalian cells. Am J Physiol 250:C1-C17
2. Nishimura RN, Dwyer BE, Liotta K, Cole R, de Vellis J (1986) Induction of stress proteins in astrocytes. Trans Am Soc Neurochem 17:325
3. Nishimura RN, Dwyer BE, Liotta K, Cole R, de Vellis J (1987) Heat stress response in primary rat neuronal and glial cultures. Neurology 37 (suppl) 370
4. McCarthy, KD, de Vellis J (1980) Preparation of separate astroglial and oligodendroglial cell cultures from rat cerebral tissue. J Cell Biol 85:890-902.
5. Laemmli UK (1970) Cleavage of structural proteins during the assembly of the head of bacteriophage T4. Nature (London) 277:680-685
6. Burdon RH (]986) Heat shock and the heat shock proteins. Biochem J 240: 313-324
7. Love JD, Vivino AA, Minton KW (1986) Hydrogen peroxide toxicity may be enhanced by heat shock gene induction in _Drosophila_. J Cell Physiol ]26:60-68

Sponsored by United Cerebral Palsy Research Foundation and Veterans Administration Research Service

# PERIPHERAL NERVE GRAFTS IMPLANTED INTO RAT CNS (OPTIC NERVE) SHOW ELECTROPHORETIC PATTERNS OF RADIOLABELLED FAST AXONALLY TRANSPORTED PROTEINS SIMILAR TO THE PATTERN SEEN IN THE NORMAL HOST CNS TRACT.

G.W. Perry
Department of Physiology and Biophysics
University of Miami School of Medicine
Miami, Florida 33101, U.S.A.

In their eloquent studies on peripheral nerve grafts implanted into rat central nervous system (CNS), Aguayo and colleagues [3,6] have demonstrated that when given an appropriate environment, mammalian CNS neurones, like other nerve cells, can regrow their axons great distances after damage. However, whether or not special components manufactured within nerve cells are also necessary to effect regeneration is still a matter of conjecture. One such group of components may be proteins that are rapidly transported down regenerating axons and appear to be selectively increased compared to other transported proteins.[1,2,4,5] If such proteins are indeed prerequisite for nerve growth, then their expression in CNS fibres growing through peripheral nerve grafts might also be expected. In these preliminary studies I report that proteins are seen in peripheral nerve grafts implanted into the rat eye which appear very similar to fast axonally transported proteins seen normally in the host CNS, and are presumably conveyed along CNS fibres growing within the graft.

Under Nembutal anaesthsia the rat optic nerve was almost completely severed at the point it exists the sclera, and one end of a tibial nerve graft from the same rat was inserted into the sclera to partially replace the optic nerve. The grafts were left in place for 6 weeks afterwhich 50uCi of $^{35}$S-methionine was injected into both eyes for 6h. Proteins in the graft and the contralateral optic nerve were analyzed by gel electrophoresis.

Figure 1a&b shows the fluorographic patterns of labelled proteins from normal rat optic nerve (a), and from the tibial nerve graft (b). The band patterns of labelled proteins from the two nerve samples are very similar, as determined visually and by densitometric scanning (not shown). However, analysis of the expression of individual proteins must await separation using 2-D gels. To ensure that the electrophoretic patterns in Fig. 1 a&b indeed represent labelled fast transported proteins, and not locally synthesized proteins, they were compared to the electrophoretic patterns of labelled proteins locally synthesized in the nerve segments. Isolated optic and tibial nerves were incubated for 6h in media containing

NATO ASI Series, Vol. H22
Neural Development and Regeneration
Edited by A. Gorio et al.

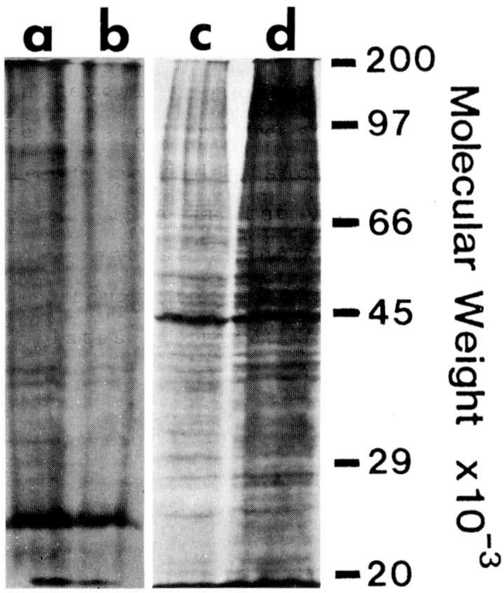


Figure 1. Fluorographic patterns of labelled transported (a & b)and locally synthesized (c & d) proteins from optic nerves (a & c) and tibial nerves (b & d). See text for further details.

$^{35}$S-methionine and the labelled proteins analyzed on 1-D gels. Fig. 1 c&d show the local synthesis patterns of labelled proteins for optic (c) and tibial (d) nerve segments. As can be seen these patterns are quite different from the transport patterns in Fig. 1 a&b. These results suggest that CNS cells in the retina, presumably the retinal ganglion cells, regrow their axons within the peripheral nerve graft and do so without major changes in the overall complement of their fast axonally transported proteins.

These studies were supported by NIH grant EY06449.

1. Benowitz LI, Shashoua VE, Yoon MG (1981) Specific changes in transported proteins during regeneration of the goldfish optic nerve. J. Neurosci. 1:300-307
2. Perry GW, Wilson DL (1981) Protein synthesis and axonal transport during nerve regeneration. J. Neurochem. 37:1203-1217
3. Richardson P, McGuinness U, Aguayo A (1980) Axons from CNS neurones regenerate into PNS grafts. Nature 284:264-265
4. Skene JHP, Willard M (1981) Changes in axonally transported proteins during regeneration in toad retinal ganglion cells. J.Cell Biol. 89:86-
5. Skene JHP, Willard M (1981) Axonally transported proteins associated with growth in rabbit central and peripheral nervous systems. J. Cell Biol. 89:96-103
6. So K, Aguayo A (1985) Lengthy regrowth of cut axons from ganglion cells after peripheral nerve transplantation into the retina of adult rats. Brain Res. 328:349-354

# DIFFERENTIATION OF A MIGRATORY BIPOTENTIAL GLIAL PROGENITOR CELL IN THE DEVELOPING RAT OPTIC NERVE

R. Small
Department of Zoology & Cell Biology
University College London
Gower Street
London WC1E 6BT

Recent evidence indicates that the progenitor cells which give rise to the myelin-forming cells of the rat optic nerve, migrate from the brain into the embryonic nerve beginning at its chiasmal end (Small, 1986; Small et al, 1987). Both oligodendrocytes which produce myelin sheaths, and type-2 astrocytes which contribute fine processes to the node (ffrench-Constant & Raff, 1986), derive from this common bipotential 'O-2A' progenitor cell (Raff et al, 1983). Widespread migration of O-2A progenitor cells from the brain appears to be a general mechanism for distributing the O-2A cell lineage to regions of CNS that become myelinated.

The optic nerve provides an almost ideal model system for examining factors which regulate the migration and differentiation of progenitor cells in vivo. The nerve is thought to contain only three types of glial cells (type-1 astrocyte, oligodendrocytes and type-2 astrocytes), ganglion cell axons but no neuronal perikarya. Type-1 astrocytes develop from a distinct precursor cell (Raff et al, 1984) that appears to be an intrinsic neuroepithelial cell of the optic stalk (Small et al, 1987). These are the first differentiated glial cells of the nerve, and they first appear at embryonic day 16 (E16). Type-1 astrocytes secrete a potent growth factor which expands the O-2A cell pool in vitro by stimulating division of progenitor cells (Noble & Murray, 1984). The O-2A progenitor cell, which is an extrinsic, migratory cell, gives rise at postnatal ages, to oligodendrocytes beginning at birth (P0=E21), and to type-2 astrocytes beginning at P8 - P10 (Miller et al, 1985).

What are the substrate requirements for progenitor cell migration and what factors cause the progenitor to stop migrating and differentiate?

NATO ASI Series, Vol. H22
Neural Development and Regeneration
Edited by A. Gorio et al.

An in vivo examination of the colonization of the optic nerve by progenitor cells provides some preliminary suggestions. The first appearance of progenitor cells in the nerve, occurs only after axons of retinal ganglion cells have reached the optic chiasm at E16. These progenitors are oriented longitudinally among the axon fascicles of the chiasmal half of the nerve and they show extensive contacts with axonal surfaces. Very few contacts have been observed between progenitor cells and type-1 astrocytes. Thus, at its first appearance the O-2A progenitor cell seems to be intimately associated with axonal surfaces and this relationship is perhaps, continued and later reflected in the functional specialization shown be the lineage for ensheathing axons. If axons guide migrating progenitor cells into the nerve, this could explain the results of earlier studies which show that lesions of the newborn rat optic nerve severely reduce the nerve's O-2A cell lineage but have minimal effects on the nerve's type-1 astrocyte population (David et al, 1984).

Upon entering the optic nerve, do progenitor cells migrate through to the retinal pole of the nerve, or do they settle and differentiate at the chiasmal pole so that progenitors arriving at later ages, progressively fill positions closer to the eye. An analysis of the initial distribution of oligodendrocytes, the first differentiated O-2A cell type, indicates that the nerve's progenitor cells are heterogeneous: some progenitor cells differentiate at the chiasmal pole while others continue their migration towards the retinal pole. The O4 antigen of oligodendrocytes (Sommer and Schachner, 1981), is first expressed at E20 by a small population of cells occurring exclusively at the nerve's chiasmal pole. Galactocerebroside (GC) is first expressed one day later, at birth, and it is also entirely restricted to cells at the nerve's chiasmal pole. Through the first post-natal week, the percentage of cells expressing O4 and GC increases, and these antigens also begin to appear on cells in the mid, and then, retinal region of the nerve. Time-lapse cinematography studies show that GC+ multipolar oligodendrocytes are nonmotile, in contrast to bipolar progenitor cells which are highly motile (Small et al, 1987). Thus, these results indicate that colonization of the nerve by nonmotile oligodendrocytes proceeds from the chiasmal region at ages when progenitor cells are still migrating into the retinal region of the nerve.

Type-2 astrocytes, the second differentiated progeny of the progenitor cell, are not detected in the nerve until about P9, and their initial distribution differs sharply with that observed for oligodendrocytes. At P9, small numbers of type-2 astrocytes appear in equal density in positions all along the nerve. P9 corresponds to an age when oligodendrocytes are evenly distributed in the nerve, and to an age when the oligodendrocytes dissociated from nerve appear studded with 10 - 20 tightly adhering cell processes. These processes show the antigenic phenotype of type-2 astrocytes: they contain glial fibrillary acidic protein (GFAP) and are A2B5+. This suggests that differentiation of type-2 astrocytes may be regulated by an interaction between oligodendrocytes and progenitor cells.

A possible explanation for the heterogeneity observed in the nerve's progenitor cell population at birth, is provided by developmental studies of type-1 astrocytes, the nerve's earliest glial cell population. The differentiation of type-1 astrocytes, as assessed by GFAP expression, begins in the embryo behind the eye at the lamina cribrosa and spreads rapidly through to the chiasmal region of the nerve in three days (Small et al, 1987). If a similar maturation gradient also applies to their secretion of growth factor (which causes proliferation of progenitor cells), then the chiasmal region of the embryonic nerve may contain relatively little or no mitogen at ages when progenitor cells first enter the nerve. Differentiation of only a subpopulation of progenitor cells at birth may indicate that progenitors differ in their dependence upon growth factor to maintain their motile, undifferentiated state.

David S, Miller RH, Patel R, Raff MC (1984) Effects of neonatal transection on glial cell development in the rat optic nerve. J Neurocytol 13:961-974

ffrench-Constant C, Raff, MC (1986) The oligodendrocyte - type-2 astrocyte cell lineage is specialized for myelination. Nature 323:335-338

Miller RH, David S, Patel R, Abney ER, Raff MC (1985) A quantitative immunohistochemical study of macroglial cell development in the rat optic nerve. Dev Biol 111:35-41

Noble M, Murray K (1984) Purified astrocytes promote the in vitro division of a bipotential glial progenitor cell: EMBO J 3:2243-2247

Raff MC, Abney ER, Miller RH (1984) Two glial cell lineages diverge pre-natally in rat optic nerve: Dev Biol 106:53-60

Raff MC, Miller RH, Noble M (1983) A glial progenitor cell that develops in vitro into an astrocyte or an oligodendrocyte depending on the culture medium. Nature 303:390-396

Small RK (1986) Evidence for migration of O-2A progenitor cells into the developing rat optic nerve: Soc for Neurosci Abstr 12: 183

Small RK, Riddle P, Noble M (1987) Evidence for migration of oligodendrocyte-type-2 astrocyte progenitor cells into the developing rat optic nerve. Nature in press

Sommer I, Schachner M (1981) Monoclonal antibodies (O1 to O4) to oligo-dendrocyte cell surfaces: Dev Biol 83: 311-327

# NEURONAL PRIMARY CULTURES - A CHARACTERIZATION

M. Söderbäck[1], E. Hansson[2], O. Tottmar[1] and L. Rönnbäck[2, 3]
Institute of Neurobiology[2]
University of Göteborg
P.O.B. 33 031
S-400 33 Göteborg
Sweden

Summary: Morphological differentiation of neurons in primary culture from various brain regions were followed. Cell aggregates were formed after seeding. Neurons, identified by immunohistochemical localization of the neuron-specific enolase (NSE), migrated from the cell-clusters during age in culture and formed networks of processes. Both aggregates and single neuronal cells showed morphological characteristics specific for the various brain regions. The results indicate the presence of specific neuronal cells in the cultures.

Dissociated neural cell cultures obtained from disruption of immature central nervous system tissue have been used to enlighten the biochemical, physiological and morphological organization of the central nervous system. Such preparations allow the visualization and study of individual neurons and small neuronal aggregates.

Cerebral cortex, striatum, hippocampus, substantia nigra and brain stem from 15-17 day-fetal rats (Sprague-Dawley strain, Alab, Sweden) were passed through an 80 µm nylon mesh into precoated poly-L-lysine Petri dishes, filled with Eagle's minimum essential medium containing 20% (v/v) fetal calf-serum, with some modifications according to Hansson (1986). 30 mM glucose and 5 µg insulin/ml were added in order to enhance the differentiation of the neuronal cells. After 24 h, the culture medium was exchanged, which led to a virtual disappearance of astroblasts. After 6 days, the cultures were treated with $10^{-5}$M cytosine arabinoside to inhibit the growth of dividing cells. The culture media were changed and the fetal calf serum concentration was reduced to 10%.

Institute of Zoophysiology[1], University of Uppsala, Uppsala, Sweden;
Dept. of Neurology[3], University of Göteborg.

NATO ASI Series, Vol. H22
Neural Development and Regeneration
Edited by A. Gorio et al.

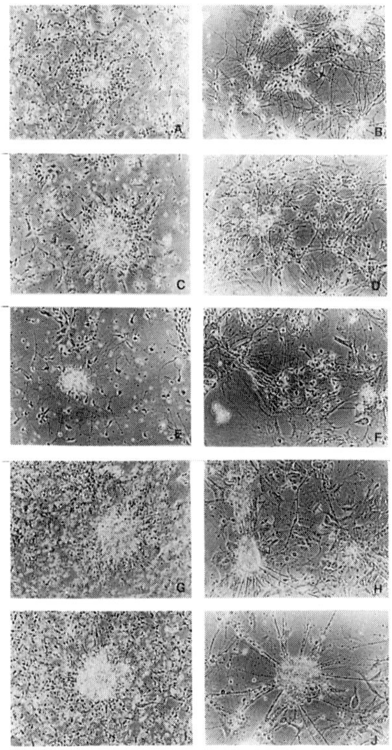

Fig. 1 A and B represent cerebral cortex, C and D striatum, E and F hippocampus, G and H substantia nigra and I and J brain stem. A, C, E, G, I are neurons grown for 2 days, and B, D, F, H, J are neurons grown for 10 days in culture. Aggregates and free neurons are seen. They differ in morphology and shape from the five brain regions.

Fig. 2 NSE positive neurons from 10 day-old primary culture of fetal substantia nigra. Unstained cells in bottom are astrocytes and mesenchymal cells.

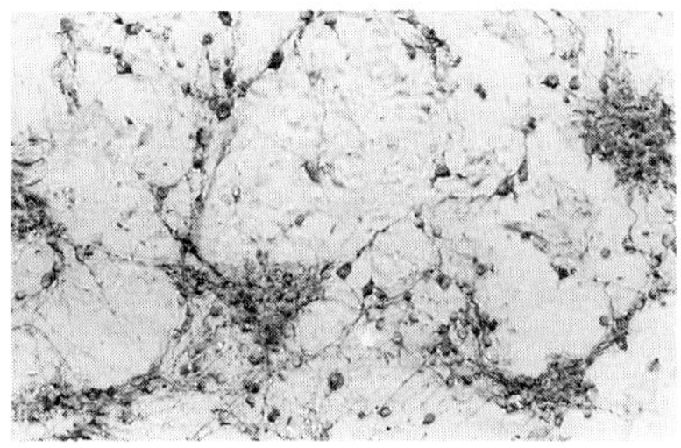

Some hours after plating, spherical aggregates were formed from cells, probably interconnecting with one another with relatively thick bundles of processes. The cells migrated from the aggregates, enlarged and developed a morphology characteristic for neurons with networks of processes. Spindle-shaped cells appeared with longer processes and pyramidal or stellate shaped cells could be found in small groups. These cells which were in majority in the cultures, stained with antibodies against neuron-specific enolase (NSE) and were considered neurons.

A minor percentage of astrocytes and mesenchymal cells were identified as well as some phagocytozing and endothelial cells.

This study received support from the Swedish Medical Research Council (project Nos. 12X-06812, 12P-7308), from the Åke Wiberg´s and Magnus Bergvall´s Foundations.

Hansson E (1986) Co-cultivation of astroglial enriched cultures from striatum and neuronal containing cultures from substantia nigra. Life Sciences 39:269-277

# Transplants of NGF-rich tissue increases survival and regeneration of axotomized cholinergic neurons in the basal forebrain.

J.E. Springer, T.J. Collier, M.Notter, R. Loy, and J.R. Sladek,Jr.
Department of Neurobiology and Anatomy
University of Rochester Medical Center
Rochester, New York 14642

## Introduction

Transections of the fimbria-fornix (F/FX) result in a loss or shrinkage of cholinergic neurons in the medial septum/vertical limb of the diagonal band (MS/VDB) possibly due to the deprivation of a retrogradely transported, target-derived trophic factor(s) in the hippocampal formation. From recent evidence reported in this and other labs, it is suggested that one of these trophic factors may be nerve growth factor or NGF (Collins and Crutcher, 1985; Hefti, 1986; Gage et al, 1986; Springer et al, 1987). Specifically, we recently reported that the receptor to NGF is actively transported in the F/FX, thus establishing a mechanism by which NGF may mediate trophic support in the septo-hippocampal pathway (Johnson et al, 1987). Further, removal of target contact by transecting the F/FX results in a loss of MS/VDB neurons which are immunoreactive to the NGF receptor (Springer et al, 1987). We also have demonstrated that aspirations of the frontoparietal and anterior cingulate cortical areas result in cell loss or shrinkage in the nucleus basalis (Springer et al, 1987).

In support of a role for NGF as a trophic factor for MS/VDB neurons, intraventricular injections of NGF can increase cell survival following axotomy (Hefti, 1986; Williams et al, 1986; Kromer, 1987). In order to provide a constant source of NGF to the axotomized neurons in the MS/VDB, we have utilized a transplantation model using intraventricular grafts of male mouse submaxillary glands. Unlike other transplantation studies where the donor tissue contains the neuronal cell population of interest, the approach of the present study is unique in that it focuses on the survival and reorganization of neurons present in the host brain.

## Methods

Female Long-Evans rats (175-225 gms) received unilateral transections of the F/FX according to the method of Springer and Loy (1985), followed by intraventricular placement of 0.3-0.5 $mm^3$ grafts of adult male mouse submaxillary glands (for transplantation procedure see Sladek and Gash, 1984). At 2-6 weeks following surgery animals were perfused and brain sections (30μm thickness) were processed for acetylcholinesterase (AChE) histochemistry, and NGF receptor immunocytochemistry. AChE and NGF receptor positive perikarya were

NATO ASI Series, Vol. H22
Neural Development and Regeneration
Edited by A. Gorio et al.

identified and counted from 18 sections throughout the ipsilateral and contralateral MS/VDB using a computer assisted image analysis system (Joyce-Loebl Magiscan).

## Results

Graft survival, as analyzed using Nissl stained sections, was found to occur in approximately 60-70% of the host animals at 3 weeks following transplantation. By 6 weeks following transplantation, graft survival was minimal. At all times analyzed, we observed a marked loss (approximately 60-70%) of AChE and NGF receptor positive cells in the MS/VDB of those animals which received F/FX and no transplant. Cell loss was limited exclusively to the ipsilateral (transected) side. However, animals which received F/FX transections and submaxillary gland grafts exhibited increased survival (~70%) of AChE and NGF receptor positive cells in the MS/VDB. This increase in cell survival was evident as late as 6 weeks following transplantation. In addition, fibers which were positive for both markers appear to course from the medial septum into the lateral septum, and in some instances penetrate the graft adjacent to the lateral septum.

In some animals the graft was removed from the host brain at 3-4 weeks following surgery and placed in a culture of PC12 cells which are known to be responsive to NGF. Within 36 hours following attachment of the graft onto the cell layer, PC12 cells were observed to differentiate and send out numerous neurites towards the direction of the submaxillary gland indicating that NGF-like activity was still present in the graft.

## Discussion

The results reported in the present study support the previous findings that transections of the F/FX result in the loss of a population of cholinergic neurons in the MS/VDB (Daitz and Powell, 1954; Gage et al, 1986; Hefti, 1986). Further, it appears that a population of these MS/VDB neurons are NGF-responsive (Springer et al, 1987). We now report that transplantation of NGF-rich tissue can influence the survival and regeneration of axotomized neurons in the MS/VDB. Specifically, we have demonstrated that grafts of male mouse submaxillary gland can increase survival of axotomized neurons in the MS/VDB which stain for AChE and are immunoreactive for the receptor to NGF. In addition, the presence of the graft appears to provide a *tropic* effect on regenerating or sprouting cholinergic fibers. Fibers which are positive for AChE and the NGF receptor were found to course into the lateral septum, an area not normally found to contain these fibers. It is possible therefore, that the graft is providing a signal which is directing and/or enhancing the growth of regenerating or sprouting fibers.

The studies previously described indicate a possible role for NGF as a trophic factor for basal forebrain cholinergic neurons. From this it has been hypothesized that a decreased availability of NGF (or a similar trophic factor) may contribute to the loss or shrinkage of cholinergic basal forebrain neurons observed in patients suffering from Alzheimer's disease (Appel, 1981: Hefti, 1983). Although there is no direct evidence to indicate that a trophic deficit may contribute to the pathogenesis of Alzheimer's disease, it is attractive to suggest that that increasing the availability of NGF may be of therapeutic value in retarding cell death associated with axotomy or neurodegenerative disorders.

## References

Appel, S.H. (1981) A unifying hypothesis for the cause of amyotropic lateral sclerosis, parkinsonism, and Alzheimer's disease. Ann. Neurol. 10:499-505.

Collins, F. and Crutcher, K.A. (1985) Neurotropic activity in the adult rat hippocampal formation: Regional distribution and increase after septal lesion. J. Neurosci. 5:2809-2814.

Daitz, H.M. and Powell, T.P.S. (1954) Studies of the connections of the fornix system. J. Neurol. Neurosurg. Psychiat. 17:75-82.

Gage, F.H., Wictorin, K., Fischer, W., Williams, L.R., Varon, S., and Bjorklund, A. (1986) Retrograde cell changes in medial septum and diagonal band following fimbria/fornix transection: Quantitative temporal analysis. Neurosci. 19(1):241-255.

Hefti, F. (1983) Alzheimer's disease caused by a lack of nerve growth factor? Ann. Neurol. 13: 109-110.

Hefti, F. (1986) Nerve growth factor promotes survival of septal cholinergic neurons after fimbrial transections. J. Neurosci. 6(8):2155-2162.

Johnson, E.M.,Jr., Taniuchi, M., Clark, H.B., Springer, J.E., Koh, S., Tayrien, M.W., and Loy, R. (1987) Demonstration of the retrograde transport of nerve growth factor receptor in the peripheral and central nervous system. J. Neurosci. 7(3):923-929.

Kromer, L. (1987) Nerve growth factor treatment after brain injury prevents neuronal death. Science, 235:214-216.

Sladek, J.R.,Jr. and Gash, D.M. (eds) (1984) Neural transplants:Development and function. Plenum Press, New York.

Springer,J.E. and Loy, R. (1985) Intrahippocampal injections of antiserum to nerve growth factor inhibit sympathohippocampal sprouting. Brain Res. Bull. 15:629-634.

Springer, J.E., Koh, S., Tayrien, M.W., and Loy, R. (1987) Basal forebrain magnocellular neurons stain for nerve growth factor receptor: Correlation with cholinergic cell bodies and effects of axotomy. J. Neurosci. Res. 17(2):111-118.

Williams, L.W., Varon, S., Peterson, G.M., Wictorin, K., Fischer, W., Bjorklund, A., and Gage, F.H. (1986) Continuous infusion of nerve growth factor prevents basal forebrain neuronal death after fimbria fornix transection. PNAS 83(23):9231-9236.

# NEUROFILAMENT PROCESSING IN DEVELOPMENT AND TRANSPLANTATION

Nancy H. Sternberger, Maceij Poltorak, William J. Freed and Ludwig A. Sternberger. University of Maryland, School of Medicine, Baltimore, MD 21201 and NIMH, Washington, D.C. 20032

In order to compare the apparently reactive phosphorylation of neurofilaments (Nf) observed in trauma and neurodegenerative disorders, we examined the expression and distribution of Nf in implants of embryonic rat cerebellum after 2 to 4 weeks survival. Donor cerebella were taken from embryos at gestational day E14 to E15 and implanted into brain parenchyma or ventricles. Immunocytochemistry with monoclonal antibodies to 5 different phospoepitopes of Nf (anti-PNf) and 5 different epitopes in non-phosphorylated Nf (anti-nPNf) (1) was done on Bouin-fixed paraffin sections using peroxidase-antiperoxidase complex from monoclonal antiperoxidase. Antibodies to other neural antigens such as myelin basic protein, glial fibrillary acidic protein and SAP, a monoclonal antibody that reacts with synapse-rich areas, were used to compare their appearance and distribution with the Nf antibodies. After 2 weeks survival, the earliest age examined, cresyl violet staining of some transplants showed the beginning of a trilaminar organization. Both PNf and nPNf epitopes were present. As in our studies of normal rat cerebellar development there was no lag in the appearance of PNf. Nf were seen in both the ventricular and parenchymal implants. By 4 weeks, transplants exhibited a high degree of internal organization. Staining patterns characteristic of cerebellum were seen with the antibodies: nPNf in Purkinje cell bodies and dendrites and PNf in basket cell axons surrounding the Purkinje cells. In summary, the transplants demonstrated cytoarchitectural features characteristic of the cerebellum. Appearance and distribution of Nf epitopes resembled that seen in normal postnatal cerebellar development and both PNf and nPNf were present at the same time in early development. In contrast to trauma and disease (2), PNf never appeared in perikarya. The rapid phosphorylation of newly formed Nf may not only indicate rapid assembly of neurofilaments but may also protect newly formed Nf against the known susceptibility of nPNf to rapid proteolysis.

Sternberger LA, Sternberger NH (1983) Monoclonal antibodies distinguish phosphorylated and non-phosphorylated forms of neurofilaments *in situ*. Proc Natl Acad Sci USA 80:6126-6130

Sternberger NH, Sternberger LA, Ulrich J (1985) Aberrant neurofilament phosphorylation in Alzheimer disease. Proc Natl Acad Sci USA 82:4274-4276

Fig. 1 A-D, 6 day cerebellum; E-H, 2 week transplant; I-L, 20 day cerebellum ; M-P, 4 week transplant. Antibodies, from left to right, nPNf, PNf, SAP and last column, cresyl violet.

NATO ASI Series, Vol. H22
Neural Development and Regeneration
Edited by A. Gorio et al.

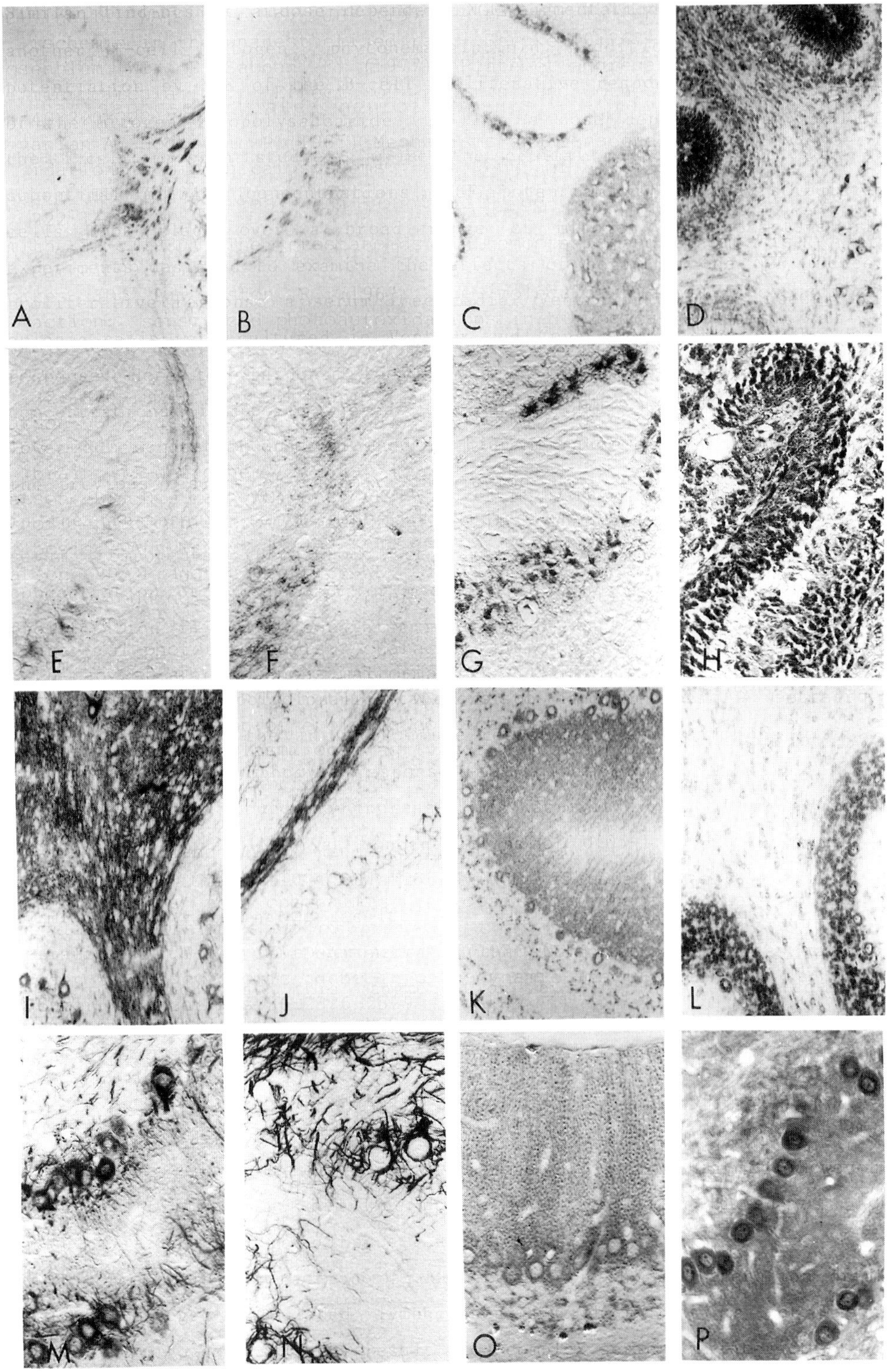
A
B
C
D
E
F
G
H
I
J
K
L
M
N
O
P

# ANTIOXIDANT ENZYMATIC ACTIVITIES AND RESISTANCE TO OXIDATIVE STRESS IN PRIMARY AND SUBCULTURED RAT ASTROGLIAL CELLS

A. Vanella, R. Avola, D.F. Condorelli, A. Campisi, A. Costa, J.R. Perez-Polo and A.M. Giuffrida Stella

Institute of Biochemistry, University of CATANIA, ITALY
Department of Human Biological Chemistry, GALVESTON, USA.

Aerobic metabolism produces potentially toxic oxygen species, such as superoxide anion radical, hydrogen peroxide and hydroxyl radical. Biochemical defences include both low molecular weight scavengers ($\alpha$-tocopherol, ascorbic acid, reduced glutathione) and enzyme systems (superoxide dismutase, catalase, glutathione peroxidase, reductase and glucose-6-phosphate dehydrogenase). Small amount of oxygen free radicals can escape to antioxidant defence causing damage to cellular constituents, such as lipid peroxidation, inactivation of enzymes, single and double DNA strand breaks. These damages could be light but constant and, if unrepaired, could accumulate with aging. It has been suggested that cell passages may represent an _in vitro_ aging model (1). The aim of the present study was to measure in rat glial cell cultures the effect of serial subcultures on the activity of some antioxidant enzymes, such as glucose-6-phosphate dehydrogenase, catalase, glutathione peroxidase and reductase. Moreover, the activity of enzymes involved in the oxidative

NATO ASI Series, Vol. H22
Neural Development and Regeneration
Edited by A. Gorio et al.

metabolism (hexokinase, lactate dehydrogenase and cytochrome oxidase) has been measured. In addition, the resistance to oxidative stress, induced by 5 mM hydrogen peroxide, was investigated in primary and subcultured rat glial cells. The measurement of the lactate dehydrogenase (LDH) released during cytolysis was used as an indicator of cellular integrity. Primary glial cell cultures were obtained from cerebral hemispheres of newborn rats as described previously (2). After one week in culture, when cells were at confluence, cultures were trypsinized and cells were submitted to serial passages up to 5 times. Some dishes were treated till confluence with 20 nM selenite. Glial cell monolayers were scraped and resuspended in PBS containing 1 mM EDTA, washed two times with 3 ml of ice-cold PBS and lysed with 50 mM phosphate buffer, pH 7.0, containing 2.5 mg/ml digitonin; centrifuged at 20,000 g and the supernatant obtained was used for the enzymatic assays. A significant decrease in glutathione peroxidase, reductase, catalase, hexokinase and lactate dehydrogenase activities was observed during the successive cell passages, but no significant difference of COX and glucose-6-phosphate dehydrogenase were found. The addition of selenite (20 nM) was inable to restore the glutathione peroxidase activity to levels occurring in primary glial cell cultures. The loss of glial fibrillary acid protein positive cells during cell passages was observed. This last result is in agreement with the findings reported by Vernadakis et al. (1).

A decrease in antioxidant enzymatic systems, found during cell passages, was accompanied by reduced cellular resistance to hydrogen peroxide. In conclusion, altered balance between the partial reduced forms of oxygen metabolism and the antioxidant enzymatic systems, caused by the various passages in rat glial cells, could play a crucial role in cell aging. Moreover, experimentally induced oxidative stress might accelerate the rate of age-related changes in subcultured glial cell cultures.

References

1) Vernadakis A., Davies D., Sakellaridis N., Mangoura D. (1986) Growth patterns of glial cells dissociated from newborn and aged mouse brain with cell passage. J Neurosci Res 15: 79-85.

2) Avola R., Serra I., Curti D., Lombardo B., Renis M., Condorelli D.F., Giuffrida A.M. (1986) Nuclear and mitochondrial DNA synthesis and energy metabolism in primary rat glial cell cultures. Neurochem Res 11: 789-800.

Acknowledgments:
Accomplished by financial supports of MPI and CNR Italy.

# ROLE OF ASCORBATE IN LAMININ ACCUMULATION, BASEMENT MEMBRANE DEPOSITION AND ACETYLCHOLINE RECEPTOR AGGREGATION ON MUSCLE.

Z. Vogel, M. Krause, N. Rosenberg, Z.Y. Xi[1], T.K. Chen[1], and M.P. Daniels[1].
Neurobiology Dept., Weizmann Institute of Science, Rehovot.

We have previously shown that embryonic brain, spinal cord and ciliary ganglia (CG) contain a low molecular weight factor (LMWF) which stimulates accumulation of collagens, including type IV (basement membrane collagen), on muscle cells in culture. The factor does this by increasing prolyl hydroxylase activity and is apparently equivalent to ascorbic acid (AA) (Kalcheim et al., 1985a,b).

Laminin is the major glycoprotein of basement membrane. Here we report that AA increases the amount of laminin immunoreactivity on the surface of cultured myotubes. Control myotubes showed a weak, diffuse or speckled staining with occasional patches containing higher concentrations of laminin (Fig. 1A). Frequently these patches were correlated with AcChR aggregates (see Daniels et al., 1984). In cultures treated with crude embryonic brain extract or with the LMWF, the surface of the myotubes was heavily stained (Fig. 1B), (the mononucleated cells were not significantly stained). Pretreatment of factor with AA-oxidase (5U/ml) sharply reduced the amount of laminin found on the myotubes (Fig. 1C), while addition of AA (50 μg/ml) to the cultures markedly increased the amount of laminin (Fig. 1D). Similarly, in cocultures of CG with muscle there was a large increase in laminin staining over the myotube surface (especially in the vicinity of explant). Although AA-oxidase inhibited the general increase in laminin staining on myotubes exposed to factor or CG, discrete areas of bright laminin staining were still observed. (Fig. 1C). These discrete areas almost always colocalized with AcChR aggregates.

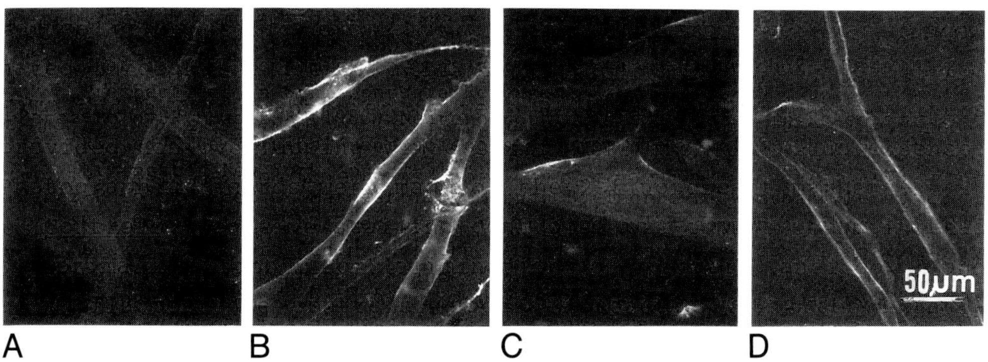


Fig. 1. One week old rat muscle cultures were treated for 1 day as described in the text and immunofluorescence stained for laminin.

[1]Lab. of Biochemical Genetics, NIH, BETHESDA, MD.

NATO ASI Series, Vol. H22
Neural Development and Regeneration
Edited by A. Gorio et al.

Electron microscopy revealed that addition of AA, the LMWF or coculture with CG (Fig. 2A) sharply increased (4- to 7-fold) the amount of basement membrane found on myotubes and the number of thick collagen fibrils in the surrounding spaces. AA-oxidase sharply inhibited these effects (Fig. 2B).

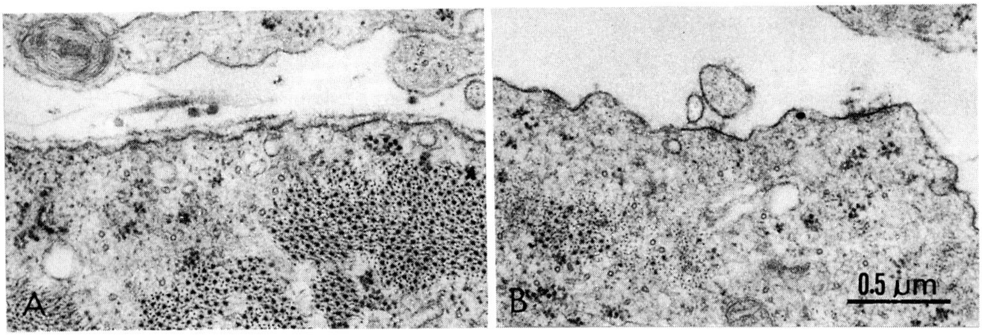


Fig. 2. One week old rat muscle cells were cocultured with CG for 2 days in the presence (B) or absence (A) of AA-oxidase, and processed for electron microscopy.

We have previously shown that AA stimulates receptor aggregation on cultured rat myotubes (Kalcheim et al., 1982). Here we report that the increased aggregation obtained by the LMWF is due largely to AA, since it is blocked by AA-oxidase. AA-oxidase also reduced the number of AcChR aggregates in CG-muscle cocultures. The substantial aggregation response which still occurred is probably accounted for by high molecular weight aggregation factor(s) released from the explants.

These results are consistent with a role for AA in the neural regulation of basement membrane formation and AcChR aggregation in muscle. (Supported by grants from the Muscular Dystrophy Association of America; U.S.-Israel Binational Science Foundation and the Minerva Foundation, Munich, Germany).

Kalcheim C, Duksin D, Bachar E, Vogel Z (1985a) Collagen stimulating factor from embryonic brain has ascorbate-like activity and stimulates prolyl hydroxylation in cultured muscle cells. Eur. J. Biochem. 146, 227-232.

Kalcheim C, Bachar E, Duksin D, Vogel Z (1985b) Ciliary ganglia and spinal cord release an ascorbate-like compound which stimulates proline hydroxylation and collagen formation in muscle cultures. Neurosci. Lett. 58, 219-224.

Daniels MP, Vigny M, Sonderegger P, Bauer HC, Vogel Z (1984) Association of laminin and other basement membrane components with regions of high acetylcholine receptor density on cultured myotubes. Int. J. Devel. Neurosci. 2, 87-99.

Kalcheim C, Vogel Z, Duksin D (1982) Embryonic brain extract induces collagen biosynthesis in cultured muscle cells: Involvement in acetylcholine receptor aggregation. Proc. Natl. Acad. Sci. USA 79, 3077-3081.

# INDEX

# NATO ASI Series H

Vol. 1: Biology and Molecular Biology of Plant-Pathogen Interactions.
Edited by J. A. Bailey. 415 pages. 1986.

Vol. 2: Glial-Neuronal Communication in Development and Regeneration.
Edited by H. H. Althaus and W. Seifert. 865 pages. 1987.

Vol. 3: Nicotinic Acetylcholine Receptor: Structure and Function.
Edited by A. Maelicke. 489 pages. 1986.

Vol. 4: Recognition in Microbe-Plant Symbiotic and Pathogenic Interactions.
Edited by B. Lugtenberg. 449 pages. 1986.

Vol. 5: Mesenchymal-Epithelial Interactions in Neural Development.
Edited by J. R. Wolff, J. Sievers, and M. Berry. 428 pages. 1987.

Vol. 6: Molecular Mechanisms of Desensitization to Signal Molecules.
Edited by T. M. Konijn, P. J. M. Van Haastert, H. Van der Starre, H. Van der Wel, and M. D. Houslay. 336 pages. 1987.

Vol. 7: Gangliosides and Modulation of Neuronal Functions.
Edited by H. Rahmann. 647 pages. 1987.

Vol. 8: Molecular and Cellular Aspects of Erythropoietin and Erythropoiesis.
Edited by I. N. Rich. 460 pages. 1987.

Vol. 9: Modification of Cell to Cell Signals During Normal and Pathological Aging.
Edited by S. Govoni and F. Battaini. 297 pages. 1987.

Vol. 10: Plant Hormone Receptors. Edited by D. Klämbt. 319 pages. 1987.

Vol. 11: Host-Parasite Cellular and Molecular Interactions in Protozoal Infections.
Edited by K.-P. Chang and D. Snary. 425 pages. 1987.

Vol. 12: The Cell Surface in Signal Transduction.
Edited by E. Wagner, H. Greppin, and B. Millet. 243 pages. 1987.

Vol. 13: Toxicology of Pesticides: Experimental, Clinical and Regulatory Perspectives.
Edited by L. G. Costa, C. L. Galli, and S. D. Murphy. 320 pages. 1987.

Vol. 14: Genetics of Translation. New Approaches.
Edited by M. F. Tuite, M. Picard, and M. Bolotin-Fukuhara. 524 pages. 1988.

Vol. 15: Photosensitisation. Molecular, Cellular and Medical Aspects.
Edited by G. Moreno, R. H. Pottier, and T. G. Truscott. 521 pages. 1988.

Vol. 16: Membrane Biogenesis. Edited by J. A. F. Op den Kamp. 477 pages. 1988.

Vol. 17: Cell to Cell Signals in Plant, Animal and Microbial Symbiosis.
Edited by S. Scannerini, D. Smith, P. Bonfante-Fasolo, and V. Gianinazzi-Pearson. 414 pages. 1988.

Vol. 18: Plant Cell Biotechnology.
Edited by M. S. S. Pais, F. Mavituna, and J. M. Novais. 540 pages. 1988.

Vol. 19: Modulation of Synaptic Transmission and Plasticity in Nervous Systems.
Edited by G. Hertting and H.-C. Spatz. 457 pages. 1988.

Vol. 20: Amino Acid Availability and Brain Function in Health and Disease.
Edited by G. Huether. 487 pages. 1988.

# NATO ASI Series H

Vol. 21: Cellular and Molecular Basis of Synaptic Transmission.
Edited by H. Zimmermann. 547 pages. 1988.

Vol. 22: Neural Development and Regeneration. Cellular and Molecular Aspects.
Edited by A. Gorio, J.R. Perez-Polo, J. de Vellis, and B. Haber. 711 pages. 1988.